CHINA POPULATION CENSUS

中国2010年人口普查资料〔中册〕

TABULATION ON THE 2010 POPULATION CENSUS OF THE PEOPLE`S REPUBLIC OF CHINA（BOOK Ⅱ）

国务院人口普查办公室
国家统计局人口和就业统计司 编

Compiled by
Population Census Office under the State Council
Department of Population and Employment Statistics
National Bureau of Statistics

中国统计出版社
China Statistics Press

中国2010年人口普查资料
〔中册〕
中国统计出版社
China Statistics Press

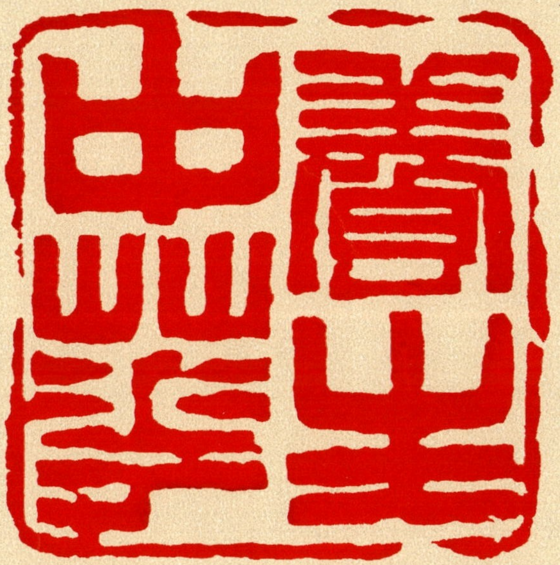

養生中華

A Canon of Chinese Health Regimens

图书在版编目（CIP）数据

养生中华：汉英对照 / 任犀然著；徐芳译．-- 北京：当代世界出版社，2012.4
ISBN 978-7-5090-0828-7

Ⅰ．①养… Ⅱ．①任… ②徐… Ⅲ．①养生（中医）–基本知识–汉、英 Ⅳ．① R212

中国版本图书馆 CIP 数据核字 (2012) 第 055028 号

ISBN 978-7-5090-0828-7

9 787509 008287 >

书　　名	养生中华
出版发行	当代世界出版社
地　　址	北京市复兴路四号
网　　址	http://www.worldpress.com.cn
电　　话	（010）83908408　83908409　83908410（传真）
出　　品	澳新春雨（北京）文化传播有限公司
经　　销	全国新华书店
责任编辑	叶晓林
版式设计	任犀然
印　　刷	北京圣彩虹制版印刷技术有限公司
规　　格	889×1194 毫米　1/12
印　　张	22
版　　次	2012 年 5 月第 1 版
印　　次	2012 年 5 月第 1 版
定　　价	600.00 元

樂天長壽辭

心理衛生近代漸盛養性修身早垂古訓人生疾病外因易防七情六欲內賊難當憤怒煩惱抑鬱悲哀神明內疚百病之階健康要道端在正心喜怒不縈於胸襟榮辱不擾乎方寸縱遇不治之疾自有回天之功毋慮毋憂即是長生聖藥常開笑口便是卻病良方養生只此真詮長壽無他奧秘昔時七十已稱稀今後百齡不足奇隨遇而安無往不樂優哉悠哉同登壽域

陳存仁撰

張大千書

序

中华民族自古以来就有重视健康的传统。中国最古老、最重要的典籍之一《尚书》中论述理想的人生幸福有五个要素，即富裕的生活，良好的道德，健康、平安，长寿，让生命善始善终。健康的生命是我们人生最可宝贵的。为了民族的健康和生生不息，中华民族创造了中华养生学。

中华养生学可以上溯到五千年以前。上古的舞蹈；吐故纳新，熊经鸟申的导引术；“节其饮食”的食养；还有神农尝百草的传说……这些都奠定了中华养生学的基础。中华养生学有几个特点：

一、讲究顺其自然。即顺应生命的自然规律，让生机盎然。

二、讲究天人相应。“顺四时而适寒暑，和喜怒而安居处，节阴阳而调刚柔。”注重社会、天时、地理与心理诸大小环境和内外因素对人的影响。

三、 强调整体辩证的养生观，追求适度与和谐。“致中和，天地位焉，万物育焉。”

四、注重防病。“不治已病治未病”，“夫唯病病，是以不病”。

《周易》说，天之大德曰生。珍惜生命，热爱生命，让身心健康是中医养生学的根本目标。

中华养生学（含中医药）数千年来为中国人民的健康事业作出了举世瞩目的贡献，也一定能为世界人民的健康事业作出重要贡献。

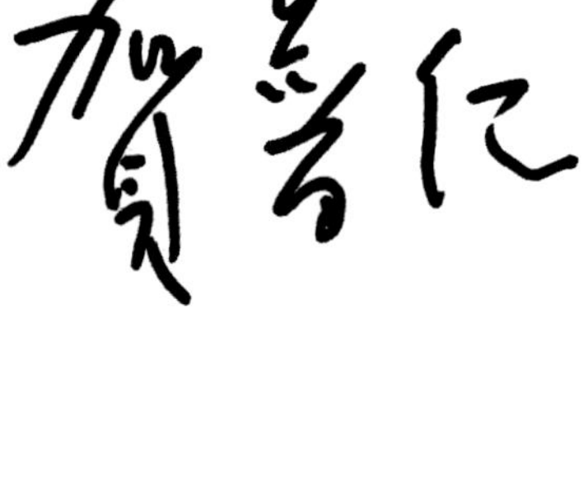

PREFACE

Since ancient times it has been the tradition of the Chinese nation to treasure health. The *Book of History*, one of the oldest and most important books of ancient China, dwells on the five essential elements for human happiness, i.e. affluence, virtue, health, safety and longevity, and advocates good quality of life throughout its journey. Health is superior to everything else. To ensure national health and permanent prosperity, the Chinese nation has developed its own theories on health preservation.

Chinese theories on health preservation date back to five thousand years ago, finding their origins in the dances of time immemorial, the imitation of the body movements of birds and bears and the control of breath, the nourishment through temperately taking in food and drinks, the legend of Shennong tasting various herbs, etc. Chinese theories on health preservation have the following characteristics:

a. They are committed to following the natural course. Their doctrine is that compliance with the natural course will ensure a blooming life.

b. They are in pursuit of harmony between humanity and nature. "It is imperative to follow the rhythm of the four seasons to adapt to heat and cold, moderating anger and elation for a tranquil life, and proportioning yin and yang to temper hardness with softness." Chinese theories on health preservation attach importance to the impact of social, meteorological, geographical and psychological factors on human beings.

c. They hold the holistic view of health maintenance, putting a premium on moderateness and harmony. "When moderation is achieved, things will be in their respective places and thrive."

d. They lay emphasis on the prevention of diseases. “It is recommended to cure the latent illnesses rather than the manifest ones.” (cited from the *Inner Canon*) “Detect the disease in advance and try to keep it off.”

Zhouyi, or the *Book of Changes*, points out that the ultimate virtue under the sky is the love for life. So in treasuring life and maintaining spiritual as well as physical health lies the fundamental goal of Chinese traditional medicine.

Chinese theories on health preservation – of which TCM is a part – have made remarkable contributions to the health of the Chinese people over thousands of years. They will also contribute greatly to the health of people in the rest of the world.

賀普仁

He Puren

目　录

Contents

壹　养生祛病　健康长寿　/ 12
I . Health Preservation and Longevity

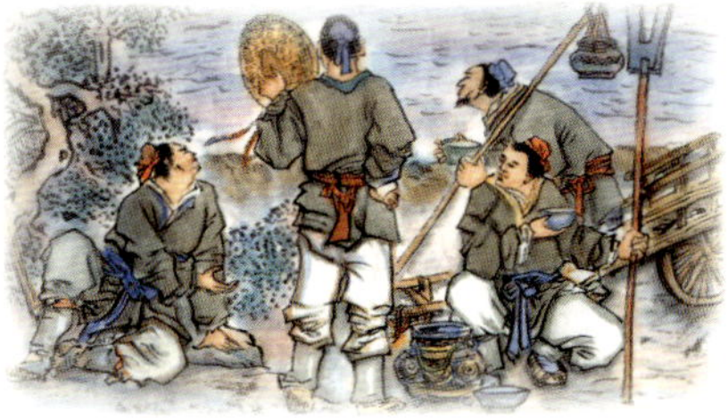

健康的八项标准　/ 14
Eight standards for health

人失去健康的四个主要原因　/ 16
Four main health-impairing factors

寿　歌　/ 19
Song of Longevity

病后调养四要点　/ 20
Four tips for better rehabilitation

贰　源远流长　/ 22
II . Time-honored Theories on Health Preservation

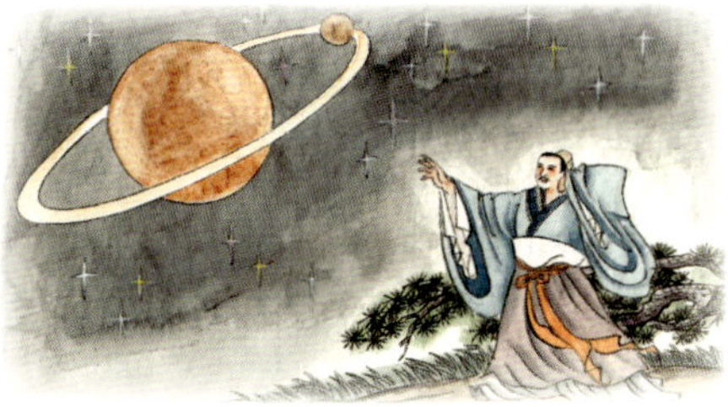

中华养生文化有三个基本特点　/ 24
Three basic characteristics of Chinese regimens

中华养生的萌芽　/ 26
The dawn of Chinese regimen

火的作用与食物养生萌芽　/ 26
The use of fire and the emergence of dietary regimen

先民懂得择居和“沐浴”　/ 27
Selecting shelters & bathing

劳动与体育养生　/ 27
Labor and physical regimens

中华养生的理论基础　/ 28
The theoretical basis of Chinese regimens

《黄帝内经》　/ 28
Inner Canon of the Yellow Emperor

叁　博大精深　/ 32
III. The Profound Culture of Chinese Regimens

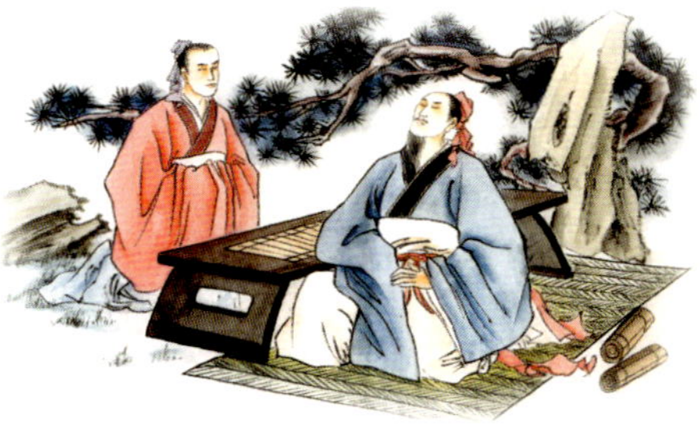

诸子百家与养生文化　/ 34
Quotes concerning health preservation of the Hundred Schools of Thought

道家养生　/ 36
Taoist regimen

道法自然　/ 36
Tao follows the law of nature.

恬惔虚无　/ 38
Spiritual tranquility

重在贵生　/ 39
Cherishing life and health

不治已病治未病　/ 42
Prevention of diseases as the best therapy.

儒家养生　/ 43
Confucian regimen

致中和　/ 43
The state of moderation

慈、俭、和、静　/ 44
Benevolence, frugality, harmony, and tranquility

君子有三戒　/ 45
Three must-nots for health preservation

仁者寿　/ 48
Benevolent people tend to live longer

佛家养生　/ 50
Buddhist regimen

调心之法　/ 52
Methods of mind cultivation

禅定与修心　/ 53
Meditation and mental equilibrium

佛家的病理观　/ 54
Buddhist pathology

身心合一　/ 56
Body and mind become one

医学养生派　/ 58
Regimen of Medicine School

中医经络　/ 60
TCM meridians and collaterals

经络在全身的分布规律　/ 61
Distribution of meridians and collaterals in the human body

十二经脉　/ 63
Twelve meridians

奇经八脉　/ 69
Eight extra channels

四时之脉 / 70
Pulse in the four seasons

医易同源 / 72
Traditional Chinese Medicine and *Book of Changes* sharing the same origin

阴阳、五行学说 / 74
Theories of yin, yang and the five elements

一天中的阴阳 / 78
Yin and yang of a day

人体的生命周期 / 80
Processes of a human life

剖析衰老的奥秘 / 82
Analysis of the mystery of aging

四种生命活动基本特征的探讨 / 83
Four basic features of life

肆 养形健身 / 84
IV . Fitness Keeping and Health Promotion

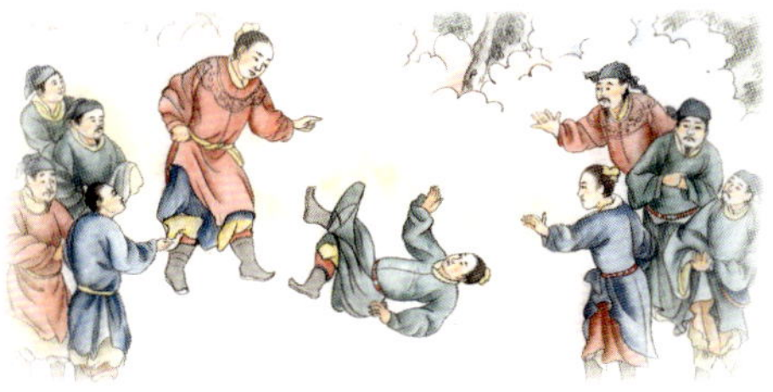

四季养生 / 86
Regimens in different seasons

春季养生 / 87
Spring regimen

夏季养生 / 89
Summer regimen

秋季养生 / 91
Autumn regimen

冬季养生 / 93
Winter regimen

调节四季情志 / 95
To regulate emotions in the four seasons

五官调护 / 96
The nursing of facial features

五官保健功法 / 97
Exercises for the health of facial features

腿、足及身体调护 / 100
Caring for legs and feet

脏与腑 / 102
Zang organs and fu organs

五脏 / 102
Five zang organs

六腑 / 103
Six fu organs

动静结合 / 105
The combination of the dynamic and the static

生命在于运动 / 105
Life lies in movement

运动原则 / 106
Principles of physical exercise

中国古代体育 / 108
Ancient Chinese sports

历代流传的养生强身功法选录 / 113
A selection of exercises for preserving and improving health handed down from past ages

易筋经 / 114
The Muscle-bone Strengthening Exercise

五禽戏 / 117
Five Animal Frolics

十二段锦 / 123
The Twelve Pieces of Brocade

延年九转法 / 126
The Nine Movements for Prolonging Life

太极拳 / 128
Tai Chi Chuan

太极八法 / 132
The Eight Methods of Tai Chi Chuan

吴式太极拳三十七式 / 140
The Thirty-Seven Movements of Wu Style Tai Chi Chuan

伍 正心养神 / 164
V. Mental Health

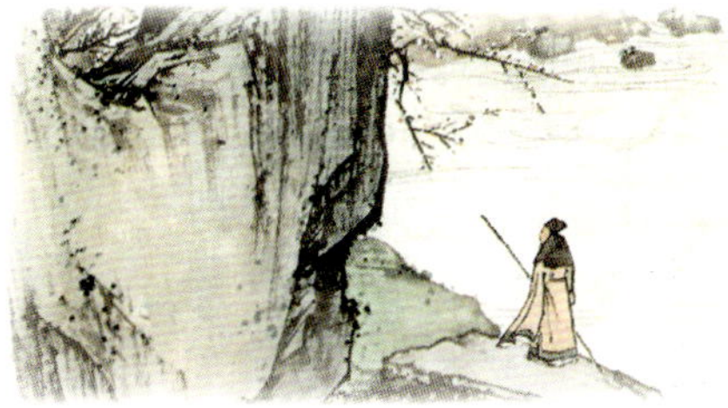

养神之道 / 166
The art of spiritual cultivation

"神"在人体居首要之位 / 166
Spirit, the premier component of human body

形神一体 / 167
Union of body and spirit

养神的方法 / 168
Methods of spiritual cultivation

养心之道 / 172
Theories of spiritual cultivation

脑力劳动也益寿 / 182
Mental labor, no damage to life span

陆　起居安适　/ 184
VI . Importance of Comfortable Living

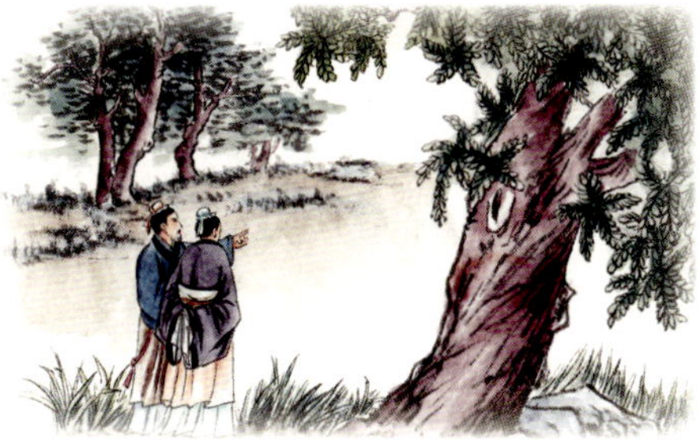

规律起居　/ 186
Keeping regular hours

安于居处　/ 188
Living in an agreeable environment

睡眠与梦境　/ 191
Sleep and dream

睡眠养生三法　/ 195
Three ways to preserve health through sleep

科学起居要注意肠中常清　/ 198
Purge your bowels of waste

肠胃运化食物图解　/ 199
Illustrations of food digestion

科学起居要防“五劳七伤”　/ 201
To avoid the “five fatigues” and “seven harms”

柒　食 养　/ 204
VII. Dietary Regimen

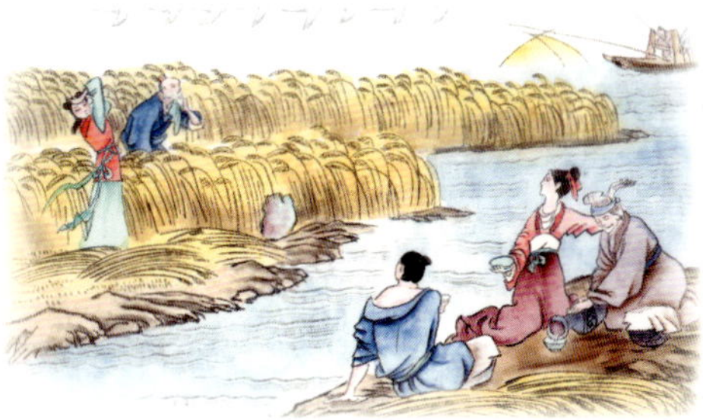

调和五味　/ 207
Balancing the “five tastes”

五谷为养　/ 207
The “five grains”, a source of nutrition

五果为助　/ 207
The “five fruits”, essential food supplements

五菜为充　/ 207
The “five vegetables”, indispensable nutrients

五畜为益　/ 207
Meat of the “five domestic animals”, health boosters

四季饮食　/ 208
Diets of the four seasons

养气、血、阴、阳的食养品　/ 210
Foods for the nourishment of qi, blood, yin, and yang

养心、肝、脾、肺、肾的食养品食物　/ 212
Foods for the nourishment of heart, liver, spleen, lungs and kidneys

养筋、骨、肤、发、齿的食养品常用食物　/ 213
Foods for the nourishment of tendons, bones, skin, hair and teeth

饮食有节　/ 214
Moderate diet

催人早衰的物质　/ 215
Substances inducing premature aging

必须注意食品养生之禁忌　/ 216
Important dietary taboos

饮水　/ 217
The intake of water

食物——人体的生化之源　/ 218
Food, the source of energy for the body

“谨和五味”　/ 219
Balancing the “five tastes”

茶道养生　/ 220
The health-preserving effects of tea

捌　房室养生　/ 226
VIII. Preserving Health through Sex Life

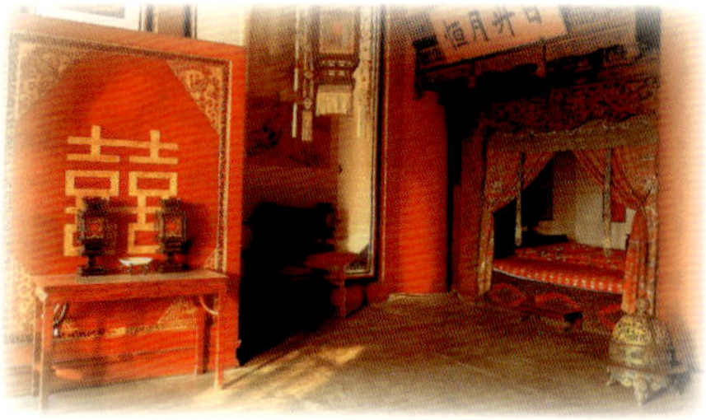

房室养生　/ 228
Preserving health through sex life

玖　食用本草　/ 236
IX . Consumption of Chinese Herbs

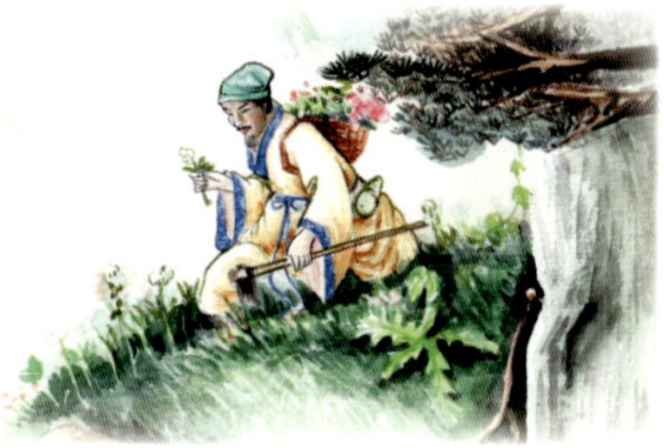

稻　/ 238
Rice

小麦　/ 238
Wheat

小米　/ 239
Millet

雀麦　/ 239
Oat

玉米 / 240
Maize

高粱 / 240
Sorghum

萝卜 / 241
Radish

黑豆 / 241
Black soybean

绿豆 / 242
Mung bean

芝麻 / 242
Sesame

白菜 / 243
Chinese cabbage

韭菜 / 243
Leek

芹菜 / 244
Celery

菠菜 / 244
Spinach

黄瓜 / 245
Cucumber

茄子 / 245
Eggplant

胡萝卜 / 246
Carrot

莴笋 / 246
Lettuce

木耳 / 247
Black fungus

山药 / 247
Yam

大葱 / 248
Scallion

姜 / 248
Ginger

番茄 / 249
Tomato

番薯 / 249
Sweet potato

冬瓜 / 250
Wax gourd

豆腐 / 250
Tofu

洋葱 / 251
Onion

鸡蛋 / 251
Eggs

藕 / 252
Lotus root

海带 / 252
Kelp

苹果 / 253
Apple

梨 / 253
Pear

柑 / 254
Tangerine

桃子 / 254
Peach

葡萄 / 255
Grape

香蕉 / 255
Banana

西瓜 / 256
Watermelon

荔枝 / 256
Litchi

栗子 / 257
Chestnut

枣 / 257
Date

猪肉 / 258
Pork

牛肉 / 258
Beef

羊肉 / 259
Mutton

鸡肉 / 259
Chicken

后记 / 260
Afterword

壹　养生祛病　健康长寿

I. Health Preservation and Longevity

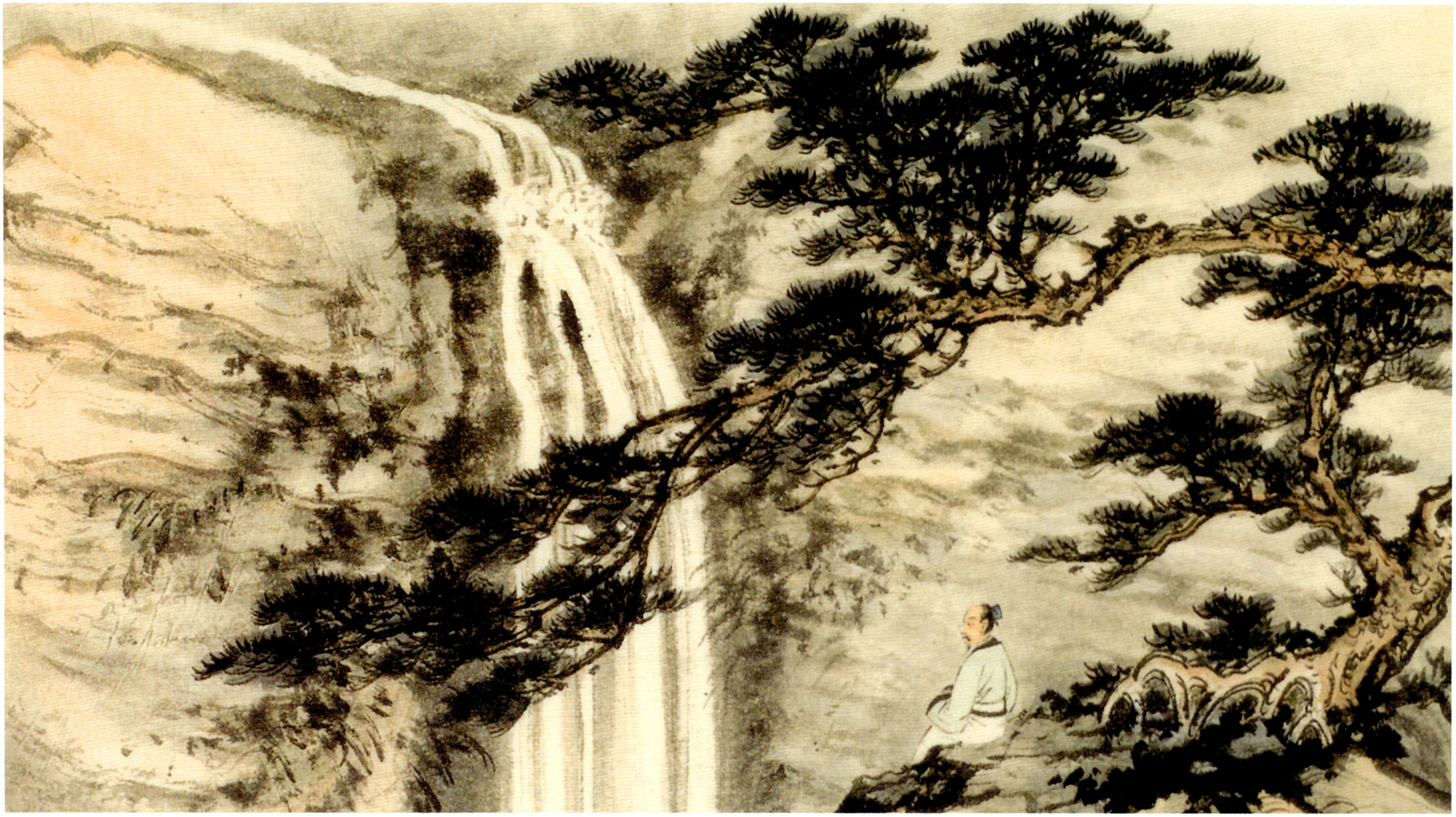

随着社会的进步，越来越多的人开始关注健康，重视养生。健康是生活幸福的基础，了解什么是健康，懂得养生保健的原则和方法，有益于防病祛病，健康长寿。

With the progress of human societies, more and more people have begun to value health preservation. As health is the basis of a happy life, to know what good health means and how to achieve it through regimens will help us to prevent diseases and live a long life.

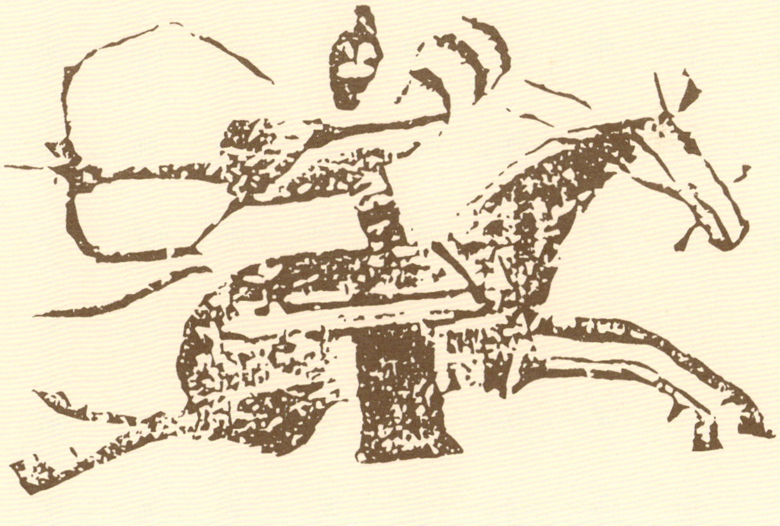

健康的八项标准

Eight standards for health

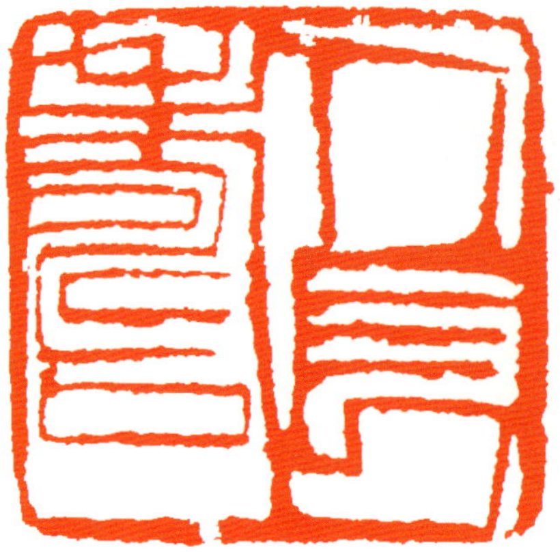

人们在追求健康时，首先应了解什么是真正的健康。世界卫生组织（WHO）对“健康”有明确的定义。

一是健康不仅是没有伤病，而且是躯体上、精神上健康，有良好的社会适应能力，有足够充沛的精力，能从容不迫地应对日常生活和工作压力，且不因此感到过分的紧张。

二是处事乐观，态度积极，乐于承担责任，事无巨细不挑剔。

三是善于休息，睡眠良好，应变能力强，能适应环境的各种变化。

四是能够抵抗一般性感冒和传染病。

五是体重适中，身材匀称，站立时头、肩、臂位置协调，眼睛明亮，反应敏锐，眼睑不发炎。

六是牙齿清洁，无空洞，无痛感，牙龈颜色正常，无出血现象。

七是头发有光泽，无头屑。肌肉、皮肤富有弹性，走路感觉轻松。

八是有健康的人格和良好的道德品质。

While we pursue health, we must first understand what the real health is. World Health Organization (WHO) has defined “health” clearly.

Firstly, health refers not only to no injury or disease, but also to health in body and mind. A healthy person is adaptable, energetic, able to cope with daily things and work stress calmly, and never too nervous.

Secondly, a healthy person is optimistic and positive in attitude, willing to take responsibilities, and not fussy or particular about trifles.

Thirdly, a healthy person is able to rest and sleep well, flexible and adaptable to various changes in the environment.

Fourthly, a healthy person can resist common cold and common infectious diseases.

Fifthly, a healthy person has an adequate weight and a shapely figure. In a standing position, his head, shoulders and arms are symmetrical. His eyes are bright and responsive, and his eyelids do not have inflammation.

Sixthly, a healthy person’s teeth are clean without holes or pain, and the gum color is normal without bleeding points.

Seventhly, a healthy person’s hair is shiny without dandruff. His muscles and skin are elastic. He walks in an easy manner.

Eighthly, a healthy person should have a good personality and sound moral character.

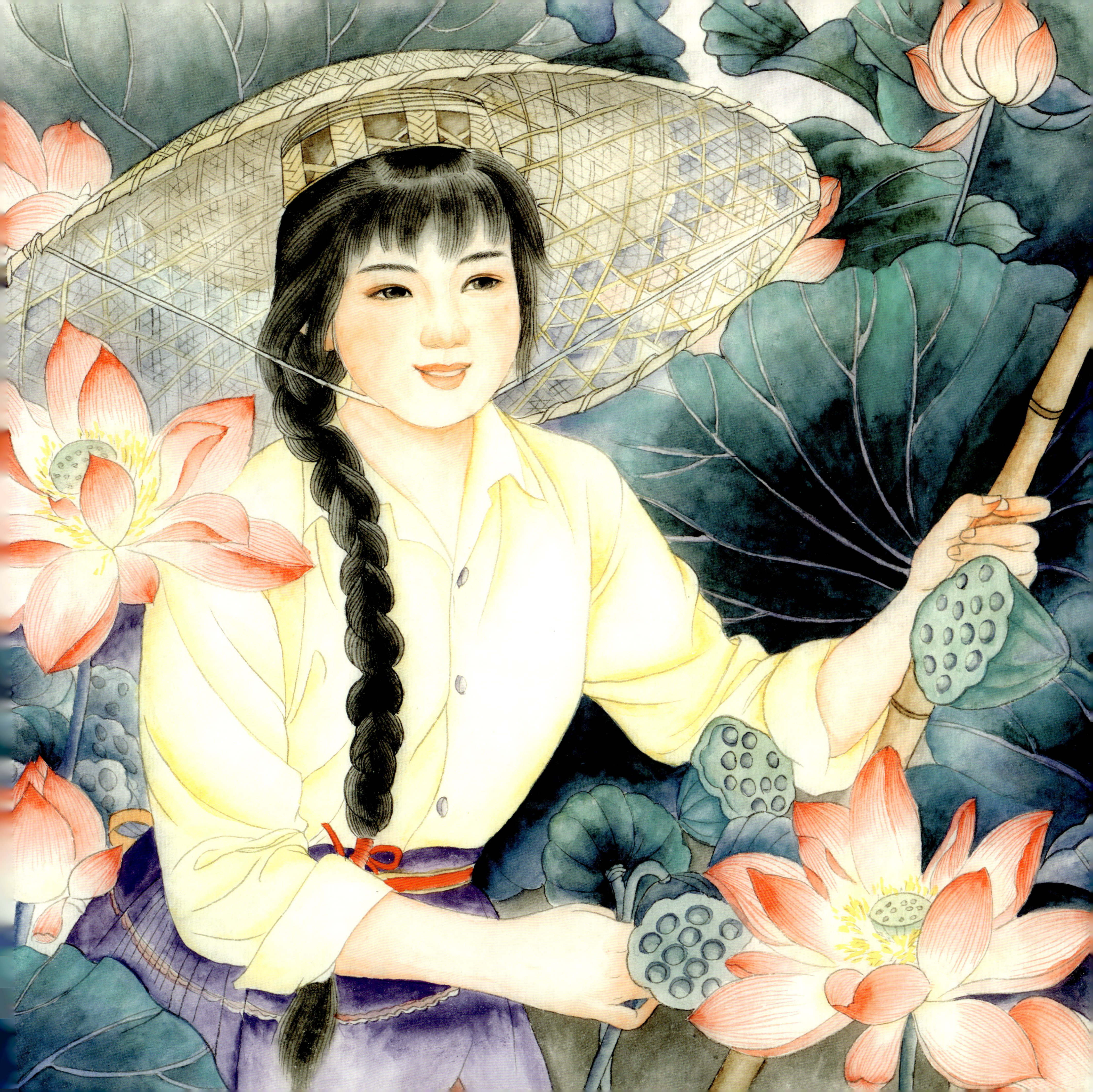

人失去健康的四个主要原因

Four main health-impairing factors

中医学认为，保持健康就需要学会养生，人们生病、早衰的主要原因在于不懂养生。

人失去健康有以下四个主要原因：

1. 起居不合规律

规律而节制的生活，对于防止和抵御疾病的发生、获得健康具有十分重要的意义。饮食不节（过饥、过饱、偏食，饮食过冷、过热、过辣、过咸、过酸、过油腻）、饮酒过多、劳逸失常、房劳过度等，都可造成脏腑功能失调，精气受损，进而导致疾病，加速衰老。

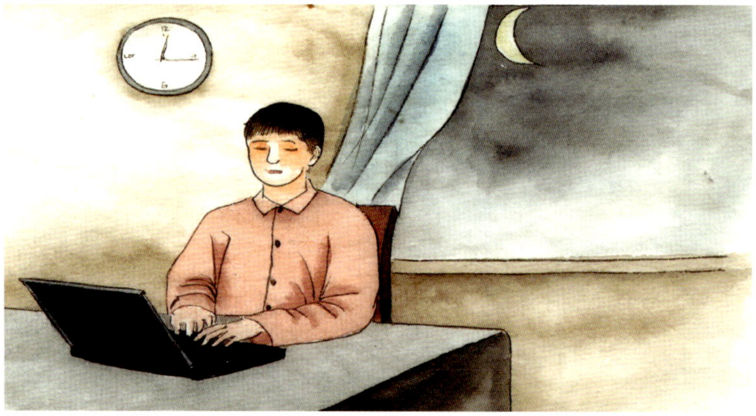

劳累过度

Over exhaustion

2. 情绪失于调节

若情志失调，七情太过（过喜、过怒、过忧、过思、过悲、过恐、过惊），就会引起人体气血不和，阴阳失调，脏腑功能发生紊乱，造成各种病变，导致早衰。

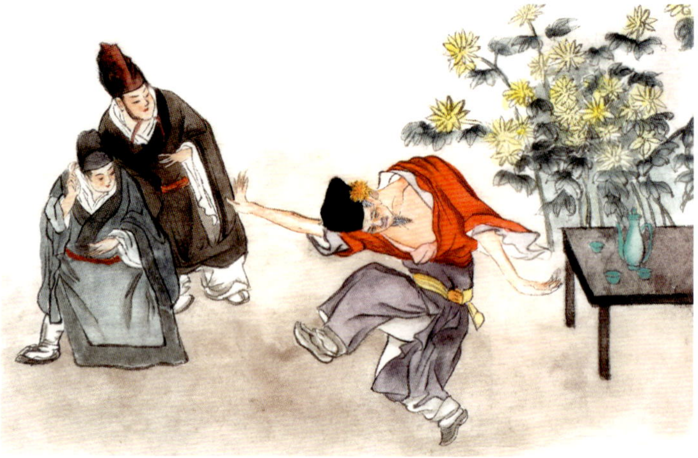

情志失调

Mental imbalance

Chinese traditional medicine believes that the main reason for health is regimen, and the root causes of diseases and premature aging lie in not understanding regimen.

1. No regular living

Aregular and moderate life is of great significance to prevent and resist diseases. Intemperance in eating (eating too little or too much, picky about food, eating too cold, hot, spicy, salty, sour and greasy food), drinking too much, disorder of work and rest, excessive sex, etc. can cause dysfunctional organs, and damage one's vigor, which further leads to diseases and accelerates aging.

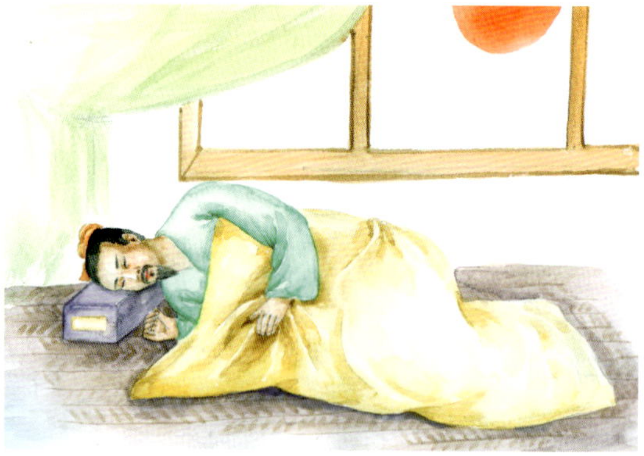

作息不规律

Irregular life

2. The maladjustment of emotions

If emotions are maladjusted, or any of the seven emotions goes to extremes (too happy, angry, worried, broody, sad, afraid, or scared), the qi and blood, the yin and yang of the body will be unbalanced, and the function of organs will be disorderly, resulting in various diseases and even premature aging.

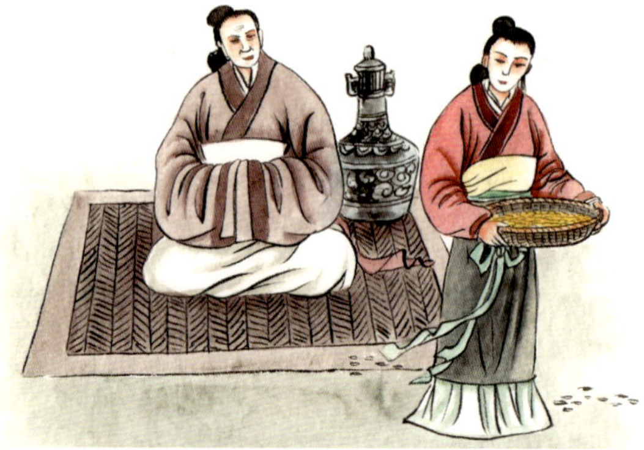

生活不和谐

Disharmonious life

3. 生活方式有问题

人的健康不是单靠强调吃什么或炼什么就可以得到的，健康是由人的整个生活方式决定的。如果生活方式有问题，积累不良习惯，就会导致疾病。

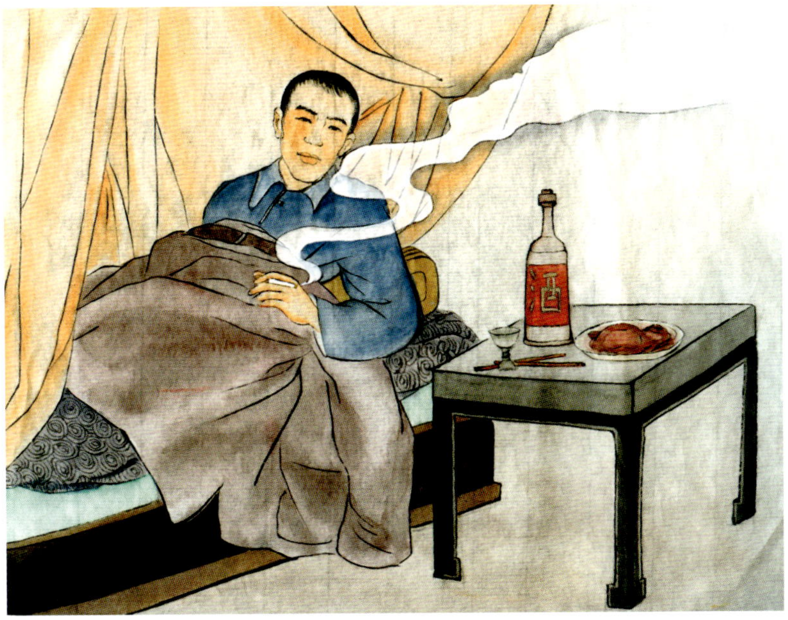

烟酒过度

Excessive smoking and drinking

4. 禀赋有强有弱

禀赋有强有弱主要指遗传因素；而体质，则是指人体在遗传性和获得性基础上表现出来的功能和形态上相对稳定的固有特征。中医学很早就认识到人的寿命与禀赋及体质强弱相关。

3. A problematic way of life

One cannot stay healthy merely by eating something or doing certain exercise, for health is determined by the whole way of life. A problematic way of life, in which bad habits are formed, will lead to illness.

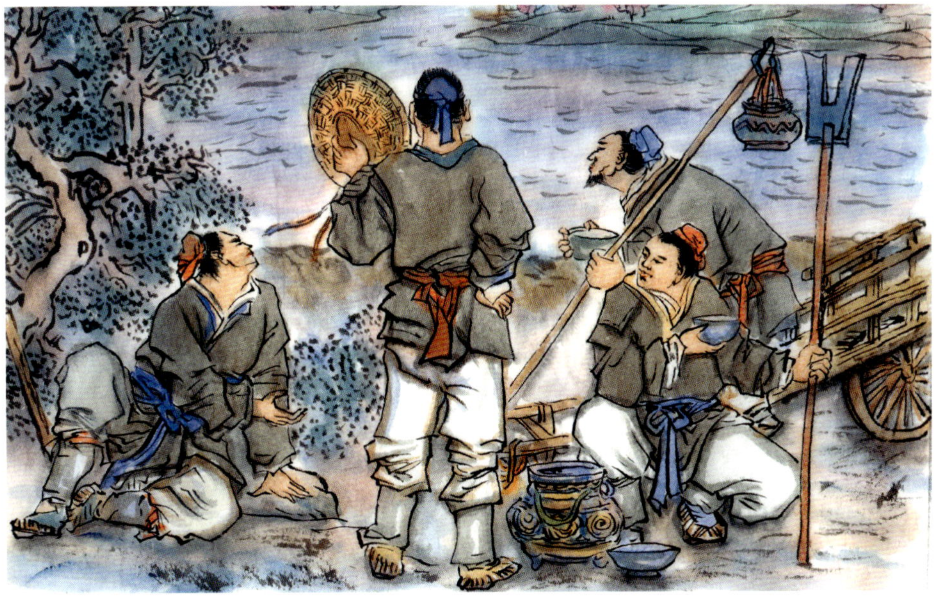

劳作有度

Moderate work

4. Strong or weak natural endowment

Strong or weak natural endowment refers primarily to genetic factors, while constitution refers to the relatively stable characteristics inherited and acquired as shown in the function and disposition of the body. Chinese traditional medicine has long recognized that one’s life span is related to one’s natural endowment and constitution.

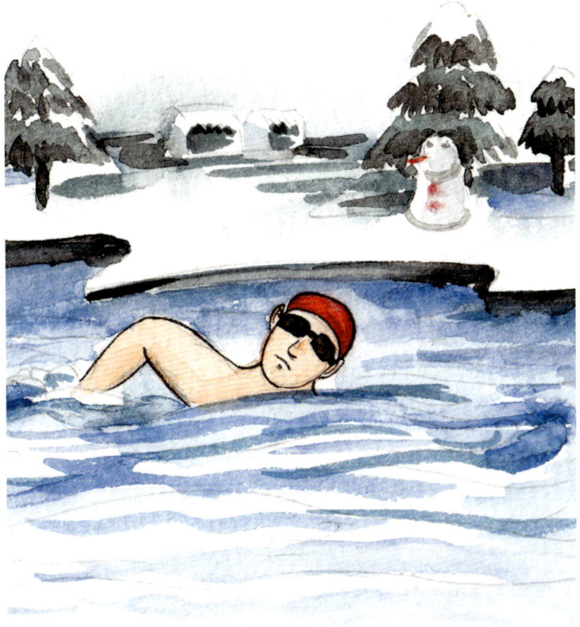

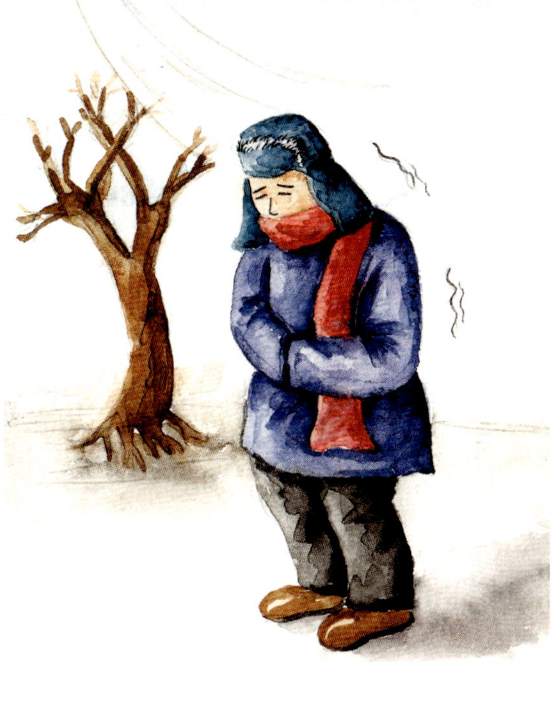

《辞海》对健康的定义是：人体各器官系统发育良好，功能正常，体质健壮，精力充沛，并具有良好的劳动效能的状态。

Ci Hai (an encyclopedic Chinese dictionary) defines “healthy” in this way: all the organs and systems in the human body have developed well and are functioning normally. The body, strong and vigorous, can perform the function of labor effectively.

人的先天禀赋不同，有的人天生抗冻，有的人天生惧寒

People are born with different constitutions. Some are resistant to cold while others are afraid of it.

欧洲人的平均寿命在公元前 4000 年为 18 岁，公元前 2000 年为 29 岁，文艺复兴时期为 35 岁，19 世纪达到 40 ~ 45 岁，20 世纪 20 年代是 55 岁，发展到 80 年代已达到 72 岁。

从我国有关历史资料查得：先秦时代中国人的平均寿命为 18 岁，东汉时为 22 岁，唐代时为 27 岁，宋代时为 30 岁，清代时为 33 岁，20 世纪 40 年代时为 35 岁，新中国成立后至 1957 年，国人人均寿命上升至 57 岁，1981 年为 68 岁，1985 年为 68.97 岁。至今已超过 73 岁。上海人均寿命期望值已达 80.98 岁（2008 年统计）。

The average life span of Europeans was 18 in 4000 BC, 29 in 2000 BC, 35 during the Renaissance, 40-45 in the 19th century, 55 in the 1920s, and 72 in the 1980s.

An examination of Chinese historical records shows that the average life span of the Chinese was 18 in the pre-Qin period, 22 in the Eastern Han Dynasty, 27 in the Tang Dynasty, 30 in the Song Dynasty, 33 in the Qing Dynasty, 35 in the 1940s, 57 during the period between 1949 and 1957, 68 in 1981, 68.97 in 1985, and above 73 at present. The average life expectancy of Shanghai citizens has reached 80.98 (2008 statistics).

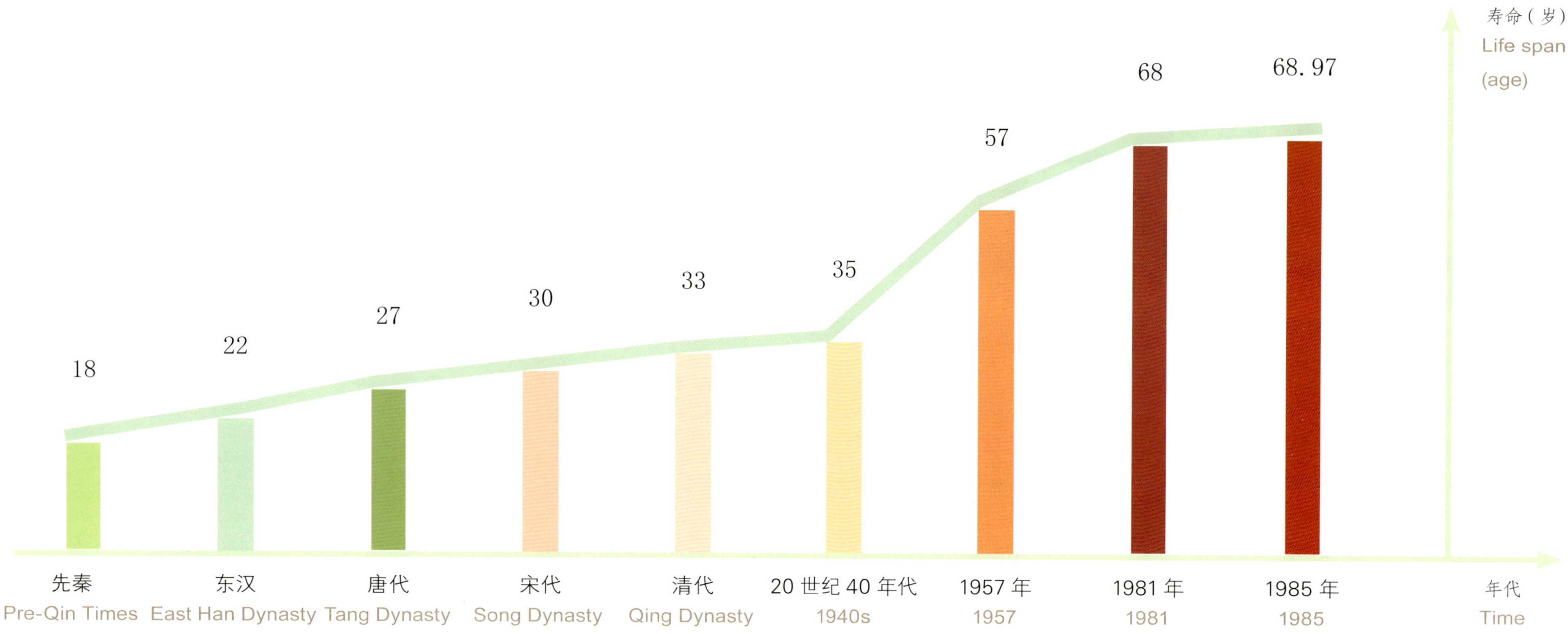

目前全世界人口的平均寿命为 66 岁，而我国人均寿命已超过 73 岁，加上百岁老人的比例在快速增长，我国总有一天可以达到“长寿之国”的标准。从个人来说，争取长命百岁的希望越来越大了，但是要使亿万国民的平均寿命增至百岁还需要大家共同努力。

At present, the average life span of the world population is 66. With an average life span above 73 and the rapid growth of the percentage of people aged 100 or above, China can be expected to become a “country of long-lived people” sooner or later. Although it is no longer difficult to attain the age of 100 for an individual, to increase the average life span of millions of Chinese citizens to 100 is a long journey that has just been started.

寿　　歌

Song of Longevity

一要寿，横逆之来欢喜受；
二要寿，灵台如镜光明透；
三要寿，艳舞妖娇如仇寇；
四要寿，夫妻恩爱常左右；
五要寿，俭朴安然常守旧；
六要寿，平生莫遣双眉皱；
七要寿，浮名不与人相斗；
八要寿，与人为善乐为友；
九要寿，谨防坐卧风穿牖；
十要寿，断酒莫教滋味厚。

寿歌大意是：一要长寿，遇到挫折愉快接受；二要长寿，心灵要如镜子光明正大；三要长寿，娇艳歌妓屏退左右；四要长寿，远离爱人如避仇寇；五要长寿，安然过着俭朴生活，一切照旧；六要长寿，平生乐观无虑无忧；七要长寿，淡泊名利不争不斗；八要长寿，与人为善，乐于为友；九要长寿，坐卧慎防风寒入户；十要长寿，戒酒还要少吃厚味。

First, take setbacks in your stride. Second, keep your mind as clean as a shining mirror. Third, keep away from coquettish singsong girls. Fourth, avoid too much sex like plague. Fifth, be contented with a frugal and uneventful life. Sixth, be optimistic and carefree. Seventh, do not compete for fame or fortune. Eighth, be kind and friendly to others. Ninth, do not sit or sleep in draft. Tenth, abstain from drinking and eating too much.

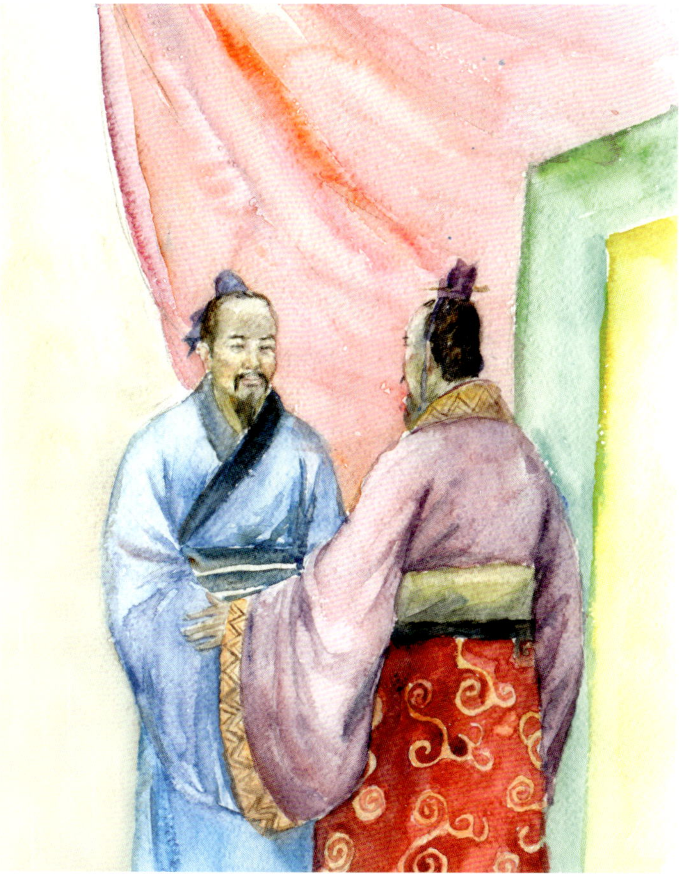

要长寿，平生乐观无虑无忧；要长寿，淡泊名利不争不斗

To attain longevity, one should be optimistic and free of anxiety and worries; to attain longevity, one should be indifferent to fame and wealth, and be non-contentious.

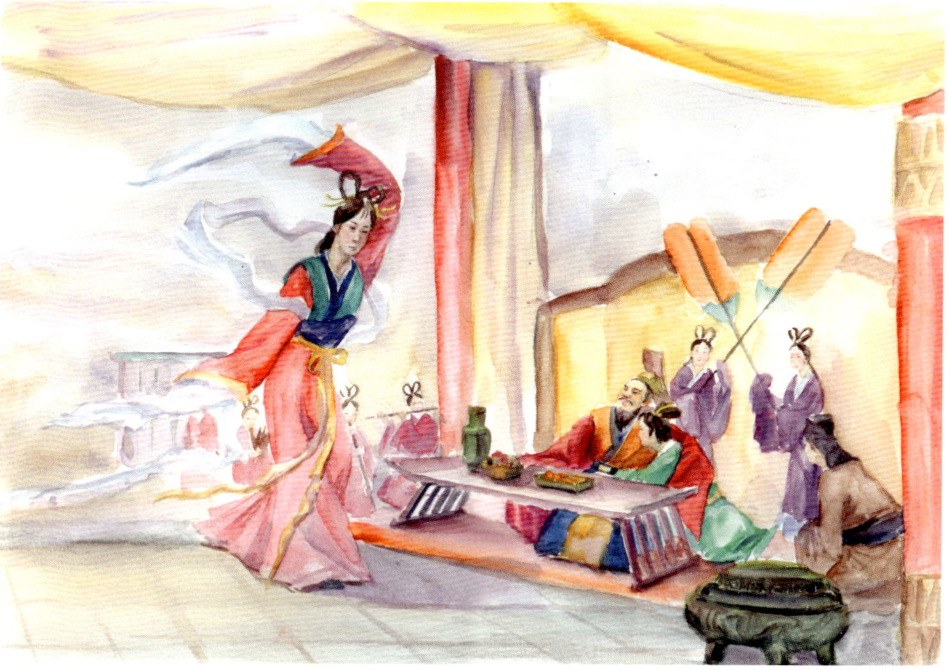

酒色无度对健康有着极大危害

Wallowing in alcohol and sex is extremely detrimental to health.

病后调养要点

Tips for better rehabilitation

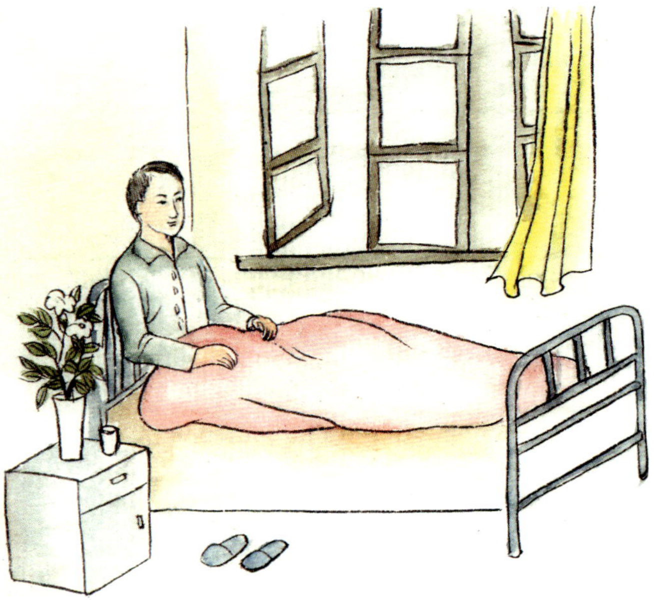

房间注意通风，保持空气新鲜。

Keep the room well-ventilated and the air fresh.

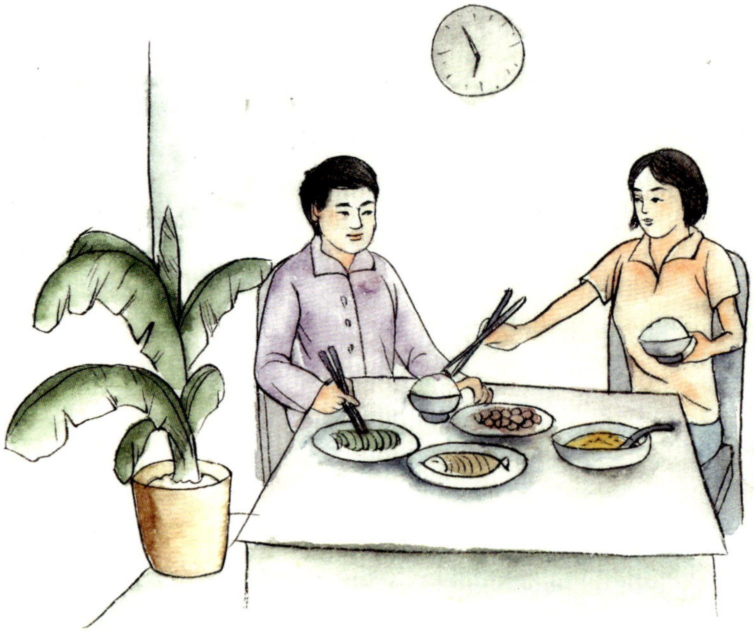

调养期间要注意加强营养，但营养搭配要合理，饮食要规律。

During the period of rehabilitation, take in enough nutrition, but reasonably so. Have meals regularly.

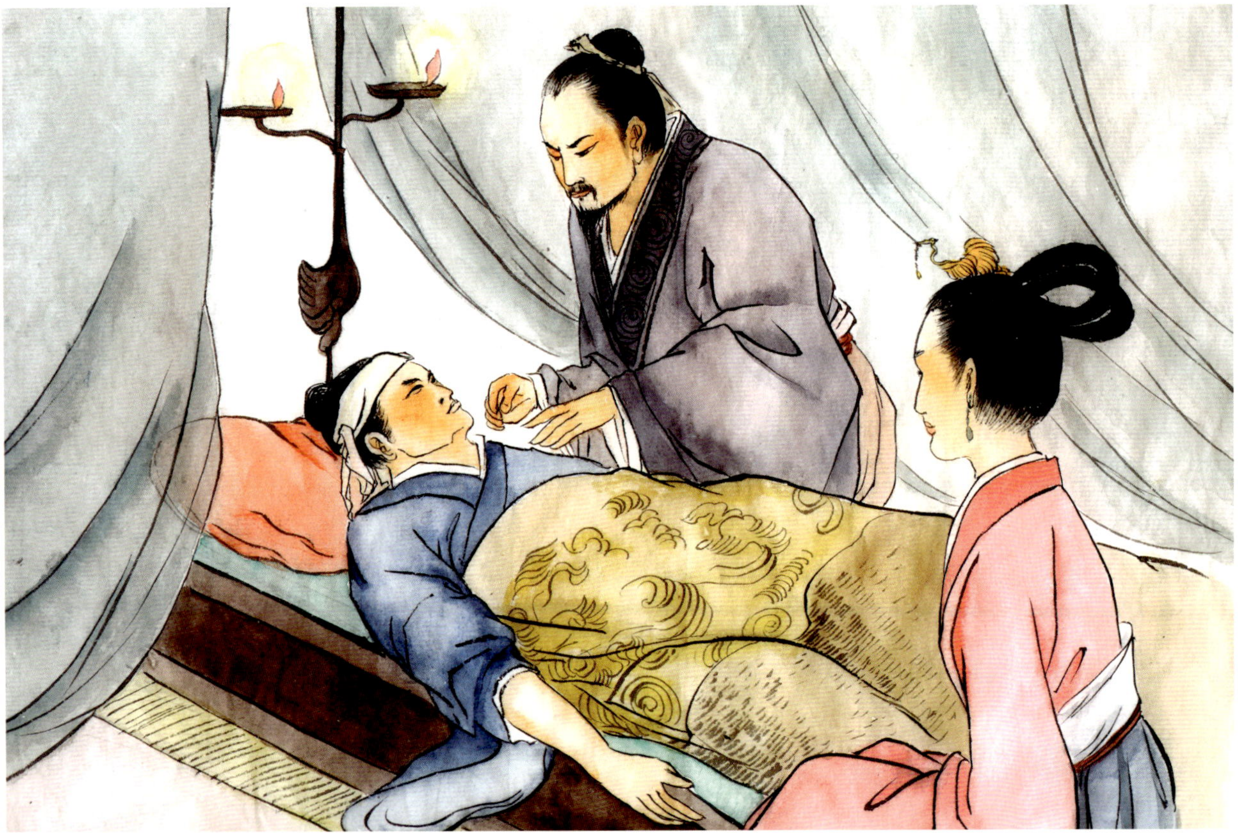

病来如山倒，病去如抽丝。

Diseases come on horseback, but go away on foot.

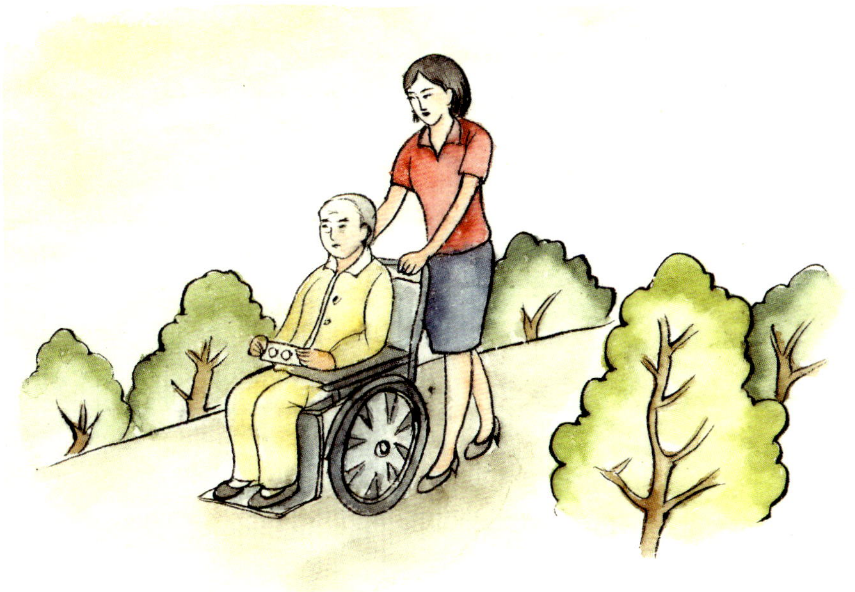

要设法解除病人的精神负担，让病人多做一些愉快的事情。

Find ways to relieve the patient of psychological burdens and tell him/her to do something enjoyable.

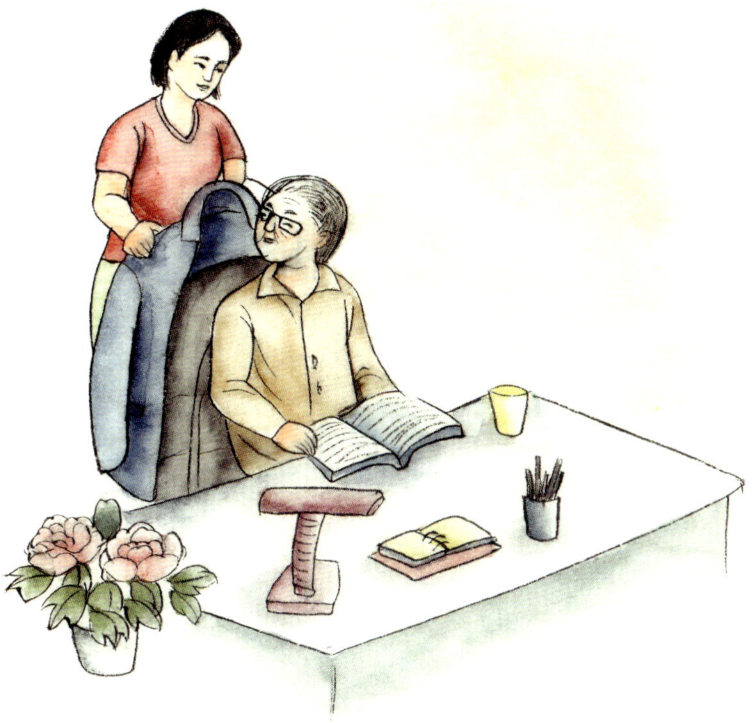

病后人的体质虚弱，易感冒。要遇寒加衣服，遇热减衣服。

As one is feeble and susceptible to colds after illness, one should be more alert to the temperature change and put on or take off clothes accordingly.

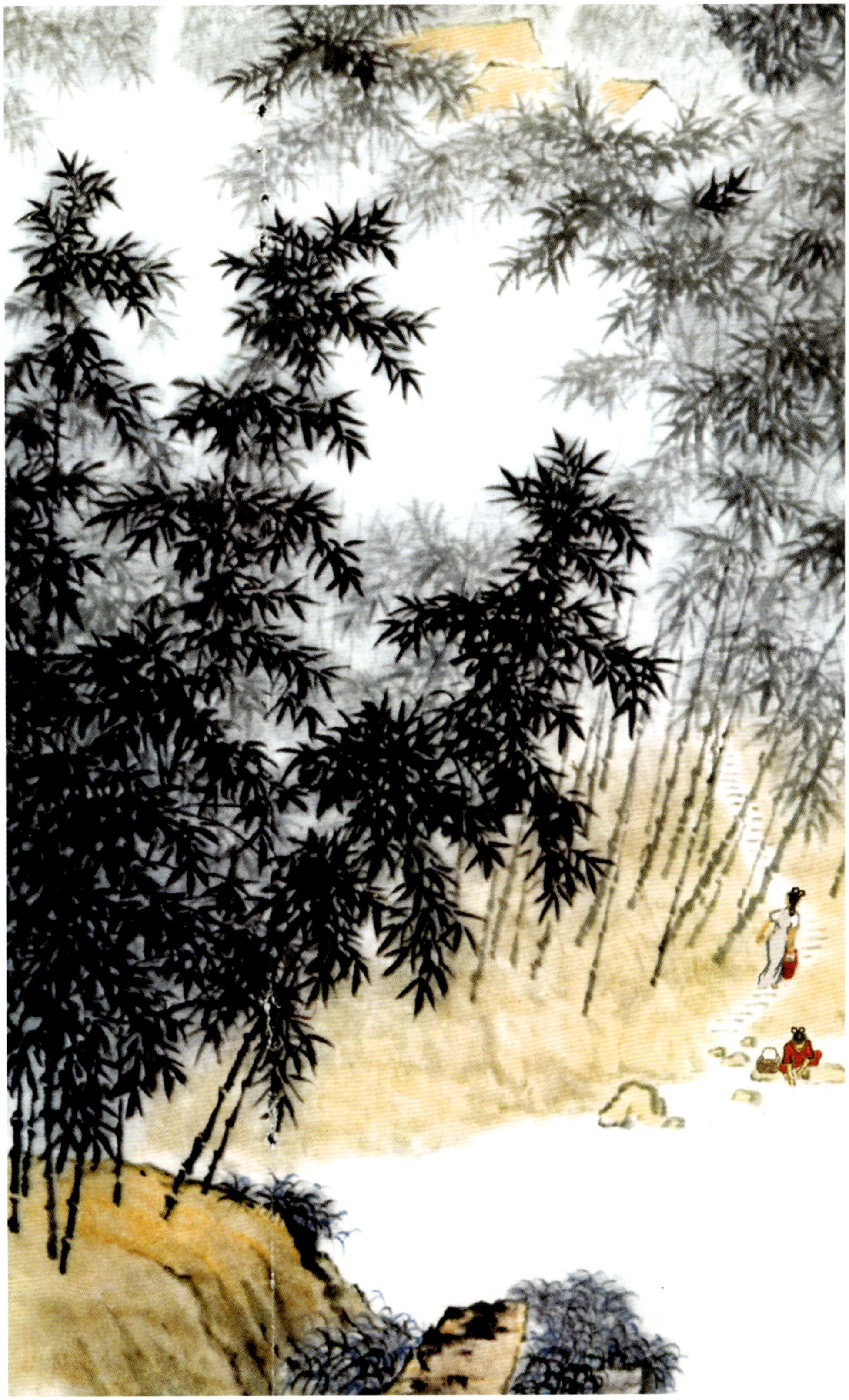

病后宜居静养图

Tranquil Living for Recovery after Illness

贰　源远流长

II. Time-honored Theories on Health Preservation

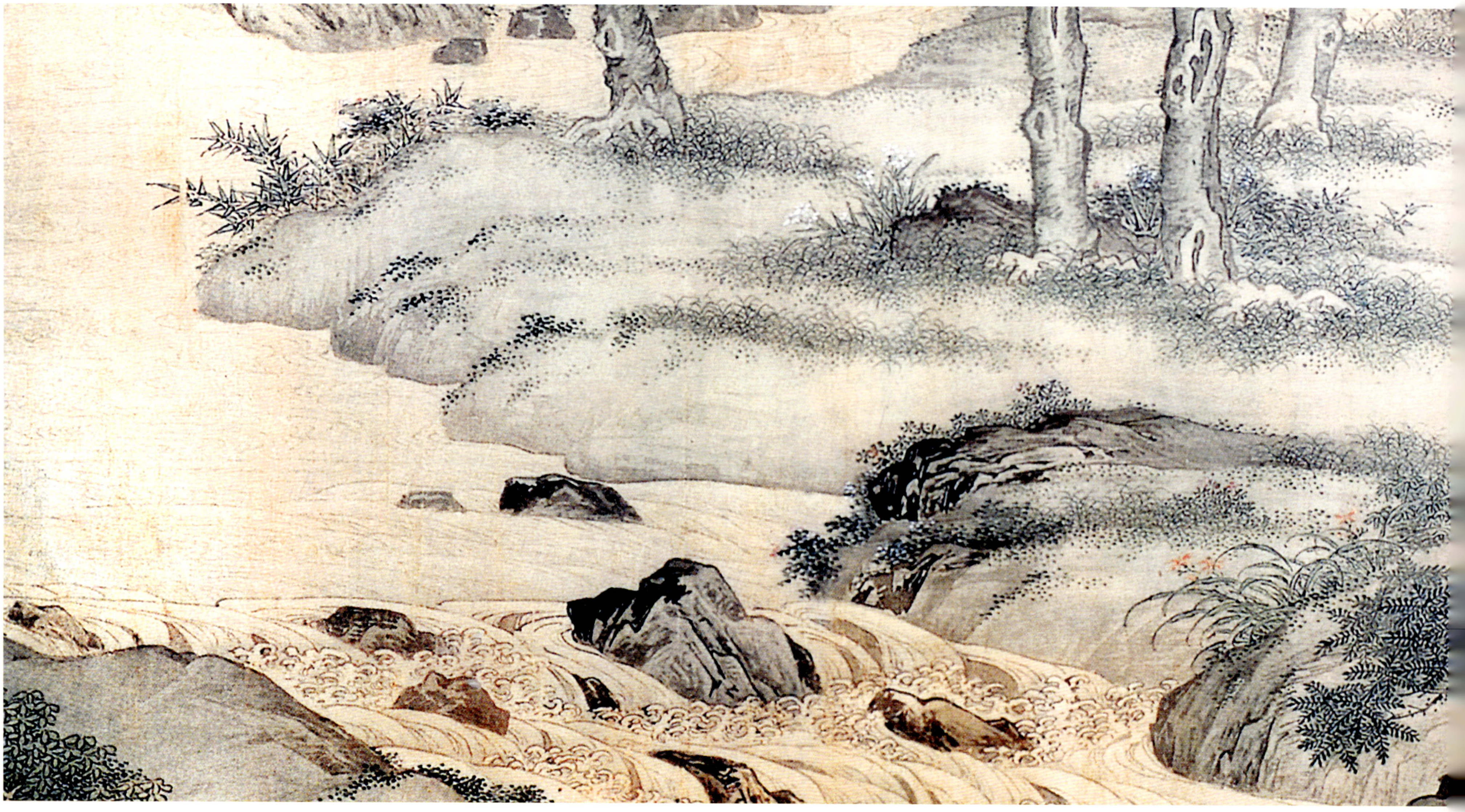

养生又称摄生，其目的是珍惜生命，保护身心，防疾祛病，健康长寿。中华民族的养生学有着悠久的历史，我们的祖先在过着茹毛饮血的生活时就已经开始摸索养生之道。先秦时期，导引术已经成熟，人们知道用吐故纳新的方法来促进身心健康。大约成书于战国时期的《黄帝内经》，更是为中华养生奠定了医学理论基础。

The purpose of Yangsheng, or 'health preservation', is to care for life, maintain both physical & psychological health, prevent and cure diseases, and conduce to longevity. Chinese theory on health preservation has a long history. Chinese people have been exploring ways of preserving health since the primitive society when people 'fed on raw meat and fowl'.Tao Yin attained maturity during the pre-Qin times, when Chinese people learnt that they could improve their physical and psychological health by 'breathing out stale air and breathe in fresh'. The Inner Canon of the Yellow Emperor, a book on Traditional Chinese Medicine completed in the Warring States Period, has laid the theoretical foundation for Chinese theories on health preservation.

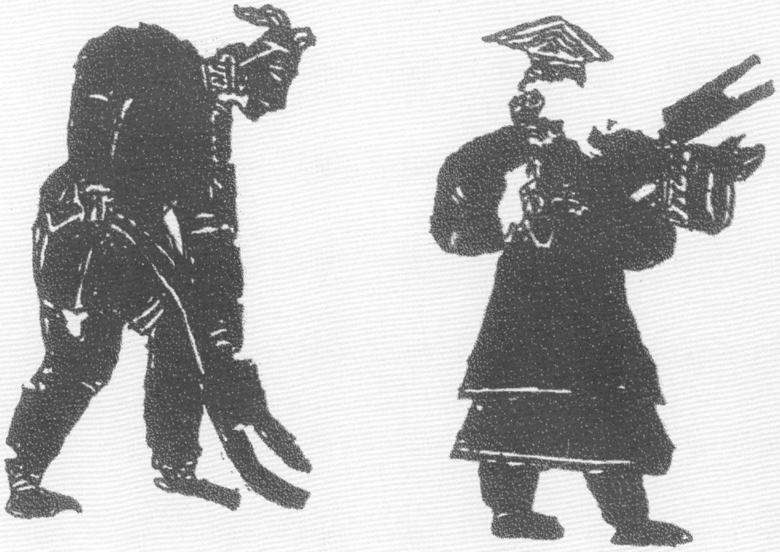

中华养生文化有三个基本特点

Three basic characteristics of Chinese regimens

中华养生是把人和自然看做一个整体来讲求生命的保养的。养生之道，是中国几千年来医疗、食疗、精神调摄和古代体育等养生文化的总和。总体来说，中华养生文化有三个基本特点：

一、"天人合一"的整体观。即认为人体这一系统与客观自然环境系统是统一的。

二、形神合养的一体观。重视养神与养形的关系和精气神在人体中的作用。

三、阴阳和谐的辩证观。注意阴阳平衡，劳作有度，动静结合。

Chinese regimens view human and nature as a whole to preserve health. The culture of Chinese regimens is the summation of Chinese traditional theories on medicine, food therapy, "psychological tune-up", as well as ancient sports and exercises. Generally speaking, Chinese regimens have three basic characteristics:

1. The holistic view which holds that the Heaven and humanity are one. In other words, the system of human body and the system of nature are concordant.

2. The totality concept which puts a premium on the parallel nourishment of body and spirit. In other words, the relationship between mental and physical health is emphasized and the role of the spirit in the body is highly valued.

3. The dialectical view of harmony between yin and yang, which attaches importance to the harmony between opposites, e.g. work and rest, movement and relaxation, etc.

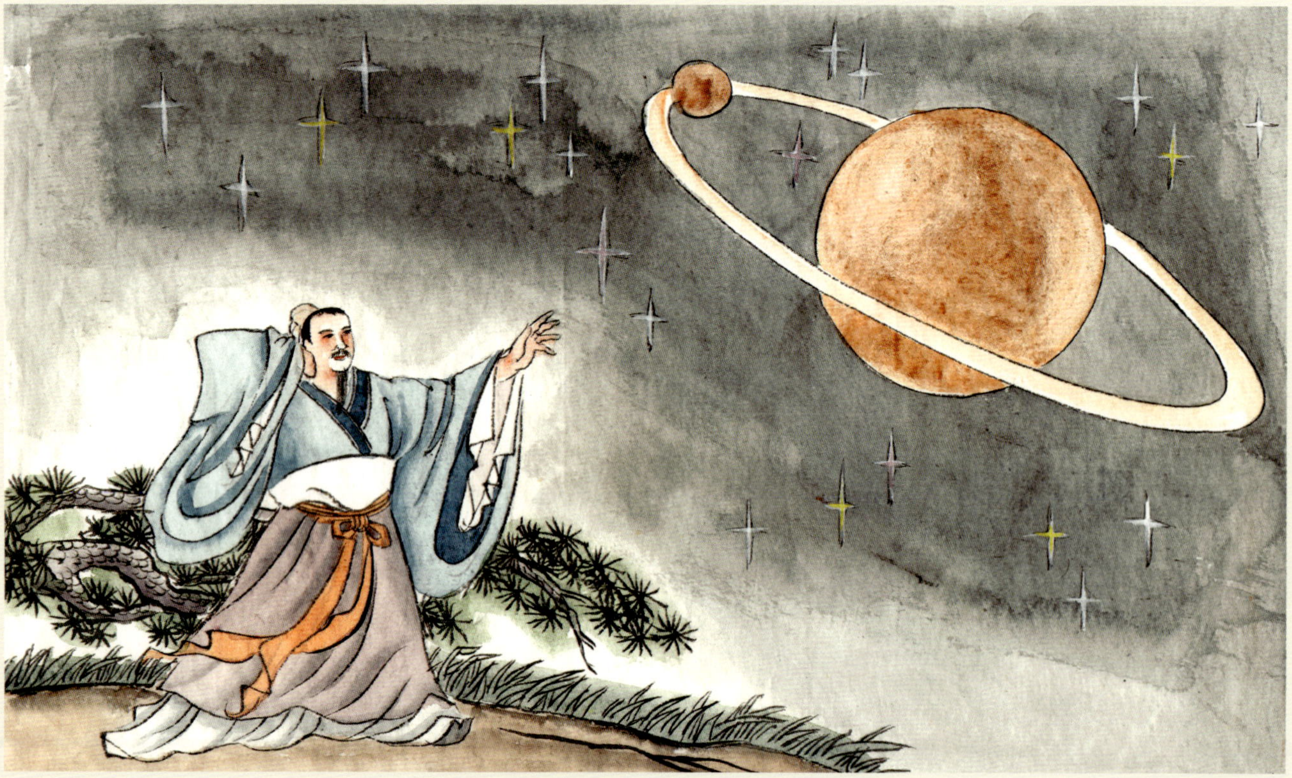

"天人合一"的整体观

The union of Heaven and humanity

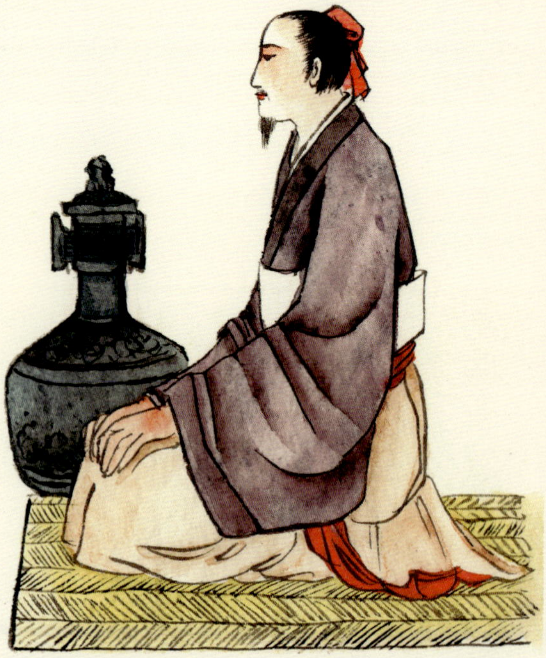

形神合养的一体观

A holistic approach to the nourishment of body and spirit

阴阳和谐的辩证观

The dialectical view of harmony between yin and yang

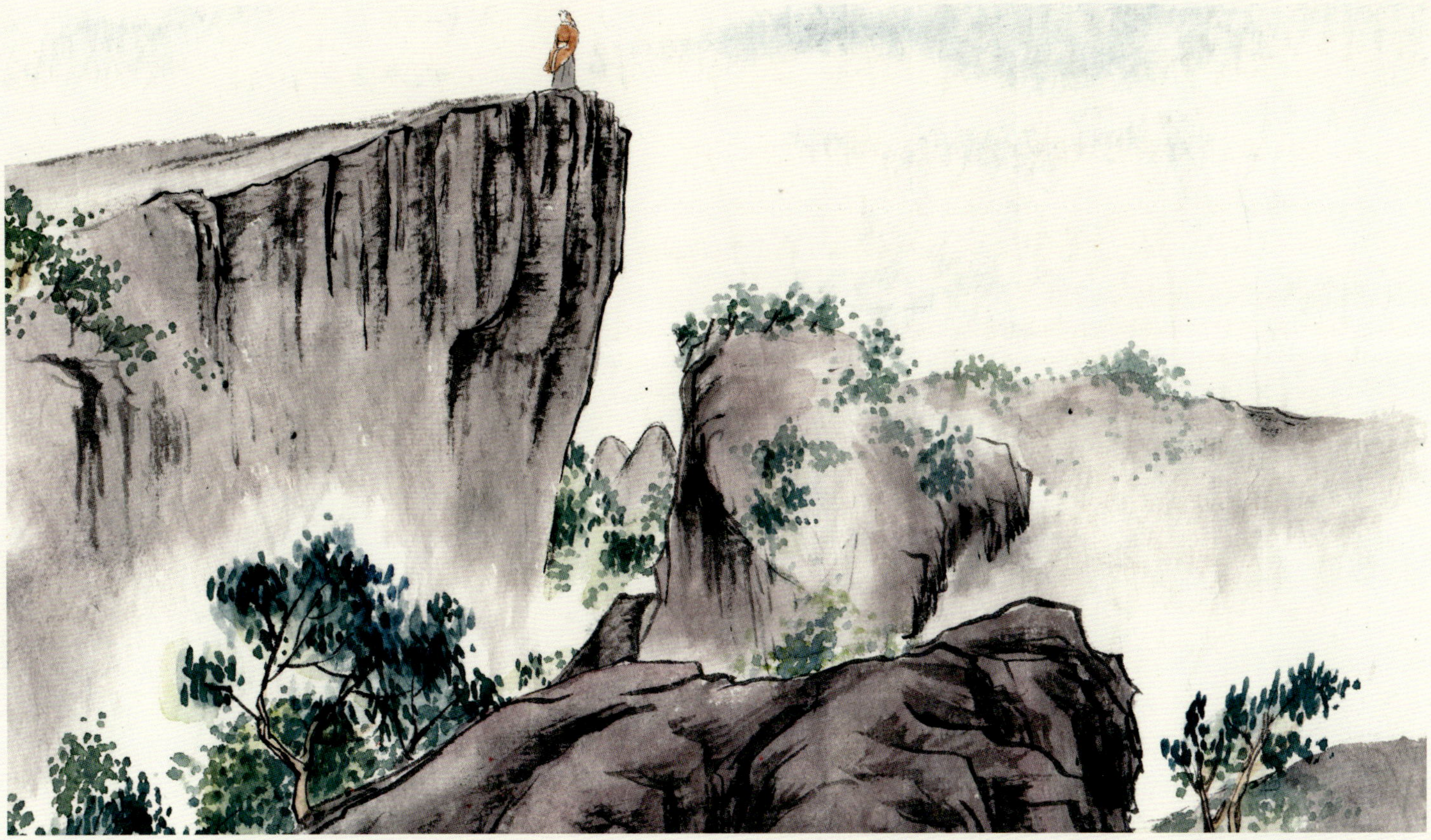

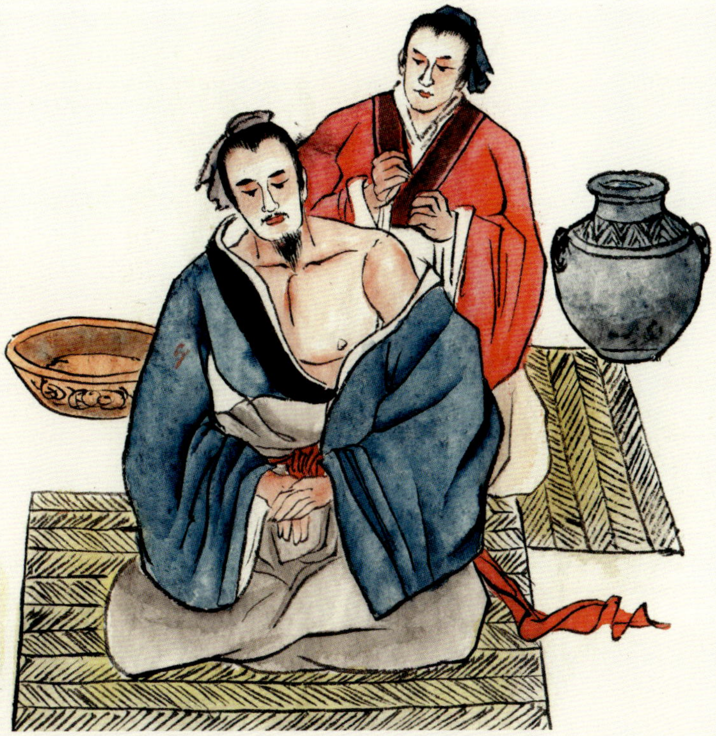

医疗、食疗、精气神调摄

Medicine, nourishment, spiritual conditioning

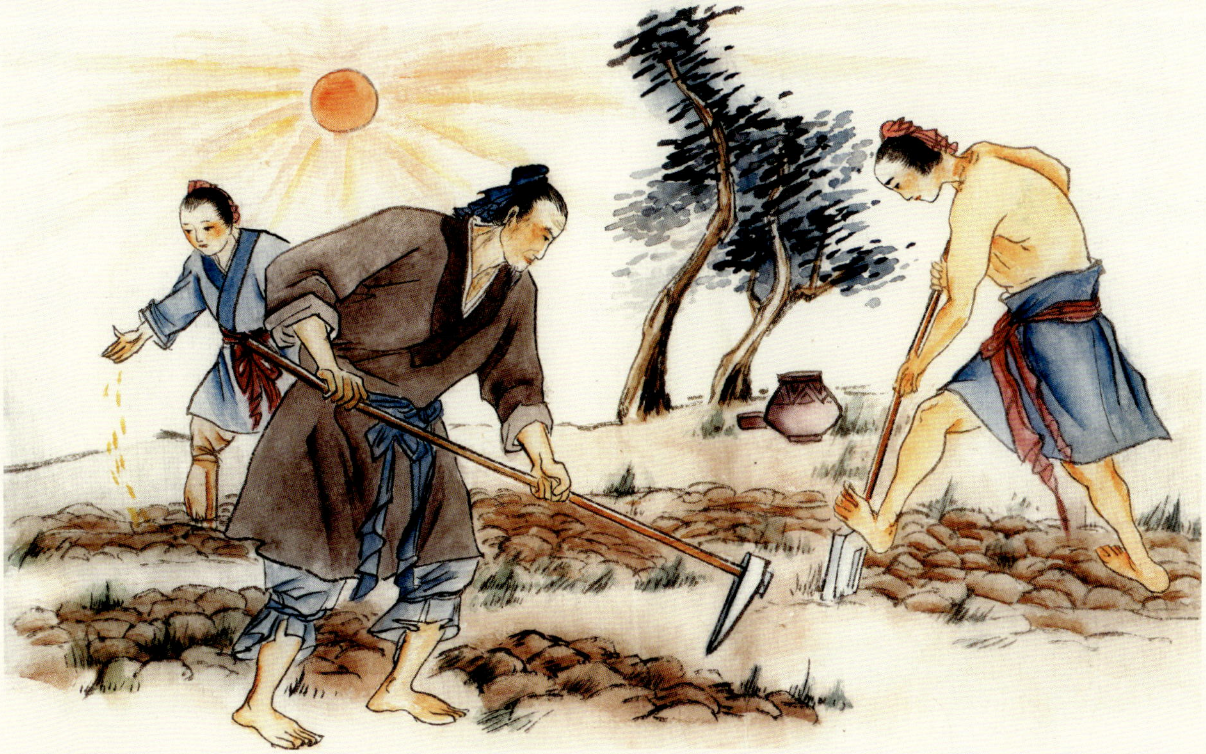

劳作有度，动静结合。

Work/rest balance

中华养生的萌芽

The dawn of Chinese regimen

从原始部落时期到公元前 21 世纪的夏朝，我们的祖先在适应和改造大自然的漫长过程中，谋求生存和发展。他们创造觅食工具、择居筑巢以避风寒防野兽、烤制熟食，积累了许多保护、滋养生命的经验。

From the primitive tribal times to the Xia Dynasty (circa 21st century BC) our ancestors managed to sustain themselves and evolve through adapting to nature and changing it. In this long process they learned to make tools, choose shelters and build dwellings so as to keep beasts off, stay away from cold and roast raw foods. As a result, our ancestors gained increasingly large amount of experience for the protection and nourishment of life.

火的作用与食物养生萌芽

The use of fire and the emergence of dietary regimen

火不仅可以帮助人照明、御寒，还帮助人类结束了“茹毛饮血”的生活，提高了人体对食物的消化吸收质量，防止了一些肠道疾病的发生。“民以食为天”，先民们为了生存，必须猎取食物，由食用偶然发现的食品到主动寻找食物，经过了相当长时间的经验积累，逐步了解了一些食物的养生作用，人类养生文明悄然萌芽。医学史上所称“医食同源”也即指此。

Besides offering our ancestors light and heat, fire put an end to their uncouth way of living, which can be vividly described as “drinking blood and eating hair”. In addition to helping the human body to digest and absorb food, the use of fire contributed to the reduction of incidence of intestinal diseases. As the saying goes, food is the top priority for people. In order to survive, our ancestors had to hunt for food, shifting from accidental encounter to voluntary pursuit. The accumulation of experience over time gave rise to the promotion of health through nourishment. In the history of traditional Chinese medicine, medical treatment and food nourishment are regarded as sharing one origin. From then on, civilization in the form of regimen made its incipient appearance.

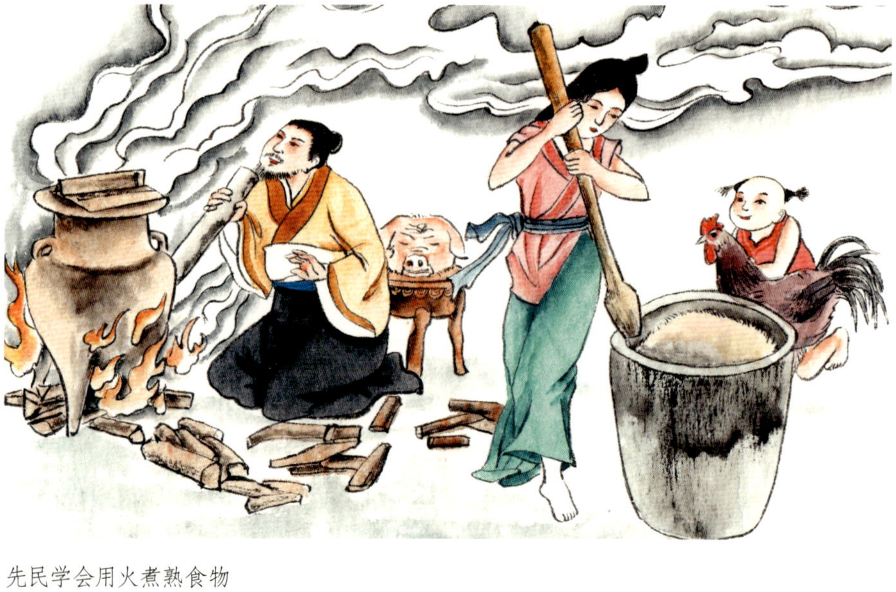

先民学会用火煮熟食物

The ancient people learnt to use fire to cook food

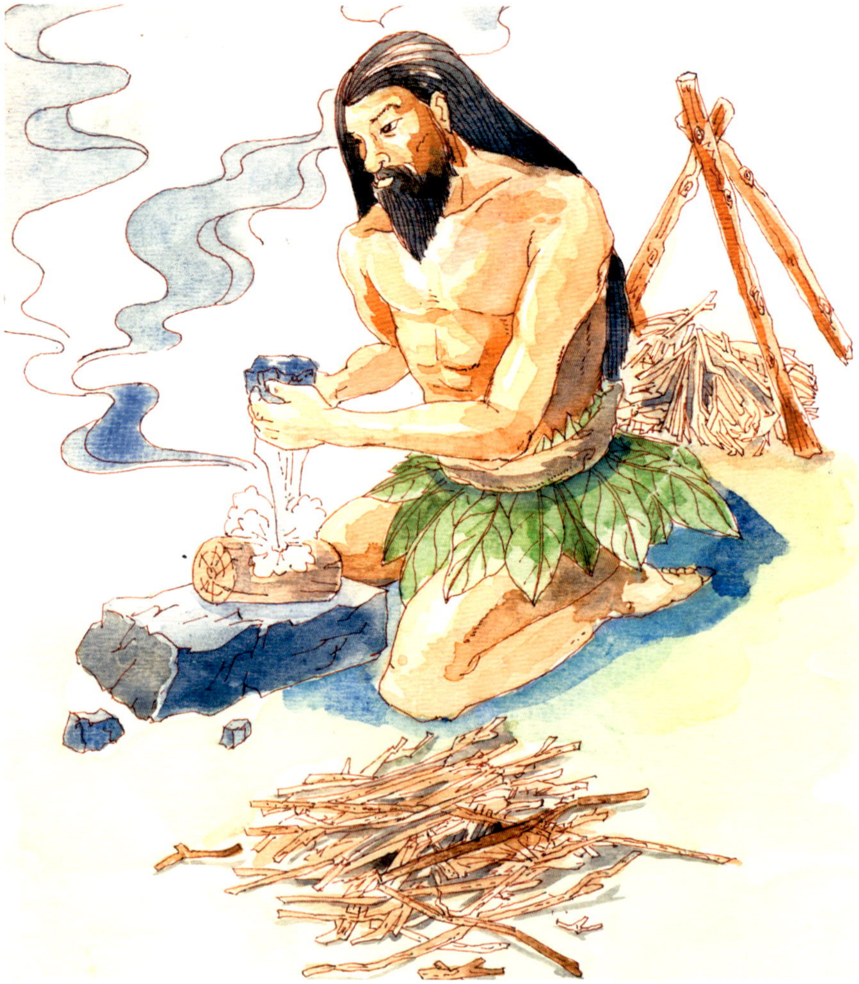

先民钻木取火

The ancient people learnt to drill wood to make fire

先民们在用火取暖的过程中，还慢慢地掌握了一些简单的“火疗”技能，比如灸、熨等，他们用这些技能治病养生。

While employing fire for heat, our ancestors came up with some simple skills for the maintenance of health and treatment of diseases with fire, which can be called “fire therapy”, e.g. moxibustion and the applying of hot irons or compresses.

先民懂得择居和“沐浴”

Selecting shelters & bathing

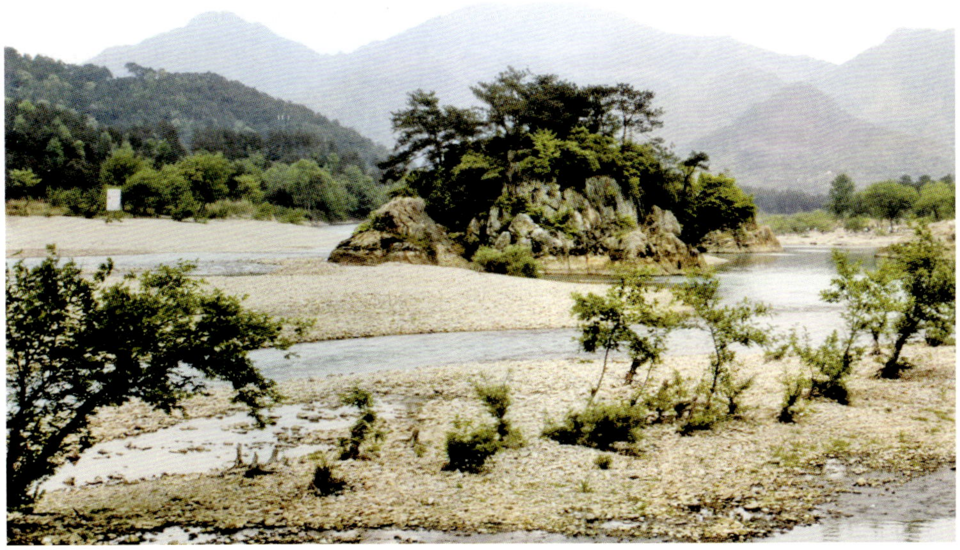

在出土的殷商时期的甲骨文中，已经有“沐”（洗头发）、“浴”（洗澡）等和卫生有关的文字。

我们的祖先原来在有肥美水土及充足食物的河谷一带群聚而居，若是遇到自然灾害，被迫迁徙，他们就会依据这些条件有选择地居留。在《诗经·大雅·公刘》一篇中就有“观其流泉”的描写。

劳动与体育养生

Labor and physical regimens

早期人类通过劳动寻找食物、火种，他们发明简单的工具，建造房舍，满足了最基本的吃、穿、住、用、行等生存需求。劳动在帮助人类改善生活的同时，又促使人类开拓了眼界，增长了智慧，增强了体质，延长了寿命。劳动之余，先民们载歌载舞庆祝丰收，由舞蹈产生了宣导养生（宣导，又称导引，吐纳，晋代以后所谓养生功）。体育养生出现了。

By securing food and fire, and then by making tools and lodgings, primitive people managed to meet their basic needs for making a living. In addition to improving people's livelihood, labor helped to enlarge their visions, sharpen their wisdom and enhance their physique. All of this contributed to longer life spans. People danced and sang in celebration of harvests, which resulted in the emergence of breath conditioning – the approach for improvement of health through exhalation and inhalation that evolved into Qigong in the Jin Dynasty (265-420 AD) and later on. Thus regimen through physical exercise appeared and a primitive regimen culture began to take shape.

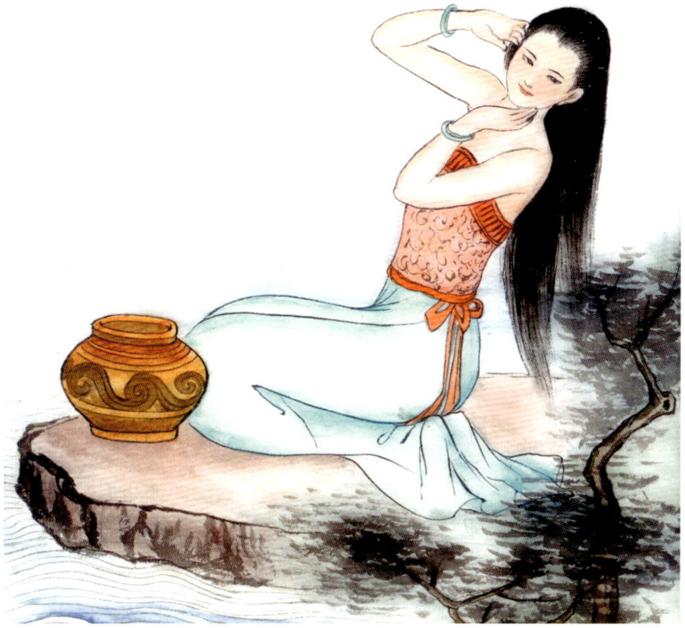

先民沐浴

Bathing

On the unearthed oracle bones of the Shang Dynasty (circa 17th-11th century BC), characters with the meanings of washing the face and taking a bath can be detected. This can give us a glimpse of our ancestors' hygienic practices.

Our ancestors used to gather and live along rivers, the basins of which could provide them with moist fertile land and abundant food. In the case of natural disasters and displacement, people had to seek shelters where they could find basic living conditions. A typical scene was captured in the "Ode of Gong Liu" in *The Book of Songs* which described one of our ancestors' explorations for favorable living conditions along a river under the leadership of Gong Liu, the chief of the tribe.

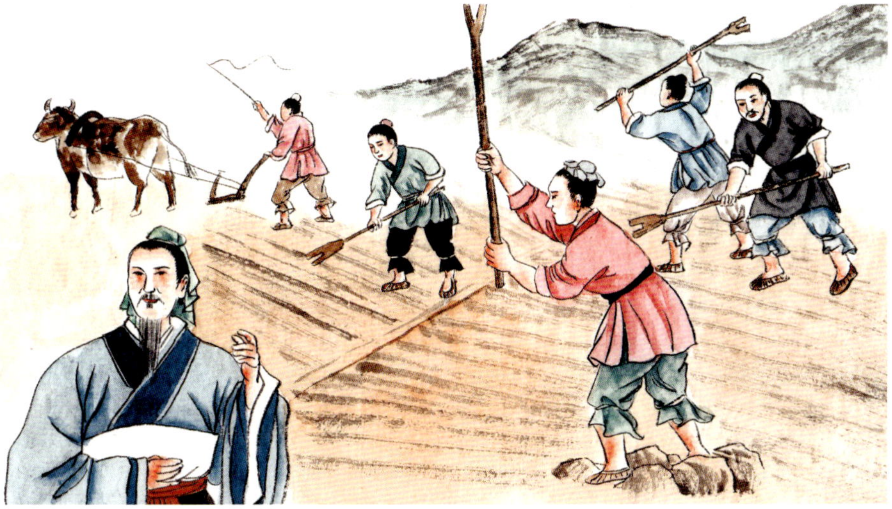

养生源于劳动

Methods of health preservation originated from labor.

中华养生的理论基础

The theoretical basis of Chinese regimens

《黄帝内经》

Inner Canon of the Yellow Emperor

在中华养生史上，《黄帝内经》一书的出现是一个里程碑。它奠定了中华养生学的基础，确立了“天人相应”的养生原则。

In the history of Chinese regimen, the compilation of the *Inner Canon of the Yellow Emperor* is a milestone. It is this book that laid the foundation for Chinese regimen. The *Inner Canon of the Yellow Emperor* established the regimen principle that man and heaven are consonant with each other.

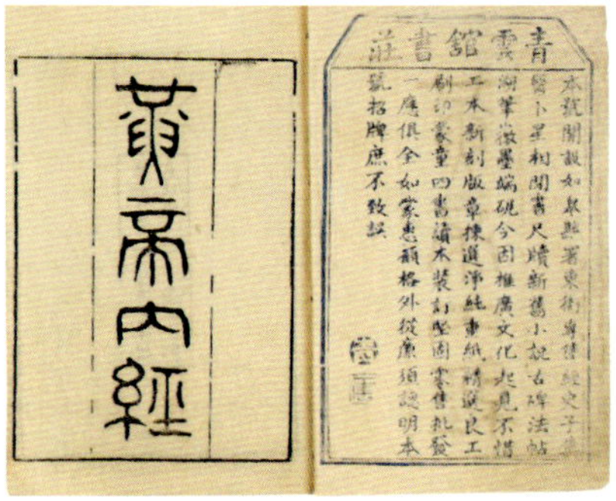

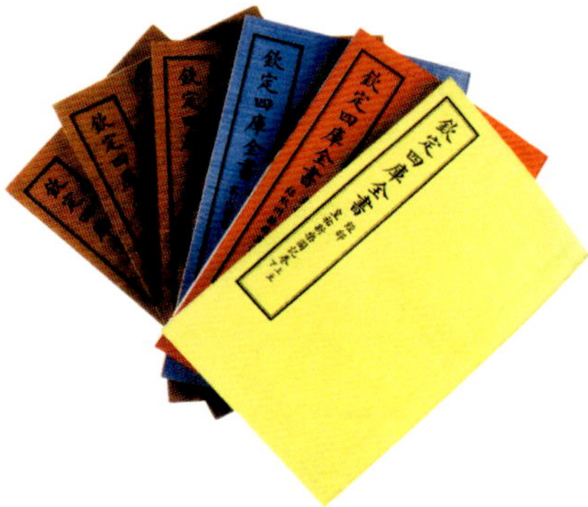

《黄帝内经》书影

Inner Canon of the Yellow Emperor

黄帝与岐伯

Yellow Emperor and Qibo

传说中的岐伯是我国远古轩辕黄帝时期的重要人物，是历史上著名医学家。据说他的著述很多，但多已失传，仅留残著。后人根据他的残著整理编辑成《黄帝内经》，流传至今。因此，岐伯也被称为中华医学的鼻祖。

《黄帝内经》认为“人以天地之气生，四时之法成”，所以养生的要旨是“顺四时而适寒暑，和喜怒而安居处，节阴阳而调刚柔”（《灵枢・本神篇》），要“春夏养阳，秋冬养阴”。人如果能顺应四时的变化，就能益寿延年。

Qibo, a legendary figure dating back to the period of Yellow Emperor, was both a remarkable medical practitioner and a prolific author of medical works, most of which, however, got missing over time. The remnants of his works were compiled into a book entitled the *Inner Canon of the Yellow Emperor*, and Qibo has ever since been called the progenitor of Chinese medicine.

It is postulated in the *Inner Canon* that humans come into being as a representation of *qi* (meaning air, vital force in Chinese) from heaven and earth, and that they are supposed to comply with the rhythm of the four seasons. The essence of maintenance of health lies in following the rhythm of the four seasons to adapt to heat and cold, moderating anger and elation for a tranquil life, and proportioning yin and yang to temper hardness with softness. It is imperative to “nurture yang in spring and summer while supporting yin in autumn and winter.” A person acting in accordance with the rhythm of seasons is likely to enjoy a long life.

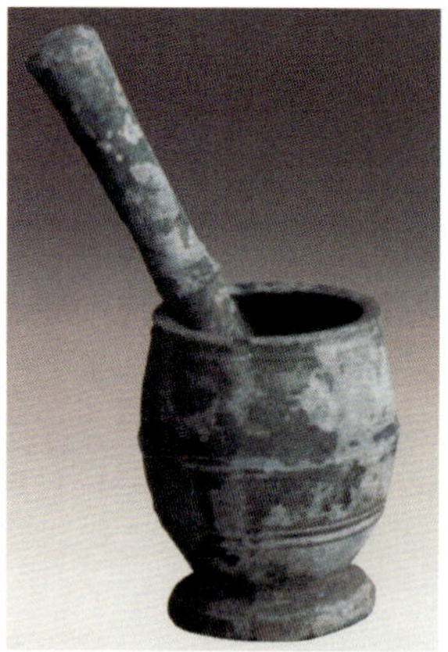

西周　铜药臼

Western Zhou Dynasty
Bronze medicine mortar

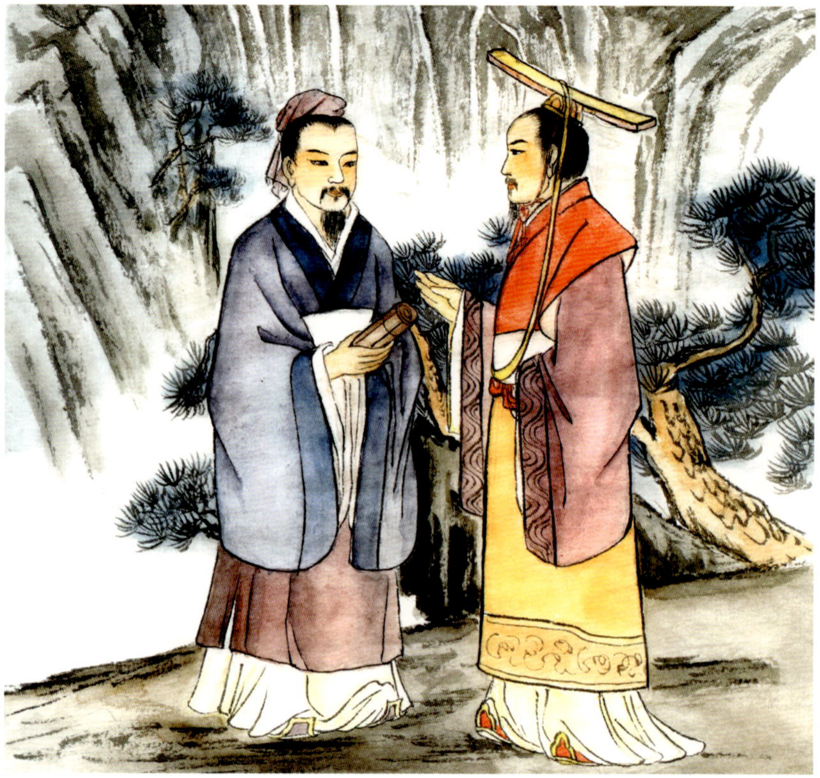

黄帝与岐伯

Yellow Emperor and Qibo

精、气、神为人身三宝

The three treasures in a human body: essence, qi, and spirit

《黄帝内经》认为精是构成人体的基本物质，精又是人体生命活动的原始动力。气，指精微物质，又指脏腑活动的能力。神为生命活动现象的总称，是一切生命活动的集中表现。由是，精、气、神谓之为人身“三宝”。

It is postulated in the *Inner Canon* that essence is the fundamental substance of which the human body consists. Essence constitutes the primary driving force for life activities of the human body. Qi refers to infinitesimal substance and the capabilities of the viscera. Spirit is the aggregate of the phenomena of life activities and the epitome of all life activities. Essence, qi and spirit are called “the three gems” of the human body.

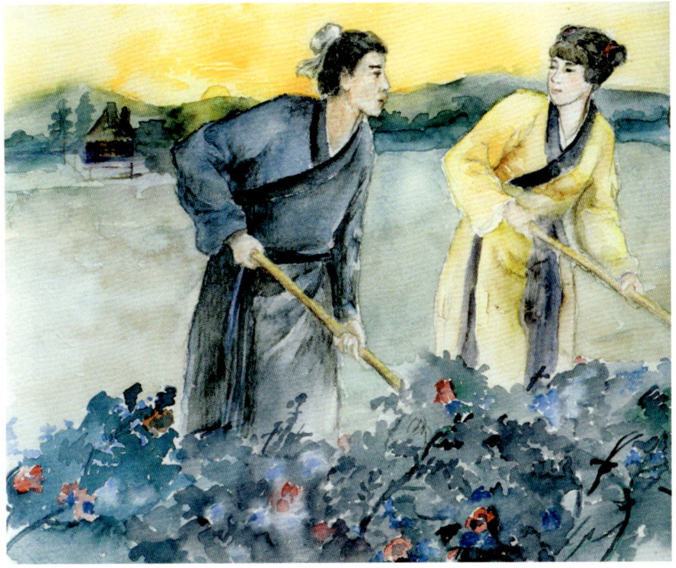

精气神之一

Essence, qi, and spirit

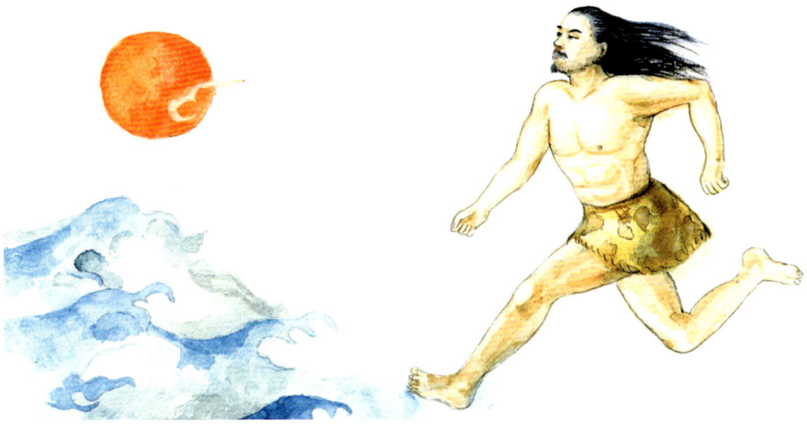

精气神之三

Essence, qi, and spirit

《黄帝内经》保留了战国以前有效的养生方法和原则，提出了食养与食疗、动静结合、形体锻炼等养生方法。

The *Inner Canon* helps to preserve the effective approaches and principles of regimen before the Warring States Period, and puts forward such concepts as nourishment with food vs. food therapy, the combination of movements and relaxation, exercising the body for strength and health, etc.

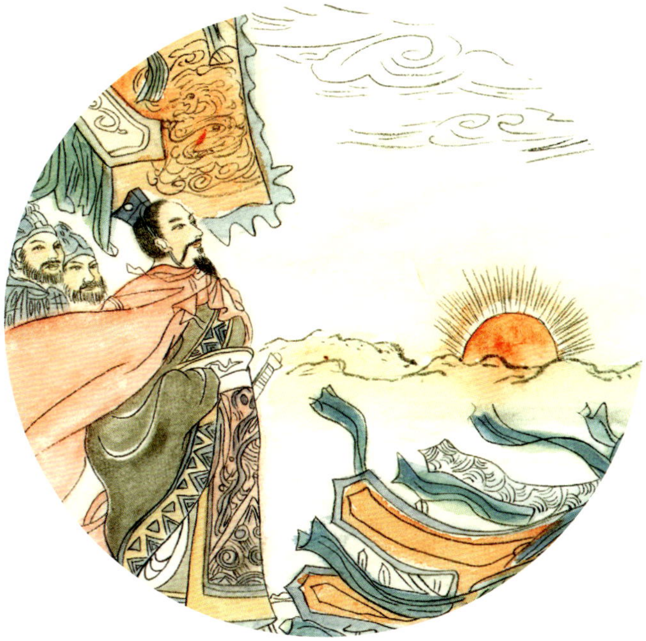

精气神之二

Essence, qi, and spirit

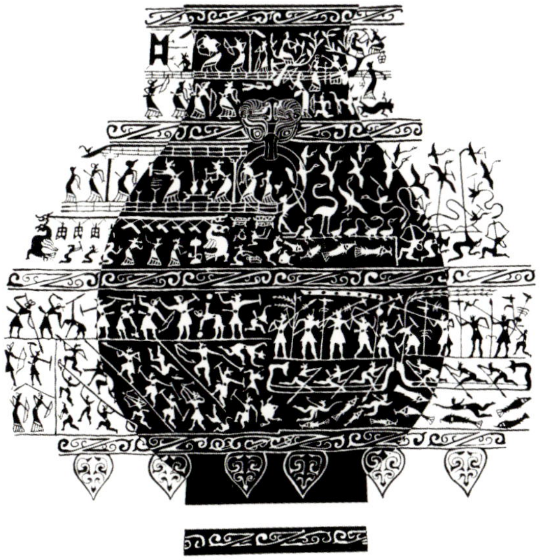

战国　宴乐狩猎攻战图

The Warring States Period　Banquet, hunting and combat

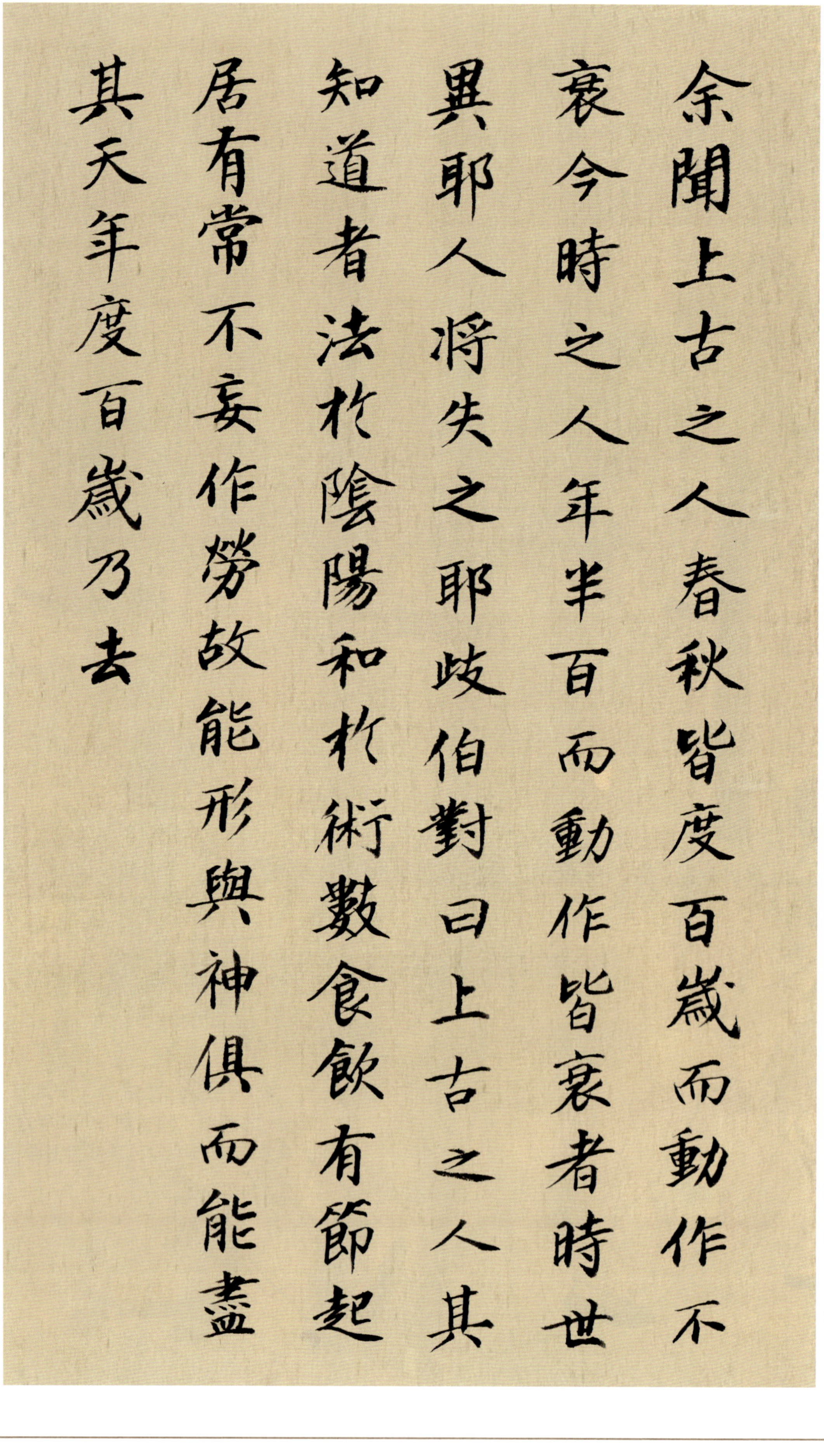

《黄帝内经·素问》

Inner Canon of the YellowEmperor : Suwen

这是中医学第一部经典《黄帝内经》关于人如何做到健康长寿的论述，也是中华养生学的理论基础。

This is the explanation of how a human being can achieve health and longevity from the first classic of TCM, the *Inner Canon of the Yellow Emperor*, and it is also the foundation of Chinese traditional theories on health preservation.

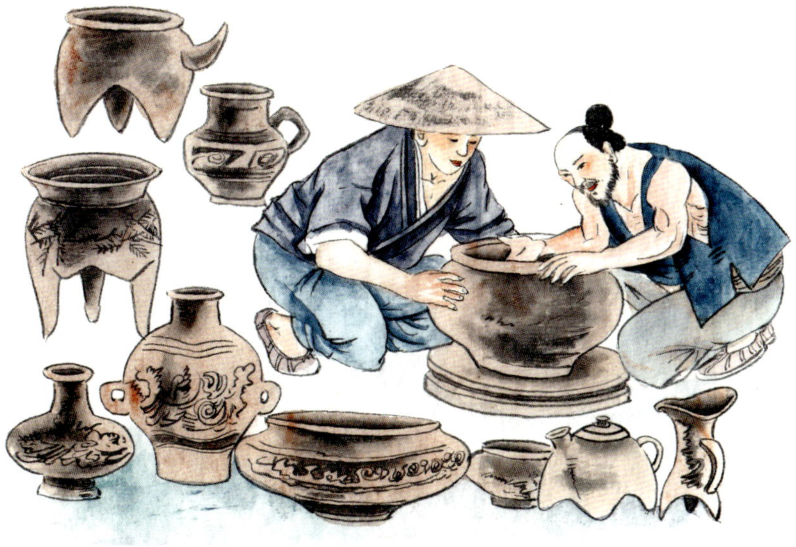

上古之人，春秋皆度百岁，而动作不衰
Ancient people lived beyond the age of a hundred without showing any sign of decrepitude in their movement or conduct.

余闻上古之人，春秋皆度百岁，而动作不衰；今时之人，年半百而动作皆衰者，时世异耶，人将失之耶？岐伯对曰：上古之人，其知道者，法于阴阳，和于术数，食饮有节，起居有常，不妄作劳，故能形与神俱，而尽终其天年，度百岁乃去。今时之人不然也，以酒为浆，以妄为常，醉以入房，以欲竭其精，以耗散其真，不知持满，不时御神，务快其心，逆于生乐，起居无节，故半百而衰也。

夫上古圣人之教下也，皆谓之虚邪贼风，避之有时。恬惔虚无，真气从之，精神内守，病安从来？是以志闲而少欲，心安而不惧，形劳而不倦，气从以顺，各从其欲，皆得所愿。故美其食，任其服，乐其俗，高下不相慕，其民故曰朴。是以嗜欲不能劳其目，淫邪不能惑其心，愚智贤不肖，不惧于物，故合于道。所以能年皆度百岁而动作不衰者，以其德全不危也。

〖白话〗我听说上古时代的人，其寿命都超过了一百岁，而动作举止仍然没有衰老的迹象；现在的人，则年过半百，就显得非常衰老，是时代不同的原因呢，还是人类自己把生命丢失了呢？歧伯回答说：上古时代的人，懂得养生规律的，师法阴阳，知道养生的具体方法，饮食有节制，起居有规律，不作无益之事损害身体，所以形体与精神协调统一，而能够活到应活的年龄，超过了一百岁才死去。如今的人却不是这样，他们把酒作为日常饮料，以混乱的生活为正常，醉酒之后进行房事，想要竭尽精气，耗散真元，不知谨慎小心，不按规律进行思维活动，一味放纵自己的心愿，违背养生之道，生活没有规律，所以人到五十便过早地衰老了。

上古时代的圣人教育百姓，都说对一切邪气风寒，要及时避开。恬静淡泊无欲无为，真气就会产生，精神就不会散失，这样一来，疾病怎么能产生呢？放松精神减少欲望，心绪安定不惊不惧，形体劳而不倦，血气流畅不滞，如此则能随心所欲，实现自己的愿望。不挑剔饮食，不讲究穿着，随乡入俗，安分守己，其民风就称得上淳朴。因此嗜好和欲望不能损害自己的眼睛；淫欲和邪念不能迷惑自己的内心，无论是愚蠢、聪明，还是贤明、无能，只要对外界事物无所动心，就合乎养生之道。所以那些活到一百多岁仍然不显衰老的人，就是由于懂得养生之道的缘故。

I am told that ancient people lived beyond the age of a hundred without showing any sign of decrepitude in their movement or conduct. Today's people, however, look senile once they are over fifty. Is this because times are different? Or have human beings lost their long lives because of their own fault?

The following is Qibo's answer:

Ancient people understood the laws for the preservation of health and followed the rules of yin and yang. Also familiar with the specific methods for preserving health, they were temperate in their diet and lived according to a regular routine, without doing anything harmful to their health. As a result, their achieved concord and unity in both form and spirit, and were able to attain the due life span, which is beyond a hundred. This is not the case among today's people. They drink every day and mistake the abnormal for the normal. They have sex when drunk, which drains their essential pneuma (jingqi) and dissipates their vital spirit (zhenyuan). Instead of acting prudently and thinking rationally, they spare no effort to satisfy their desires. Because of their violation of the rules for preserving health and disorderly way of life, they begin to age prematurely at fifty.

Ancient sages taught people to promptly avoid all evil influence and cold. To live a tranquil life without pursuing fame and fortune will generate true vitality (zhenqi) and prevent the spirit from dissipating. If so, how could one fall ill? Relax yourself and reduce your desires, calm your thoughts and be free of fear and panic, apply yourself to work without getting tired, and ensure that your blood and vital energy circulate smoothly. Thus you will be able to do as you like and fulfill your wishes. Don't be particular about food or clothing. Do in Rome as the Romans do, and act in a way proper to your status. If everybody does so, the social mores can be said to be simple and honest. Thus your hobbies and desires will not harm your eyes, and no lust or evil thought will lead your mind astray. No matter if you are wise or not, able or incompetent, to remain unperturbed by anything around you will be in keeping with the way to preserve health. It is because of the understanding of that way that some people have lived beyond the age of a hundred without showing any sign of decrepitude.

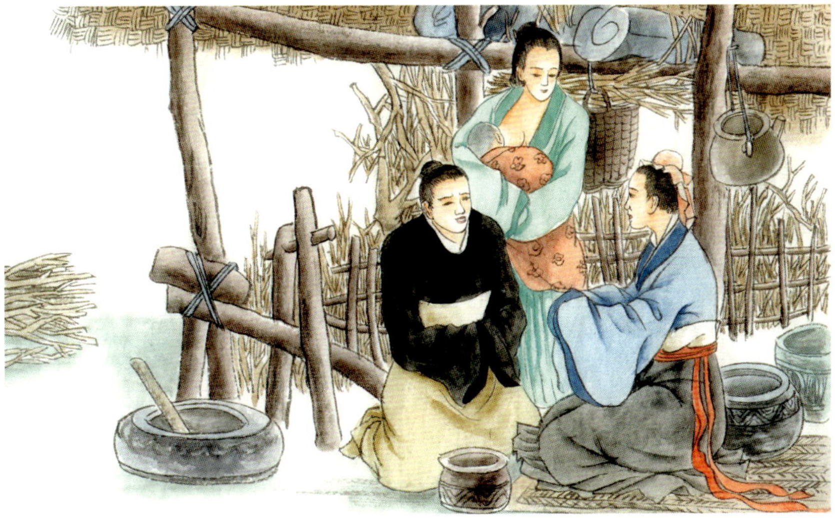

上古时代圣人教育百姓
An ancient sage advising people on health

叁　博大精深

III.　The Profound Culture of Chinese Regimens

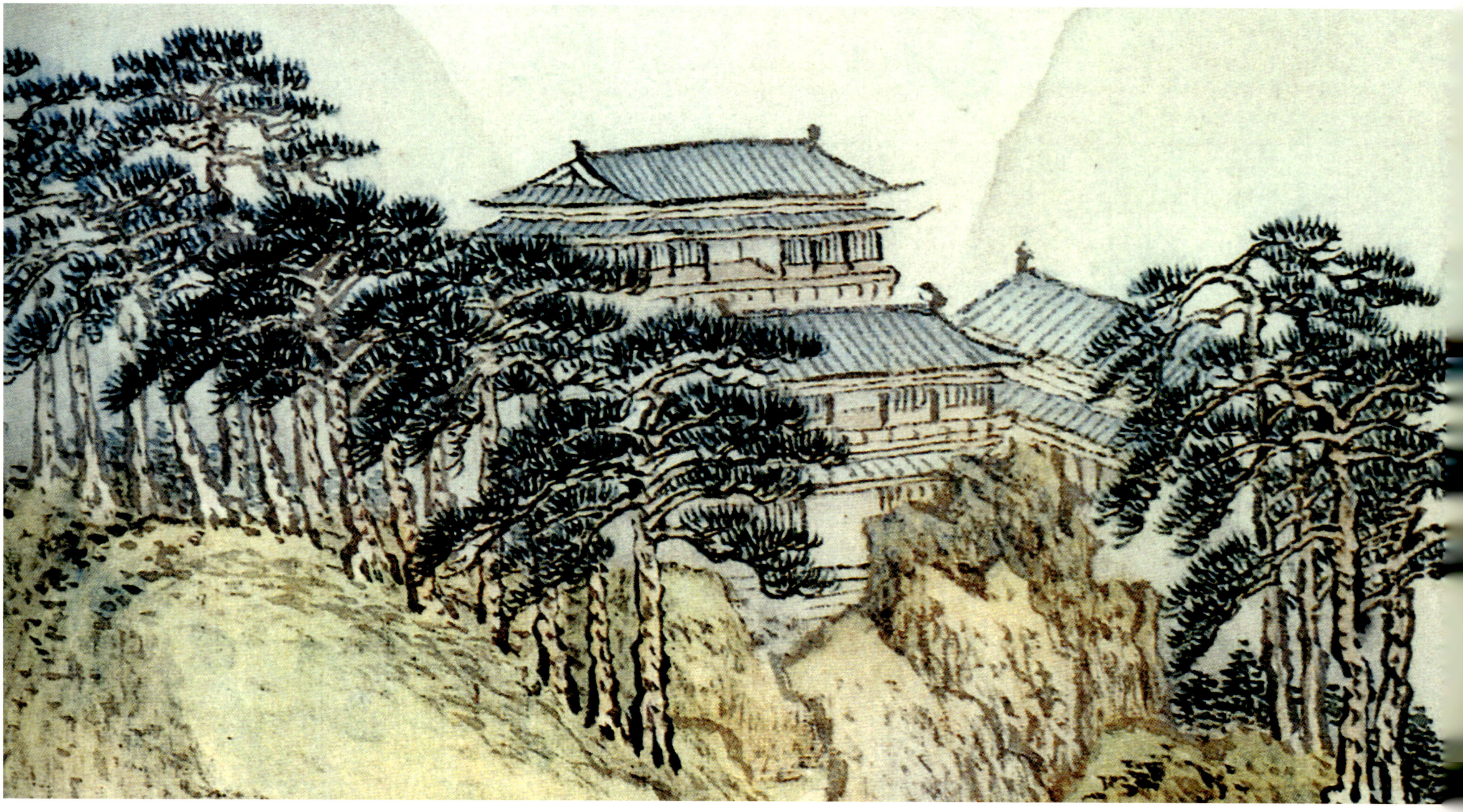

早在先秦时期，中华养生学就已经十分丰富。由狩猎活动、欢庆舞蹈和作息调节发展出了导引术；顺应自然、保养精神形成了道家养生；加强修养、自强自律形成了儒家养生。《黄帝内经》及汉以后两千多年的中国医学、养生学可谓博大精深。

Chinese theory on health preservation had already attained prosperity in the pre-Qin times (the times before 221 BC). Tao Yin, a series of breathing exercises, originated from hunting and festive dances; the Taoist theory on health preservation was derived from Chinese people's efforts to be in line with Nature and to conserve health; and the Confucian theory on health preservation consisted in self-cultivation and self-discipline. Chinese medicine and theories on health preservation in the over 2,000 years since the completion of the Inner Canon of the Yellow Emperor and the Han Dynasty (206 BC-220 AD) are very rich and profound.

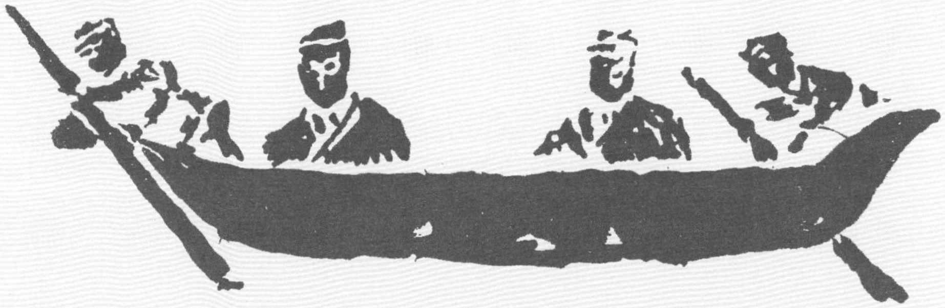

诸子百家与养生文化

Quotes concerning health preservation of the Hundred Schools of Thought

先秦学术界风起云涌，产生了儒家、道家、法家、名家、墨家、阴阳家、纵横家、兵家、农家，以及小说家的诸子百家。各学术流派分别对医学和养生学产生了不同程度的影响。

The turbulent academia before the Qin Dynasty was rife with various schools of thought: Confucianism, Taoism, Legalism, the School of Names or Logicians, Mohism, Yinyang School, Lobbyism, Militarism, Agriculturist School, Talking Shop School, to name just a few. These schools of thought have, more or less, exerted their influence on medicine and regimen.

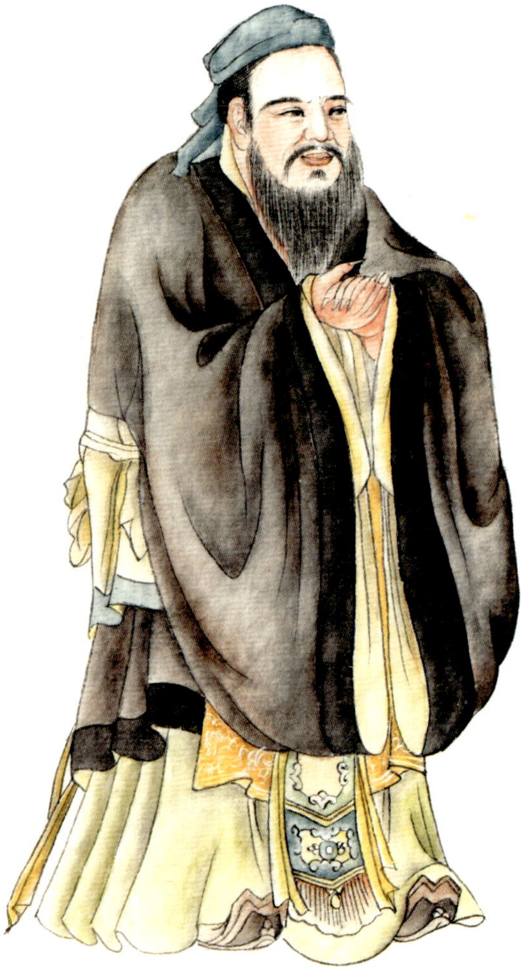

孔子
Confucius

【孔子名言】

A famous quote from Confucius

孟武伯问孝，子曰："父母唯其疾之忧。"

〖语解〗父母最担心的是孩子生病。健康最为重要。

Meng Wubo asked about filial piety. Confucius said, "Behave in such a way that your parents have no anxiety about you, except your health."

儒家学说的全部内容可以用"三纲领、八条目"六个字来概括。"三纲领"即"在明明德，在新民，在止于至善"。明白了"止于至善"，才能坚定信念，克服私欲，使内心平静，遇事安详，思虑周到，从而求得真知正道。"道"就是修身养性的至高点。

The entire Confucian philosophy can be generalized into "three principles" and "eight steps". The "three principles" are "to illustrate the illustrious virtue, to renovate the people, and to rest in the highest excellence". Only when you know that you should not rest until the highest excellence can you acquire a firm belief, overcome your selfish desires, quiet your mind, and deal with affairs in a serene and thoughtful manner, thereby attaining true knowledge and Tao, which is the acme of self-cultivation.

【老子名言】

A famous quote from Lao Tzu

（顺其自然）是谓深根固柢、长生久视之道。

〖语解〗顺其自然是健康长寿的正道。

To live in harmony with nature is the best way leading to health and longevity.

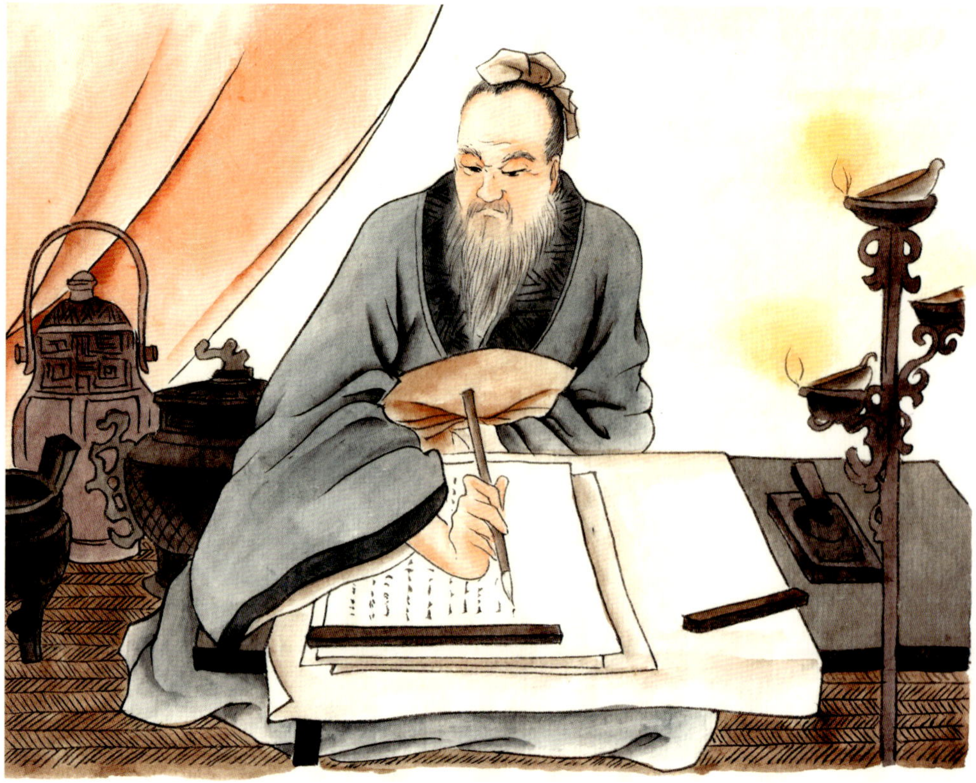

老子
Lao Tzu

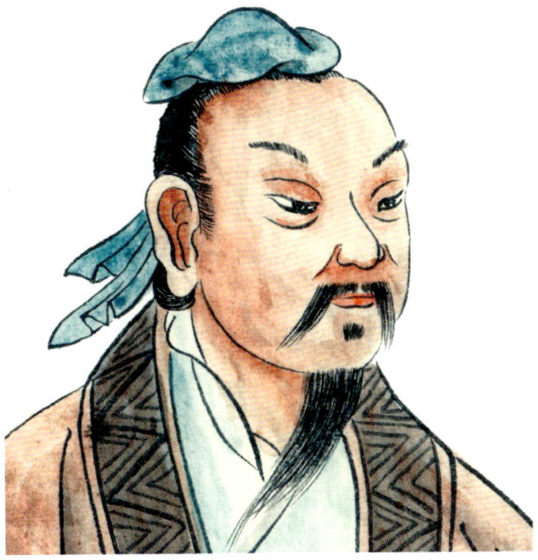

庄子 Chuang Tzu

【庄子名言】

A famous quote from Chuang Tzu

夫形全精复，与天为一。

〖语解〗保全形体、恢复精神，便能与自然合二为一。

Preserve your body and restore your spirit, and you will be one with nature.

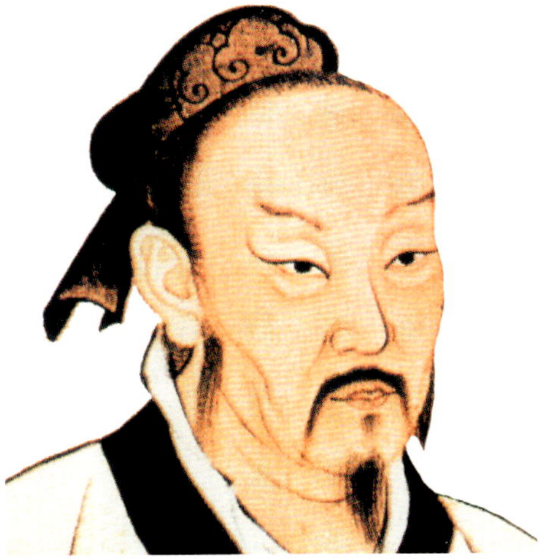

孟子 Meng Tzu

【孟子名言】

A famous quote from Mencius

吾善养吾浩然之气。

〖语解〗我善于培养我的浩然正气。

I am good at cultivating my noble spirit.

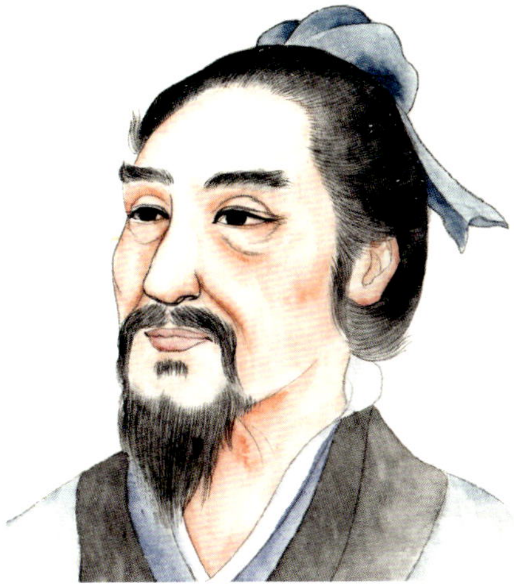

墨子 Mo Tzu

【墨子名言】

A famous quote from Mozi

志不强者，智不达；言不行者，行不果。

〖语解〗意志不坚强的人，就不能把智慧变为行动；光说不做，就不会有收获。

Without a strong will one cannot put wisdom into action; without practicing what one preaches, one cannot achieve anything.

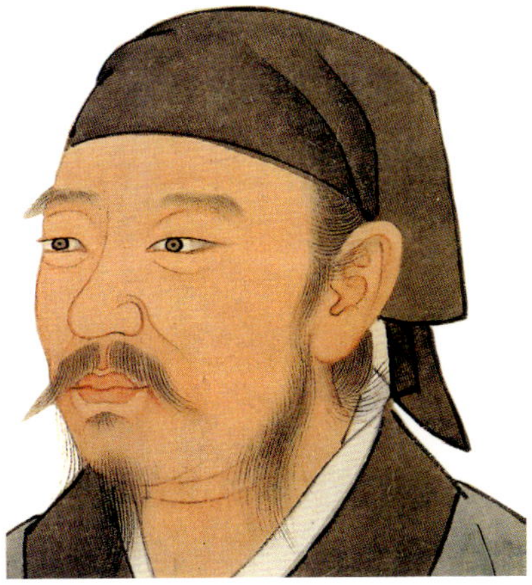

荀子 Xun Tzu

【荀子名言】

A famous quote from Xun Zi

恶以不闻为善。

〖语解〗坏事知道得越少越好。（荀子此言宜于养心。）

Keep your knowledge of evil things to a minimum. (This is good advice for mental cultivation.)

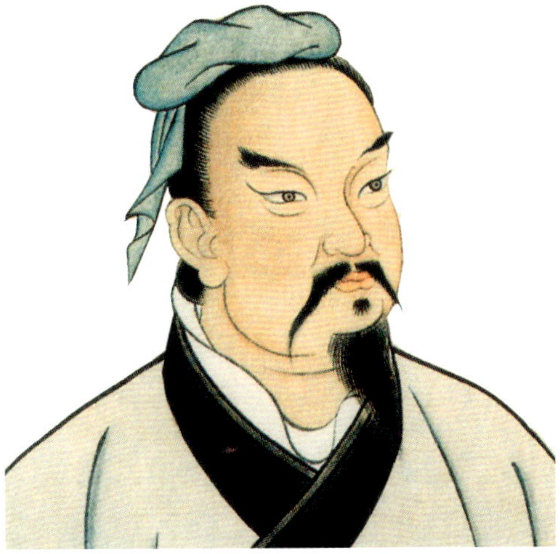

孙子 Sun Tzu

【孙子名言】

A famous quote from Sun Tzu

知己知彼，百战不殆。

Know the enemy and know yourself, and you can fight a hundred battles without defeat.

〖语解〗此语用于养生时，是说对于病症要真切了解，才能手到病除。

Explication: for health preservation, this means that one cannot cure a disease without understanding it thoroughly.

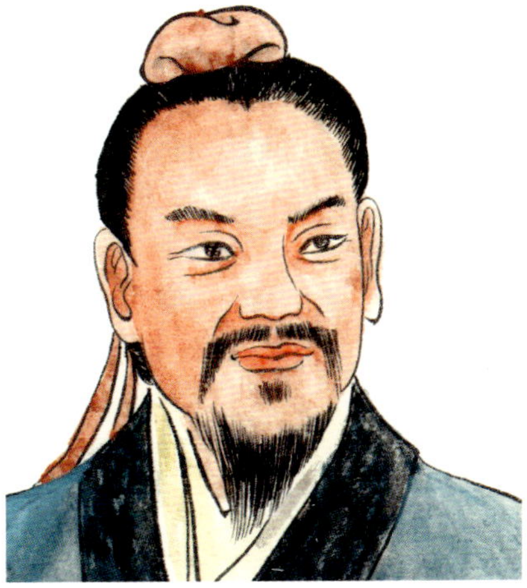

韩非子 Han Fei Tzu

【韩非子名言】

A famous quote from Han Feizi

千里之堤，毁于蚁穴。

One ant hole may cause the collapse of a thousand-li dike.

〖语解〗此语用于养生时，是说养生要从细节做起。

Explication: for health preservation, this means that one should start from the details.

道家养生

Taoist regimen

道家学说的创始人是春秋时代的老子，代表作是《道德经》。战国初期的庄周，继承和发扬了老子的思想，传世有《庄子》一书，故道家思想又称“老庄哲学”。道家的宗旨是追求顺其自然。通过养生、避世、清心、寡欲等方式达到祛病延年的目的。许多道士又是著名医药学家、养生家。

The progenitor of Taoism was Lao Tzu of the Spring and Autumn period, who authored *Tao Te Ching*, the masterpiece of Taoism. Zhuang Zhou, a follower of Lao Tzu of in the early ages of the Warring States Period, carried the ideas of Lao Tzu forward and wrote the book entitled *Chuang Tzu*. As a result, Taoism was also called the philosophy of Lao-Zhuang. The tenet of Taoism is to follow the natural course. Taoists sought to keep diseases off and achieve longevity by promoting health, retiring from society and abstaining from indulgences. Many Taoists turned out to be well-known medical practitioners and regimen experts.

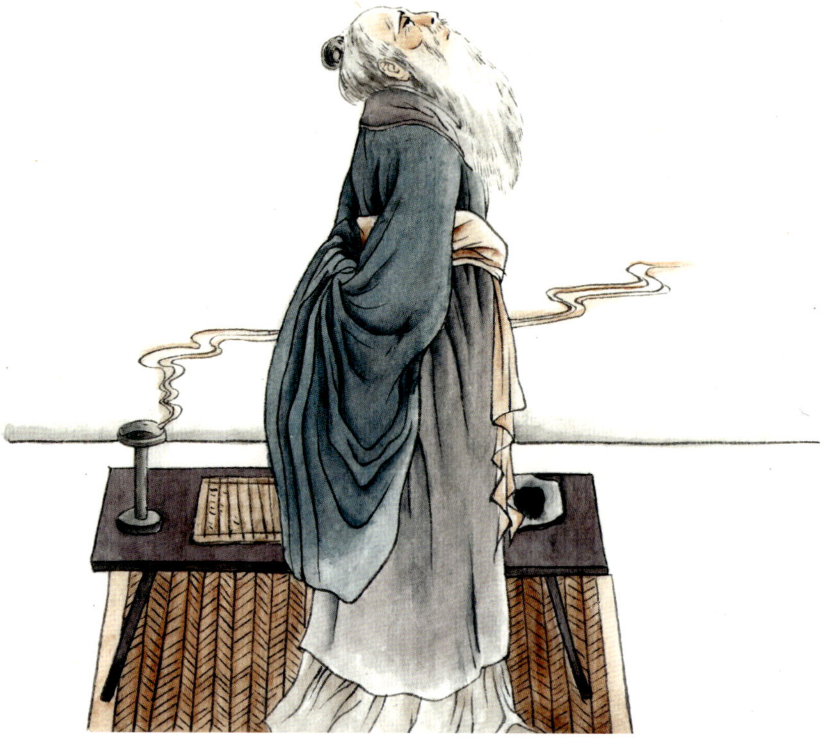

老子

Lao Tzu

道法自然

Tao follows the law of nature.

“道”体现了生命的本源和运动变化的法则。《道德经》指出：“人法地，地法天，天法道，道法自然。”老子的“道法自然”是通过对社会和自然的观察和思考得来的，这一观念被称为“生态智慧”。所谓得“道”即长生，违“道”即短寿，“道”与“生”是相守相保、辩证统一的，人们的生命活动要符合自然规律的变化，这样才能健康长寿。

Tao (literally meaning way) represents the essence of life and the rules of life activities. In *Tao Te Ching* it is postulated that humans imitate earth, earth imitates heaven, heaven imitates Tao while Tao imitates Nature. The assertion that Tao imitates Nature is derived from observation of and meditation on antagonisms in nature and society. This concept is called ecological wisdom. Acquisition of Tao means longevity while defiance of Tao entails short life. Tao and life are mutually protective and supportive. Such a dialectical view calls on people to live in compliance with natural laws so as to maintain health and achieve longevity.

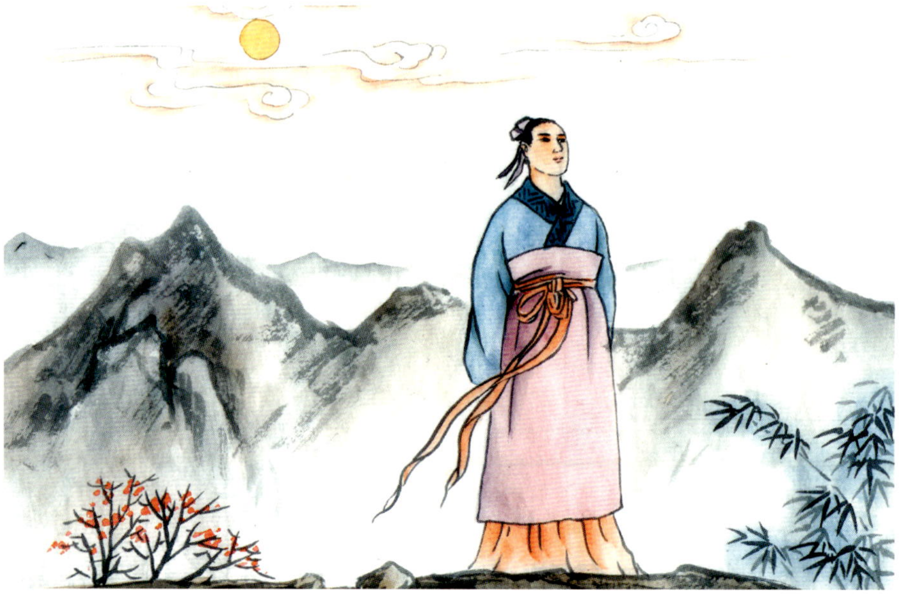

人法地，地法天

Human beings follow the law of the earth, while the earth follows that of heaven.

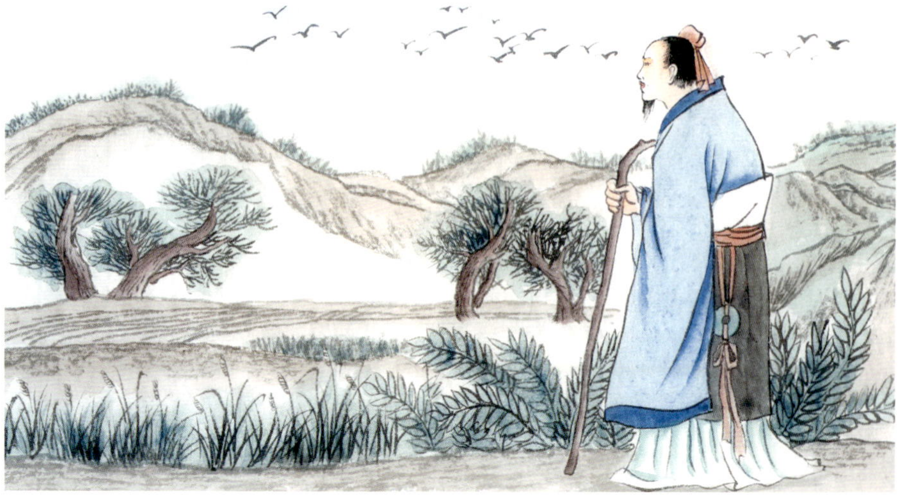

道法自然

Tao follows the law of nature.

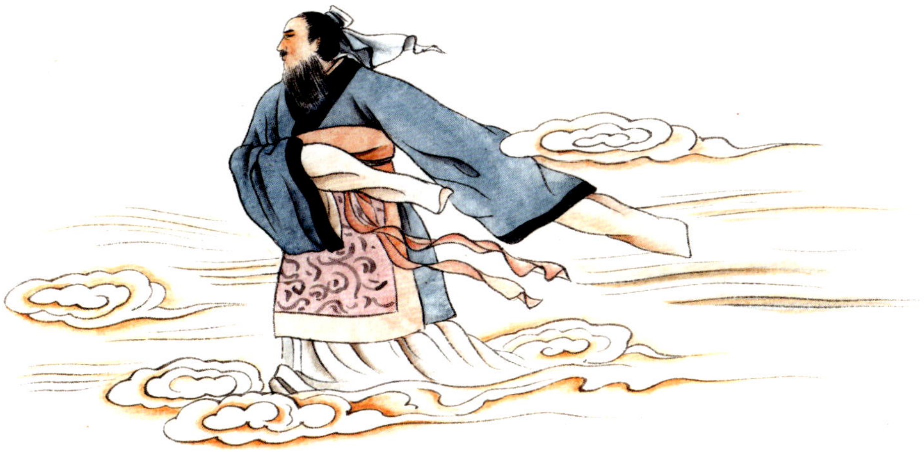

列子御风

Liezi riding the wind

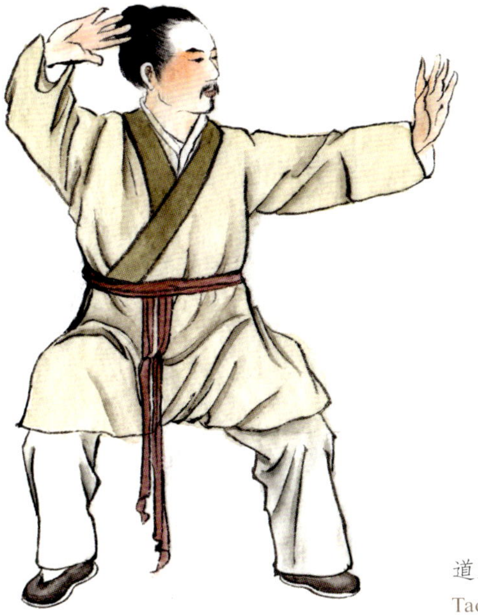

道家功法

Taoist exercises

道家相信人的生死是可以由自己掌握的。与宿命论不同，道家否定了听天由命的消极思想，在修养的路上不断地探索着自主命运的路。道家认为人类能够认识并运用自然规律来认识、改造自身，达到“长生久视”的目的。

The doctrine of Taoism advocates that man can control life and death on his own, renouncing the pessimistic approach of putting life at destiny's disposal. In contrast to the view of predestination, Taoism seeks unceasingly to explore the path of taking life into man's own hands. Taoism holds that human beings can comprehend and employ natural laws to know more about themselves and improve themselves so as to achieve health and longevity.

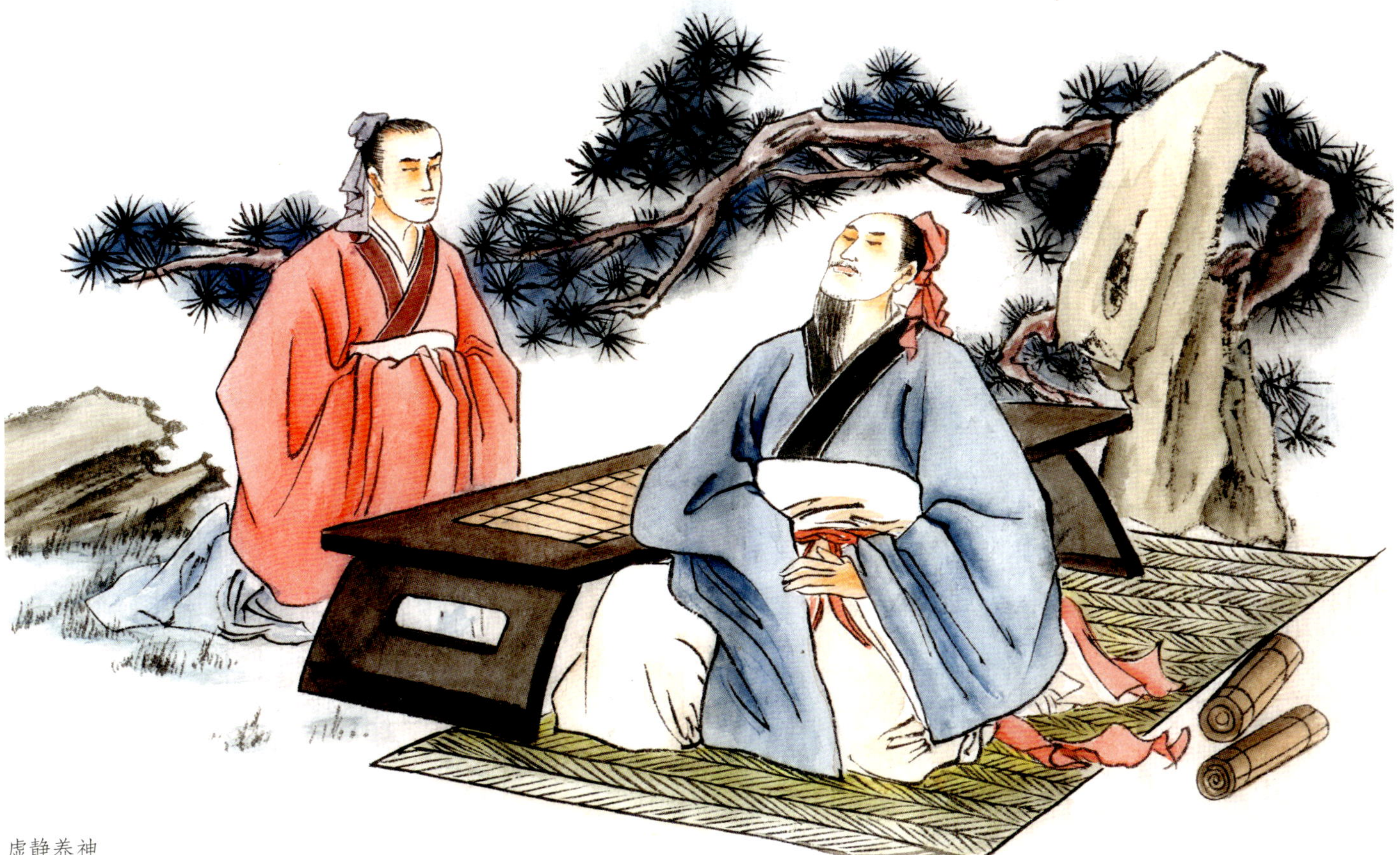

虚静养神

Tranquility nourishes the mind

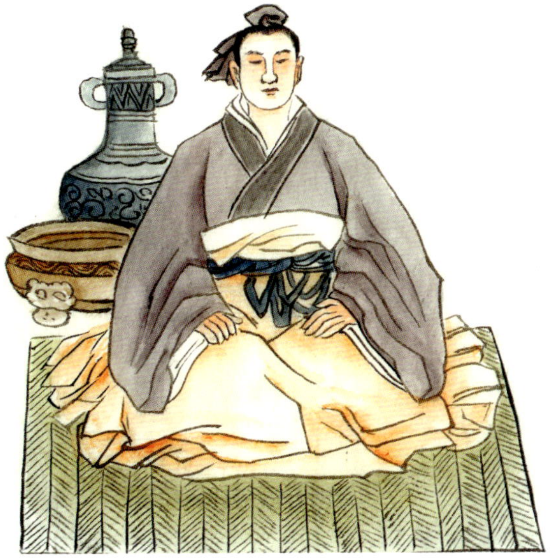

清静无为

Keep the body still and the mind at peace

恬惔虚无

Spiritual tranquility

老子主张清静虚无，意在通过柔弱无为、虚静自守来排除干扰，以达到返朴归真的目的。“道”的本质规律就是自然无为。因此，人应当心慈于物，与人为善，以近于道。老子对于“道”的理解是要“以柔克刚”、“有无相生”，即“贵柔”。中国传统的健身术也是以柔见长，如导引、气功、太极拳等。庄子主张形神相守以尽养天年，倡导“去物欲以养形，致虚静以养神”。

Lao Tzu was an advocate of tranquil mindset and nihilistic views, keeping away external distractions and turning back to simplicity through remaining pliable, taking no action and restraining oneself. The essence of Tao consists in naturalness and non-action. To get closer to Tao, a person is supposed to be benevolent towards creatures and kind to other people. In accordance with the teachings of Lao Tzu, being and non-being are conducive to each other while hardness is to be tempered with softness. Tao puts a premium on softness. Traditional Chinese regimen is permeated with softness, as can be seen in breath conditioning, Qigong, shadow boxing, etc. Chuang Tzu called on people to enjoy their lives allotted by divine providence through the maintenance of both body and spirit. In his words, it is recommended to nurture the body by renouncing desires and nurture the spirit with tranquility.

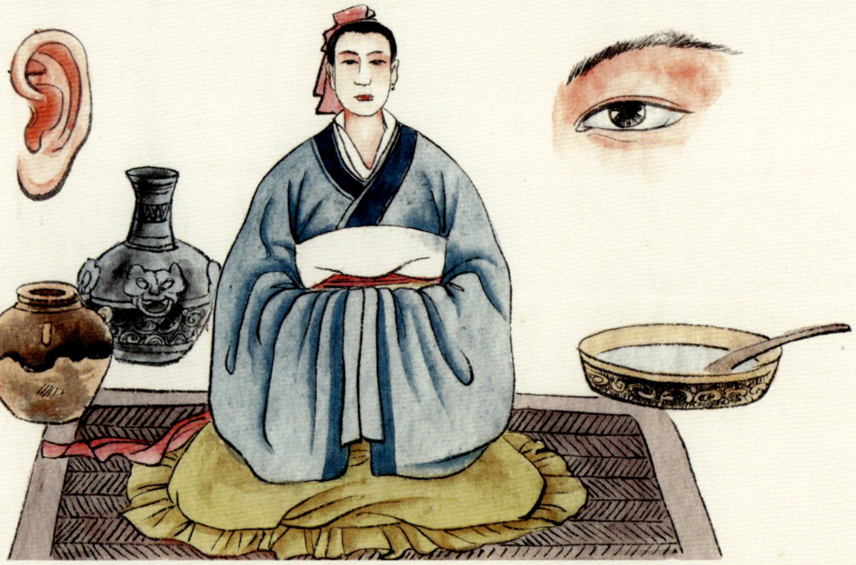

道家养生讲求全神保真

Taoism emphasizes the harmony of spirit and body

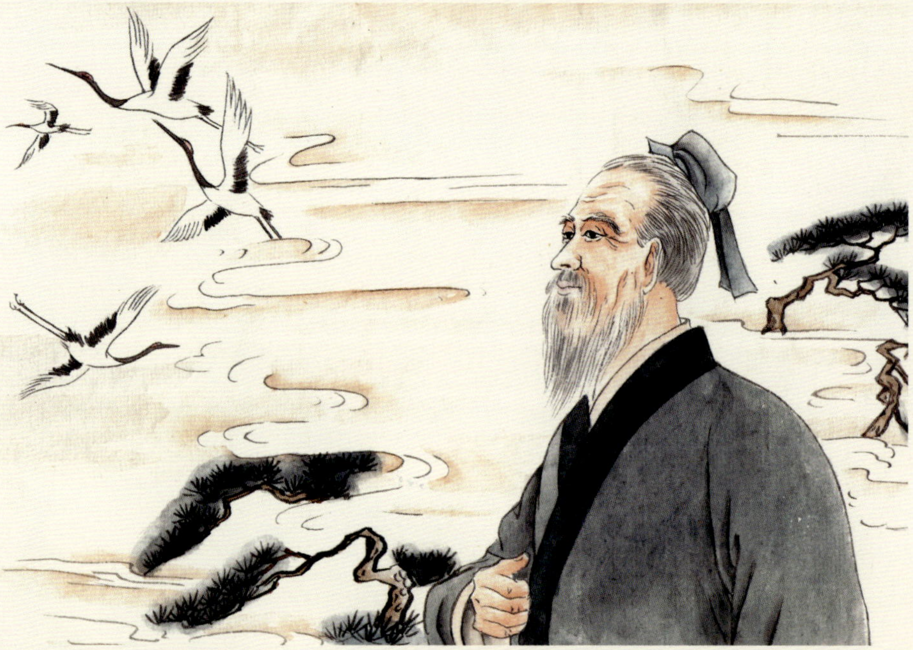

道家崇尚自然，创立了一套顺乎自然的气功养生方法。《庄子·刻意篇》中的“吹呴呼吸，吐故纳新，熊经鸟申”就是典型例子。所谓“吹呴呼吸”即是一种顺乎自然，使真气来至，废气排出的调气法，也是一种模仿自然界禽兽活动的导引方法。

Thanks to their veneration for Nature, Taoists managed to invent a set of regimen approaches called Qigong, which imitated natural phenomena. One typical example can be seen in one chapter of *Chuang Tzu*, which incites people to condition breath by inhaling fresh air while exhaling spent air in addition to imitating the limb movements of bears and birds. The conditioning of breath is an approach that accords with the natural process of taking in what is fresh and giving off what is spent. Imitation of the movements of birds and animals can also enrich the approaches to health maintenance.

重在贵生

Cherishing life and health

“重在贵生”的思想鼓励人们乐生重生、颐养天年。道家在养生手段和原则方面，形成了性命双修、形神兼养、众术合修的修炼观。总之追求延年益寿是医道相通的纽带，道家医论直接影响着中医养生学的发展。

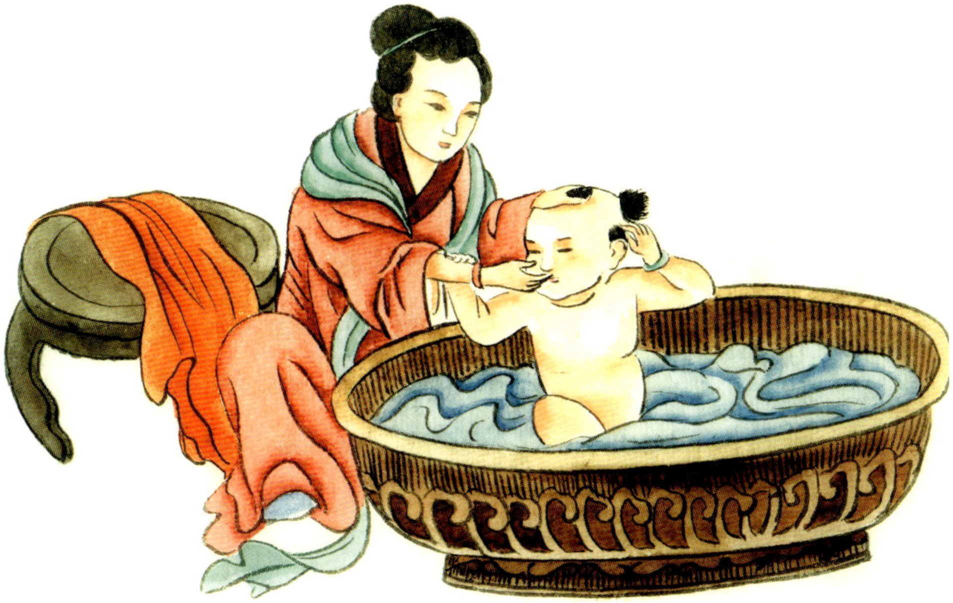

重在贵生
Cherishing life and health

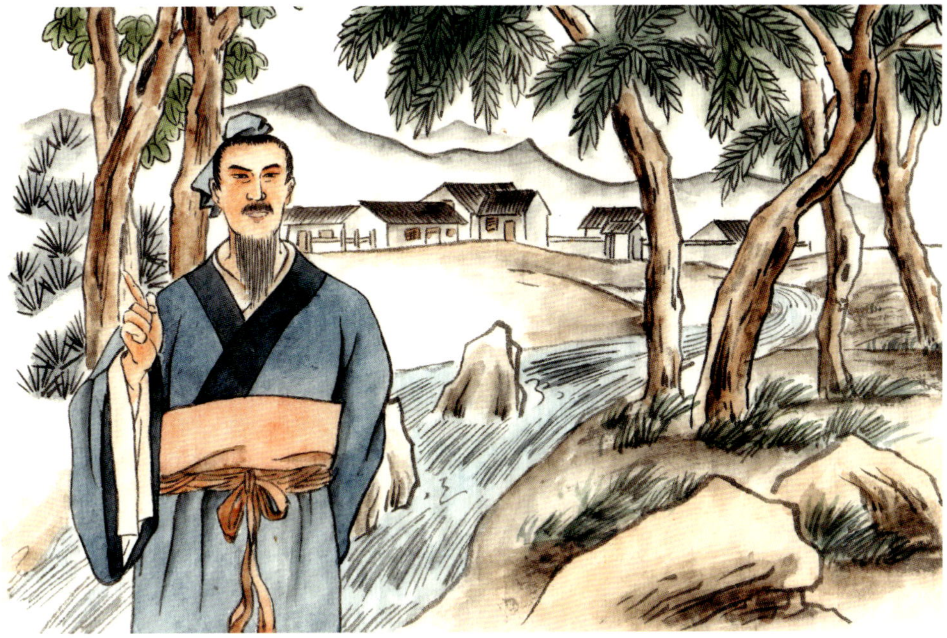

崇尚自然
Veneration for Nature

The viewpoint of putting a premium on regimen encourages people to take delight in life, cherish life and live to the full of life. In terms of the approaches and principles of regimen, Taoism advocates the parallel tempering of human nature and human life, the combined improvement on body and spirit, the practice of diversified methods, etc. In a word, the pursuit of longevity constitutes the band linking medicine and Taoism while the doctrines of Taoism regarding medicine have exerted a direct influence on the development of regimen within the scope of Chinese medicine.

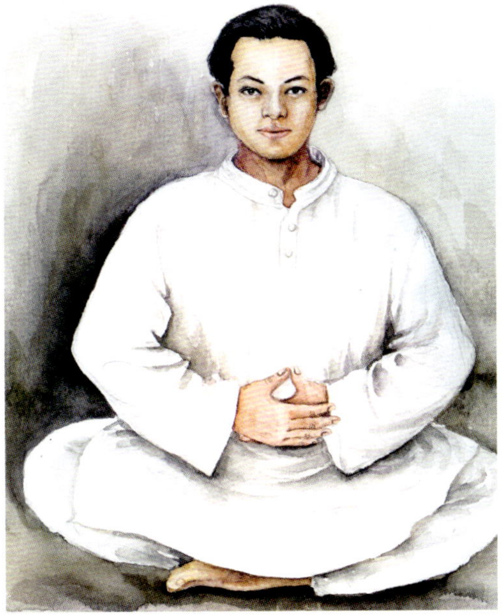

吐故纳新
Get rid of the stale and absorb the new

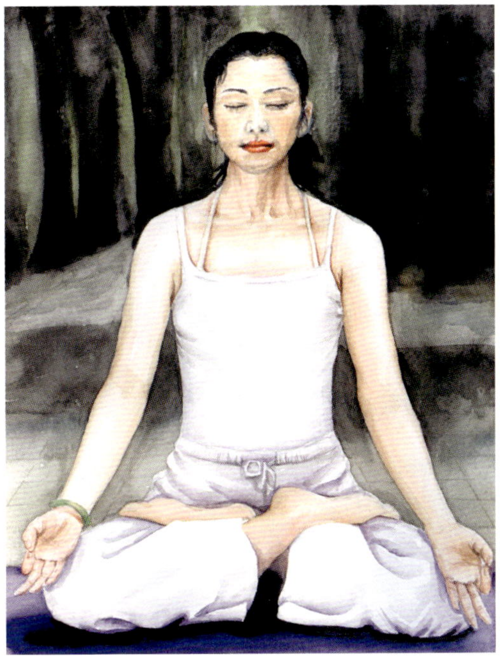

静坐调息
Sit still and regulate the breathing

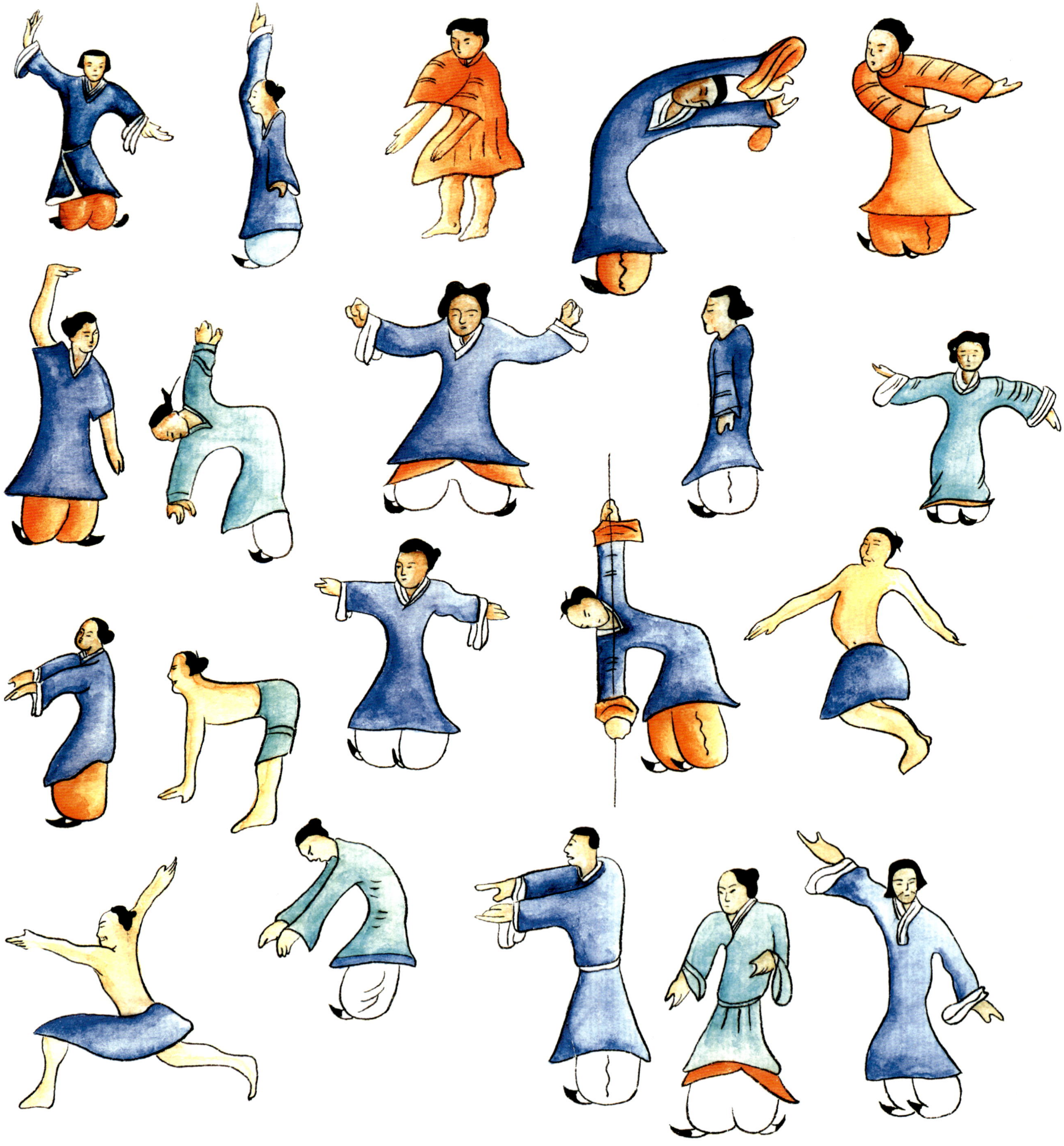

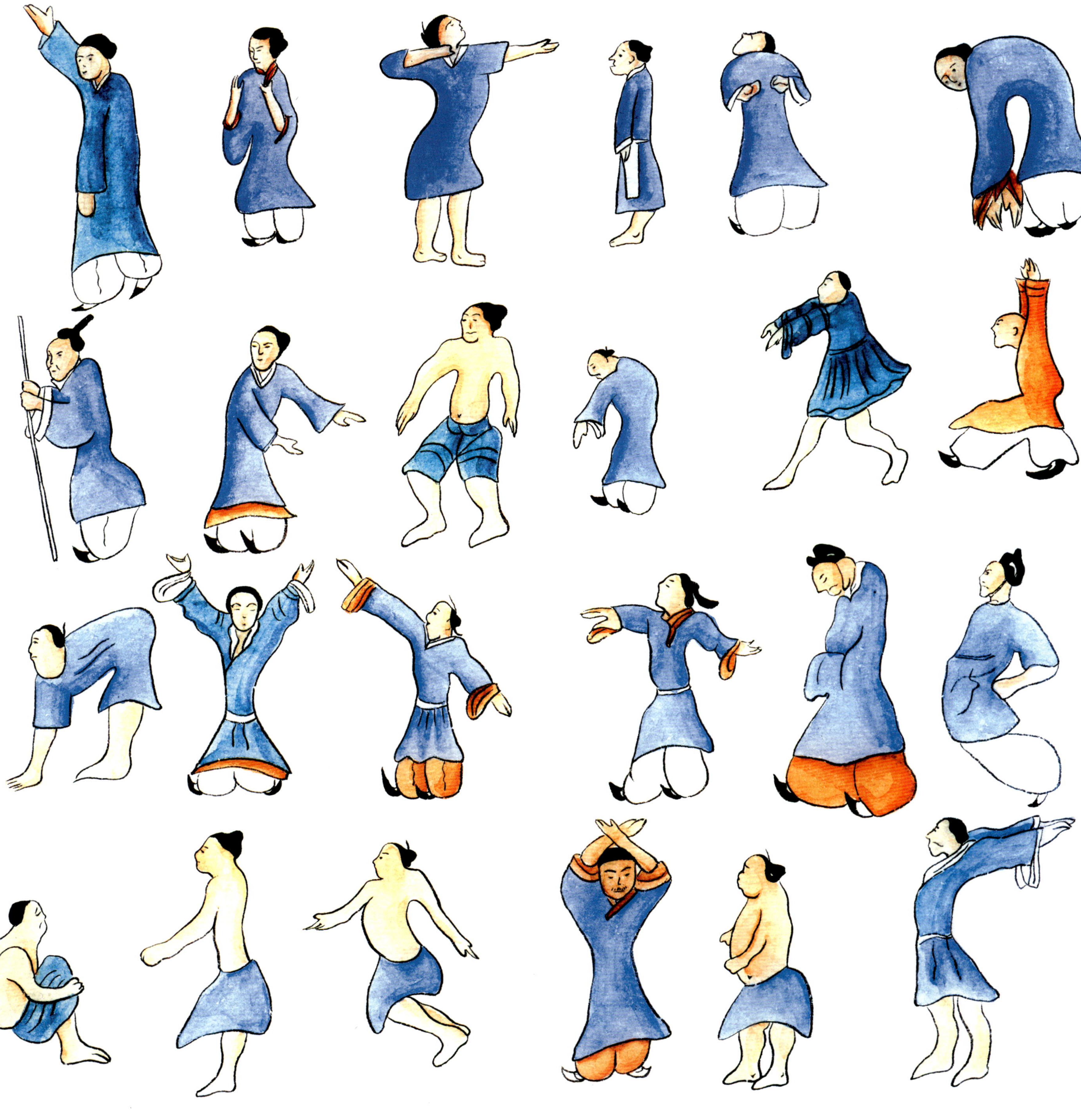

不治已病治未病

Prevention of diseases as the best therapy.

老子说：“为之于未有，治之于未乱。”（《老子·六十四章》）。《黄帝内经》云：“不治已病治未病，不治已乱治未乱。”（《素问·四气调神大论》）这种“治未病”的思想（“治未病”实际上包含养生与预防的思想），正是道家朴素的辩证法思想与医疗经验相结合的产物。

In Chapter 64 of his booklet Lao Tzu recommended people to “do it before it happens, sort it out before it breaks down.” Obviously, this is an echo of the idea in the *Inner Canon* which recommends people to “cure an ailment before it develops and sort out a trouble before it brews.” In essence, the idea of curing an ailment before it develops covers both maintenance of health and prevention of diseases. Such an idea came into being when the primitive dialectical idea of Taoism was wed to medical practice.

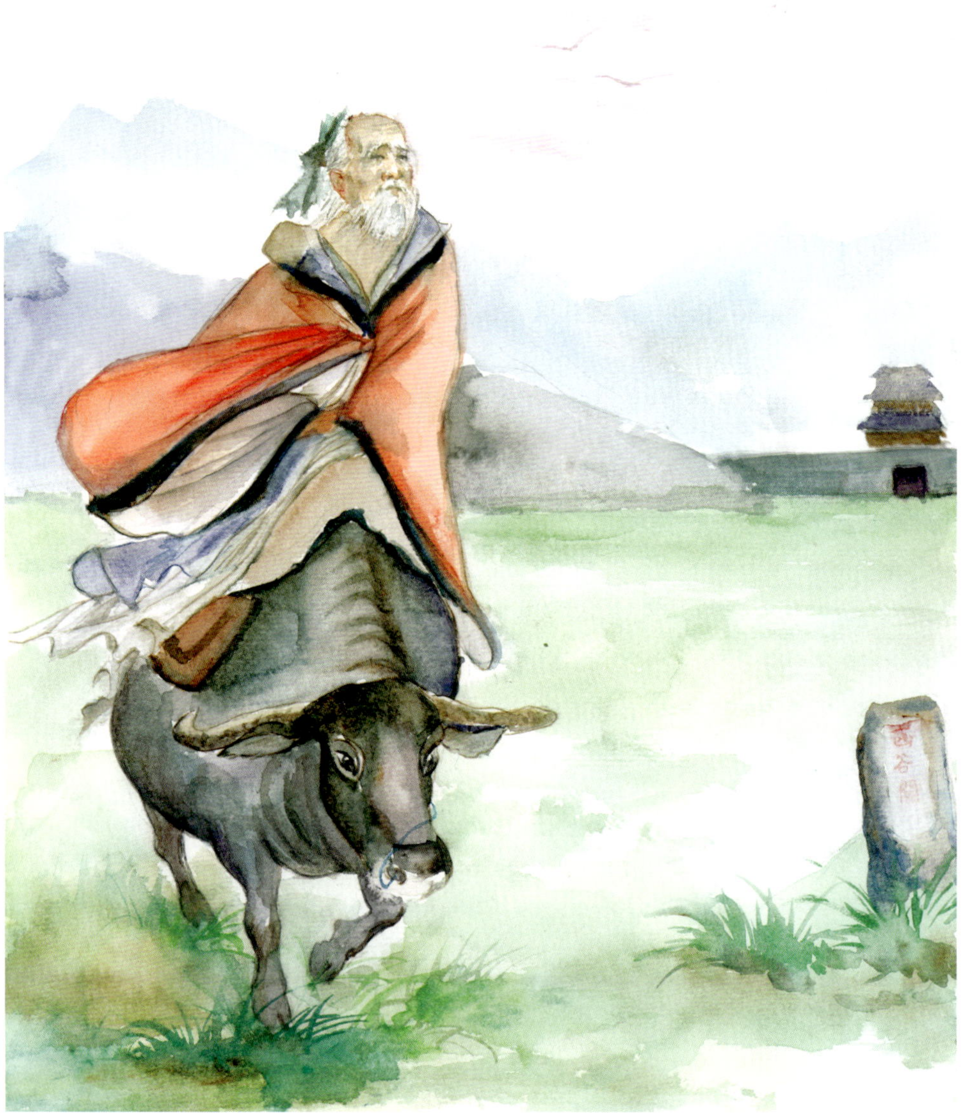

老子
Lao Tzu

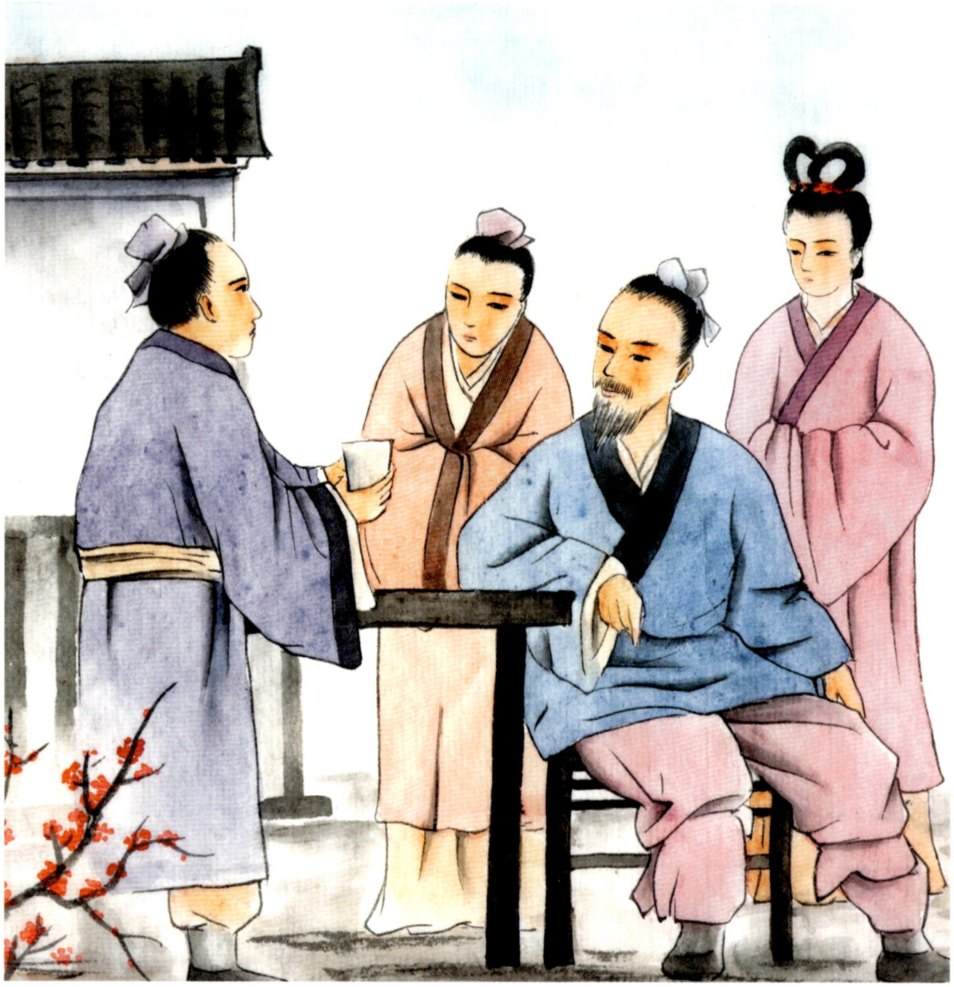

不治已病治未病
Prevention of diseases is the best therapy.

儒家养生

Confucian regimen

以孔孟为代表的儒家学派，对我国的历史文化产生了莫大的影响，儒家的“中和观”对中医养生学影响最深。

Spearheaded by Confucius and Mencius, Confucianism exerted profound influence on Chinese history and culture, with the idea of moderation being its greatest influence on Chinese medicine.

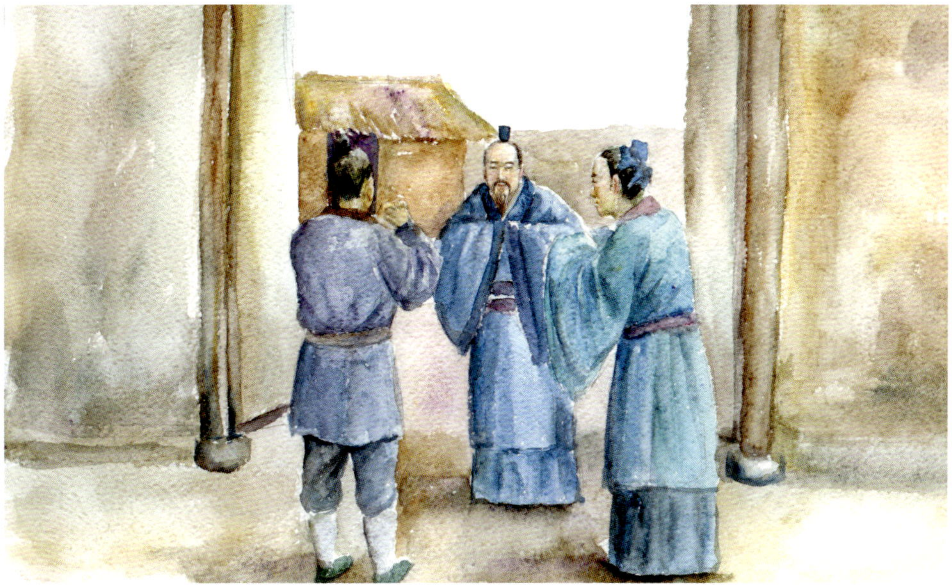

以中和之道做人

To apply the principle of moderation to daily life

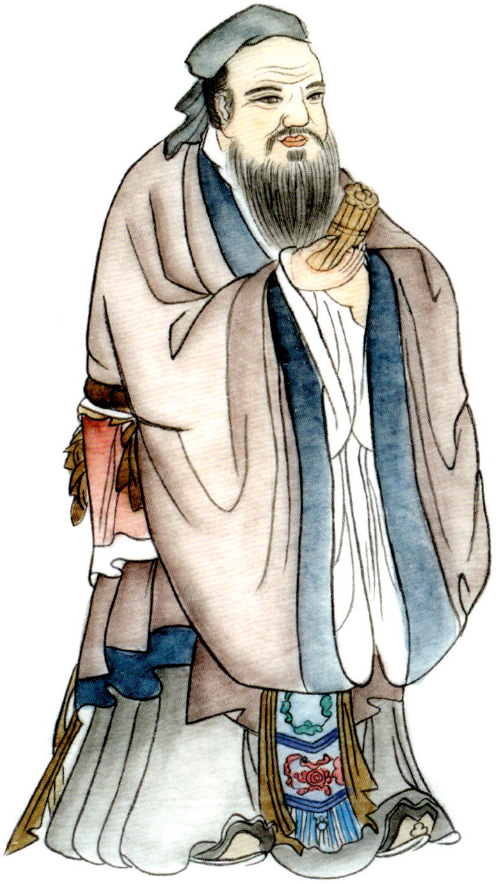

孔子像

Portrait of Confucius

致中和

The state of moderation

《中庸》指出：“喜怒哀乐之未发，谓之中；发而皆中节，谓之和。中也者，天下之大本也。和也者，天下之达道也。致中和，天地位焉，万物育焉”。

The Doctrine of the Mean points out: “Emotions brew and are pent in at first. When they are released to an intermediate extent, the state is called moderation. The pent-in emotions arise from the base of heaven and earth while moderation is the smooth path to bliss under heaven. When moderation is achieved, things will be in their respective places and thrive.”

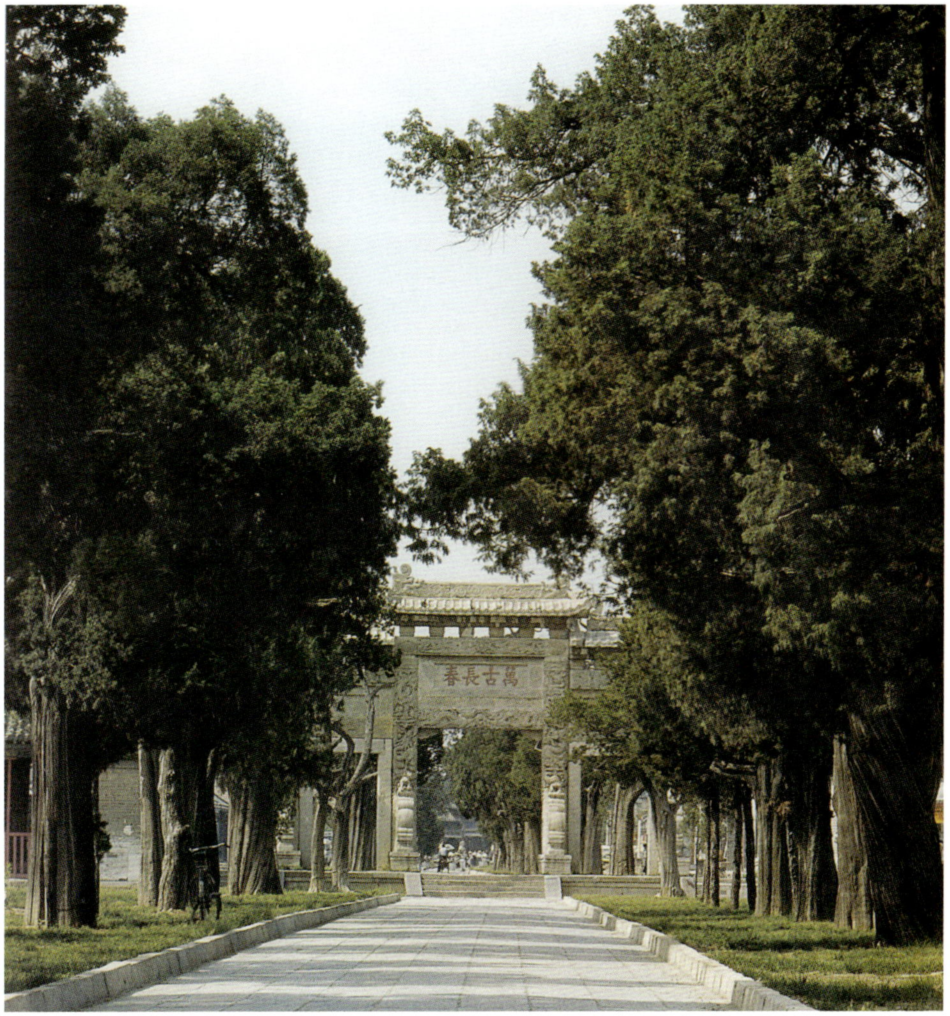

孔林万古长春坊

Forever Spring Gateway in Confucian Woods

宋代严用和在《济生方》中说道："善摄生者，谨于和调，一饮一食，使入于胃中，随消随化，则无滞留之患。""善摄生者，无犯日月之忌，无失岁时之和"（《千金要方》），"人生如天地，和煦则春，惨郁则秋"，"能中和者必久寿"。

〖白话〗：宋代严用和在他所著的《济生方》一书中说道："善于养生的人，一定是认真地调理自己，每一饮一食，进入胃中之后，要使之好好消化，就没有积食致病的问题了。"《千金要方》一书也说，"善于养生的人，不要触犯了日月阴阳的忌讳，也不要失去岁时四季的和谐"。人生就像大自然一样，和谐温暖就像春天，如果悲凉抑郁就像秋天。

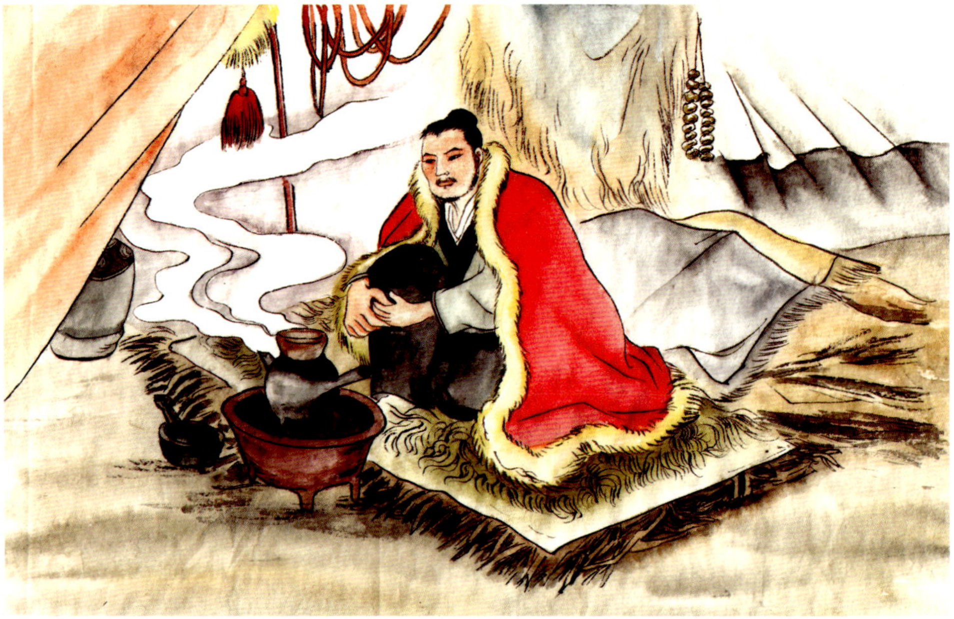

调和饮食图

Illustration of dietary arrangement

慈、俭、和、静

Benevolence, frugality, harmony, and tranquility

后来清人在总结养生经验时说："昔人谈致寿之道有四：曰慈、曰俭、曰和、曰静"（《妙香室丛话》）；孔子提倡修身养性，注重道德修养，孟子更是重视"养心"："养心莫善于寡欲。其为人也寡欲，虽有不存焉者，寡矣；其为人也多欲，虽有存焉者，寡矣。"

As the author of *Miscellaneous Talks in the Fragrant Room* remarked, "people before us found out four key points for longevity: benevolence, frugality, accord, and tranquility." Confucius advised people to temper their human nature, i.e. improve on their morals in addition to maintaining physical health. Mencius laid exclusive emphasis on cultivating the mind: The best way to cultivate the mind is to restrict the desires. A person with few desires will not lose much of his kindness while a person with a lot of desires will keep little of his kindness.

Yan Yonghe, a regimen expert of the Song Dynasty (960-1279 AD), remarked in his book *Treatise on Enhancing Life* that "he who is good at health maintenance and improvement is prudent and moderate in drinking and eating so that whatever he takes in is digested and absorbed in good time, leaving nothing stagnant in the stomach." These words are the echo of remarks by another regimen expert Sun Simiao of Tang Dynasty (618-907 AD), who in his *Prescriptions Worth a Thousand Gold for Emergencies* wrote: "He who is good at health maintenance and improvement never acts in defiance of the oracles from the Sun and the Moon, nor does he seek variance with the rhythm of seasons. People of subsequent ages came up with similar enlightenments: "Life moves on the way heaven and earth do. Temperance is conducive to the warmth of spring while depletion leads to the distress in autumn." "He who is mild and temperate is likely to live long."

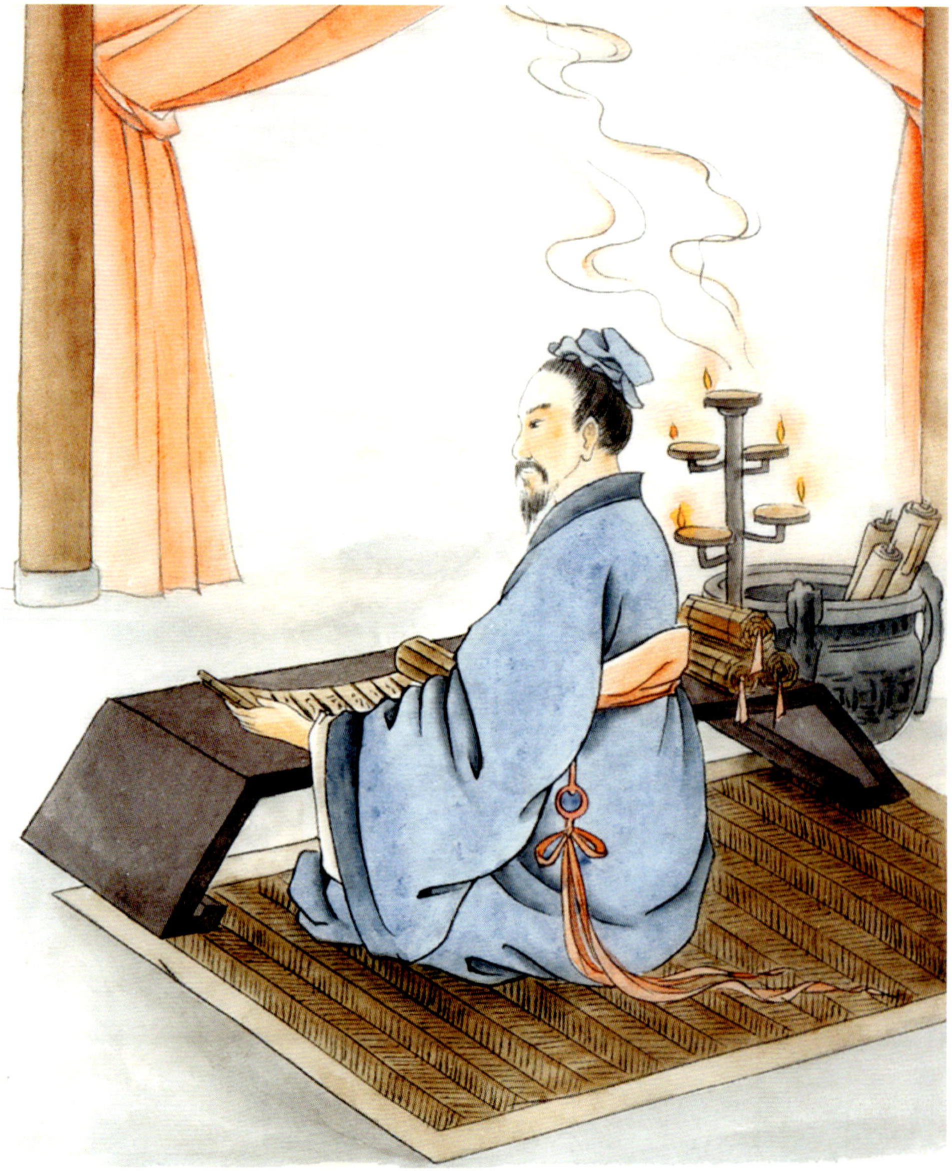

慈、俭、和、静

Benevolence, frugality, accord, and tranquility

君子有三戒

Three must-nots for health preservation

孔子还提出了“三戒”，说：“君子有三戒：少之时，血气未定，戒之在色；及其壮也，血气方刚，戒之在斗；及其老也，血气既衰，戒之在得。”（《论语·季氏》）

Confucius put forward three admonitions in *Analects*, the collection of his remarks: “A virtuous man should be on guard against three things: in puberty, when blood and *qi* tend to be turbulent, he is supposed to guard against sensuality; in his prime, when blood and *qi* tend to be robust, he is supposed to guard against pugnacity; in twilight of life, when blood and *qi* tend to lose vigor, he is supposed to guard against greed.”

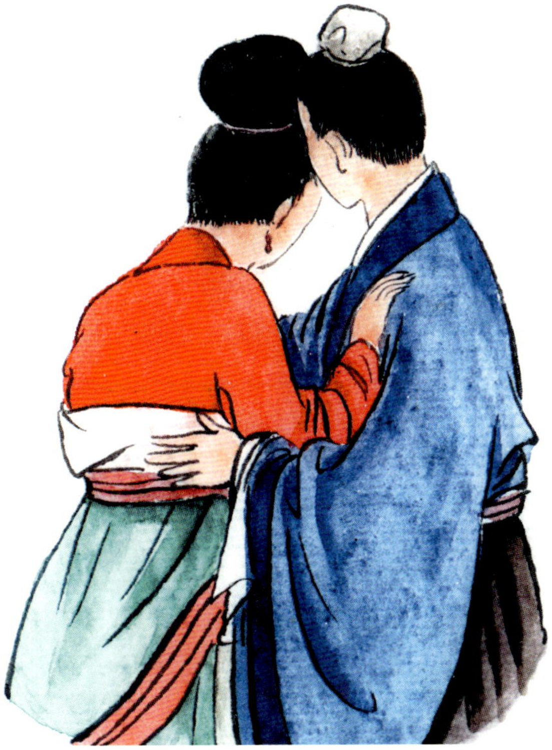

少年戒色

In puberty, he is supposed to guard against sensuality.

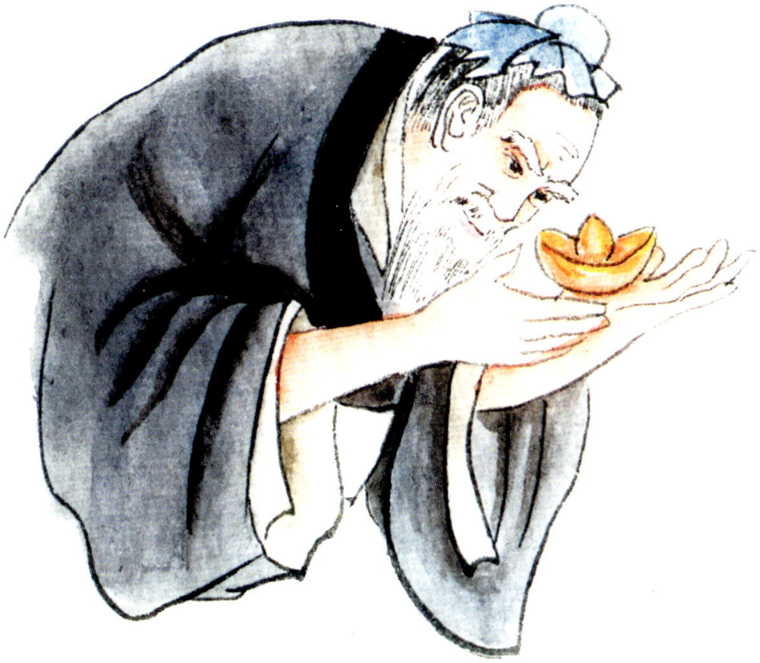

老年戒贪

In twilight of life, he is supposed to guard against greed.

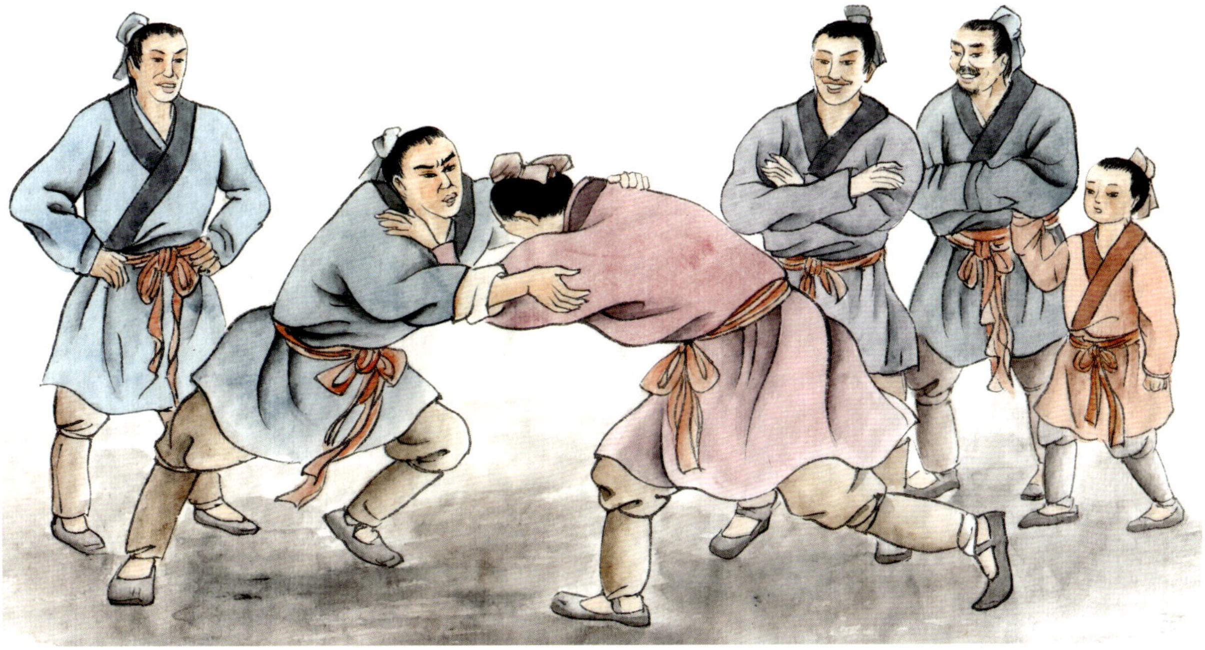

中年戒斗

In his prime, he is supposed to guard against pugnacity.

学习孔子的良好生活习惯

Learn from Confucius' good life habits

孔子终年 73 岁，人生七十古来稀，在古代，孔子是长寿的人了。他的长寿与他良好的生活方式密不可分。孔子在饮食方面，力行节俭，同时非常注意饮食卫生。他有“八不食”的习惯，从现代饮食保健观来看，非常科学。

“八不食”可以分为三类：一是色味方面，颜色不好的不食，变味了的不食；二是质量方面，粮食陈旧的不食，鱼和肉不新鲜的不食，不合时令的蔬菜不食；三是烹制方面，烹调不当的食物不食，调料不当的饭菜不食，从市场上买回的酒和熟肉不食。这八不食，对饮食卫生的要求很全面。孔子身体力行，从而避免了饮食不当所致的疾病。

此外，孔子说：“食不语，寝不言。”他对饮食方式也很有讲究。他还提倡：“食不厌精，脍不厌细。”“食”指粮食，“脍”指切碎了的鱼或肉。就是说，要多吃经过精心烹制加工过的粮食，鱼肉则是切得越细越好。这是很有道理的，一般老年人的牙齿不好，肠胃消化功能也相对较弱，粗糙食物不易咀嚼，还容易引起消化不良症。孔子认为老年人应吃适合自己身体的食物。

An old Chinese saying goes, “Few have reached the age of seventy since ancient times.” Confucius, who died at the age of 73, was considered to have lived a long life. His longevity had much to do with his sensible diet in his late years. He advocated frugality in eating, and was highly particular about food hygiene. In his twilight years, he formed the habit of “avoiding eight kinds of food”, which is highly scientific even from a modern point of view.

The “eight kinds of food” to avoid fall into three categories. The first has to do with color and taste: food whose original color or taste has been changed should not be eaten. The second has to do with quality: old rice, stale fish or meat, and vegetables out of season should not be eaten. The third has to do with cooking: improperly cooked or seasoned food and wine or cooked meat bought at the market should not be eaten. These cover a comprehensive range of issues in food hygiene. By putting these rules into practice, Confucius avoided falling sick from eating improperly.

Confucius also said, “One should keep silent when eating and lying in bed to sleep.” This suggests that he was also quite particular about table manners. He also said, “One should not object to eating rice of the finest quality, or fish or meat that is finely minced.” In other words, one should eat a lot of such rice, fish and meat. There is a good reason for this suggestion, for elderly people tend to be weak in teeth and stomach so that coarse food, which is hard to chew, is likely to cause indigestion. Confucius encouraged elderly people to eat delicious, well-prepared food, which can stimulate appetite.

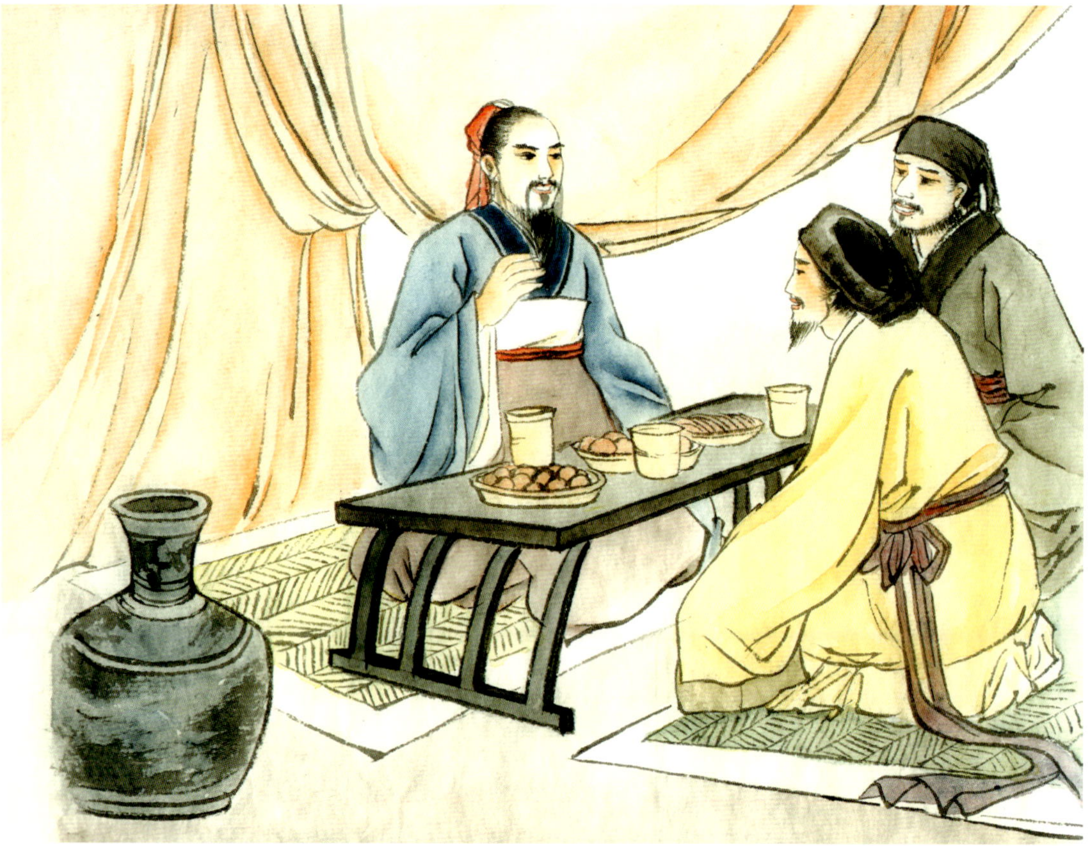

孔子讲“八不食”

Confucius explaining the “eight kinds of food” to avoid

孔子的音乐养生

Confucius' use of music for preserving health

音乐可以引起呼吸、血压、心跳及血流量的变化，不同节奏的音乐作用于人体可以调节人的生理节奏。医学验定，音乐有解压、提神、促进睡眠等功效。

儒家学派的音乐美学思想对中国传统音乐影响重大而深远。孔子酷爱音乐，精通音律，经常用音乐调节情绪，抒发心志，在抚琴咏歌的过程中，让自己的精神与音乐融会贯通。据史书记载，除丧事外"孔子无一日不歌"。孔子正是通过音乐达到放松精神，养生延年的目的的。

孔子认为人的修养开始于诗，完善于乐，其"美善合一"的主张奠定了儒家音乐的美学基础。由孔子亲自编订的《乐经》，在群众中广为流传。在孔子看来，音乐有净化心灵，使人保持良好精神状态的作用，人应多听曲调优美，积极向上的音乐。但同时也要注意，靡靡之音会销蚀人的意志、使人堕落。

Medical research has confirmed that music can relieve strain, refresh the mind, and improve sleep. Physiologically speaking, music can relieve strain and pain by causing changes in respiration, blood pressure, heartbeat, and blood flow. Psychologically speaking, music with different rhythms can regulate physiological rhythms such as pulse and respiration.

The Confucian aesthetic ideas on music have profound influence on the development of traditional Chinese music. Confucius was good at using music to regulate his mood and express his feelings. He loved music and was well versed in temperament. According to historical records, Confucius "sang every day" except during mourning periods. In his opinion, a person's self-cultivation should start from poetry and attain perfection in music. His aesthetic belief in the "unity of beauty and goodness" formed the foundation of the Confucian aesthetic ideas on music. Confucius was so highly musical that he often infused his spirit into music when playing the *qin* and singing. He also compiled *Classic of Music*, which was circulated among the masses. Confucius believed that people should listen to melodious and upbeat music, for decadent music would corrupt one's will and soul, leading to degeneration. Music is capable of purifying the mind and bringing about a healthy mental state. Thus Confucius used music to relax himself, preserve health, and prolong his life.

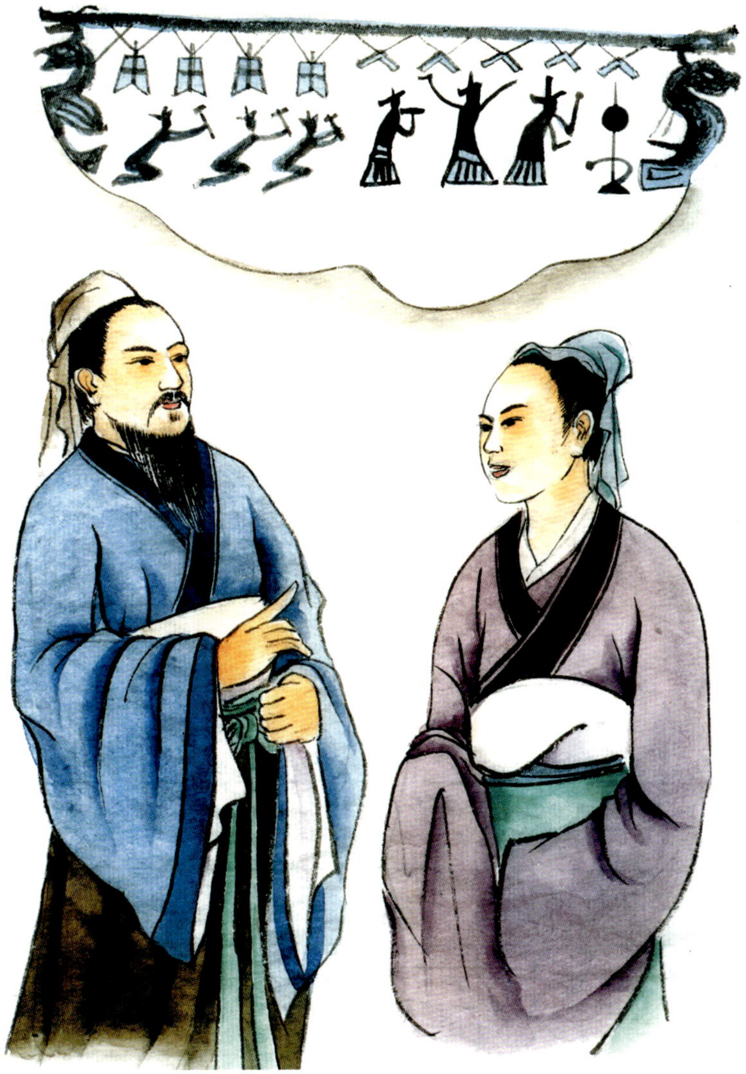

孔子讲"音乐养生"

Confucius explaining "regimen through music"

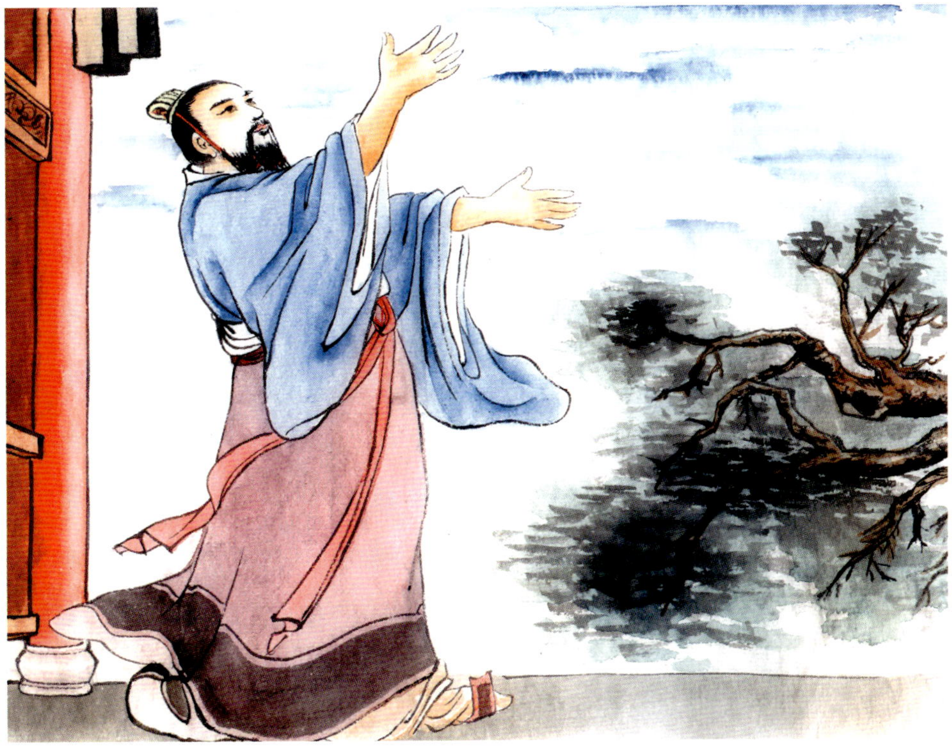

孔子每日唱歌

Confucius singing every day

仁者寿

Benevolent people tend to live longer

孔子学说的道德核心是“仁”，认为“德润身”、“仁者寿”，仁爱厚德的人会拥有良好的心态，身心健康。儒家学说的三纲领提出“在明明德，在新民，在止于至善”，要求人坚定信仰，克服七情六欲各种杂念，使内心清净，最终获得真知正道，达到仁的境界。

The core concept of Confucianism is benevolence. It is his assertion that moral virtue is conducive to good health and that benevolent people tend to live long. The Three Basic Precepts of Confucianism postulates that it is imperative to aggrandize radiant virtues and educate people so that they are willing to proceed towards supreme good. In other words, it is imperative to be firm in one's faith and hold off the distraction of various desires and the agitation of various moods. Only by securing inner cleanness and serenity, can one get access to truth and the right way, arriving at the realm of benevolence.

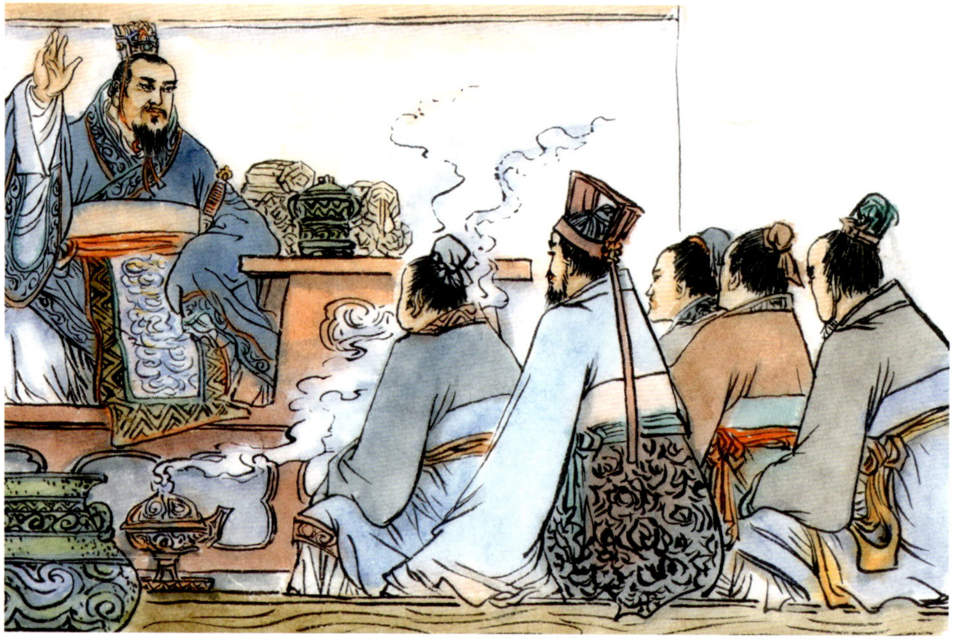

孔子讲“仁爱者长寿”
Confucius explaining “benevolent people tend to live longer”

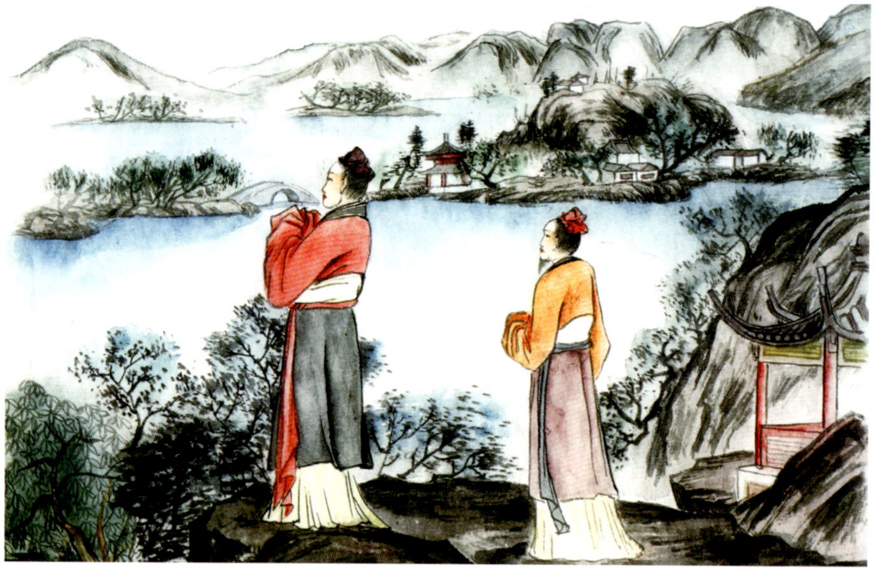

智者乐水，仁者乐山。
The wise love water, while the benevolent love mountains.

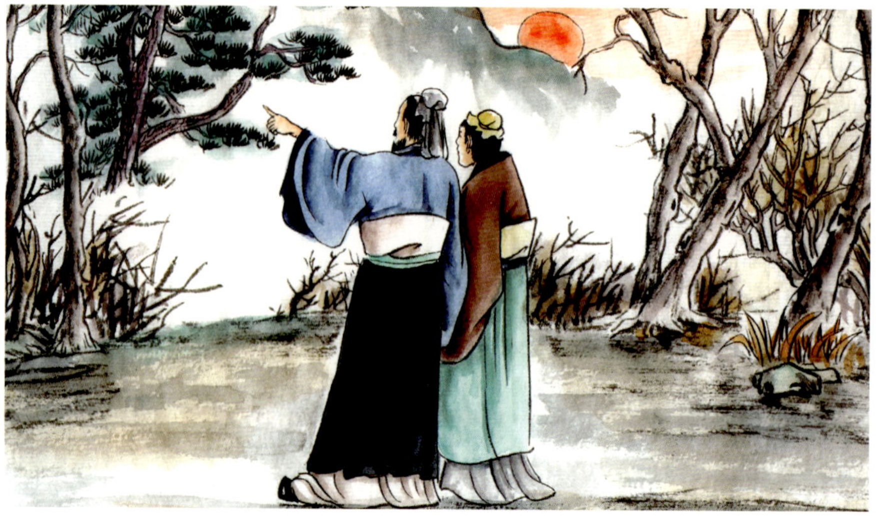

智者动，仁者静，智者乐，仁者寿。
The wise like actions, while the benevolent like tranquility; the wise tend to be contented, while the benevolent tend to live a long life.

孔子认为“大德者必得其寿”。因此，人们应该努力净化自己的心灵，提高自己的思想修养。孔子一生以乐学养生，在行为修养、情感修养、性格修养方面，强调“恭、宽、信、敏、惠”，并把中庸作为人修养自身的总原则。“中”即中和，“庸”即用、常，人应“用中和为常道”，控制好情感思绪，“乐而不淫，哀而不伤”，言行举止恰到好处。

Confucius said, “Virtue nourishes health, and the benevolent can live a long life.” He also said, “A highly virtuous person must be blessed with a long life.” Therefore, we should all try to purify our minds and cultivate our moral character. Throughout his life, Confucius preserved health by the pursuit of learning. In terms of the cultivation of conduct, emotions and character, he emphasized “respect, tolerance, faithfulness, sagacity and generosity”. According to Confucius, the general principle for self-cultivation is zhongyong (the doctrine of the mean), in which zhong means “moderation” and yong means “use” and “constancy”. *Zhongyong* means “to use moderation constantly”, i.e. to understand that during self-cultivation “going too far is as bad as not going far enough”. The quality of zhongyong is supposed to be shown by “pleasure not carried to the point of debauch and grief not carried to the point of self-injury”.

儒家把生命看成实现理想的载体，认为仁德的人乐观大度，没有忧愁。在先秦时代，孔子之所以享有 73 岁高寿，是因为他非常注重饮食卫生，坚持食养的原则和注意饮食宜忌。他主张“食不厌精，脍不厌细”，顺应四时，在饮食卫生方面提出“八不食”的膳食禁忌。除了他科学地遵循养生之道外，博学多才，还精通“六艺”（礼、乐、射、御、书、数），这些都有利于他的健康长寿。

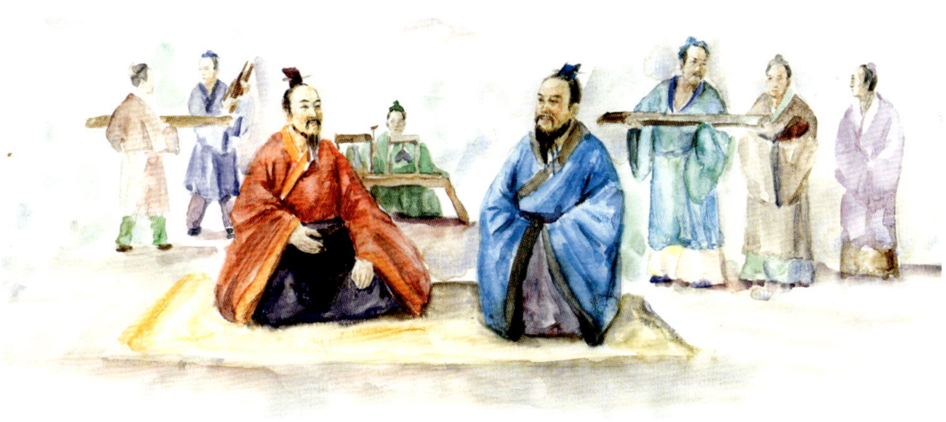

习礼，习音乐

Protocol and music

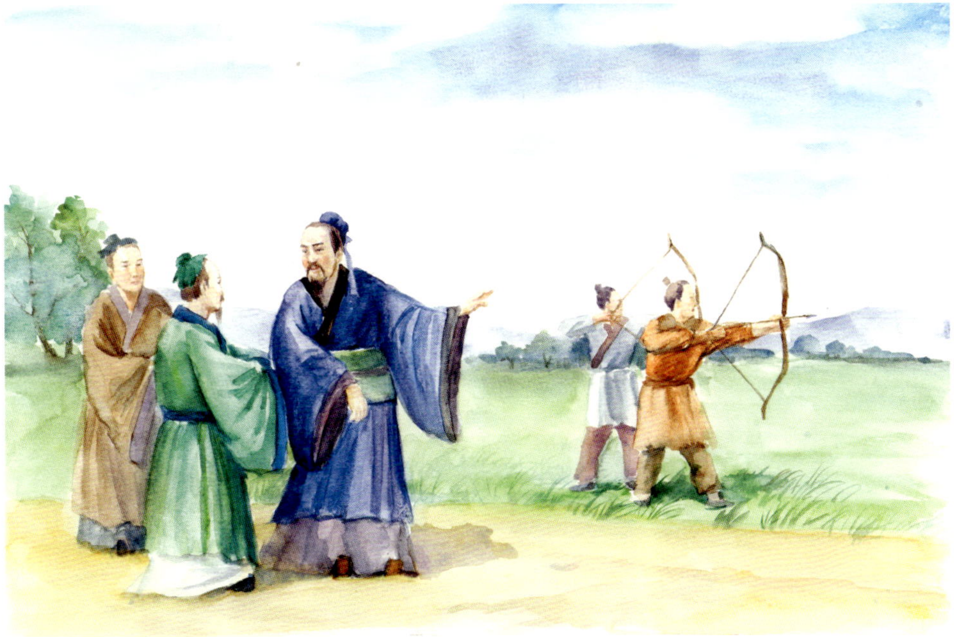

射箭

Archery

In the doctrine of Confucianism, body is regarded as the vehicle for achieving ideals. Benevolent and virtuous people are generous-minded and optimistic, immune from worries and concerns. Confucius lived to be seventy-three, a venerable age for people of the pre-Qin period (i.e. before 221 B.C.). He put forward the principles and rules for health-giving food nourishment. He advised people to take in fine and delicate instead of coarse and rough food. He put forth eight kinds of undesirable or inadvisable foods. He advised people not to eat anything out of season. In addition, he was a versatile scholar, well-versed in six arts, i.e. protocol, music, archery, driving and riding, calligraphy and arithmetic. All this contributed to his longevity.

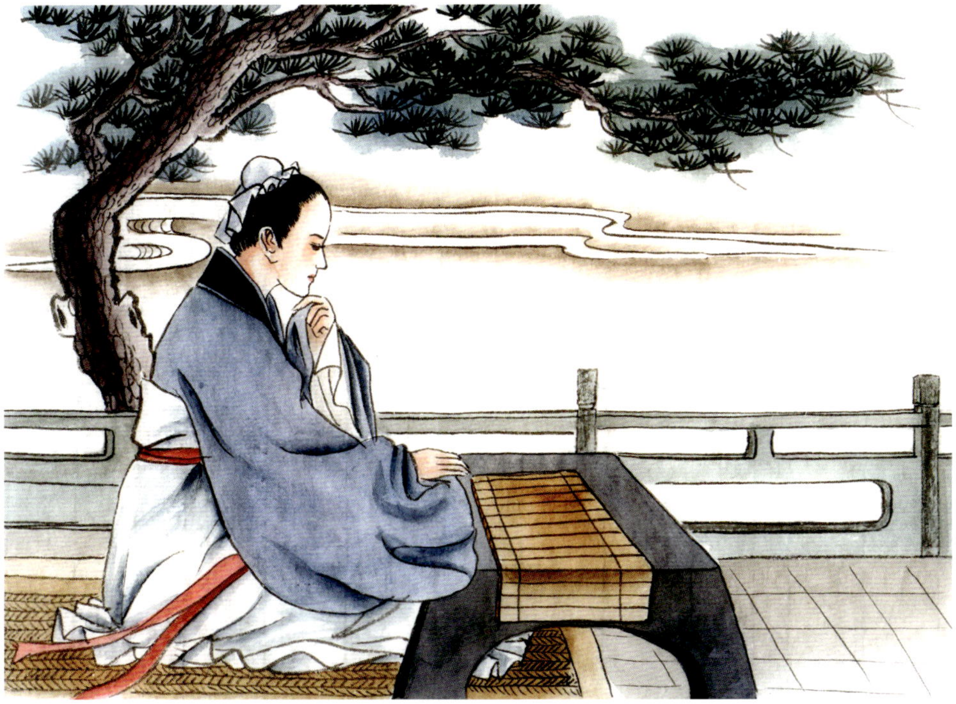

读书，数学

Calligraphy and arithmetic

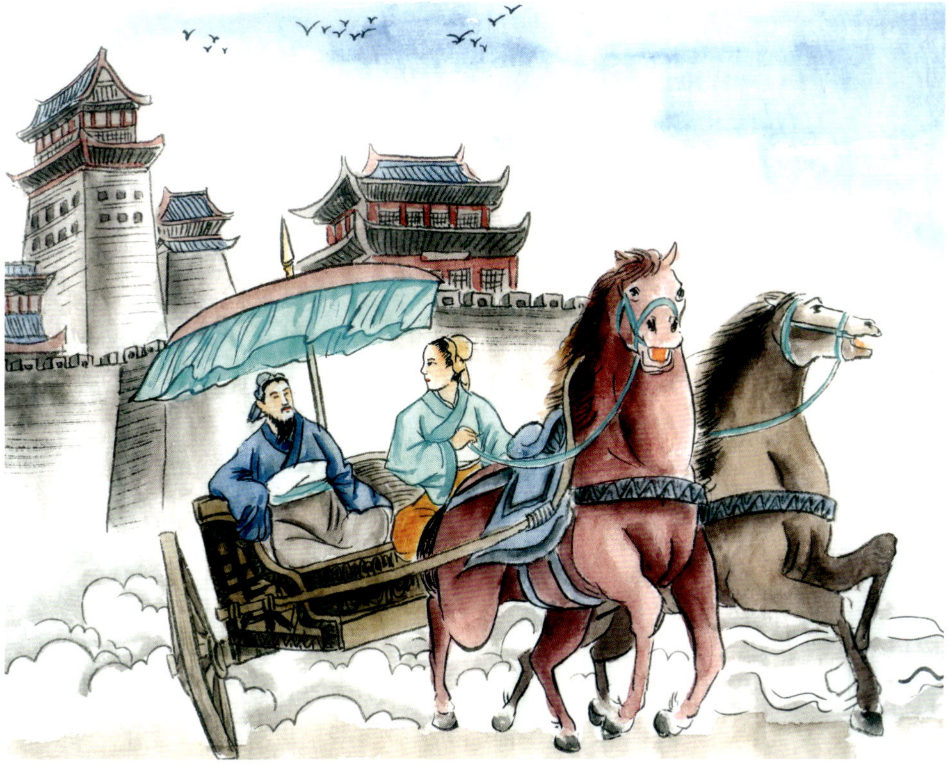

御（驾车）

Driving and riding

佛家养生

Buddhist regimen

佛教产生于印度，经由中亚传入中国新疆地区，并于西汉末年传入内地。由于佛教在传入中国后，起初与黄老学派混同一起为大众接受。因此，佛家养生法早期多附于道家养生法之中，直至隋唐时期，才成为一个独立的养生流派。孙思邈的《千金药方》收录了古天竺国的按摩导引法；而如达摩易筋经、天台宗六妙法门等为人耳熟能详的养生法也都属佛家养生法。佛家注重“禅定”（静虑为禅，心意不乱地静思为禅定）、“顿悟”，在养生理论上以“见性”为主，在养生方法上以静养为长。

Buddhism spread to China via Central Asia from ancient India, its place of origin. Buddhism first arrived at the region that is now Xinjiang and then spread to the interior in the end of the Western Han Dynasty (206 BC- 9 AD). In the initial stage of its introduction into China, Buddhism was treated as a companion to the doctrines of Yellow Emperor and Lao Tzu. The regimen of Buddhism, for a time, was attached to the regimen of Taoism. After the Sui and Tang Dynasties, the regimen of Buddhism began its work as an independent school of regimen.In his *Prescriptions Worth a Thousand Gold for Emergencies,* Sun Simiao registered the health-promoting approaches in ancient India, such as message, extending of limbs and control of breath. In the terminology of the regimen of Buddhism we can find such approaches as tendon-easing skills of Bodhidharma, Six Smart Approaches of Tiantai, etc. Buddhism put a premium on quietude and meditation, sudden perception. The regimen of Buddhism, for its part, lays theoretical emphasis on the perception of nature while its approaches are characterized by quietude.

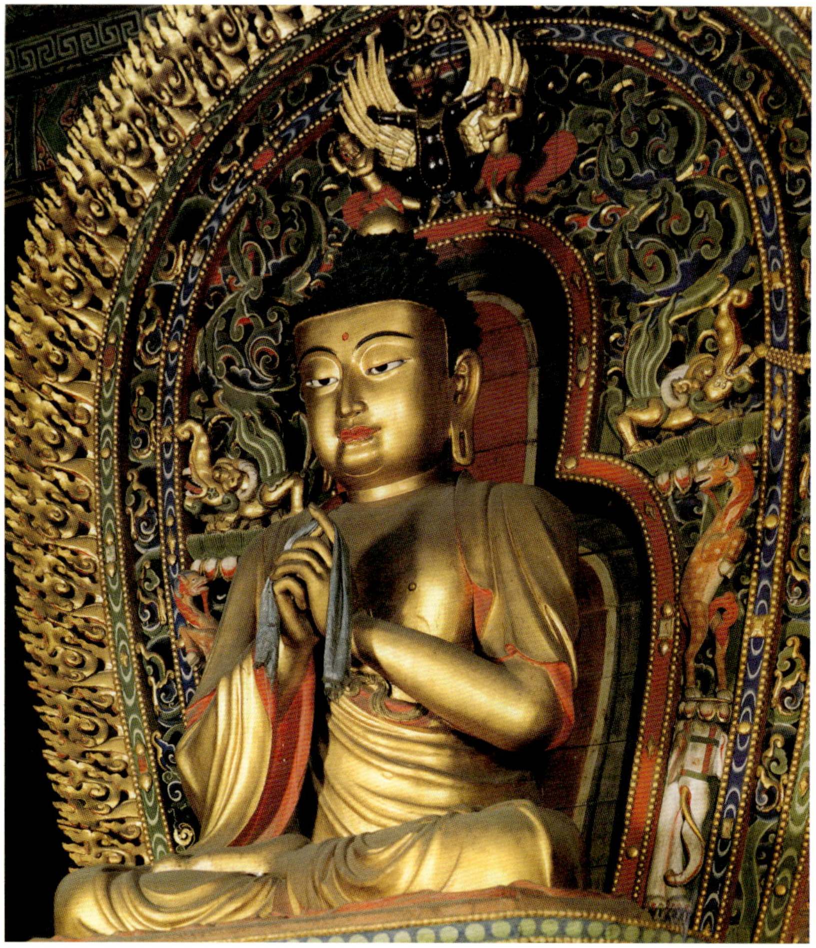

大雄宝殿佛祖像
The statue of Sakyamuni Buddha in the Mahavira Hall

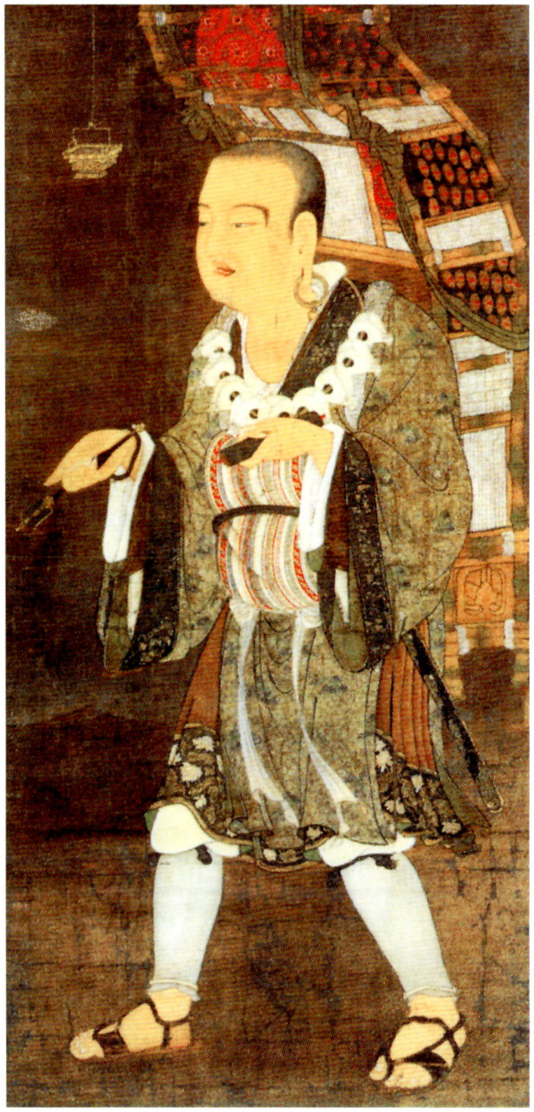

玄奘像
Portrait of Xuanzang

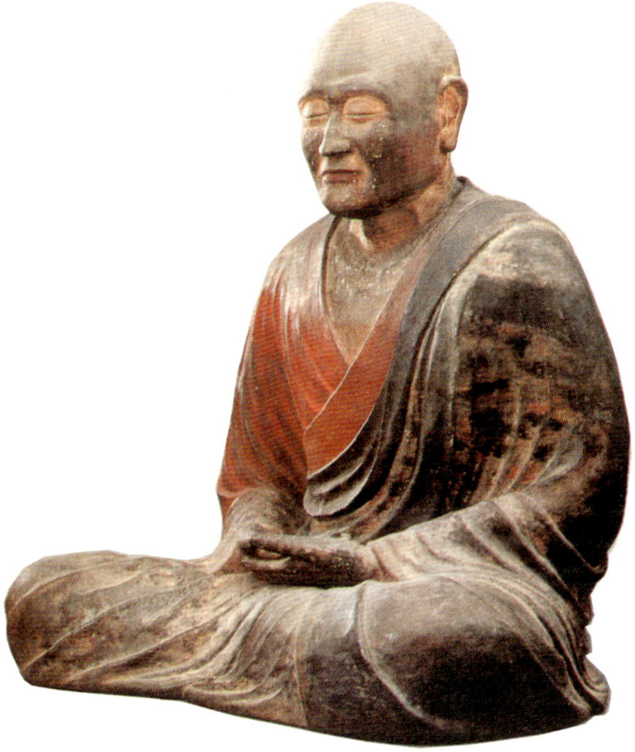

干漆夹苎鉴真像
Painted statue of Jianzhen

佛家认为凡事皆有因果，人的生理健康和心理活动、生活习惯以及人所处的环境，都有密切联系。佛家养生法把调心当做养生的根本，强调治心、修身养性。

Buddhism is good at cultivating the mind and attaches importance to the tempering of nature. Buddhism asserts that there is a cause-effect link between events. So the regimen of Buddhism puts a premium on the living environment, habits, psychological activities and their impact on physiological conditions. In all this, cultivating the mind is at the core of Buddhist regimen.

什么是调心呢?

调心，就是通过调整神经系统功能，协调人体机能的应激能力和敏感度，来提高机体的修复和抗病能力，促进身心健康。佛教特别注重内心清净，并通过各种法门对心态进行调整。由于将事物的差异归结为心念不同，佛教特别注重内心清净，用各种法门调整人的心态，认为可以用静坐来调伏人的妄念。调心时，要做到安定无杂，意念归一，让大脑逐渐进入入静状态。

What is the cultivating of the mind?

In cultivating of the mind, a person consciously adjusts the functions of the nervous system, coordinating the reflex actions and reducing the responsiveness of the body, so as to improve the body's restoring and illness-resisting capabilities. Buddhism puts a premium on internal cleanness and quietude, offering many approaches to adjust the state of mind. Buddhism asserts that differences between things are to be attributed to the turns of their minds and the fancies can be mollified through remaining quietly seated. The purpose of cultivating of the mind is to keep whims off and keep the mind centered so that the brain can actively enter a quiet state.

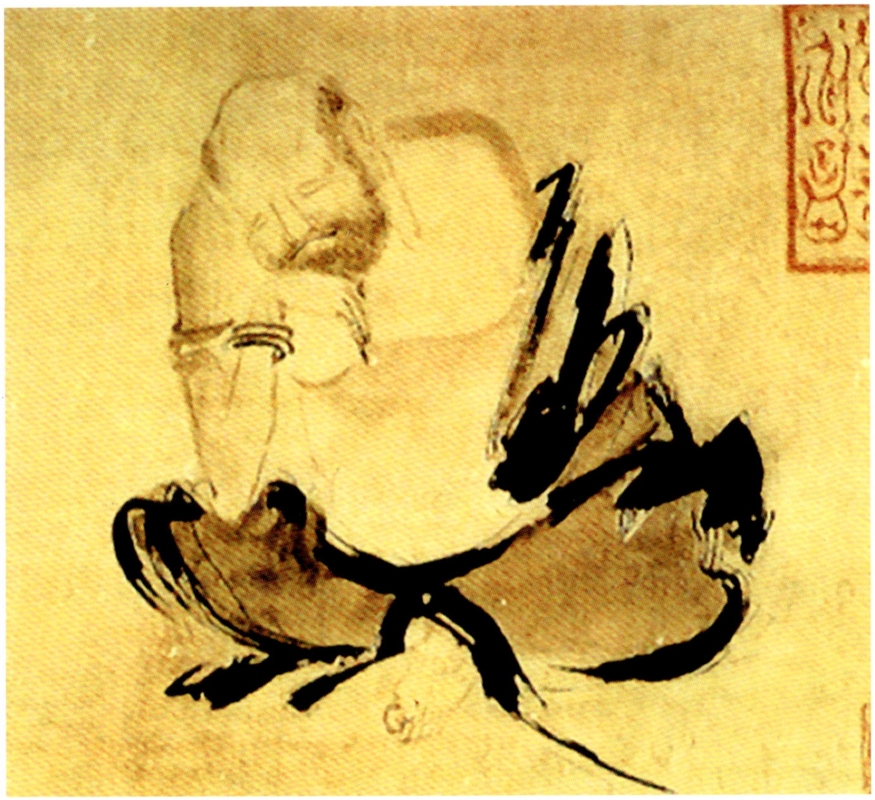

二祖调心图

Two Masters in Mental Cultivation

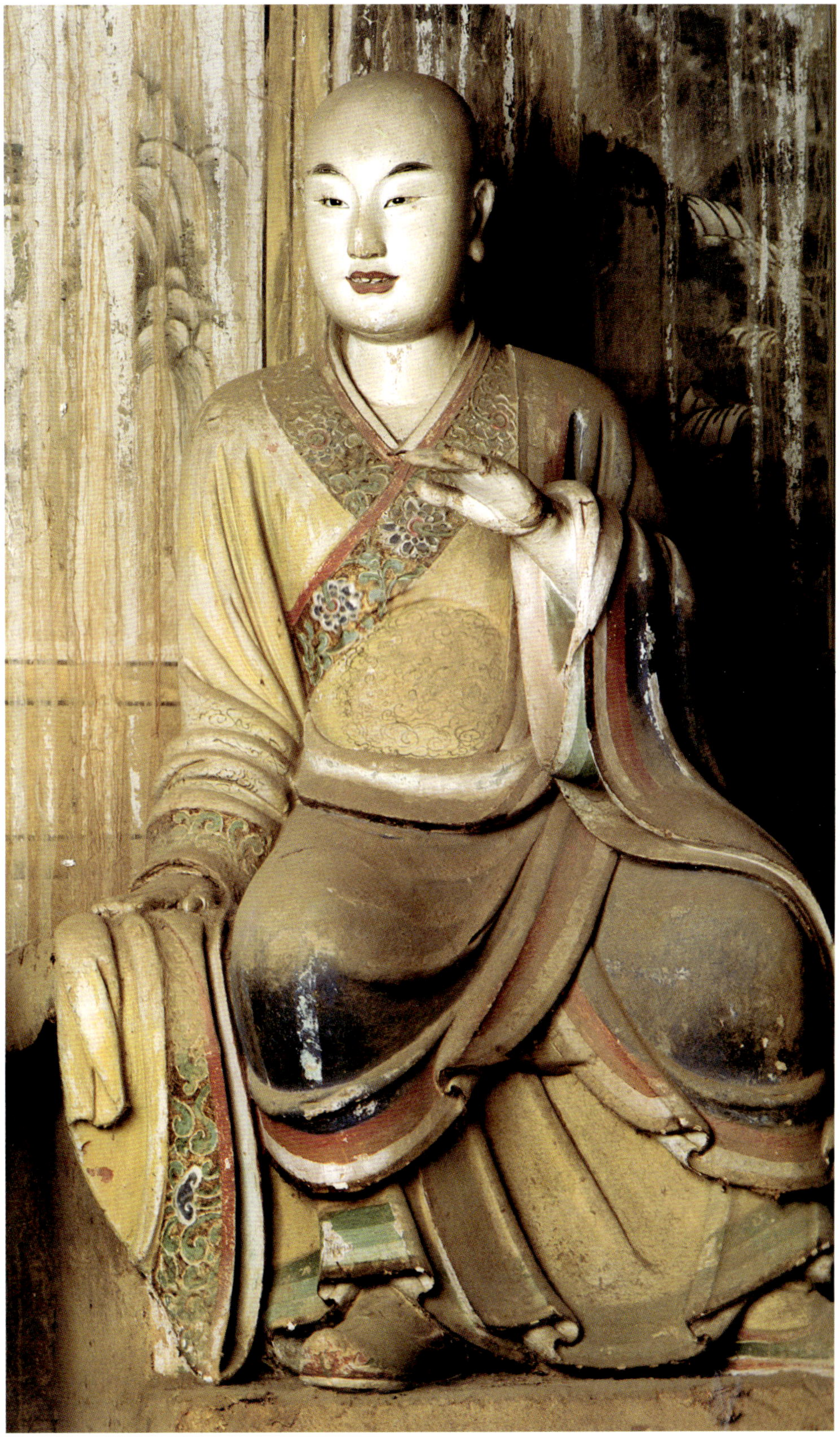

罗汉像

Statue of Arhat

调心之法

Methods of mind cultivation

佛家倡导布施、持戒、坚忍、精进、禅定，强调节制对酒、食、财的欲望，调心的最终目的是让人的心灵不再被烦恼困缚。

人们按照自己的方式、方法经营着人生，在烦乱喧嚣的现实中，有人丧失了平常心，心生烦恼、心气浮乱。如果能调伏自心，那么所有美好的事情自然会汇聚而来，这就是禅定的妙用。

In keeping with the spirit of Buddhism, it is recommended to practice almsgiving, resist temptation, persevere, endeavor diligently, seek quietude and engage in meditation. Buddhism lays emphasis on restricting desires for alcohol, food and money, freeing man's psychological activities from the fetters of boredom, which is the ultimate goal of cultivating the mind.

Everyone plans and manages his life in his own way. In this highly competitive world, most of us have forgone the serenity of mind and are haunted by boredom and vanity. The ingenious application of Quietude and Meditation If we can cultivate our mind, blessings will follow naturally.

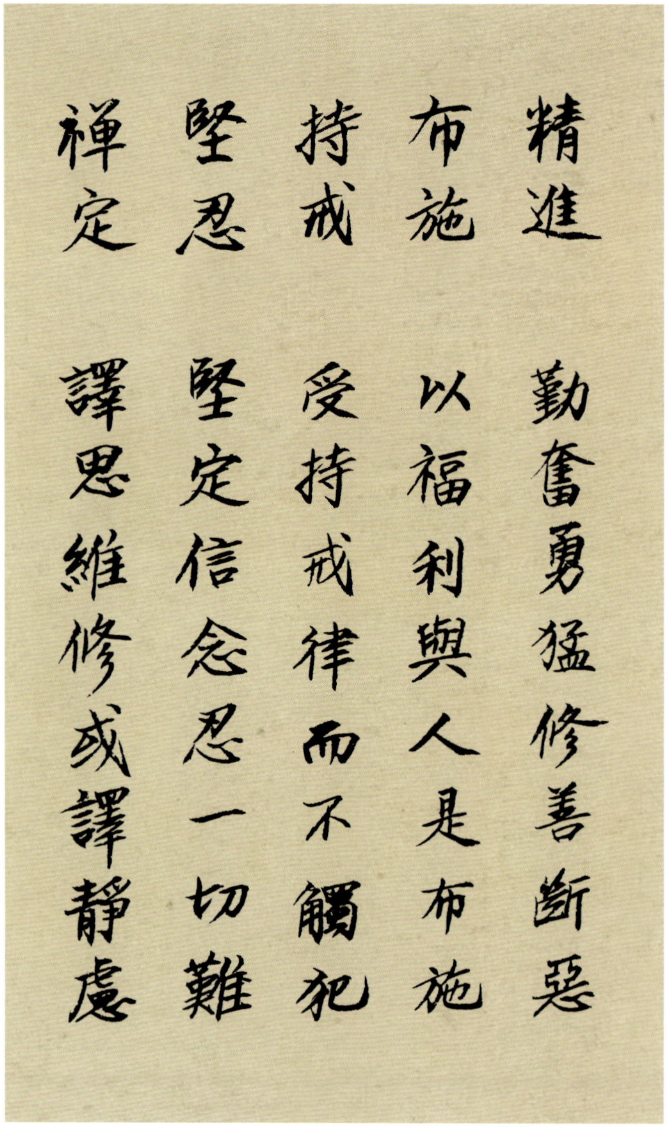

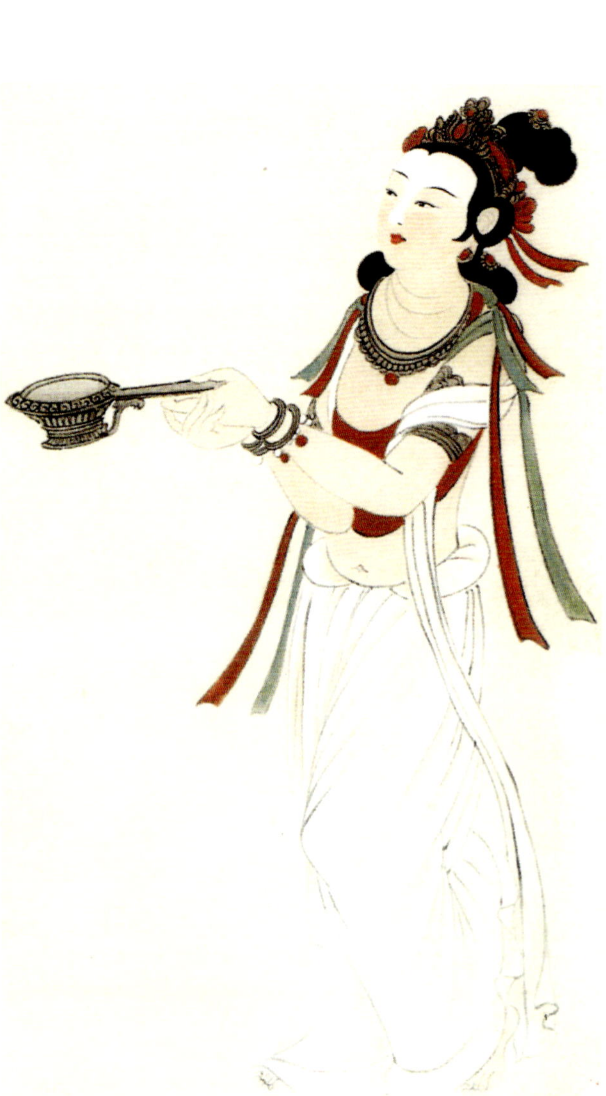

布施

Almsgiving

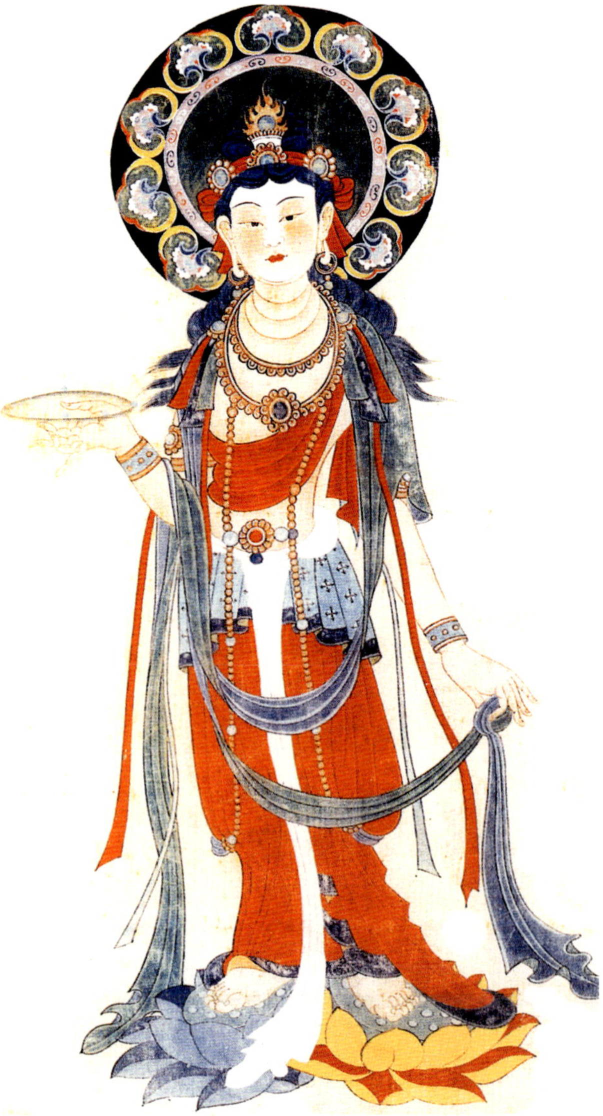

持戒

Resisting temptation

禅定与修心

Meditation and mental equilibrium

佛家认为，保持心态的平稳是长寿的关键。佛学修持心性是要获得智慧的圆满，断除一切烦恼，平衡心态。并以此开导人乐观地看待生命中的无常。禅定是佛教养生的要诀，人人都可以通过修禅来清静自心，防止贪、嗔、痴产生的病态心理，达到怯病强身，怡情养性的目的。

Buddhism sees the key to longevity in keeping the mind tranquil. To cultivate the mind is to fulfill complete wisdom and dispose of any harassment so as to secure a balanced mind. Buddhist doctrine advises people to take an optimistic look at the erratic changes of life. Quietude and meditation constitute the exclusive approach of Buddhist regimen while everyone can achieve cleanness and serenity of mind through meditation, holding off unwholesome psychological activities and physiological disorders. By such means, people can keep ailments at bay and cultivate their dispositions and inclinations.

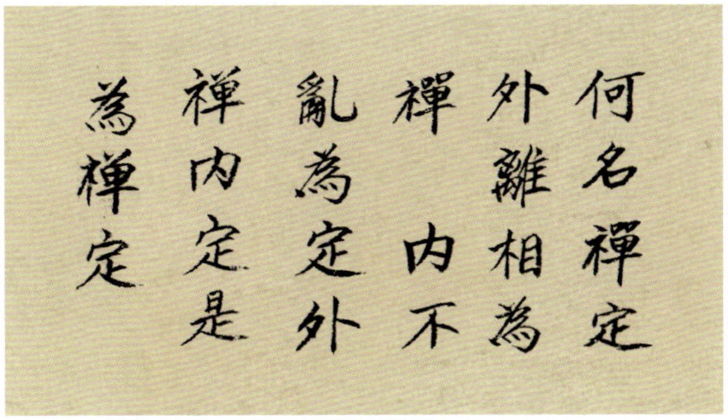

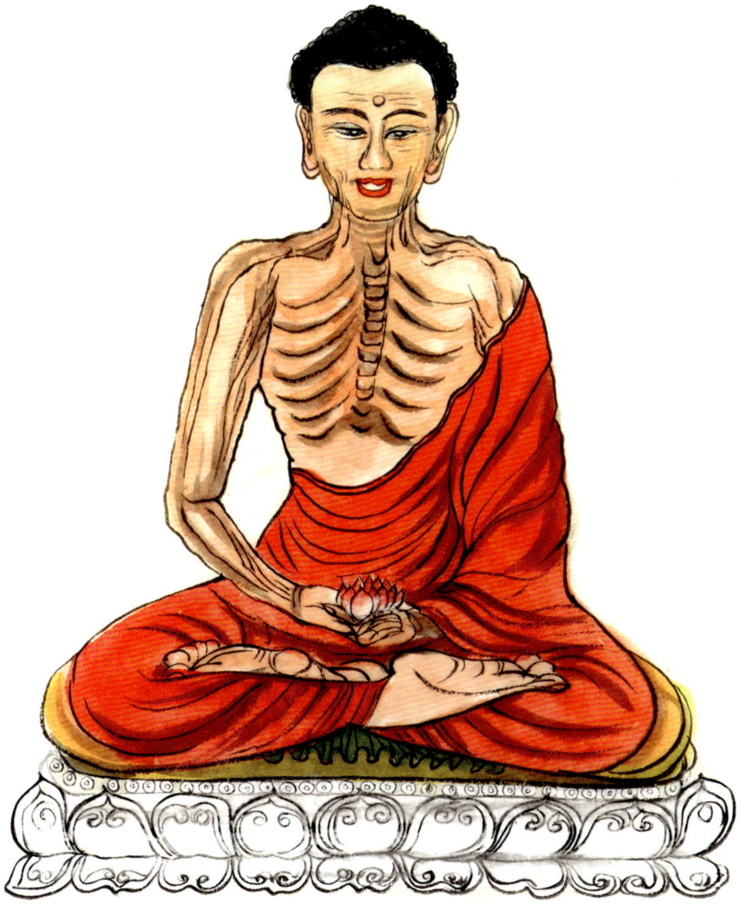

坚忍

Perseverance

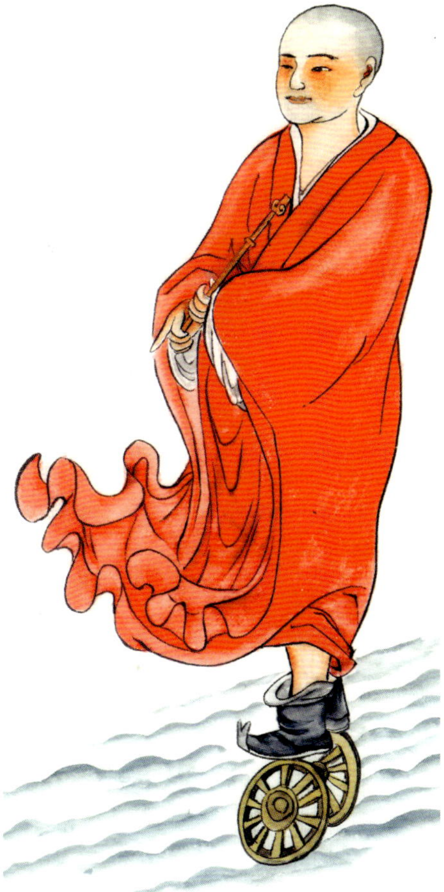

精进

Diligent endeavor

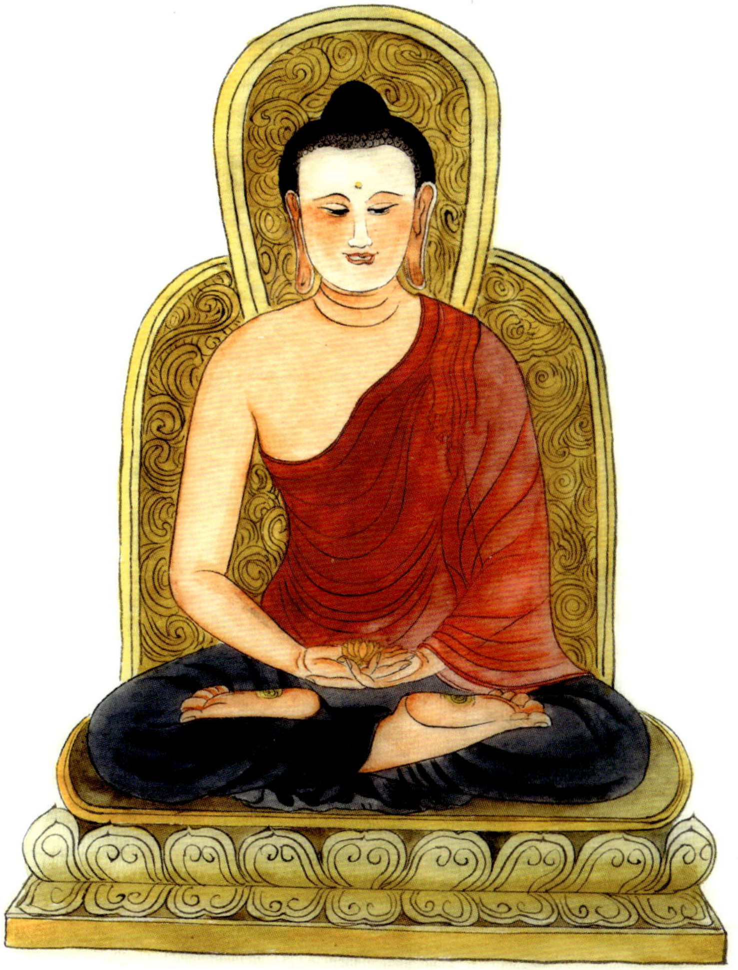

禅定

Meditation

佛家的病理观

Buddhist pathology

佛教认为食药、运动按摩和禅定等都有益于养生，而人生病无非有两种原因：一是地水火风四大病象不调，引起机体病变。二是贪、嗔、痴产生的病态心理导致生理机能紊乱。

Buddhist doctrine asserts that food nourishment, treatment of disease with drugs, physical exercises, message, quietude and meditation are all conducive to maintenance of health. Ailments come from two sources. One is the disorder of the four natural elements – earth, water, fire, wind – that results in the body's unwholesome changes. The other is the unsound psychological activities such as greed, irritation and obsession that cause functional disorders.

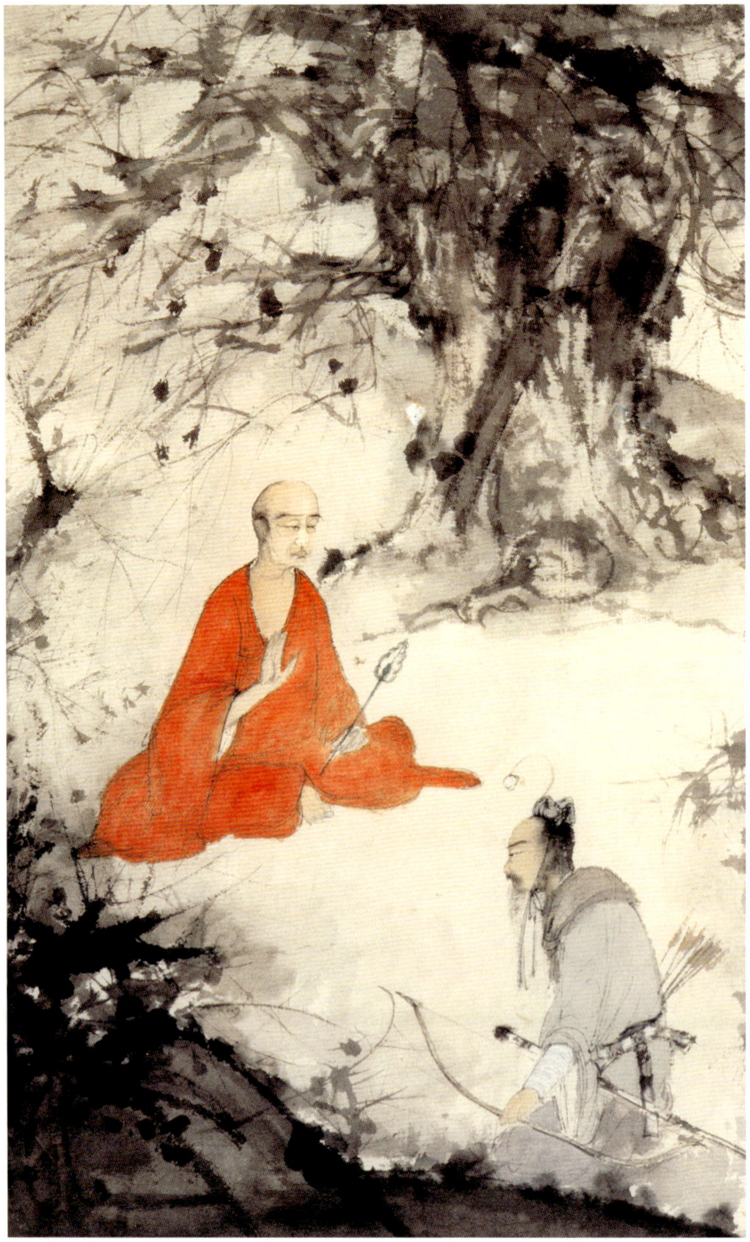

石勒问道图

Shi Le Asking about the Tao

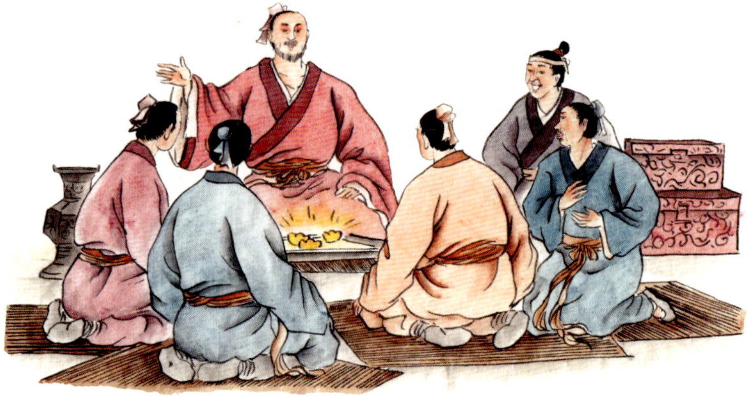

贪

Greed

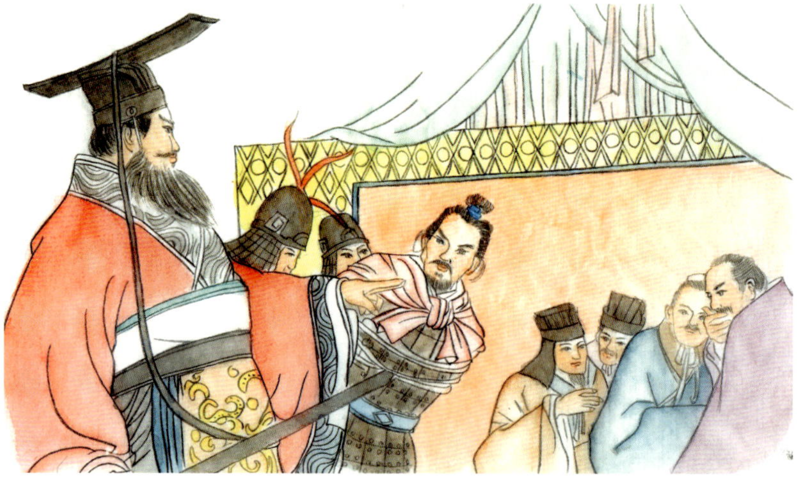

嗔

Irritation

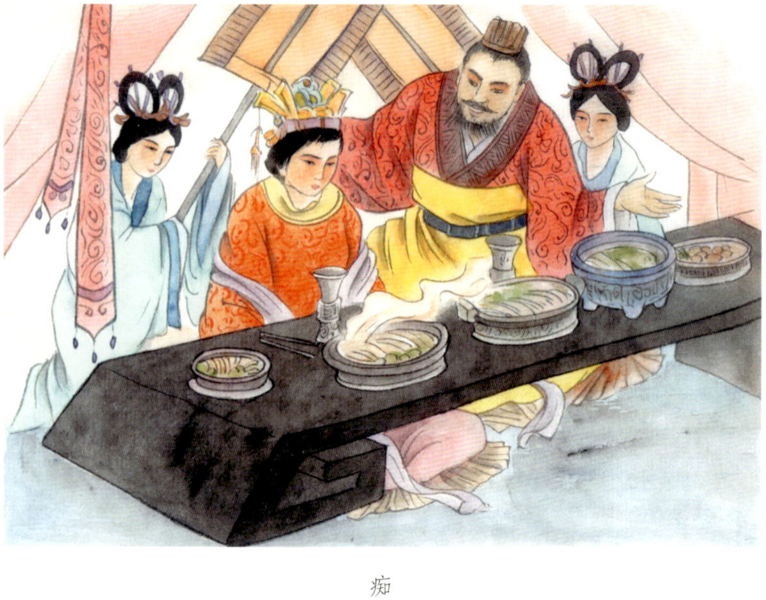

痴

Obsession

拥有平常心

To achieve a balanced mind

拥有平常心是：要平衡心态就必须排除杂念，专心为生活而活，坦然面对利害得失，无忧无虑。

To achieve a balanced mind we must hold off external distractions and live for life's sake, regarding pains and gains with a carefree mind .

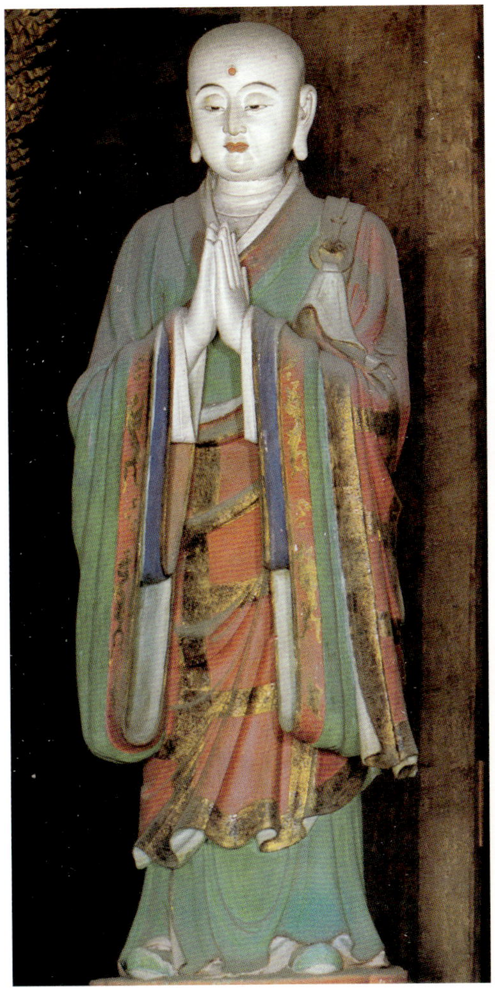

佛像

Statue of Buddha

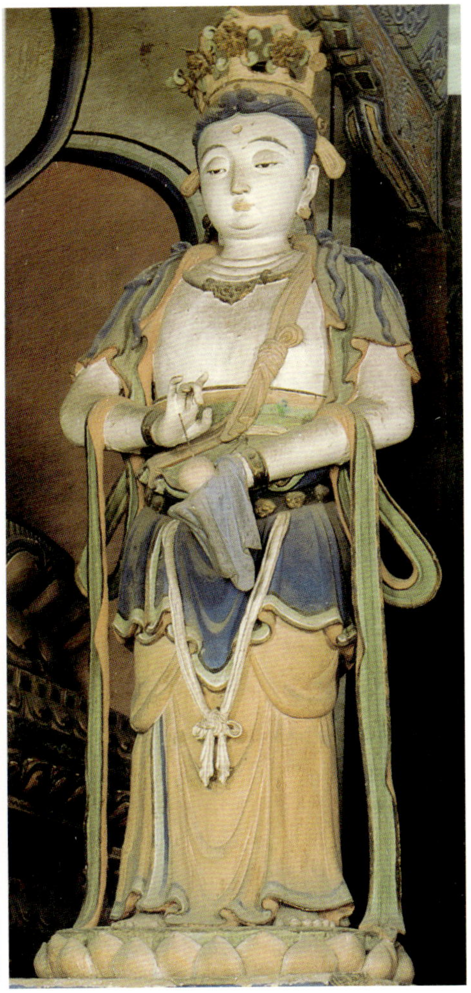

佛像

Statue of Buddha

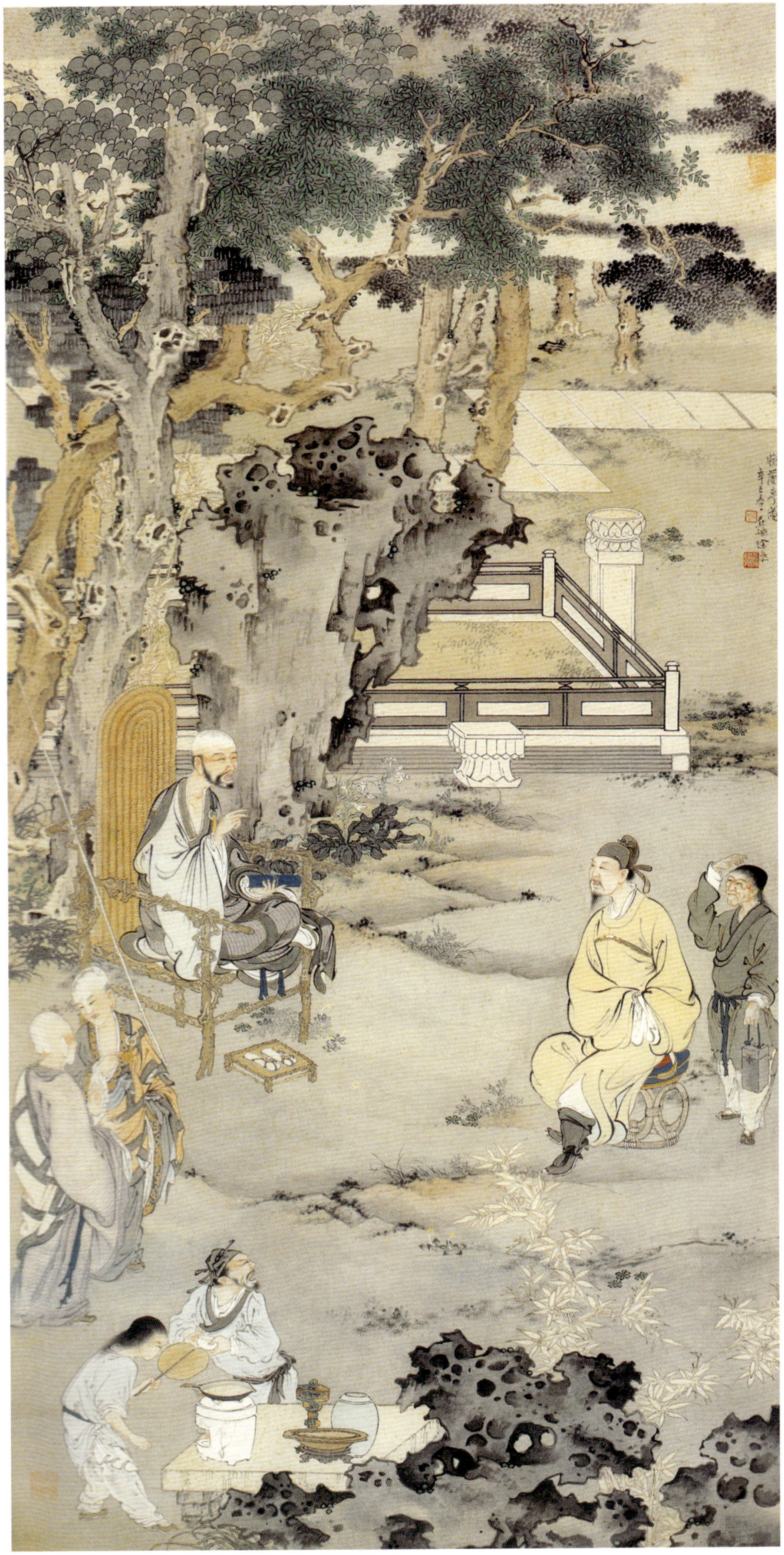

谈禅图

Discussing Zen

身心合一

Body and mind become one

人的心念意识情绪对人的影响最大，也最难调伏。禅定中，要时时检察身、息、心三者是否调和。调伏妄想乱念，使心不过度安逸，调和心念沉浮之相，使心的宽急松紧适当，最终达到万念归一：心气合一、声气合一、身心合一、意念归一。

Mindset and emotions have a remarkable impact on the person and it is extremely difficult to overcome them. In the process of meditation, we can consciously coordinate the body, breath and mind, rein in fancies and whims, keep the mind free from agitation and focus our mind on one point. The process can be summarized as follows: Mind and breath become one. Voice and breath become one. Body and mind become one. All notions become one.

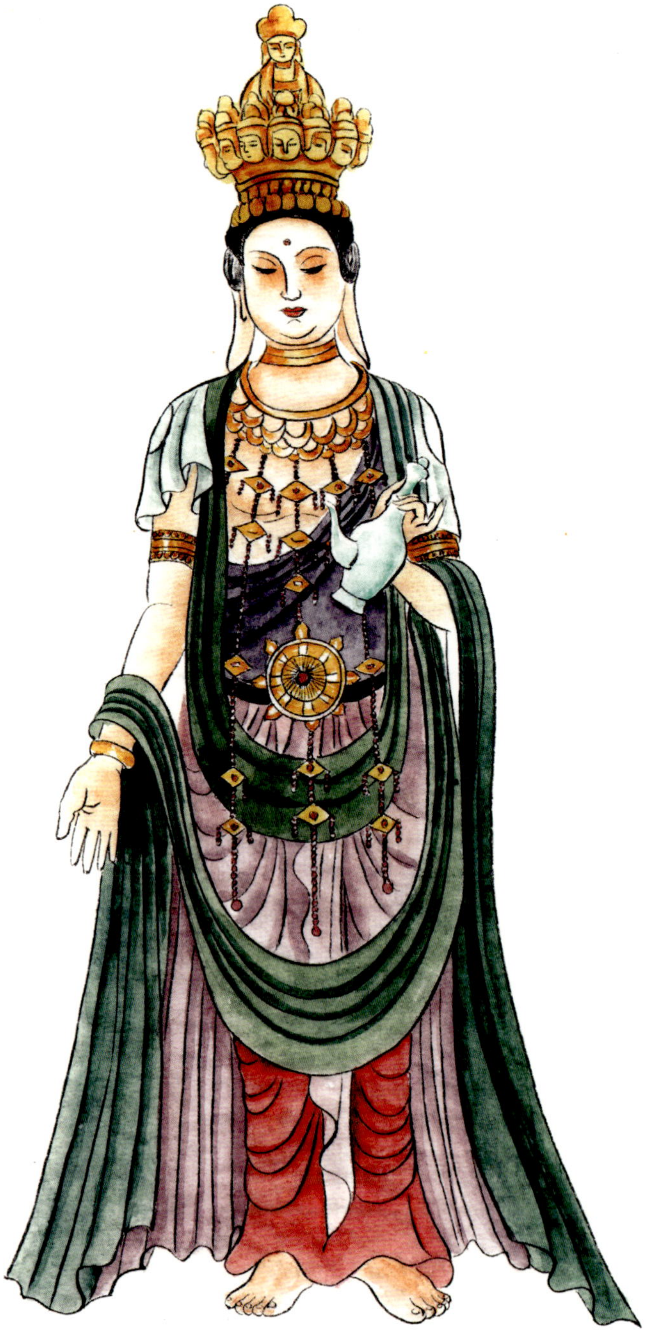

菩萨像

Portrait of Bodhisattva

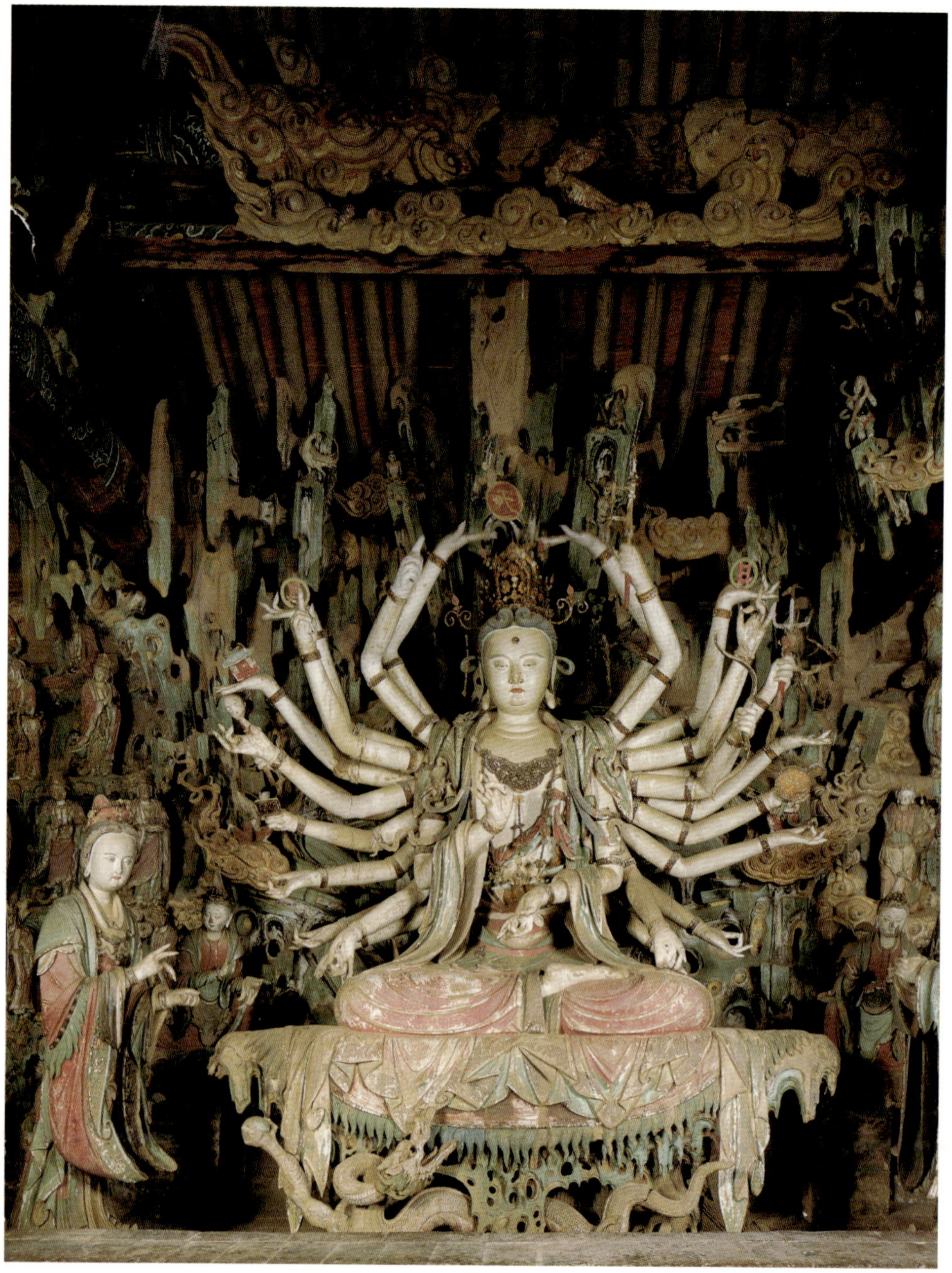

千手观音

Avalokitesvara with a Thousand Arms

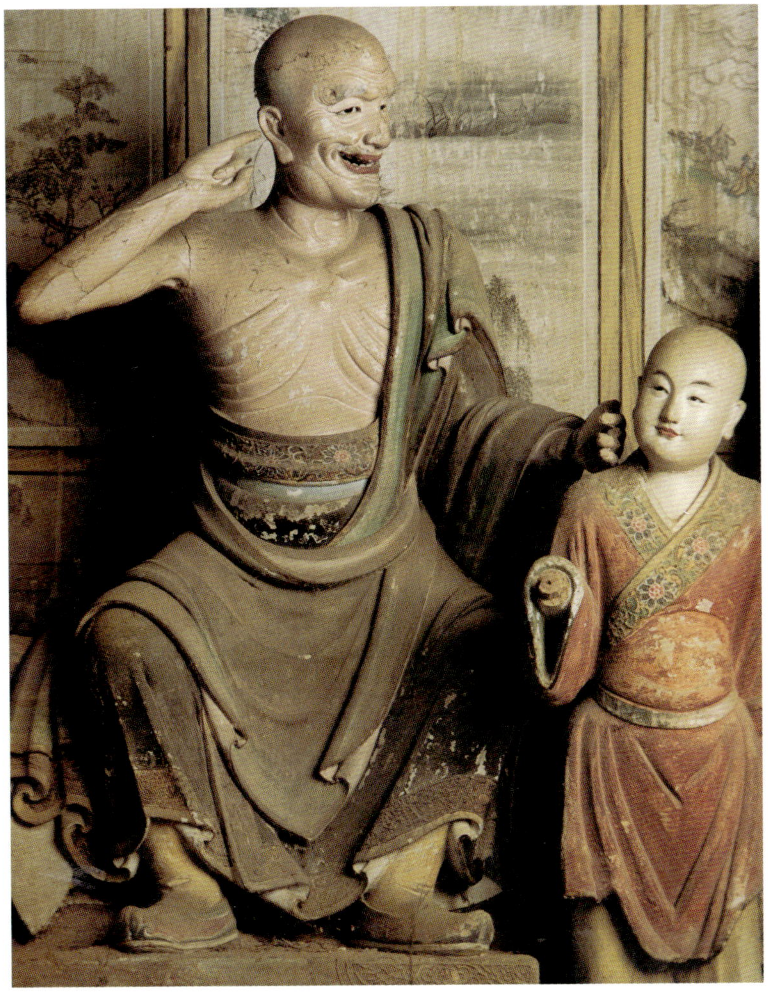

罗汉像
Statue of Arhat

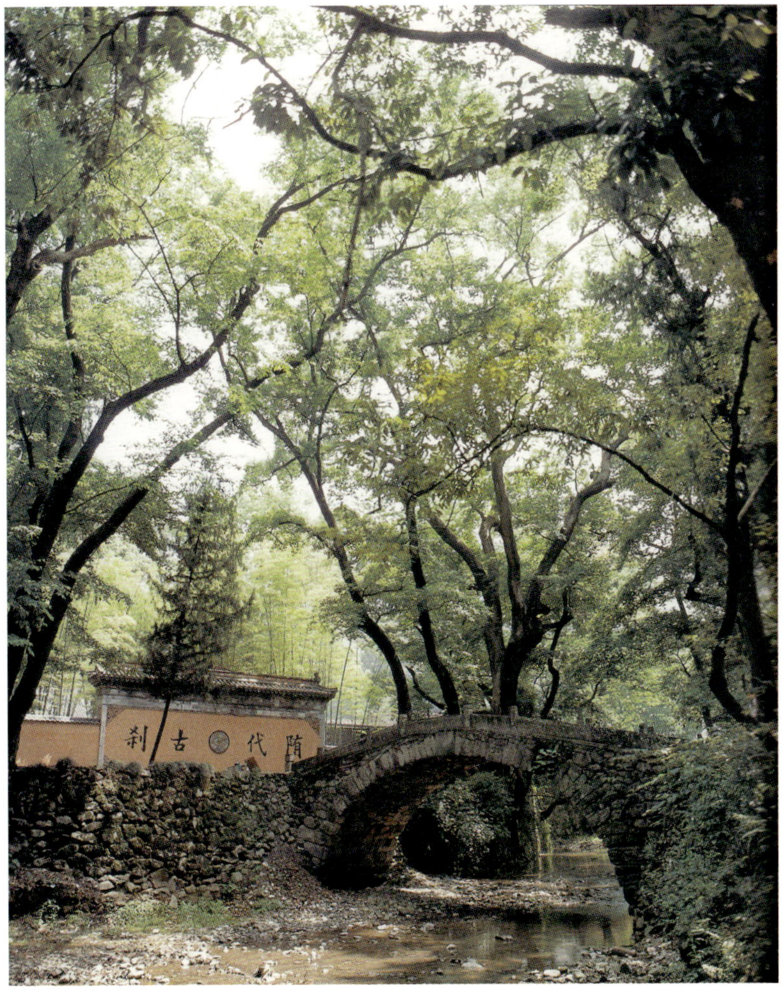

隋代古刹
A temple of the Sui Dynasty

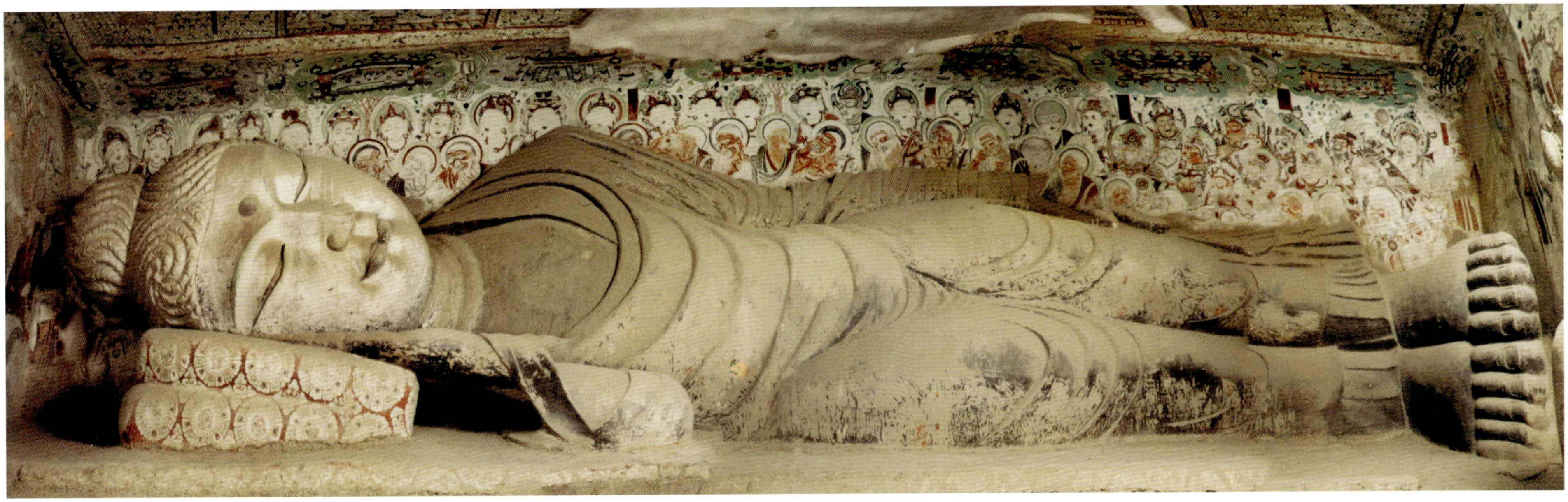

佛祖涅槃像
The nirvana of Buddha

医学养生派

Regimen of Medicine School

医家养生派是除上述三大流派以外的养生派别，是以药物、饮食为主要养生手段的养生流派。在医家养生派中，又有许多细的分支，以饮食调养为主者称为食养派，以药物调补为主者称为药养派。

必须指出的是，所谓养生流派，只是为了研究和继承的方便，根据各家的特点，采用医学史上通常划分流派的方法划分的。各流派之间并无绝然区别，唐代儒、佛、道各家互相交融，许多养生家及养生著作也是兼收并蓄、相互渗透的。

Aside from the above-mentioned three schools of regimen, there is another school: the medical regimen, which lays emphasis on medicines and foodstuff. This school has many sub-schools. Roughly speaking, the branch that values food nourishment is called food-based maintenance branch while the branch that values use of drug is called drug-oriented maintenance branch.

It must be pointed that the above-mentioned schools of regimen are categorized according to their individual characteristics and in keeping with traditional categorization of schools of thoughts. Though arbitrary to a certain extent, such categorization is convenient for study and presentation, without any implication that they are definitely different from each other. During the Tang Dynasty, Confucianism, Buddhism and Taoism tended to merge. Traditionally many regimen experts as well as their written works tended to borrow from each other and embrace common sense in this sphere.

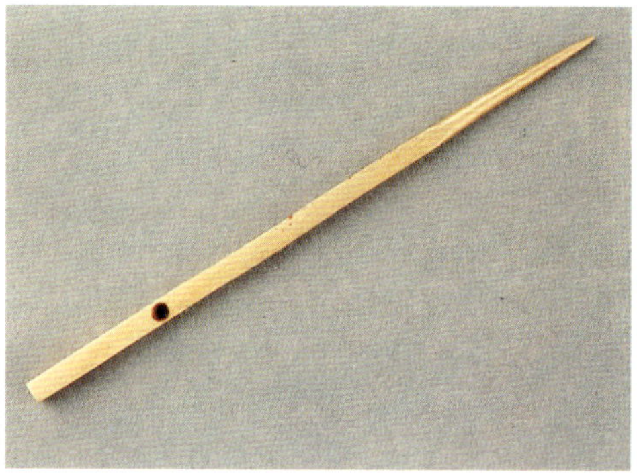

汉　金医针

Han Dynasty Gold medical needle

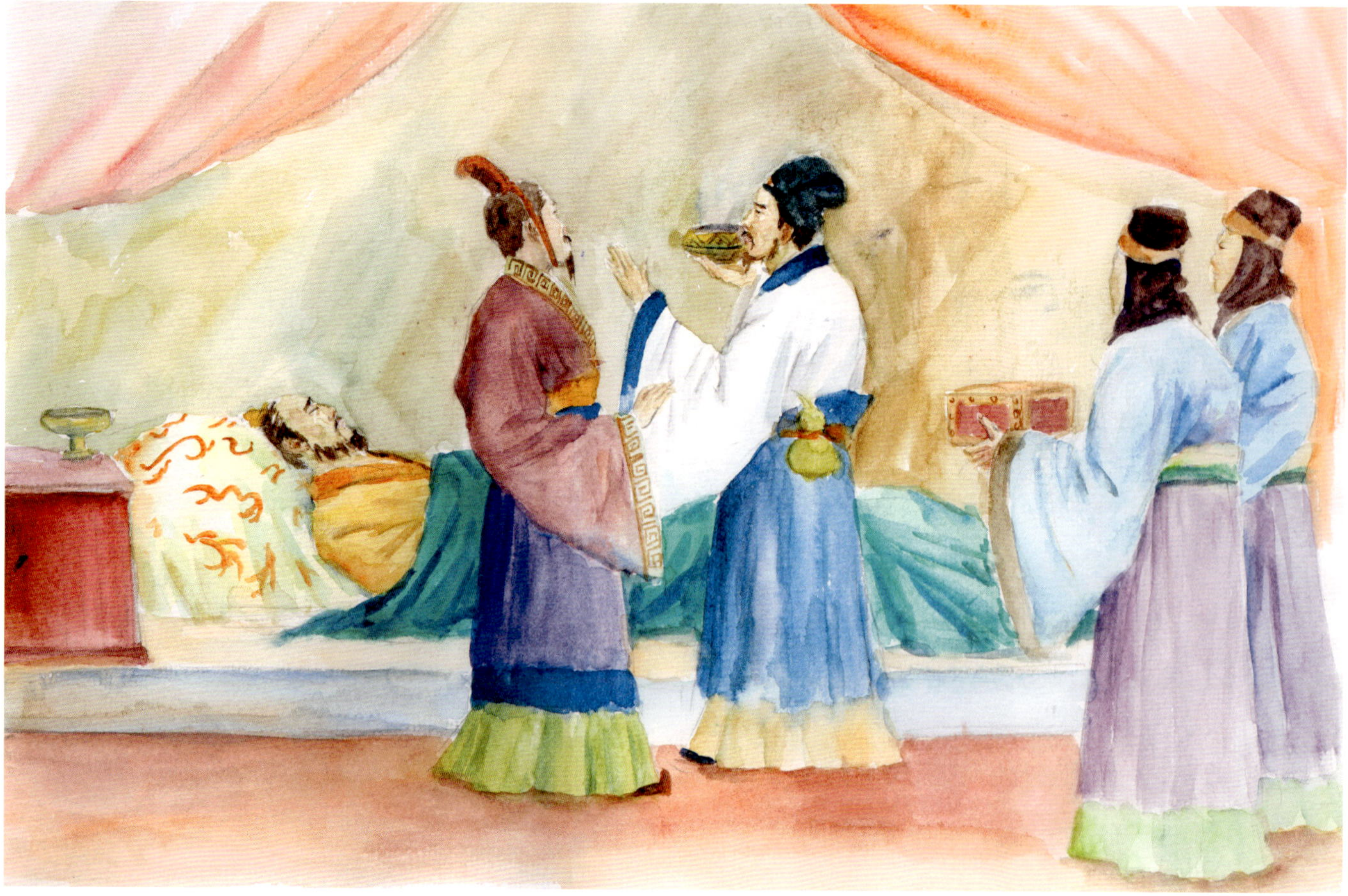

药物、饮食养生

Herbal and dietary regimens

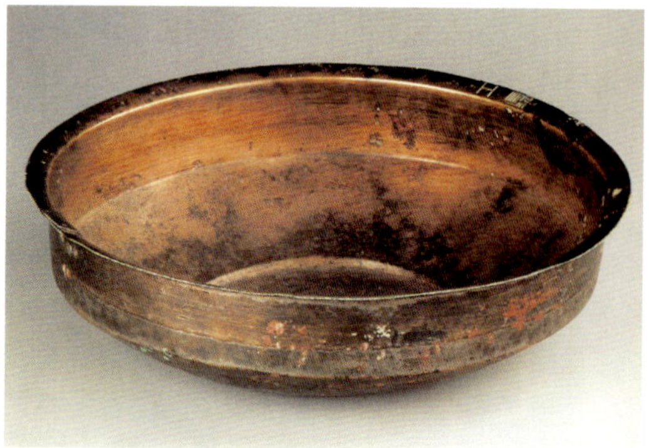

汉　"医工"铜盆

Han Dynasty Doctor's copper basin

扁鹊（前 407 年—前 310 年）创造了切脉诊断法，被后世奉为“脉学之宗”。

Bian Que (407-310 BC) laid the foundation for the pulse-feeling diagnostic method and pioneered TCM.

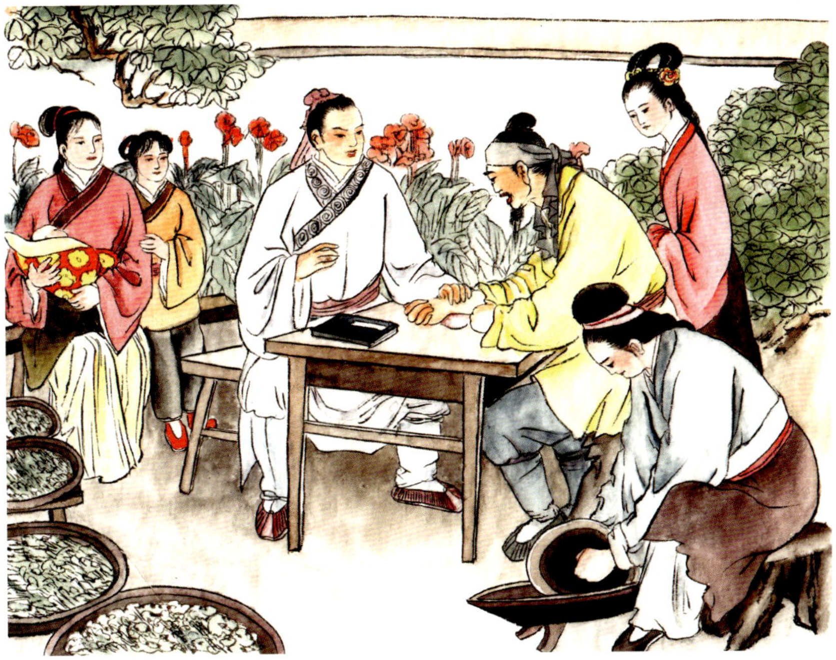

张仲景，东汉末年著名医学家，被称为医圣。其传世巨著《伤寒杂病论》是后世学者研习中医的必备经典。

Zhang Zhongjing, honored as the 'sage of medicine', was a prestigious physician of the late Eastern Han Dynasty. His magnum opus is *Shang Han Za Bing Lun* (*Treatise on Cold Diseases and Miscellaneous Diseases*), which is a must for all students of TCM.

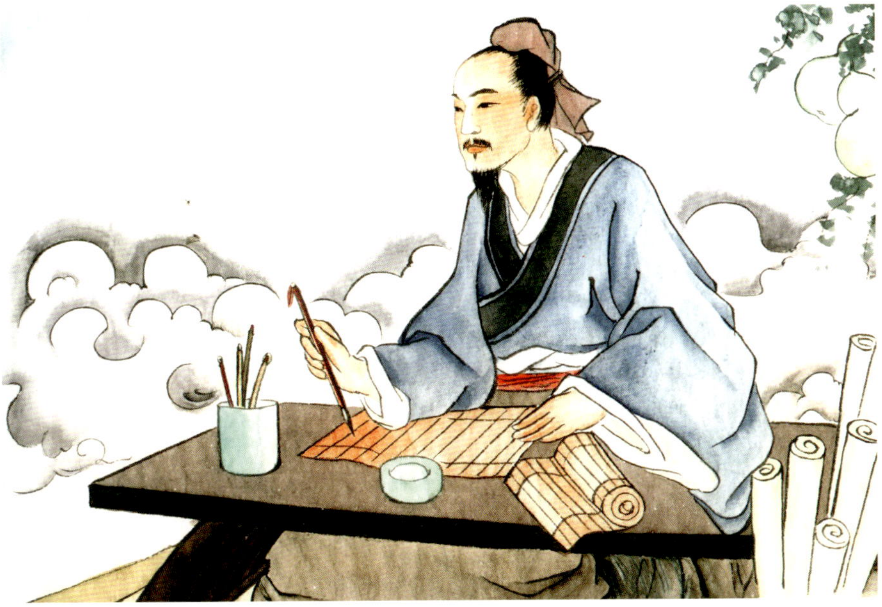

陶弘景 (456 年—536 年)，中国南朝齐、梁时期的道教思想家、医药家、炼丹家、文学家。

Tao Hongjing (456-536) was a Taoist thinker, physician, alchemist and writer of the period of Qi and Liang during the Southern and Northern Dynasties.

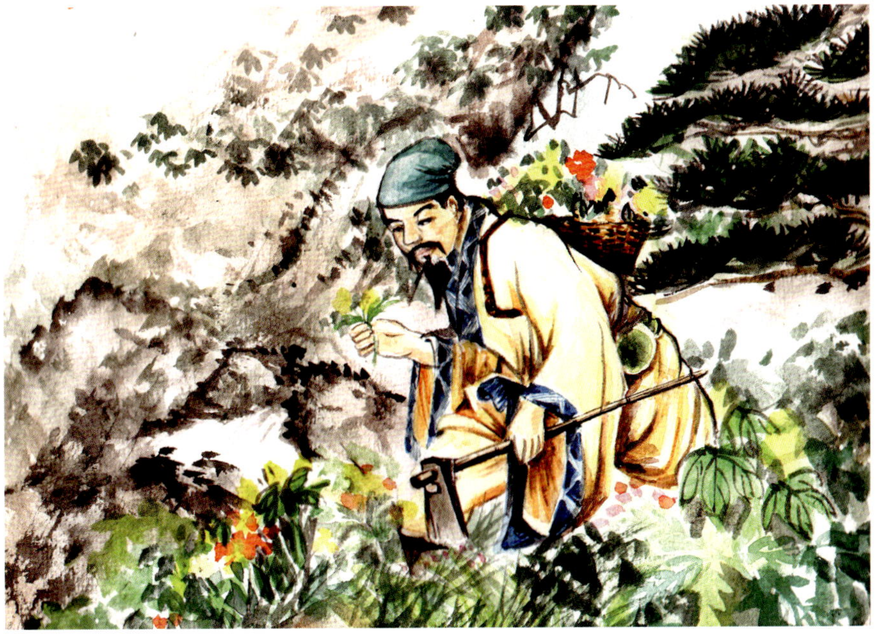

孙思邈，北周时期人，生于 581 年，卒于 682 年，享年 102 岁（有考证称其活了 141 岁）。他是中国医德思想的创始人，被西方称为“医学论之父”，是与希波克拉底齐名的世界三大医德名人之一，被后世尊为“药王”。

Sun Simiao was born in 581 during the Northern Zhou Dynasty and died at the age of 102 (or at 141 according to some textual research) in 682. He was the founder of Chinese medical ethics and is honored as the “Pharmaceutical King”. In the West he is known as the “Father of Medical Theory” and, along with Hippocrates, as one of the world's three greatest pioneers of medical ethics.

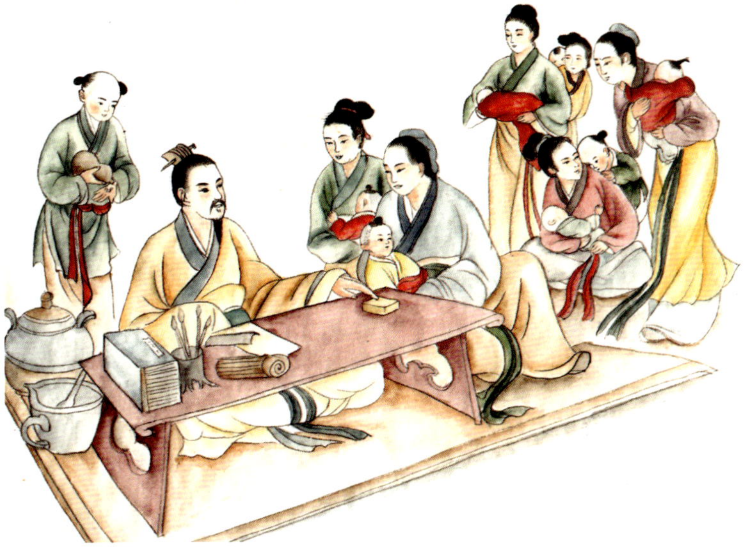

中医经络

TCM meridians and collaterals

经络是经脉和络脉的总称。人体上有一些纵贯全身的路线，古人称之为经脉；在这些大干线上有一些分支，分支上又有更细小的分支，古人称这些分支为络脉。

Jingluo is a general term for jingmai (meridians) and luomai (collaterals). The longitudinal channels through the body were called 'meridians' by ancient people. The branches and sub-branches of these main channels were called 'collaterals'.

经络总览图
TCM meridians and collaterals

经络系统 Meridian and collateral system

- 经脉 Meridians
  - 正经十二（十二经脉）The twelve meridians
    - 气血的主要通道；同内在脏腑有直接的络属关系 The main channels for the circulation of qi and blood, directly related to the internal organs
    - 手三阴经 Three yin meridians of hand
      - 手太阴肺经 Lung channel of hand taiyin
      - 手厥阴心包经 Pericardium channel of hand jueyin
      - 手少阴心包经 Heart channel of hand shaoyin
    - 手三阳经 Three yang meridians of hand
      - 手阳明大肠经 Large intestine channel of hand yangming
      - 手少阳三焦经 Tri-jiao channel of hand shaoyang
      - 手太阳小肠经 Small intestine channel of hand taiyang
    - 足三阴经 Three yin meridians of foot
      - 足太阴脾经 Spleen channel of foot tayin
      - 足厥阴肝经 Liver channel of foot jueyin
      - 足少阴肾经 Kidney channel of foot shaoyin
    - 足三阳经 Three yang meridians of foot
      - 足阳明胃经 Stomach channel of foot yangming
      - 足少阳胆经 Gall bladder channel of foot shaoyang
      - 足太阳膀胱经 The urinary bladder meridian of foot
  - 奇经八脉 Eight extra channels
    - 十二经脉以外的另一些重要的经脉，包括任脉、督脉、冲脉、带脉、阴跷脉、阳跷脉、阴维脉、阳维脉，有统率、联络和调节十二经脉的作用。
    - The 'divergent channels' of the Twelve Meridians serve to strengthen the connection between the outer meridians and the inner ones.
  - 十二经别 Twelve divergent channels
    - 从十二经脉中的经脉，有加强十二经脉中相为表里的两经之间联系的作用。
    - Ther important channels besides the Twelve Meridians, such as Ren, Du, Chong, Dai, Yinqiao, Yangqiao, Yinwei and Yangwei, serve to command, connect and regulate the Twelve Meridians.
- 络脉 Collaterals
  - 十五别络 Fifteen large collaterals
    - 从十二经脉及任脉、督脉各分出一支别络，再加上脾之大络，有加强表里两经在体表的联系和渗灌气血的作用。
    - Collaterals from the Twelve Meridians, Ren Channel and Du Channel respectively, plus the major collateral of the spleen, serve to strengthen the connection between the outer meridians and the inner ones at the body surface and infuse qi and blood into tissues and organs.
  - 浮络 Superficial collaterals
    - 浮现于体表的络脉
    - Collaterals at the body surface
  - 孙络 Minute collaterals
    - 细小的络脉
    - Minute collaterals
- 十二经筋 Twelve muscle tendon channels
  - 十二经脉之气结、聚散、络于筋肉、关节的体系，有联缀四肢百骸，主司关节运动的作用。
  - The twelve muscle tendon channels form the system for gathering or dispersing the qi of the Twelve Meridians in muscles and joints. They serve to link the limbs and bones and control the movements of the joints.
- 十二皮部 Twelve epidermal areas
  - 十二经脉的功能反映于体表的部位。
  - The parts of the body surface reflecting the functions of the Twelve Meridians.

经络在全身的分布规律

Distribution of meridians and collaterals in the human body

六阴经	Six yin channels	分布于四肢内侧和胸腹。 On the inside of the limbs, the chest, and the abdomen.
六阳经	Six yang channels	分布于四肢外侧和头面、躯干。 On the outside of the limbs, the head, the face, and the torso.
三阴经	Three yin channels	上肢为手太阴肺经在前、手厥阴心包经在中、手少阴心经在后。下肢为足三阴经在足内踝以下为厥阴在前、太阴在中、少阴在后，至内踝 8 寸以上，太阴交出于厥阴之前。 In the upper limbs, Hand Absolute Yin Pericardium Meridian is in the middle, with Hand Great Yin Lung Meridian in front of it and Hand Small Yin Heart Meridian behind it. In the lower limbs, below the inner ankles, the Great Yin is in the middle, with the Absolute Yin in front of it and the Small Yin behind it; above eight cun (about 25 centimeters) from the inner ankles, the Great Yin is in front of the Absolute Yin.
三阳经	Three yang channels	上肢为手阳明大肠经在前、手少阳三焦经在中、手太阳小肠经在后。下肢为足阳明胃经在前、足少阳胆经在中、足太阳膀胱经在后。 In the upper limbs, Hand Small Yang Sanjiao Meridian is in the middle, with Hand Yang Brightness Large Intestine Meridian in front of it and Hand Great Yang Small Intestine Meridian behind it. In the lower limbs, Foot Small Yang Gallbladder Meridian is in the middle, with Foot Yang Brightness Stomach Meridian in front of it and Foot Great Yang Bladder Meridian behind it.
足少阴肾经	Kidney channel of foot shaoyin	在胸中线旁开 2 寸，腹中线旁开 0.5 寸处。 At 2 cun (about 7 centimeters) from the central axis of the chest and 0.5 cun (about 1.7 centimeters from the central axis of the abdomen.
足太阴脾经	Spleen channel of foot taiyin	行于胸中线旁开 6 寸，腹中线旁开 4 寸处。 At 6 cun (about 20 centimeters) from the central axis of the chest and 4 cun (about 13 centimeters) from the central axis of the abdomen.
足厥阴肝经	Liver channel of foot jueyin	循行规律性不强。 With no clear pattern in circulation.
足阳明胃经	Stomach channel of foot yangming	分布于胸中线旁开 4 寸，腹中线旁开 2 寸处。 At 4 cun (about 13 centimeters) from the central axis of the chest and 2 cun (about 7 centimeters) from the central axis of the abdomen.
足太阳膀胱经	Urinary bladder channel of foot taiyang	行于背部，分别于背正中线旁开 1.5 寸和 3 寸处。 On the back, at 1.5 cun (about 5 centimeters) and 3 cun (about 10 centimeters) from the central axis of the back respectively.
足少阳胆经	Gall bladder channel of foot shaoyang	分布于身体侧面。 On the flanks of the body.

人体有两个“长寿穴”

The body has a two" long point"

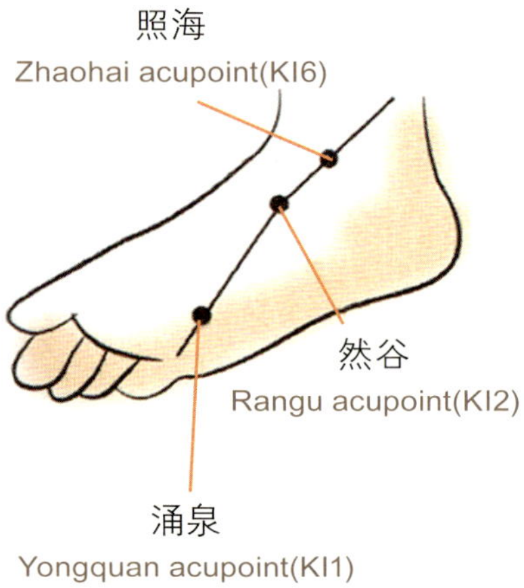

涌泉穴
Yongquan Point

肾经的一个重要穴位，经常按摩此穴，有增精益髓、补肾壮阳、强盘壮骨之功效。涌泉穴位于足底，在足掌的前三分之一处，屈趾时凹陷处便是。

(It is) an important acupuncture point, or acupoint, on the Kidney Channel. Massaging this acupoint often increases sperm productivity, nourishes marrow, tonify the kidney, enhances male sexual capacity, and strengthens sinews and bones. Yongquan Point is located at a third of the length of the sole from the toes; when you bend your toes downward, you can feel it right at the depression on the sole.

涌泉穴的保健方法

每晚睡前盘腿而坐，用双手按摩或屈指点压双足涌泉穴，以该穴位达到酸胀感觉为度，每次 50 至 100 下。

Yongquan Point Massaging Exercise

Sit cross-legged before bed every night, and rub Yongquan Points on the two soles with your hands or press them with your bent fingers 50-100 times until the acupoints feel sore.

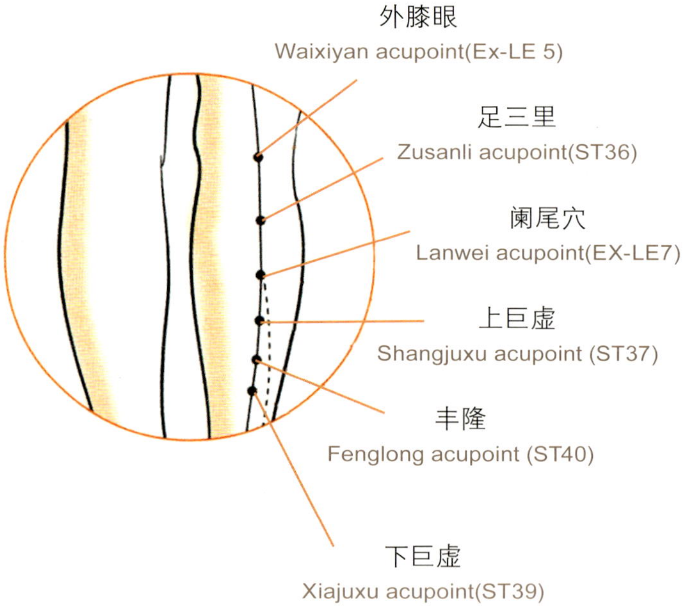

足三里穴
Zusanli Point

足三里穴是胃经的要穴，按摩此穴有助于胃部的消化吸收。

Zusanli Point is an important acupoint on the Stomach Channel. Massaging this acupoint may improve the digestive capacity of the stomach.

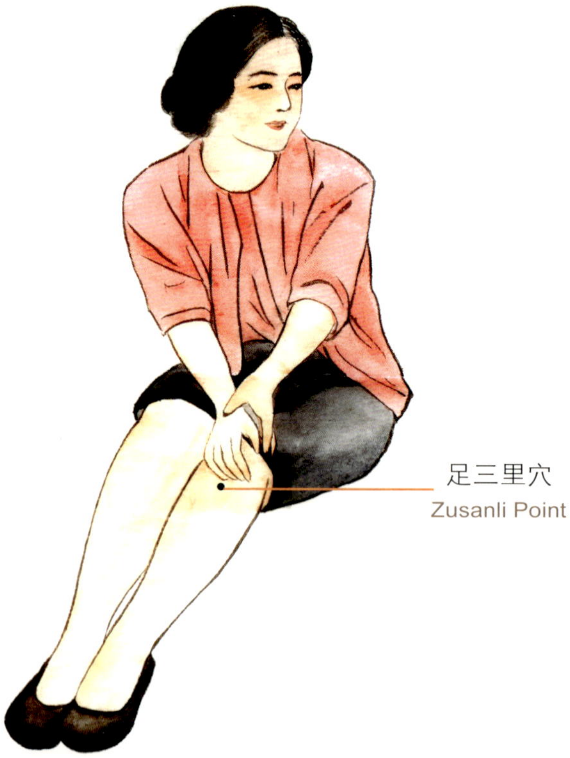

足三里穴的保健方法

每晚以指关节按压足三里，能补脾健胃，增强人体免疫功能，消除疲劳，恢复体力，使人精神焕发。

Zusanli Point Massaging Exercise

Pressing Zusanli Point with your knuckles every night may tonify the spleen, benefit the stomach, improve the immune function of the human body, relieve fatigue, help recover vigour and make you feel energized.

十二经脉

Twelve meridians

手太阴肺经

Lung channel of hand taiyin

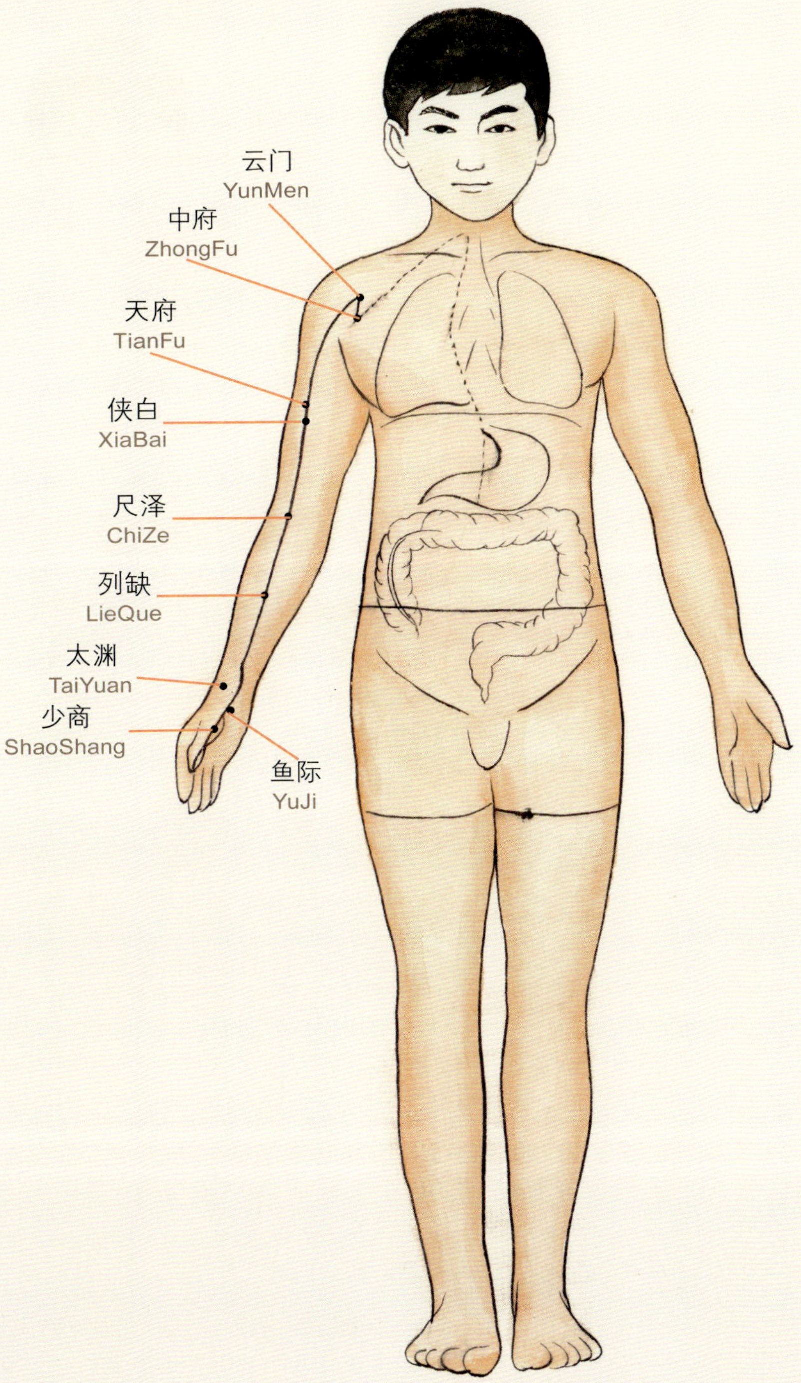

手阳明大肠经

Large intestine channel of hand yangming

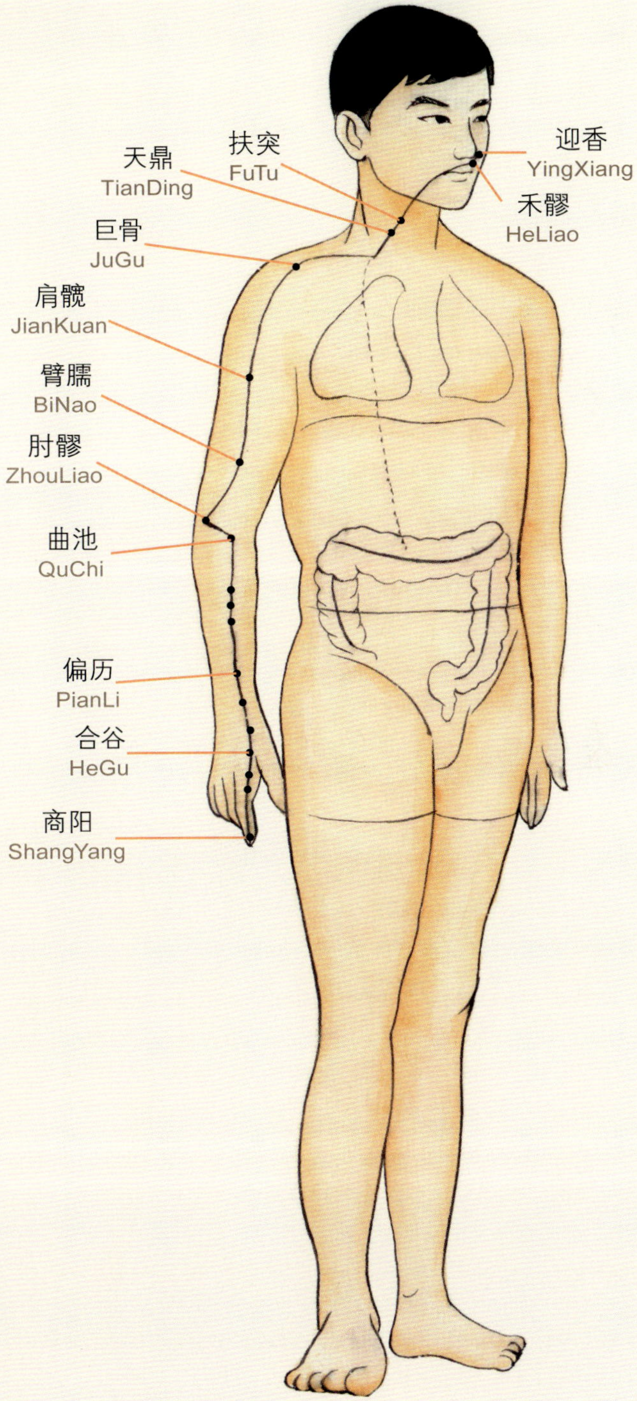

足阳明胃经

Stomach channel of foot yangming

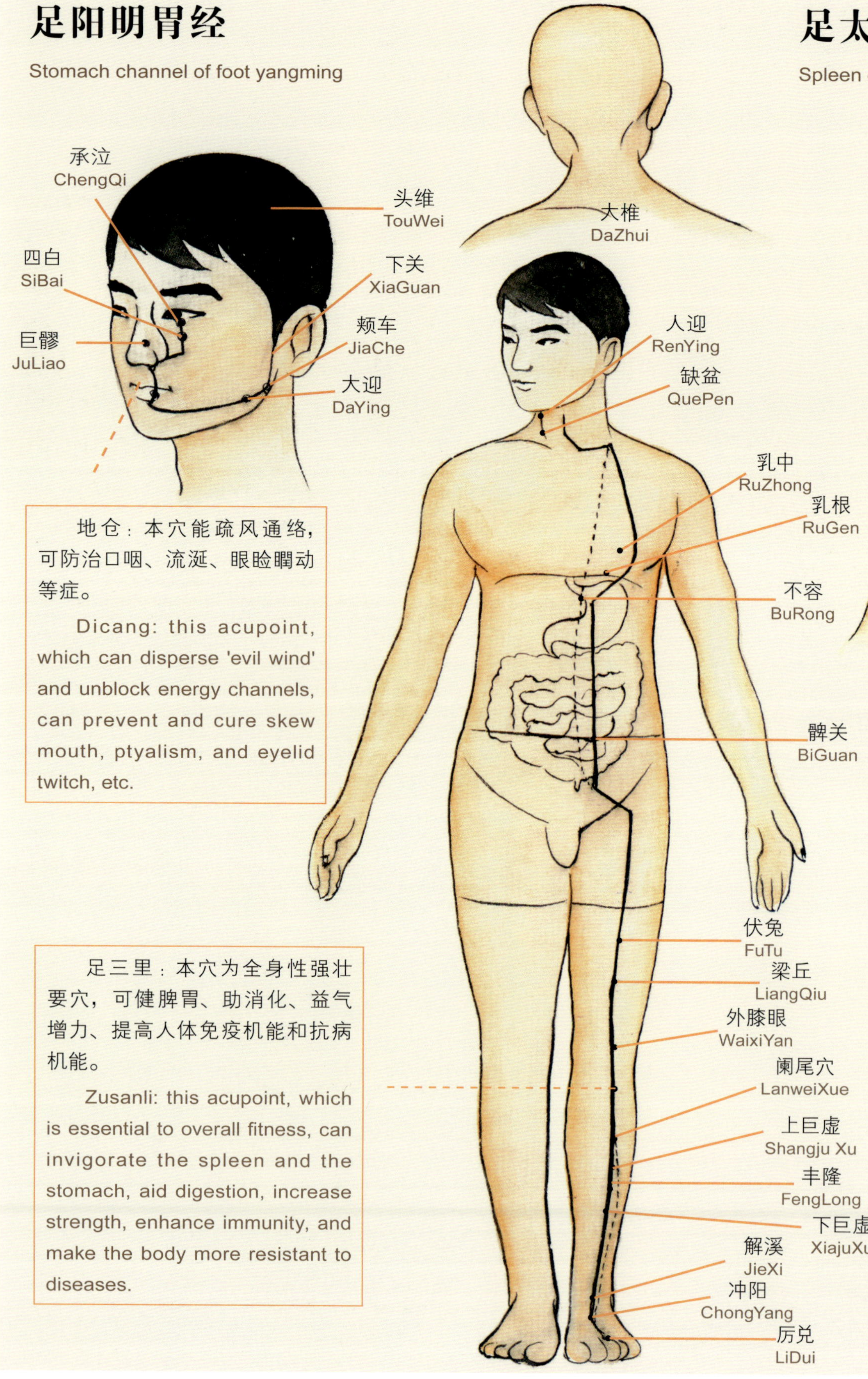

地仓：本穴能疏风通络，可防治口咽、流涎、眼睑瞤动等症。

Dicang: this acupoint, which can disperse 'evil wind' and unblock energy channels, can prevent and cure skew mouth, ptyalism, and eyelid twitch, etc.

足三里：本穴为全身性强壮要穴，可健脾胃、助消化、益气增力、提高人体免疫机能和抗病机能。

Zusanli: this acupoint, which is essential to overall fitness, can invigorate the spleen and the stomach, aid digestion, increase strength, enhance immunity, and make the body more resistant to diseases.

足太阴脾经

Spleen channel of foot taiyin

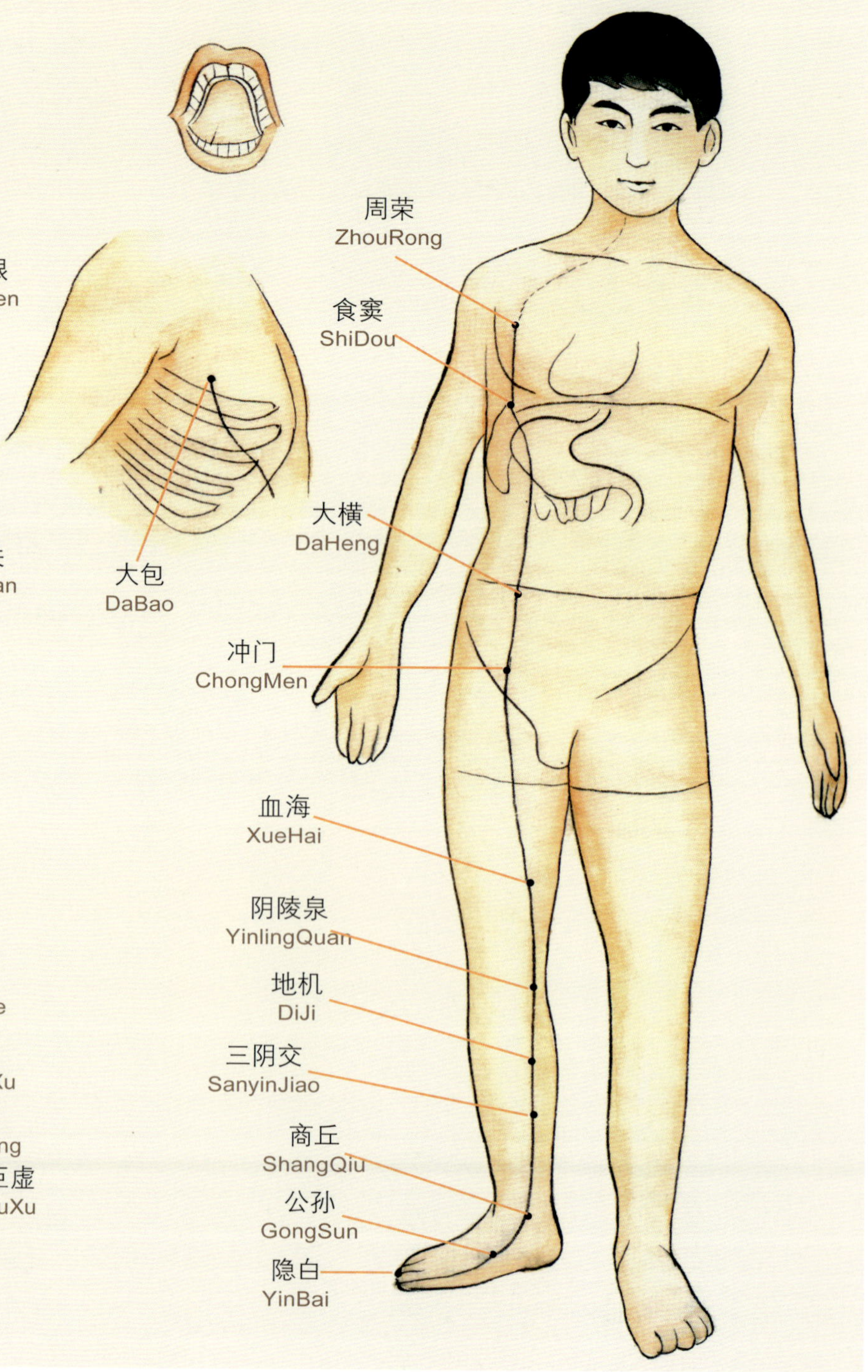

手少阴心经

Heat channel of hand shaoyin

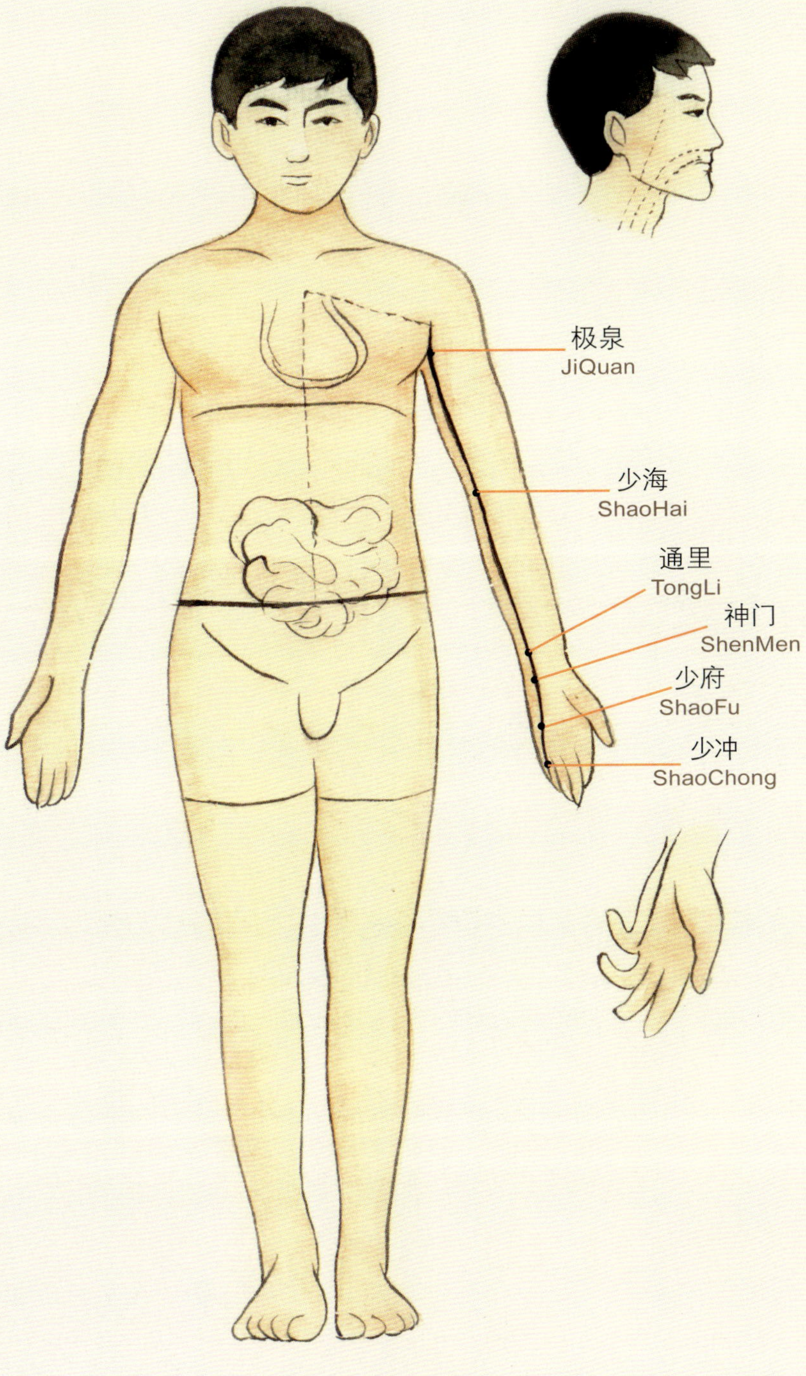

手太阳小肠经

Small intestine channel of hand taiyang

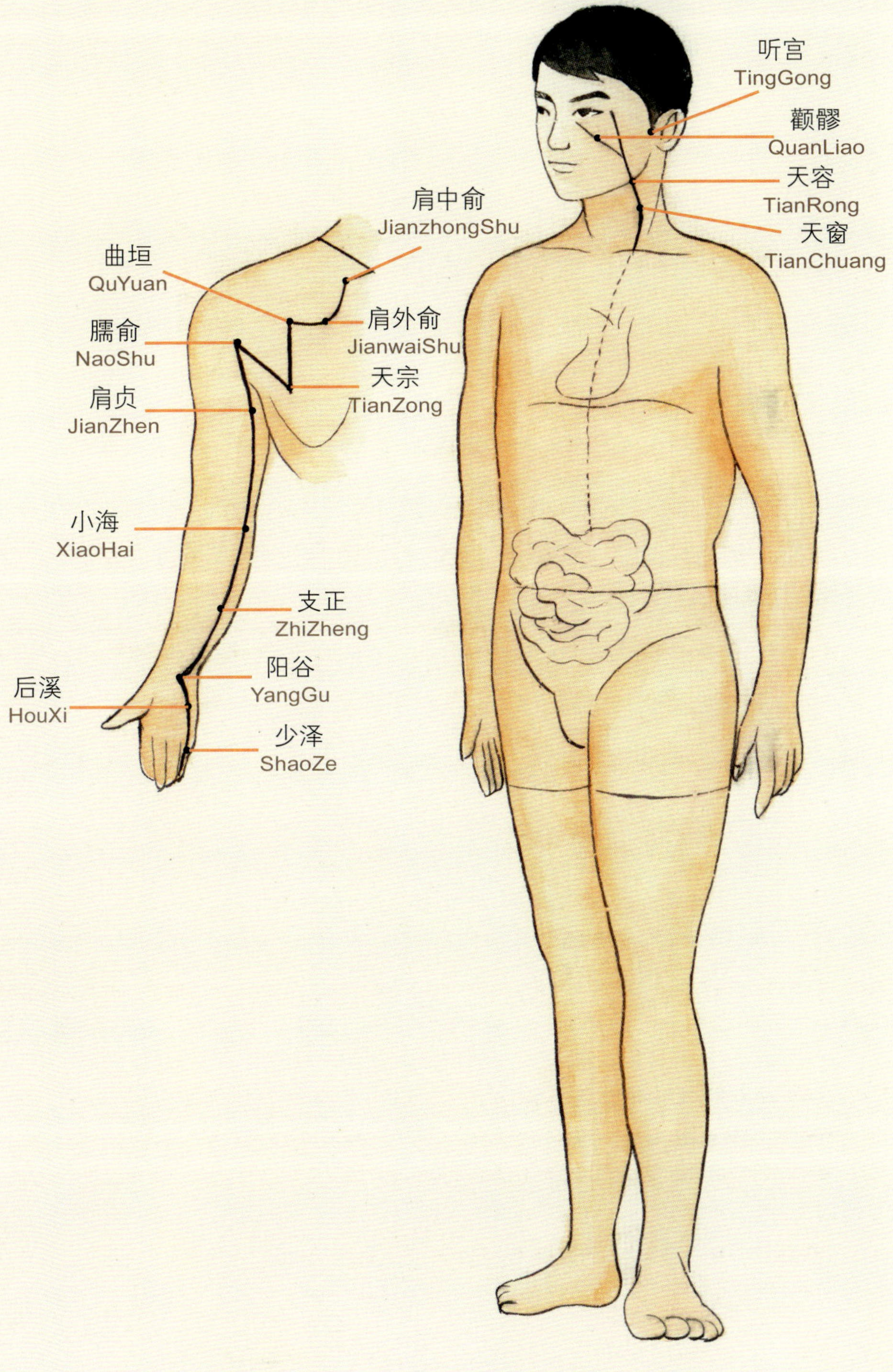

手厥阴心包经

Pericardium channel of hand jueyin

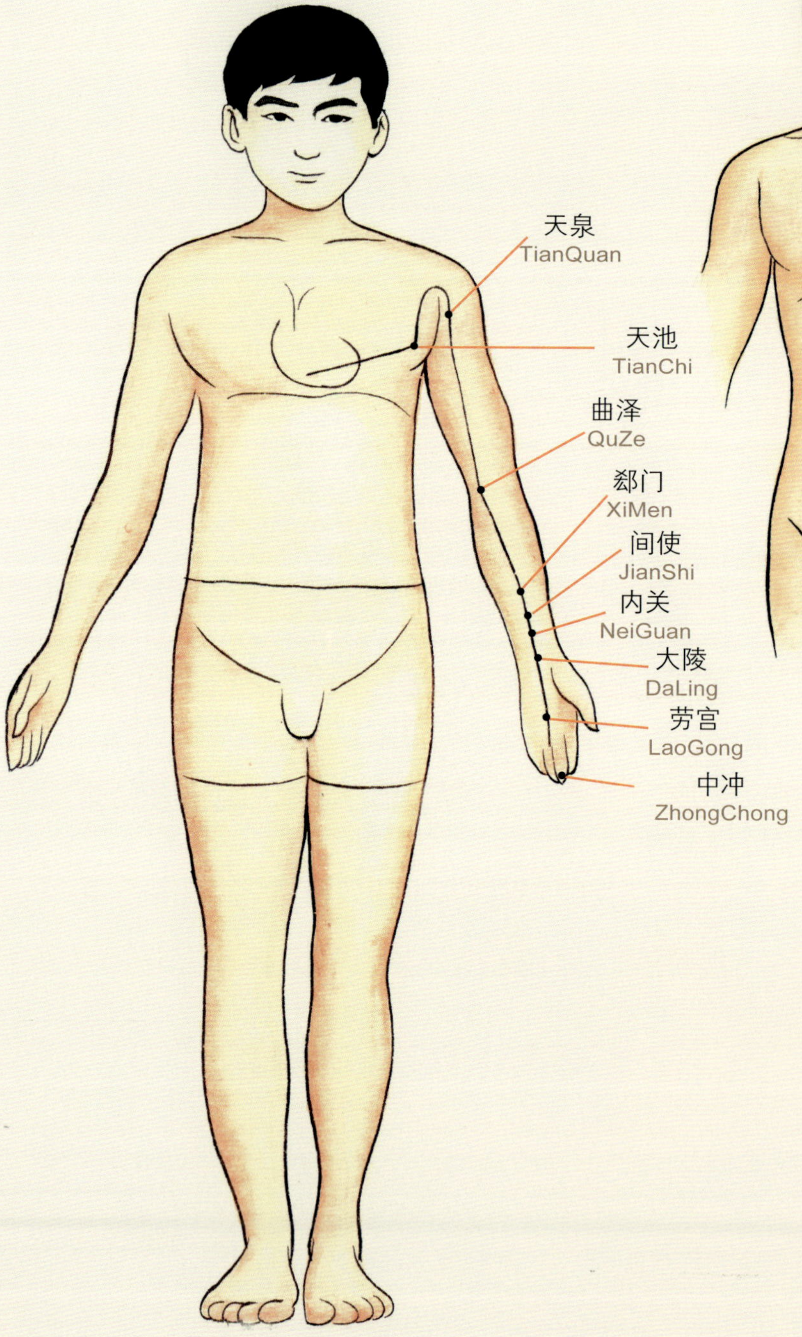

足太阳膀胱经

Urinary bladder channel of foot taiyang

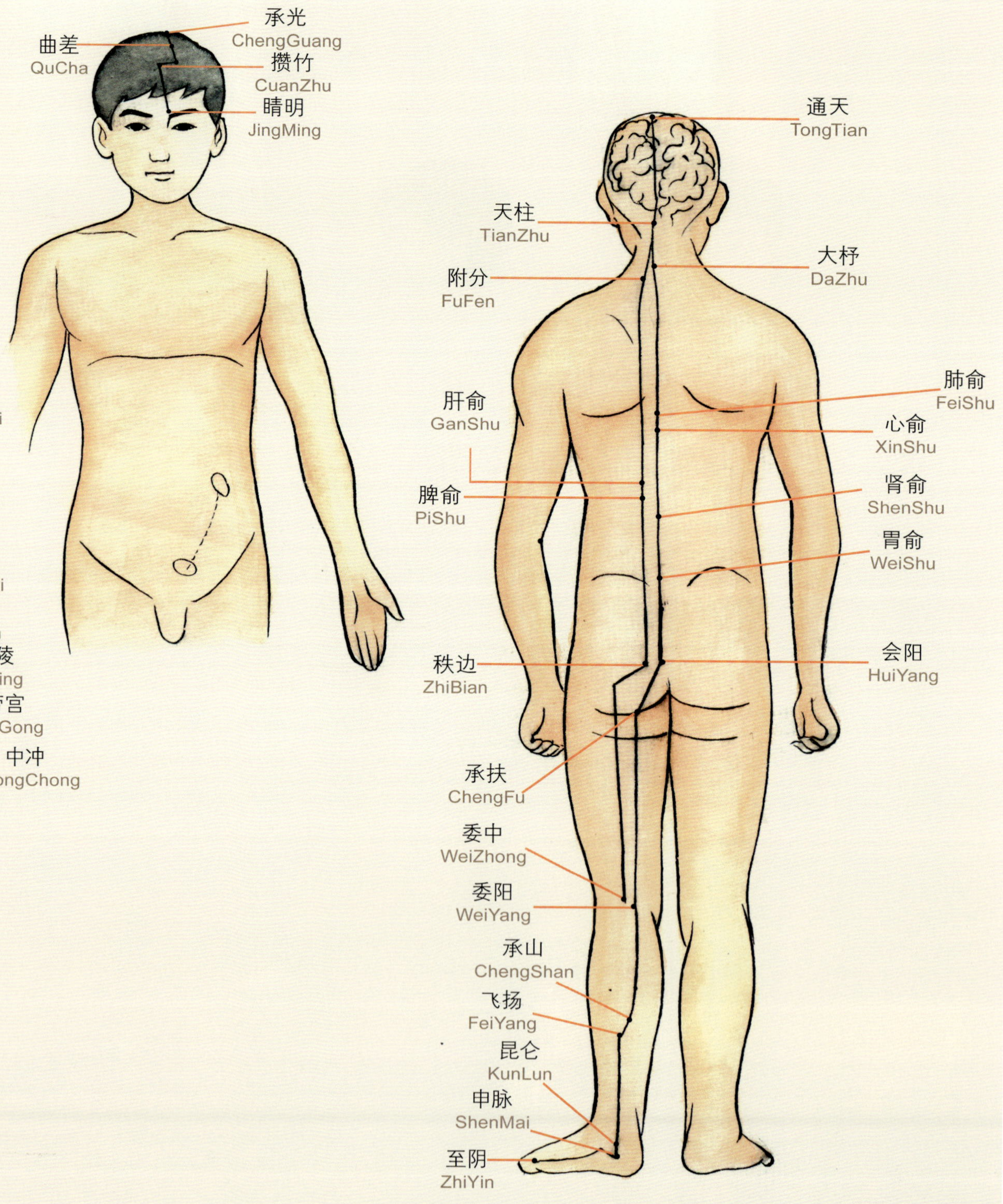

足少阴肾经

Kidney channel of foot shaoyin

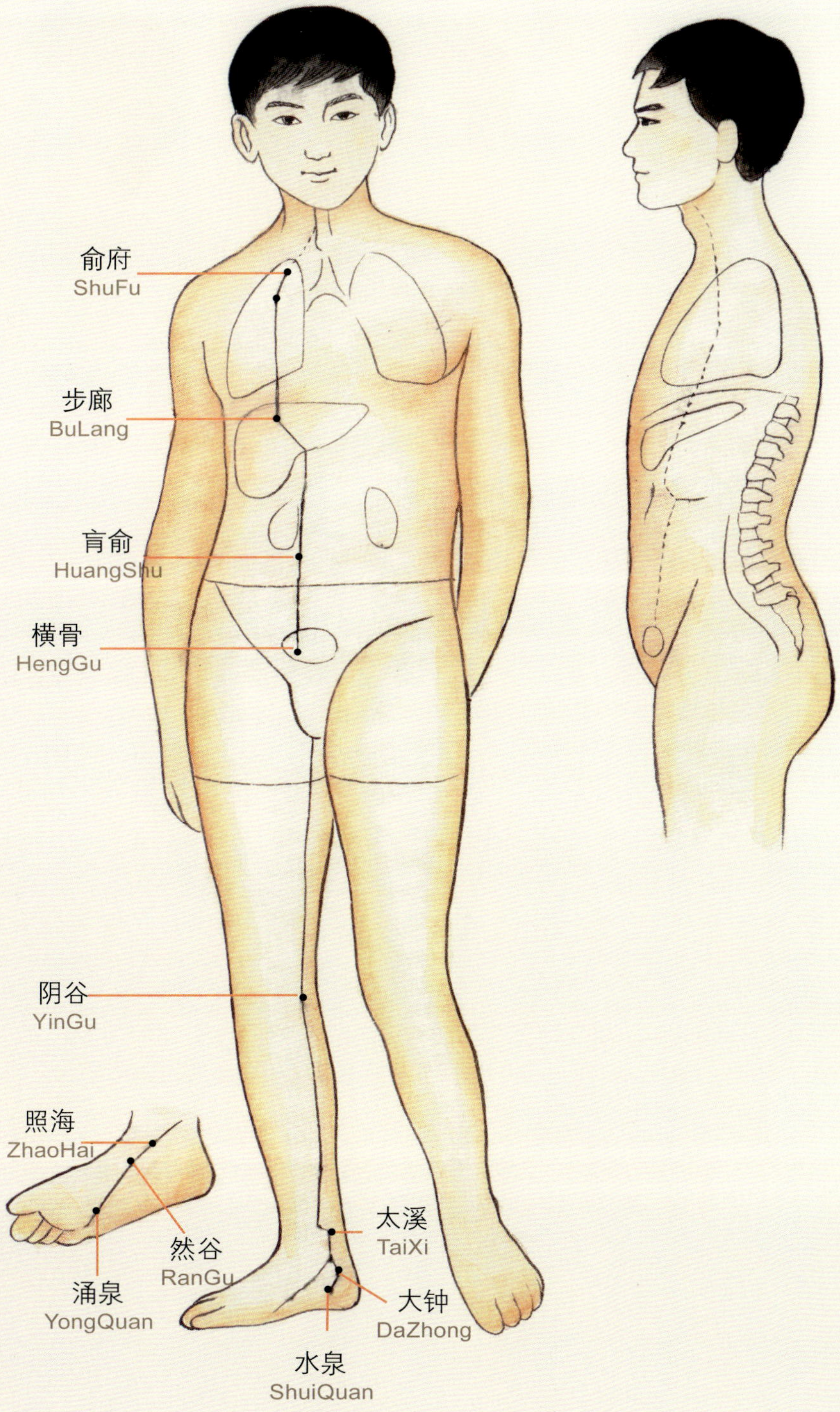

手少阳三焦经

Tri-jiao channel of hand shaoyang

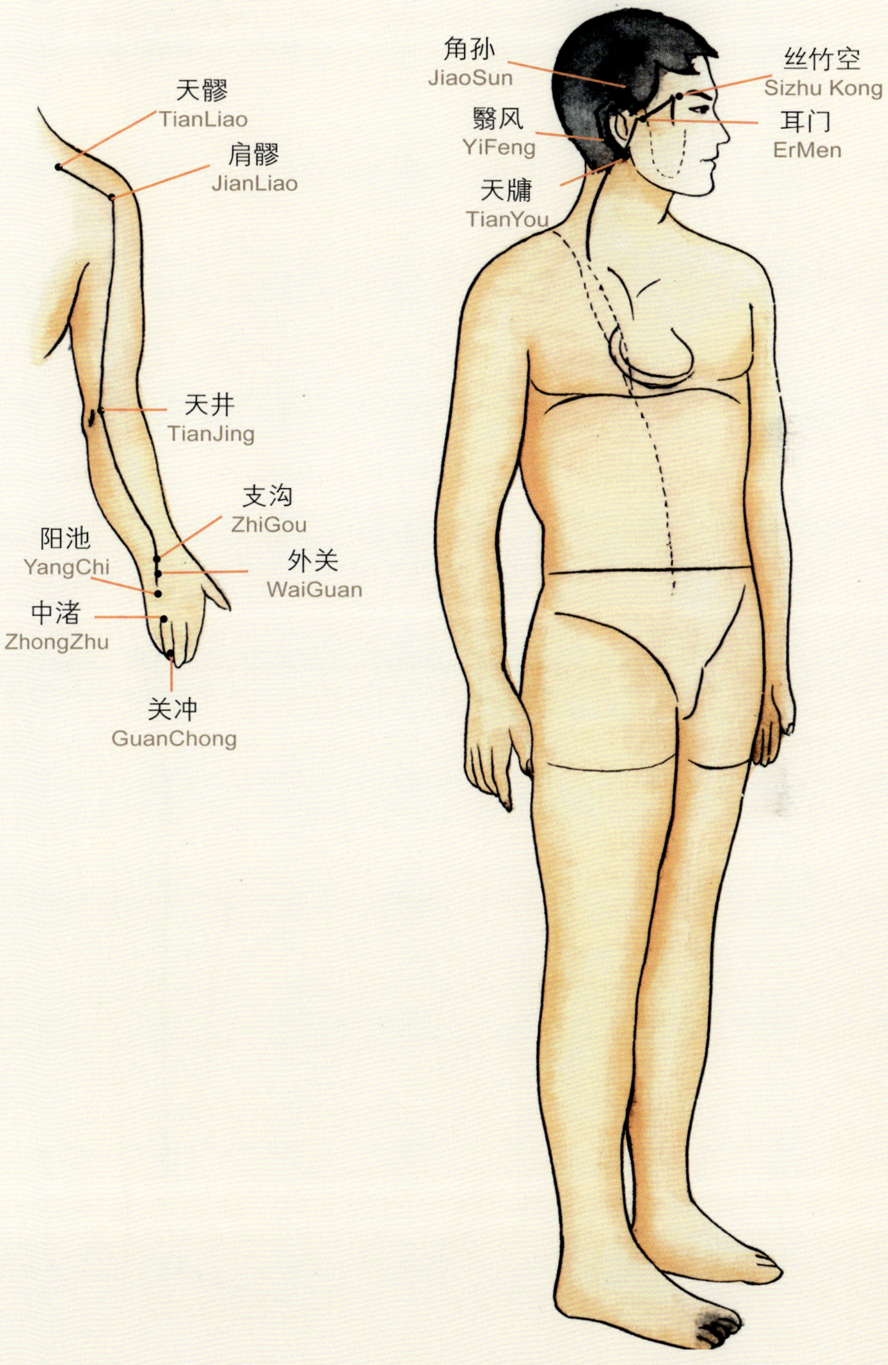

足少阳胆经

Gall bladder channel of foot shaoyang

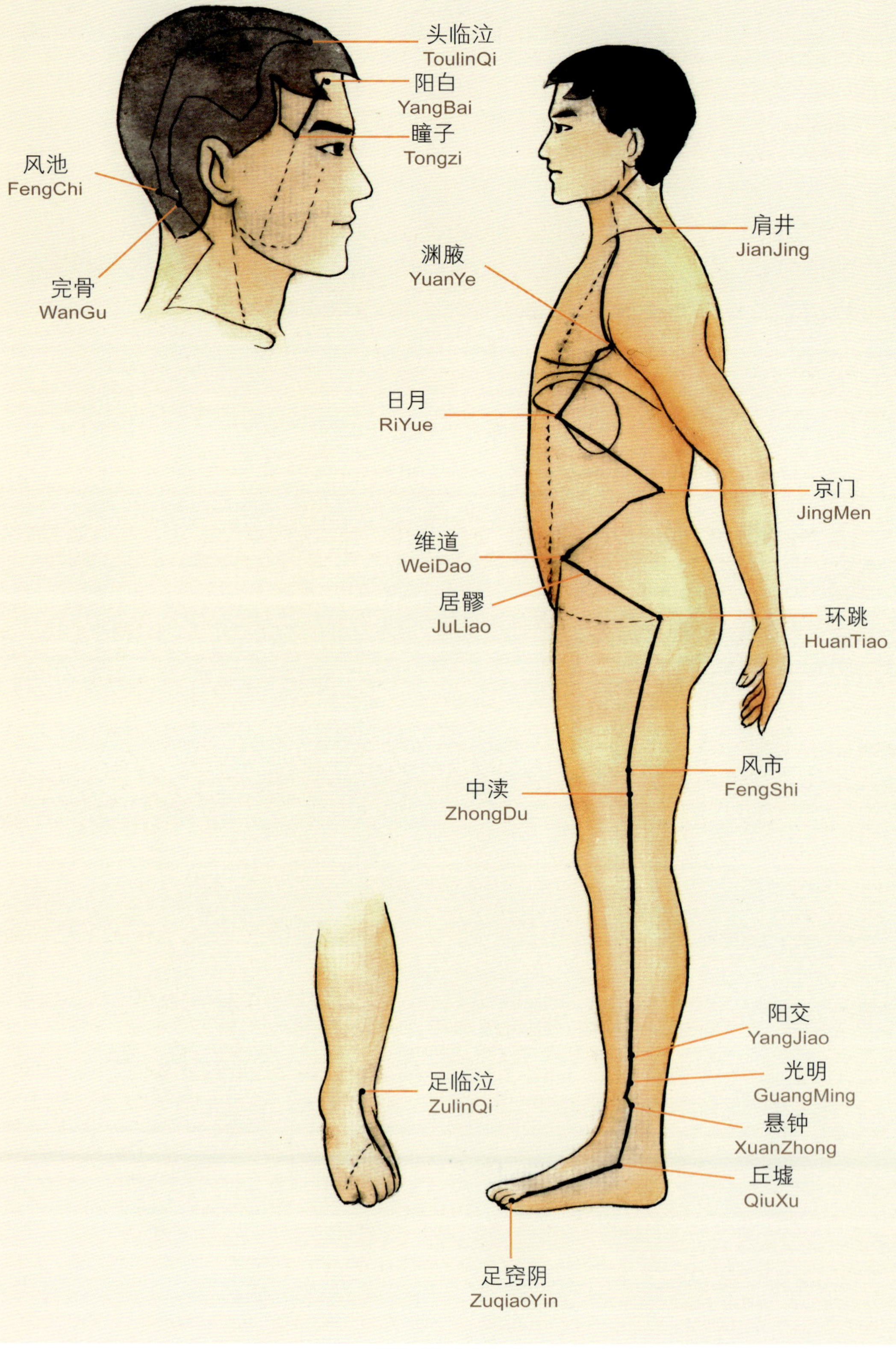

足厥阴肝经

Liver channel of foot jueyin

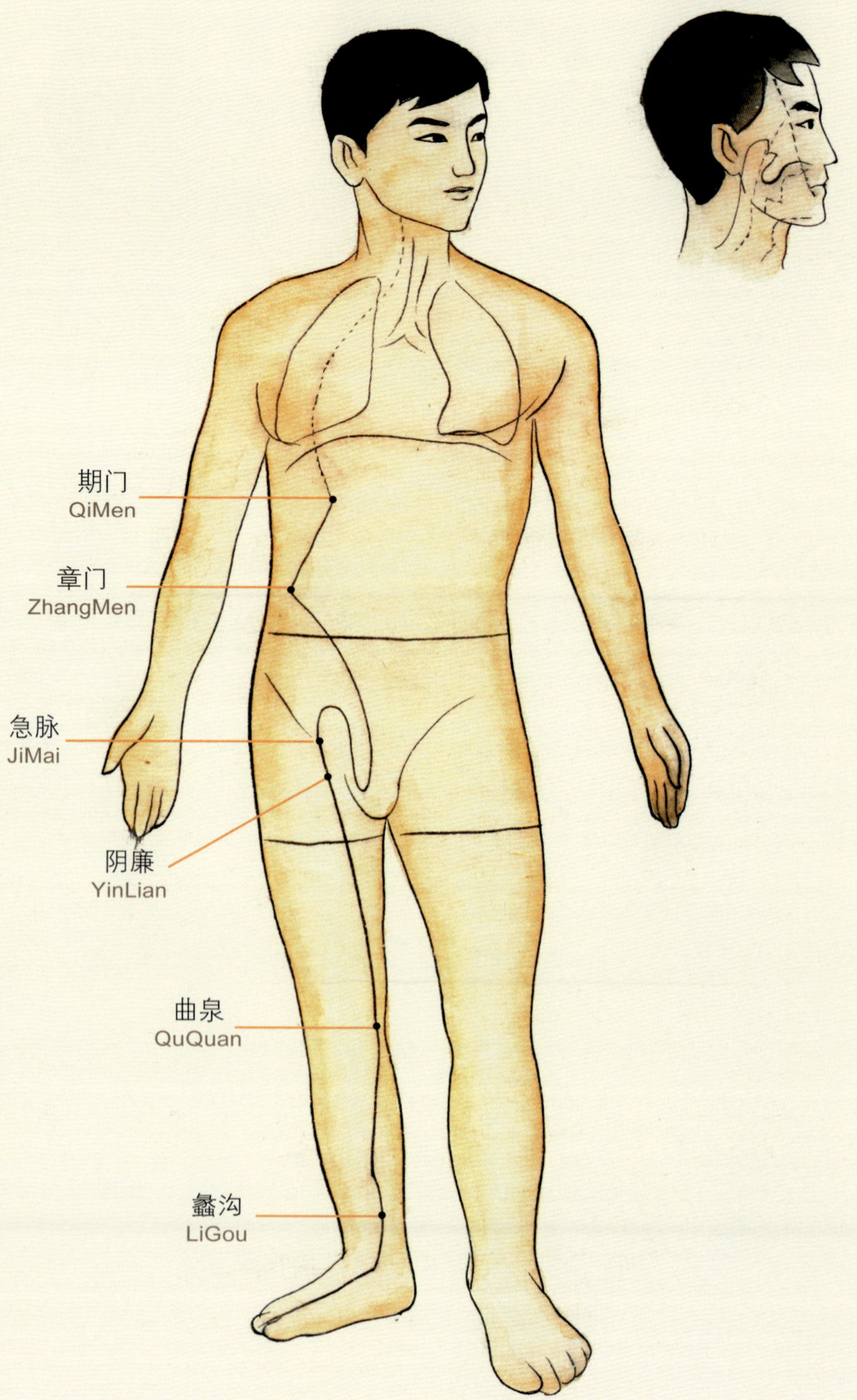

奇经八脉

Eight extra channels

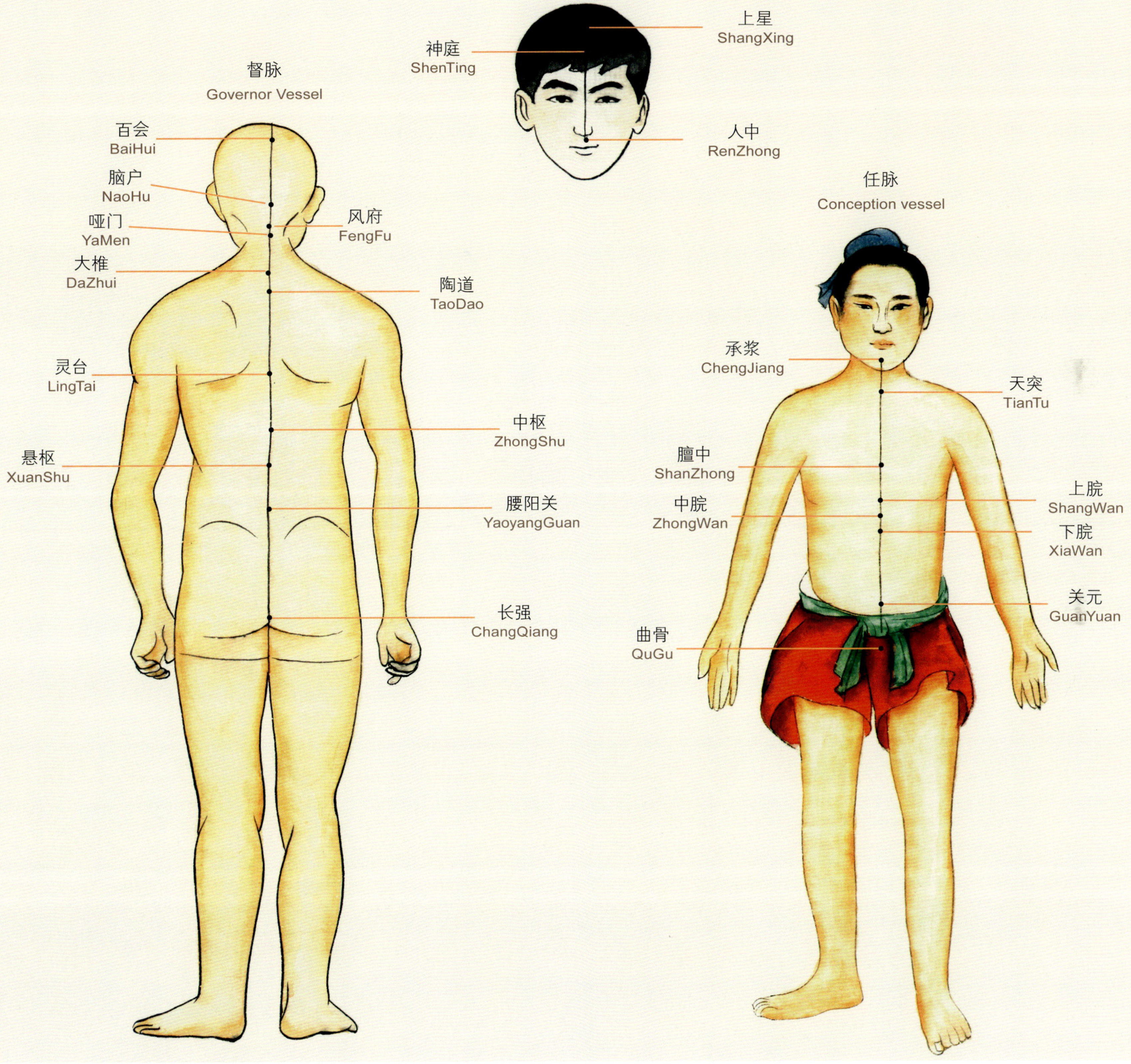

四时之脉

Pulse in the four seasons

切脉诊断法是中医望、闻、问、切四诊之一，是中国医学独有的一种诊断方法，十分神奇。其实脉象是人体信息的反映，《黄帝内经》提出自然阴阳之气随着四时而上下，人的脉象与之相应，呈现春夏秋冬的浮沉变化，可据脉象与四季相应与否来判断疾病。

Pulse palpation is one of the four diagnostic methods in Traditional Chinese Medicine, the rest three being inspection, auscultation & olfaction, and interrogation. The pulse does reveal the patient's physical conditions. The *Inner Canon of the Yellow Emperor* says that yin and yang energy in nature ebb and rise in the four seasons and that the pulse changes accordingly. Thus the correspondence between the pulse and the four seasons may be the basis for diagnosing the patient.

春弦
Stringy pulse in spring

春天阳气初升，万物开始生长，树木正待抽条，因此脉气柔软而直长，状如琴弦，故《黄帝内经》称之为弦脉。

In spring, yang energy is on the rise. Everything begins to grow. Trees are sprouting. Therefore, as reflected through pulse palpation, the pulse feels "soft, straight and long", resembling a qin string (qin is a traditional Chinese musical instrument). Hence, the *Inner Canon* refers to this type of pulse as "stringy pulse".

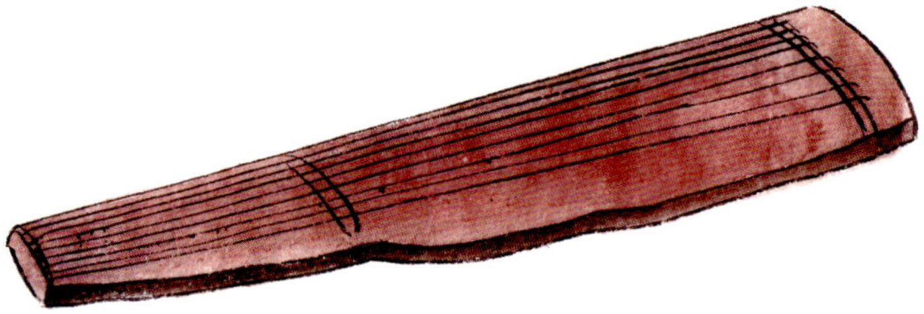

夏钩
Hook-like pulse in summer

夏天阳热之气亢盛，树木茂盛，垂枝布叶，条枝都向下弯曲好像钩子一样，故脉气来时应略快有力，去时略慢无力，《黄帝内经》称之为钩脉。

In summer, yang energy is at it peak. Trees flourish and show bent branches laden with leaves. Correspondingly, the "inner energy in the channel" (maiqi) comes fast and strong, but goes slow and weak, as manifested by the pulse. The *Inner Cannon* refers to this type of pulse as "hook-like pulse".

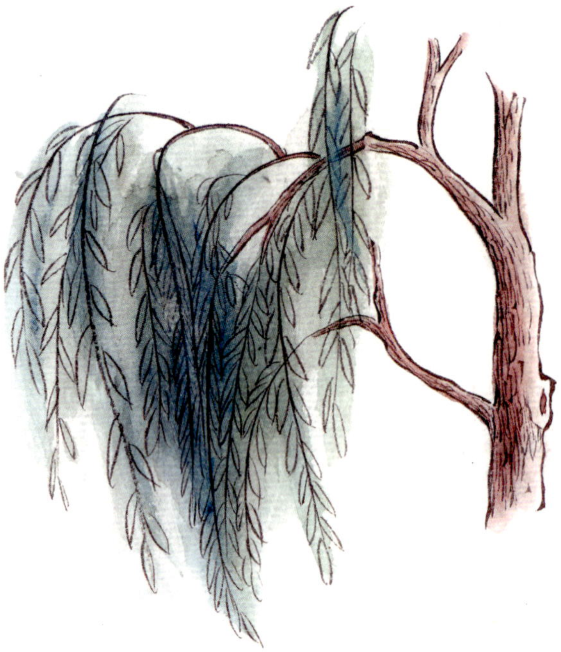

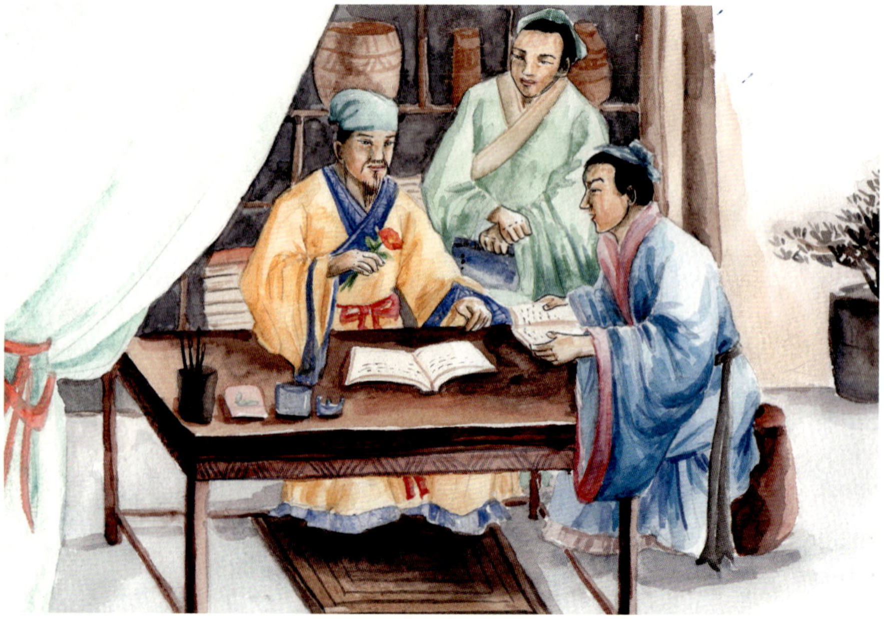

秋毛

'Hair-like' pulse in autumn

秋天阳气乍衰，万物生长至极，到了将要收成的时候，草木花叶，一般都将枯萎脱落，只有枝条还单独存在，好像人体的毫毛一样，所以脉气来时，显得轻虚带有浮象，故《黄帝内经》称之为毛脉。

In autumn, yang energy is on the decline. Flowers and leaves wither and drop off, and only branches, like hair on the human body, remain. Hence, the pulse feels feeble; though palpable by light touch, it grows faint on hard pressure. The *Inner Cannon* refers to this type of pulse as "hook-like pulse".

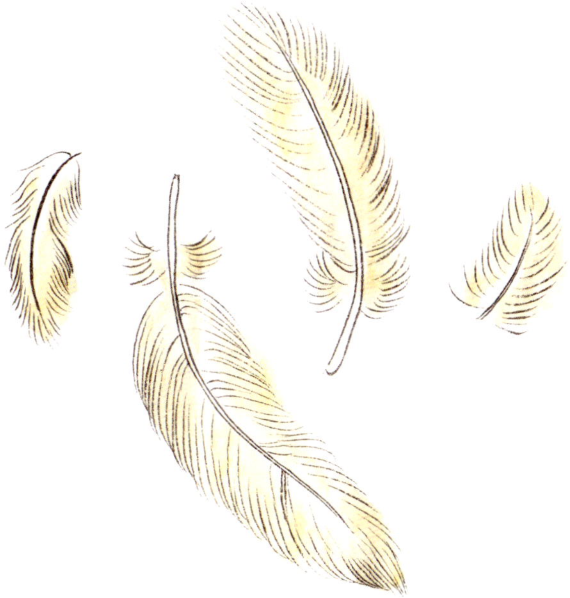

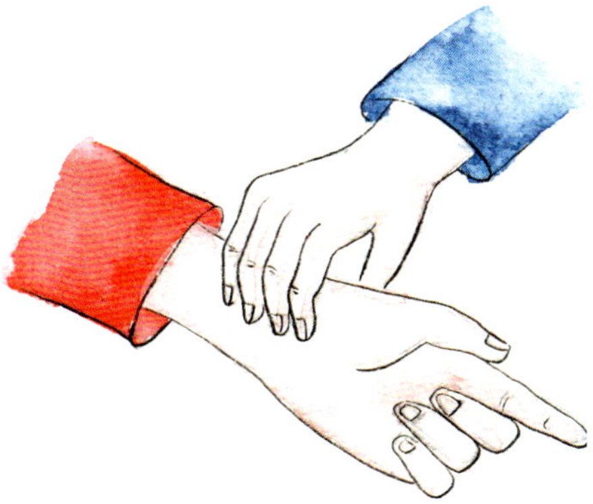

切脉是中国独创的诊断方法，近代以来西医习惯用听诊器看病，而两千多年以来，中医则用切脉法看病，即用手指按脉，根据脉象来诊断疾病。

Pulse palpation is a diagnostic method invented by the Han Chinese. It was in modern times that Western doctors developed the common practice of using the stethoscope; but Chinese doctors have been diagnosing their patients by palpating the pulse with fingers for over 2,000 years.

冬石

'Stone-like pulse' in winter

冬天阳气收敛，万物潜藏，好比水凝结成冰，如石块一样，故脉气沉伏，但应指有力，《黄帝内经》称之为石脉。

In winter, yang energy is at its lowest point. Everything is in recess. For example, water transforms into ice like stone. Correspondingly, the pulse is somewhat sinking and slippery or hard; and it grows vigorously on hard pressure. The *Inner Cannon* refers to this type of pulse as "stone-like pulse".

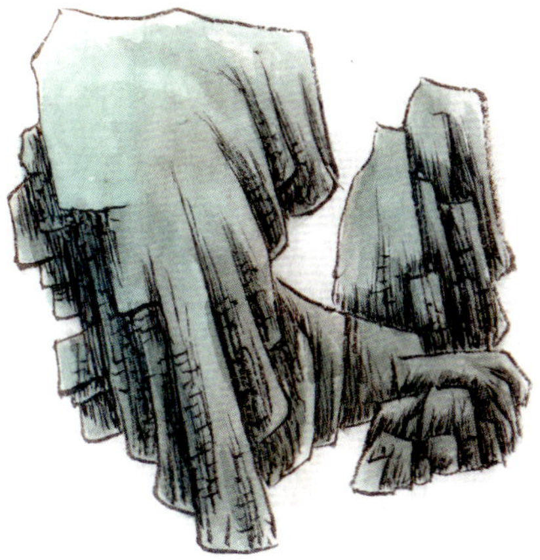

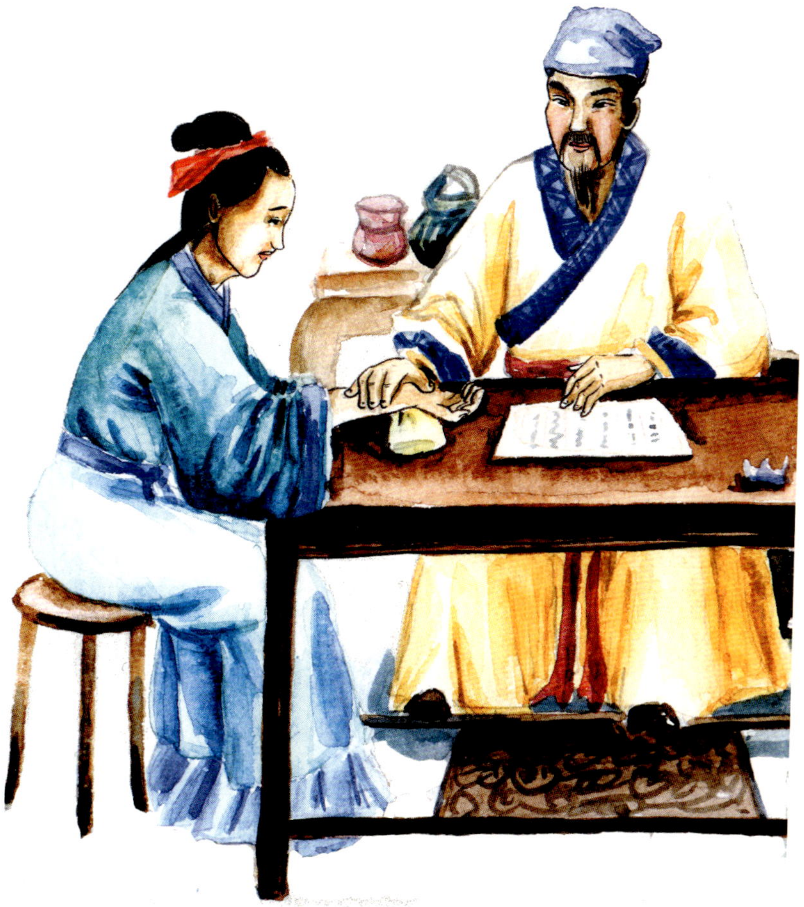

医易同源

Traditional Chinese Medicine and *Book of Changes* sharing the same origin

《易经》是阐述万物运动变化规律的具有预测学智慧的典籍，蕴涵了大量关于日常养生的理论方法，是中医养生理论的基础之一。

《易传·说卦》言“乾为首，坤为腹，震为足，巽为股，坎为身，离为目，艮为手，兑为口”，说明《易经》已把人体脏腑器官融入易学体系。孙思邈说：“不知《易》，不足以言知医。”

《易传·系辞》说“一阴一阳之谓道”。中医承袭《易经》阴阳的理论，建立了人体的阴阳学说。《易经》和中医养生学包含的武术、导引、气功等健身术密切相关，以“法于阴阳，和于术数”作为养生保健的根本方法。总之，医易是同源同理的。

Book of Changes is an ancient classic full of wisdom of predictions about the future. It studies the law of motion of everything and contains lots of theories and methods on the daily regimen, and is one of the foundations of regimen theory of Chinese traditional medicine.

Yi Zhuan: Explanation of the Sixty-Four Hexagrams points out that “the sign of Qian corresponds to the head, the sign of Kun, the belly, the sign of Zhen, the feet, the sign of Xun, the thighs, the sign of Kan, the body, the sign of Li, the eyes, the sign of Gen, the head and the sign of Dui, the mouth”, which shows that *Book of Changes* has blended human organs into Yi-ology system. Sun Simiao once said that “whoever does not know *Book of Changes* cannot say that he knows medicine.”

Notes to the Book of Changes says that Tao means the combination of yin and yang. Chinese traditional medicine inherited yin and yang theory of *Book of Changes*, and created the *yin* and *yang* concept of hidden state of the body. Based on the *Book of Changes*, the regimen theory of Chinese traditional medicine also developed a series of fitness technique, such as martial arts, physical guidance and Qigong, which follows the “law of the yin and yang, and harmonizes the art and number” as the means of regimen. In short, Chinese traditional medicine and *Book of Changes* derive from the same origin.

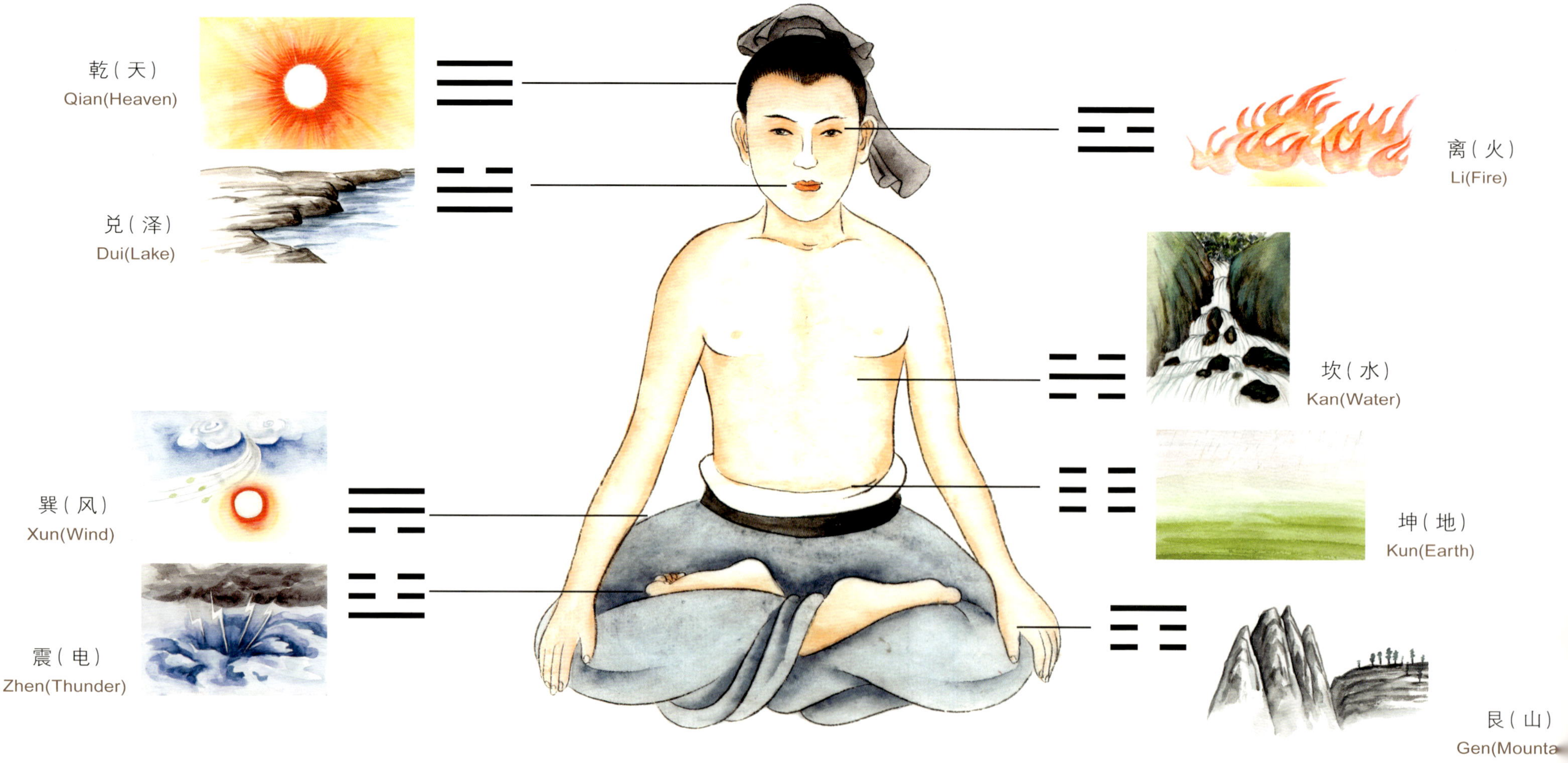

医道与生生不息的“易理”同源

Traditional Chinese Medicine shares the same origin with the *Book of Changes*, which has an everlasting influence.

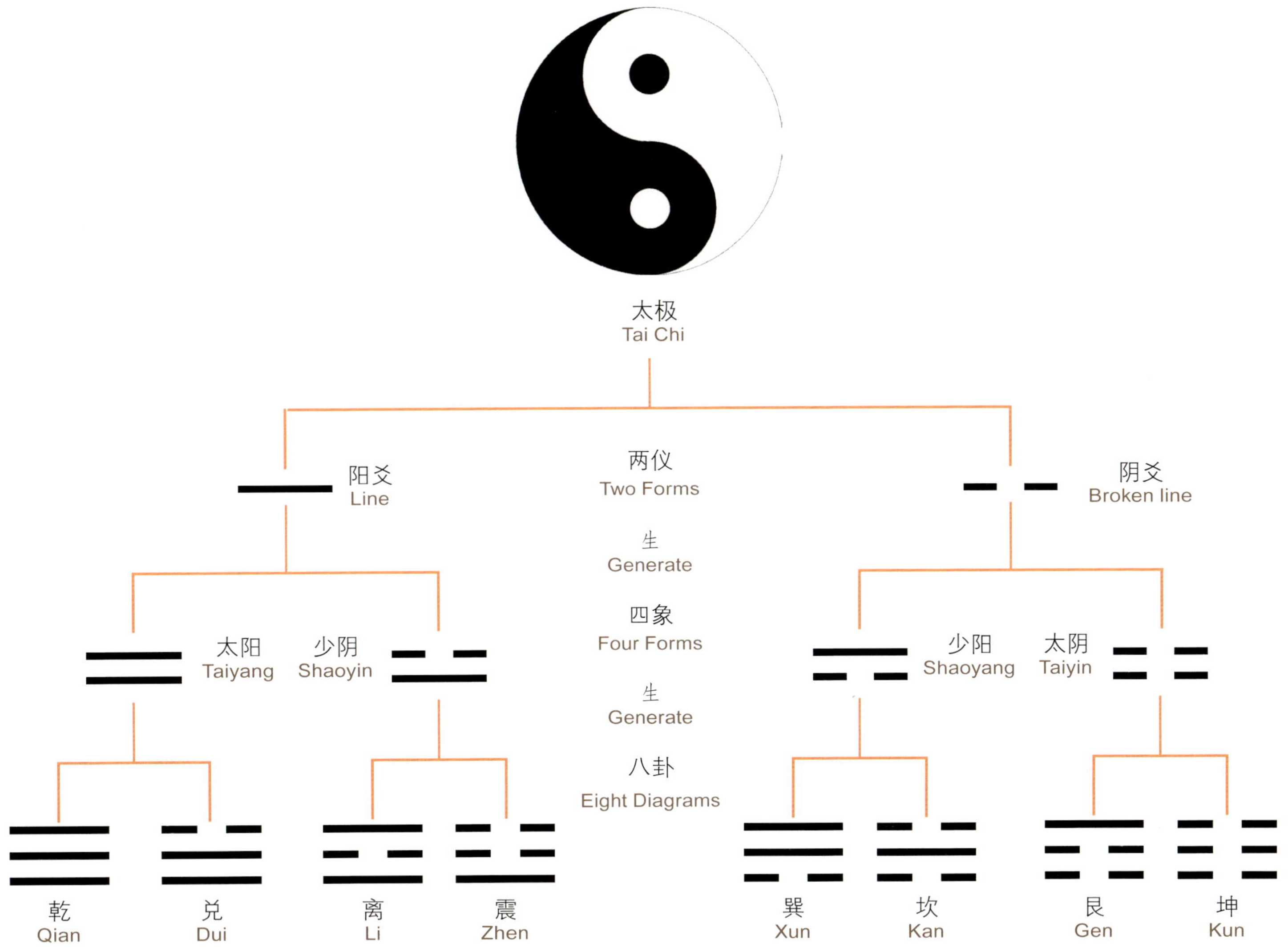

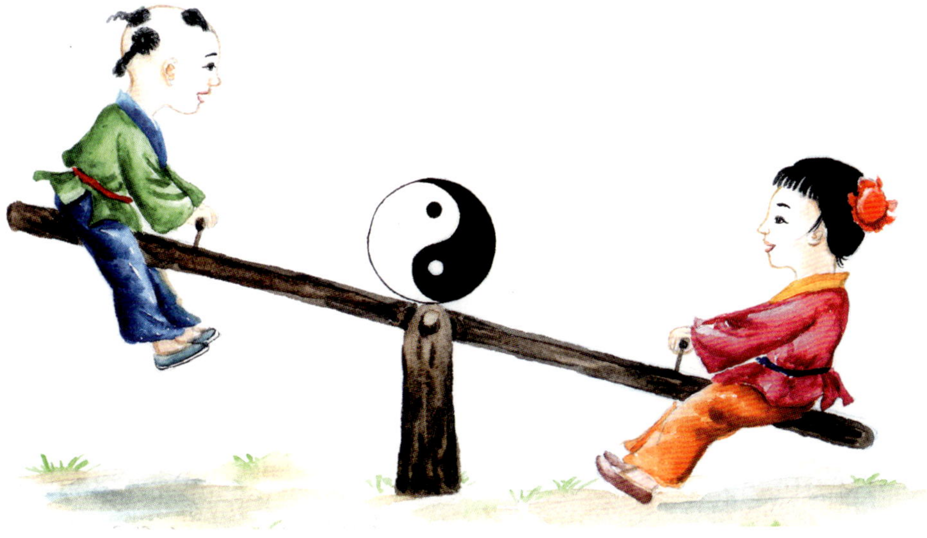

阴阳、五行学说

Theories of yin, yang and the five elements

阴阳的概念最初是非常朴素的，仅是指阳光的向背，后来逐渐引申出若干相对的概念。如：天为阳，地为阴；日为阳，月为阴；昼为阳，夜为阴；火为阳，水为阴；男为阳，女为阴。凡是活动的、无形的、向外的、向上的、温热的、明亮的、亢进的都属于阳；凡是沉静的、有形的、向内的、向下的、寒冷的、晦暗的、衰退的都属于阴。

At first, yin and yang simply referred to positions toward and against sunshine, but they gradually came to be associated with a number of opposites. For example, heaven is yang and earth is yin; the sun is yang and the moon is yin; day is yang and night is yin; fire is yang and water is yin; men are yang and women are yin. All that is moving, intangible, outward, upward, warm or hot, bright and progressing is yang; all that is still, tangible, inward, downward, cold, dark and declining is yin.

以天地而言：

In terms of heaven and earth:

阳

Yang

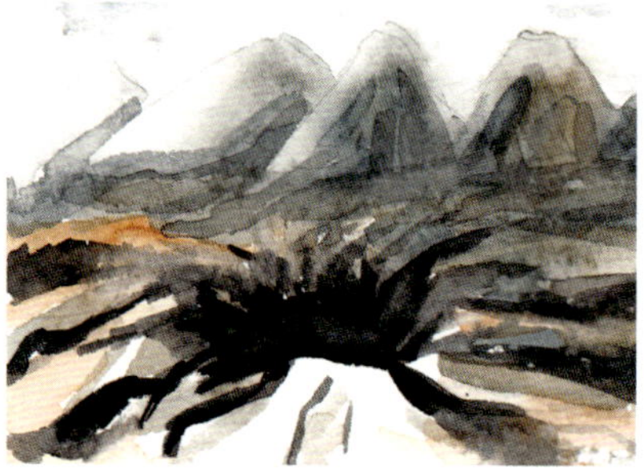

阴

Yin

以寒暑而言：

In terms of cold and heat:

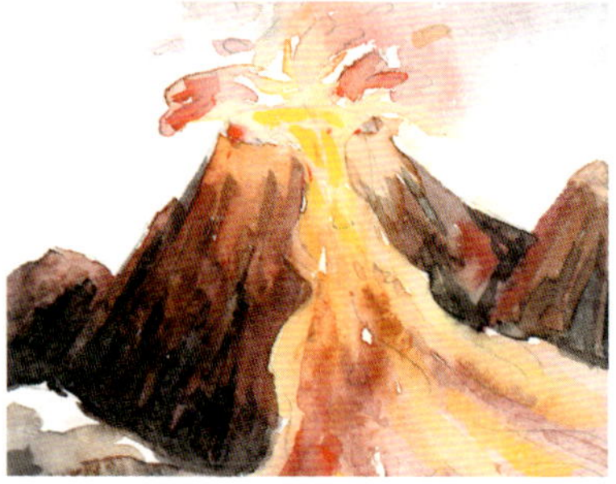

阳

Yang

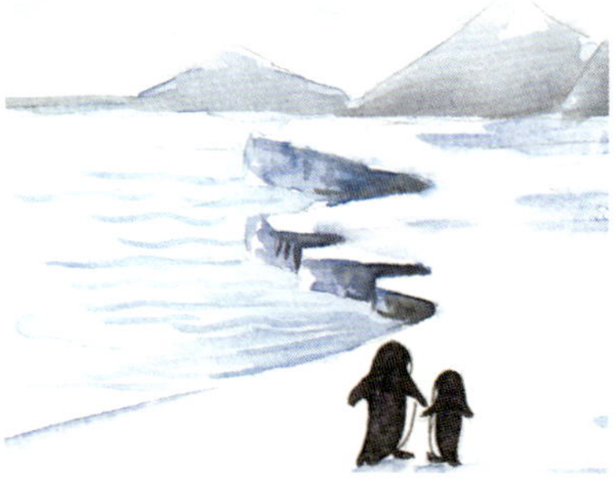

阴

Yin

以昼夜而言：

In terms of day and night:

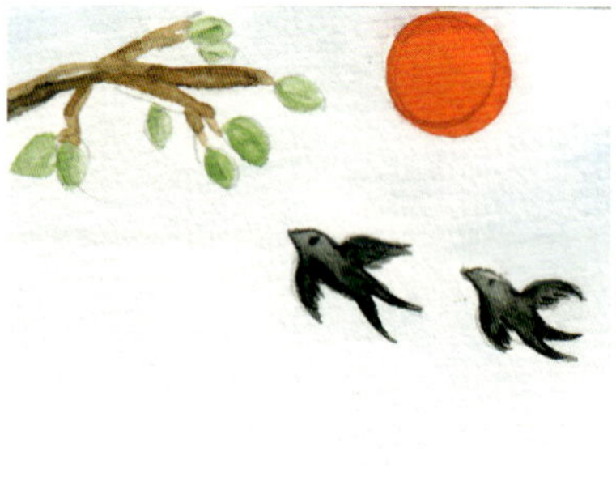

阳

Yang

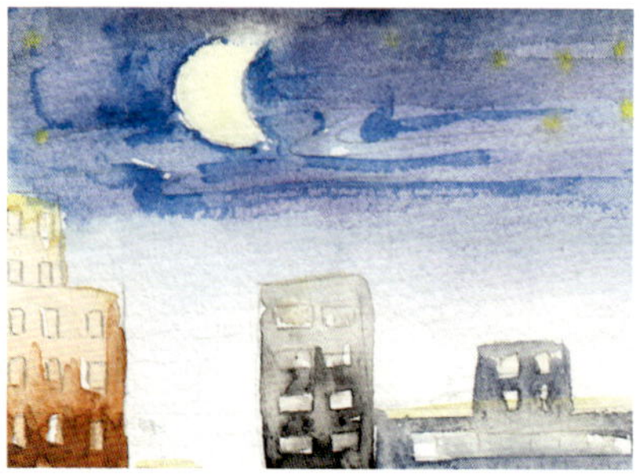

阴

Yin

以水火而言：

In terms of water and fire:

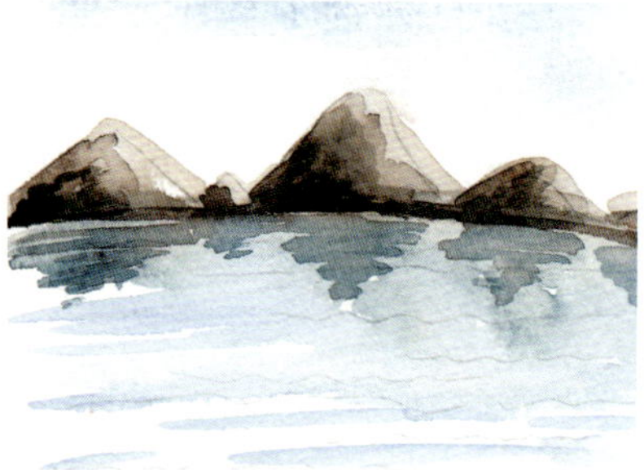

阴

Yin

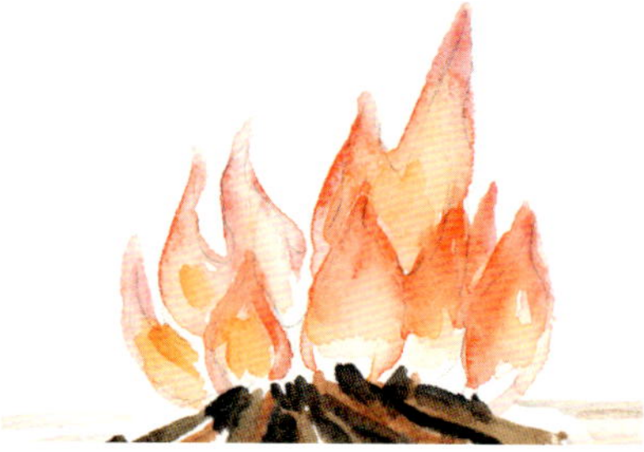

阳

Yang

以内外而言：

In terms of inside and outside:

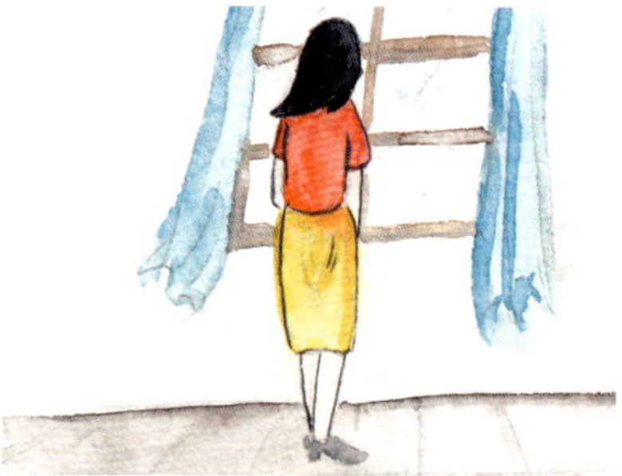

阴

Yin

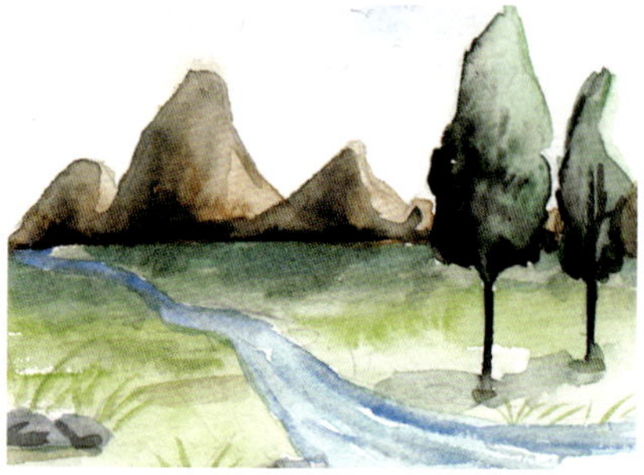

阳

Yang

以功能与物质而言：

In terms of functions and substances:

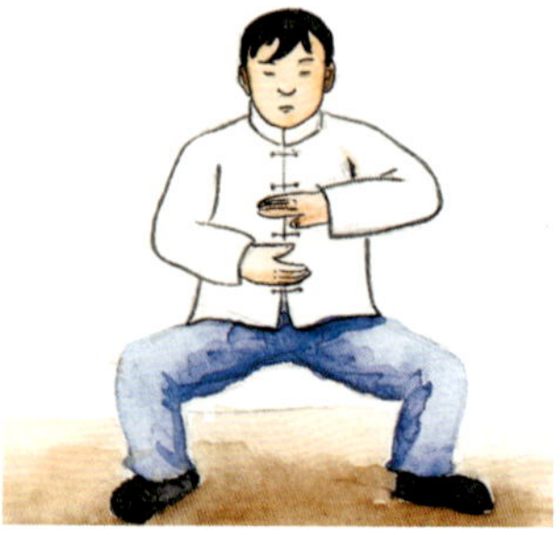

阴

Yin

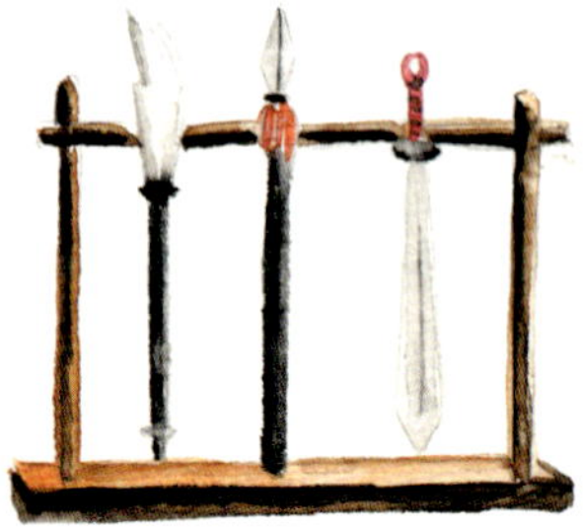

阳

Yang

《尚书·洪范》说："五行：一曰水，二曰火，三曰木，四曰金，五曰土。"《尚书》还指出，木具有生发、条达的特性，火具有炎热、向上的特性，土具有养长、化育的特性，金具有清静、收敛的特性，水具有寒冷、闭藏的特性。

According to the chapter "The Great Plan" in *Book of History*, the Five Elements are water, fire, wood, metal, and earth. Wood is characterized by growth and expansion; fire by heat and rise; earth by nurture and nourishment; metal by quietude and contraction; and water by coldness and concealment.

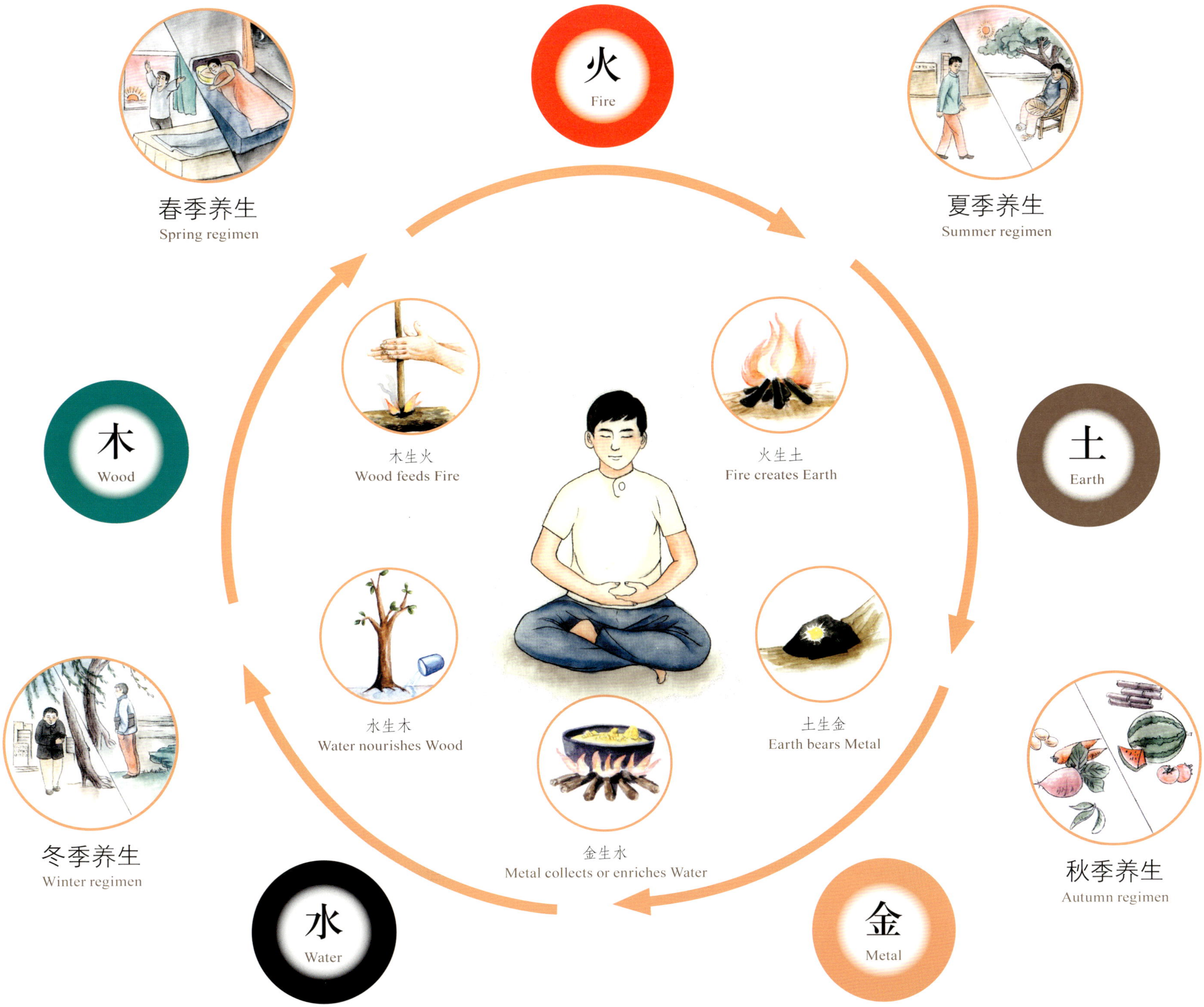

中医五行将人与自然按五种物质的功能属性归为五大类。五行的生克乘侮是五行纲目相互联系运化的法则。生克是事物运化的正常规律。生即相生，指行与行之间的相互生化，生我者为母，我生者为子，这种生化关系又称母子关系，如木生火、火生土、土生金、金生水、水生木。克即相克，指一行对另一行具有克制作用，如木克土、土克水、水克火、火克金、金克木。这种生中有克，克中有生的制化关系，维持着自然的生态平衡和人体的生理平衡。乘，即相克太过被克一行产生失常的表现，相乘的次序同于相克。侮，即相侮，是一种恃强凌弱的逆克现象，如木侮金、金侮火、火侮水、水侮土、土侮木。

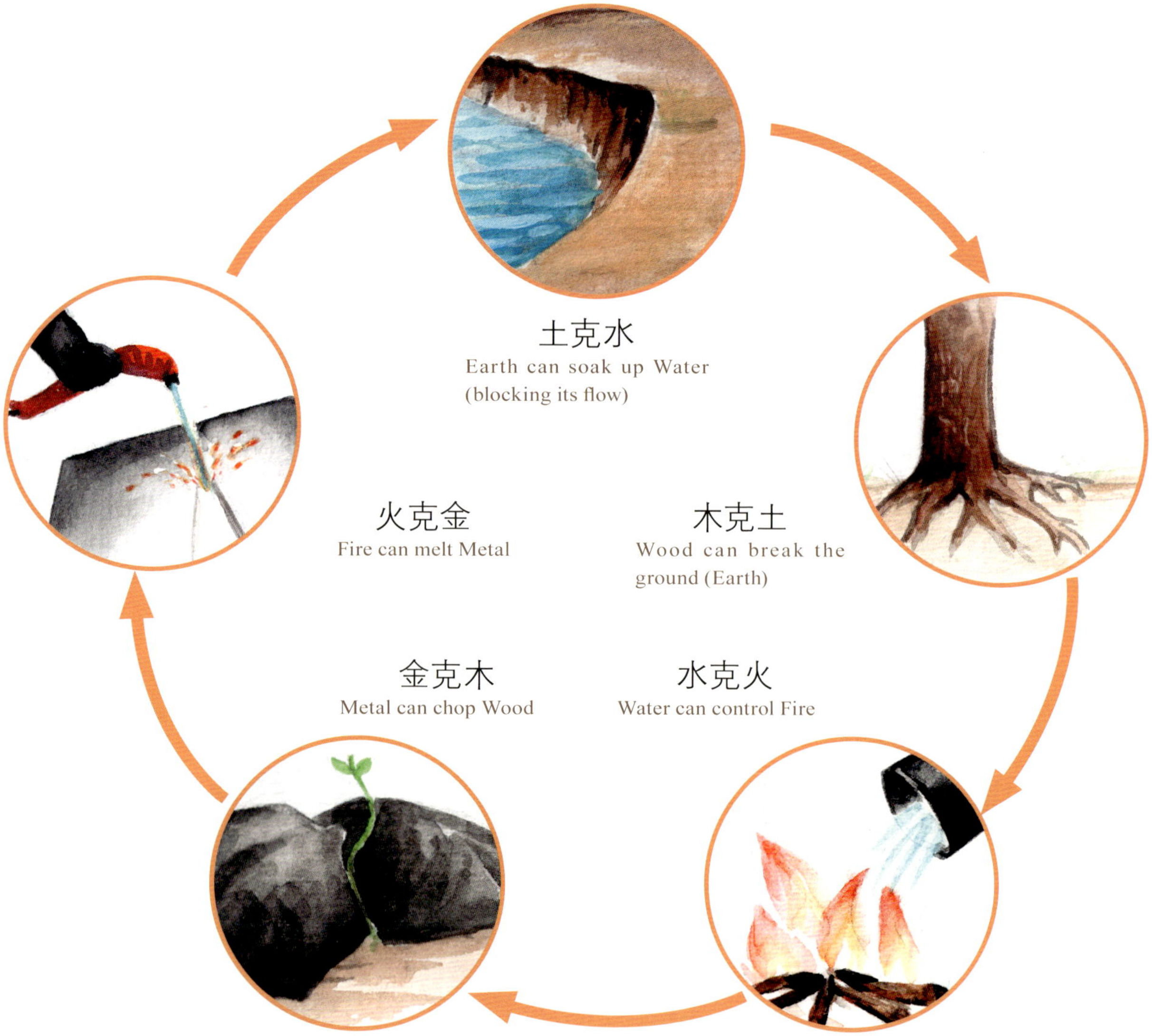

In Chinese traditional medicine, human and nature are divided into five categories according to the functions and properties of the Five Elements. *Sheng* (generating, inter-promoting, or enhancing), *ke* (control, destroying, or inter-restraining), *cheng* (taking advantage) and *wu* (rebellion) are the laws for the interaction of the Five Elements. *Sheng* and *ke* are the regular laws for the change of things, whereas *cheng* and *wu* are those for irregularity. In the sheng cycle, one element can generate, enrich, nourish or strengthen another, like the relationship between mother and child: Wood feeds Fire, Fire creates Earth, Earth bears Metal, Metal collects or enriches Water, and Water nourishes Wood. In the ke cycle, one element can control or restrain another: Wood can break the ground (Earth), Earth can soak up Water (blocking its flow), Water can control Fire, Fire can melt Metal, and Metal can chop Wood. Such coexistence of *sheng* and *ke* maintains ecological and physiological balance. *Cheng* means that a retrained element shows unusual behavior when there is too much restraint. The *cheng* cycle follows the same direction as the *ke* cycle. In the *wu* cycle, an element restrained by another can rebel against the latter: Wood can rebel against Metal, Metal against Fire, Fire against Water, Water against Earth, and Earth against Wood.

青色

肝属青色

Liver belongs to the blue

红色

心属红色

Heart belongs to the red

黄色

脾属黄色

Spleen belongs to the yellow

白色

肺属白色

Lungs belong to the white

黑色

肾属黑色

Kidneys belong to the black

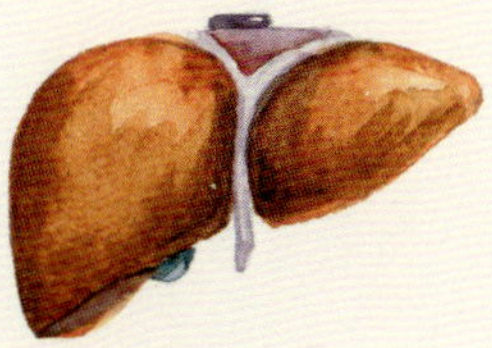

肝脏

Liver

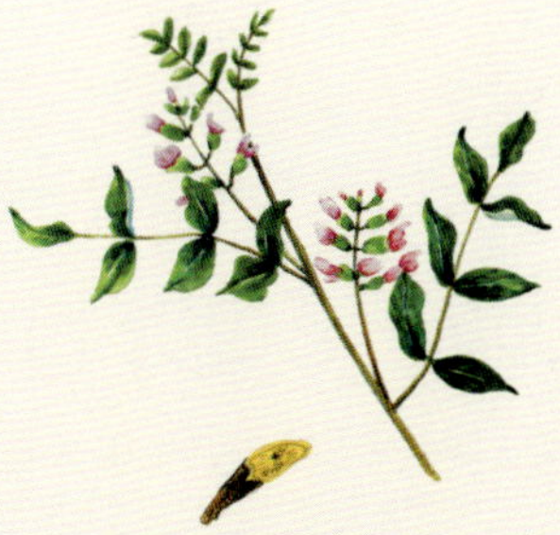

甘草补肝气郁不舒

Licorice can relieve the inhibition of the liver.

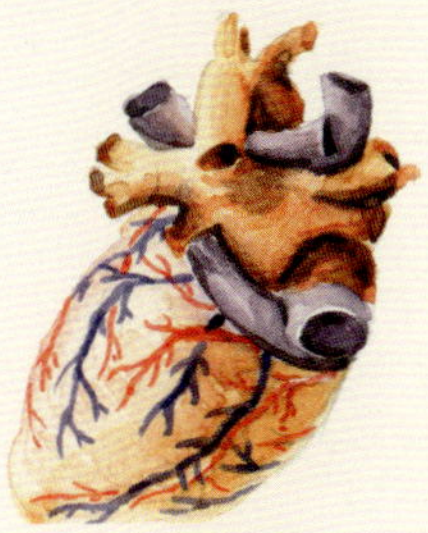

心脏

Heart

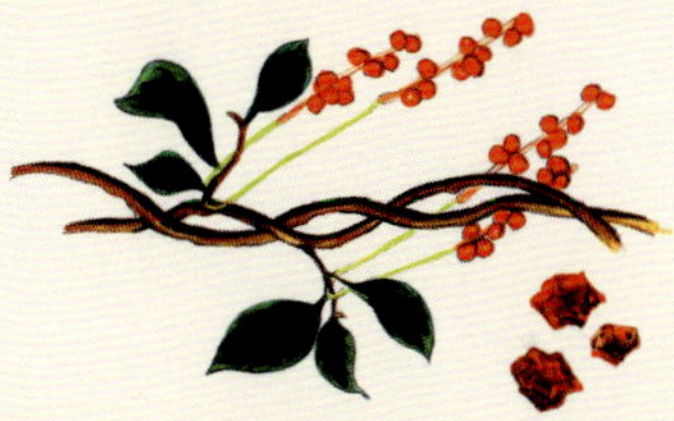

五味子补心脏气血不足

The fruit of Chinese magnolia vine can replenish qi and blood for the heart.

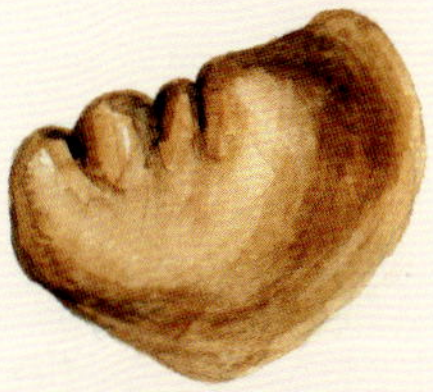

脾脏

Spleen

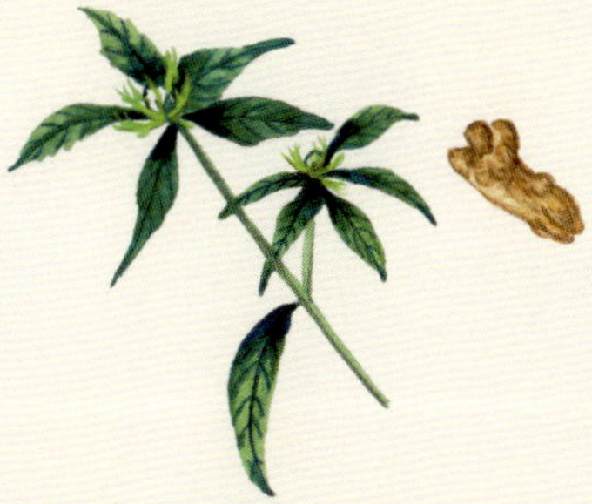

白术补脾湿邪致病

Rhizome of lagehead atractylodes can cure diseases caused by 'damp evil' in the spleen.

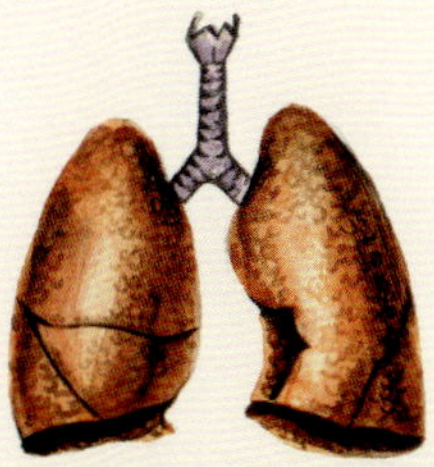

肺脏

Lung

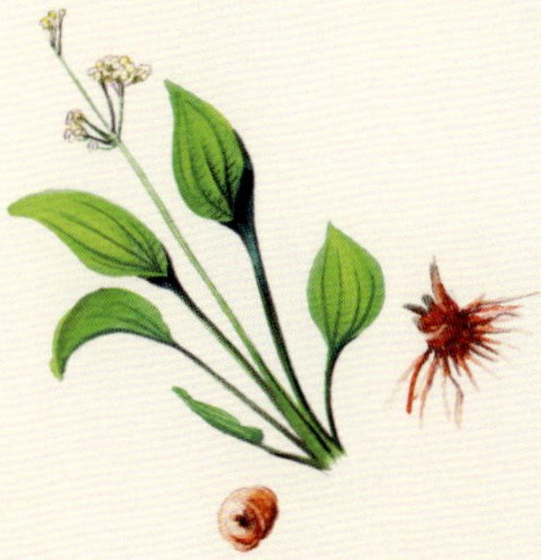

泽泻补肺气上逆

Oriental water plantain can cure the abnormal rise of lung qi.

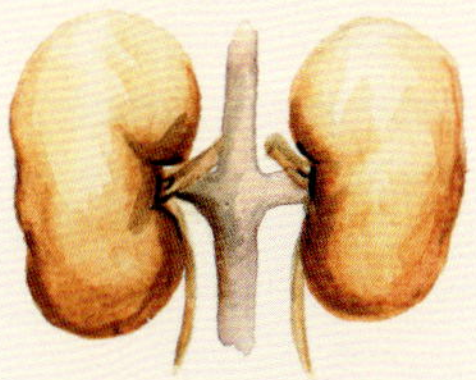

肾脏

Kidney

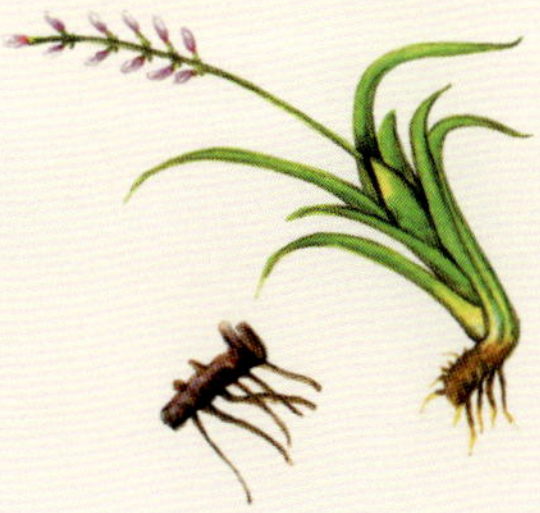

知母补肾阴虚燥

Rhizome of wind-weed can relieve the deficiency and dryness of kidney yin.

一天中的阴阳

Yin and yang of a day

人体阴阳与自然界阴阳的运动变化相通相应

Yin and yang energy in the human body corresponds with the movements of yin and yang energy in nature.

一天的阴阳变化
Changes of yin and yang in a day

人体 The human body

人身的阳气白天主司体表，到了晚上，便会收敛据守于内了。

Yang energy in the human body mainly concentrates on the skin in the daytime. But when night arrives, it converges within the human body.

自然 Nature

自然界阴阳的转变也是如此，清晨，阳气升腾，到了晚上，阳气收敛，阴气弥漫。

Yin and yang energy in Nature changes in the same way. In the morning, yang energy rises; but at night, it converges whereas yin energy predominates.

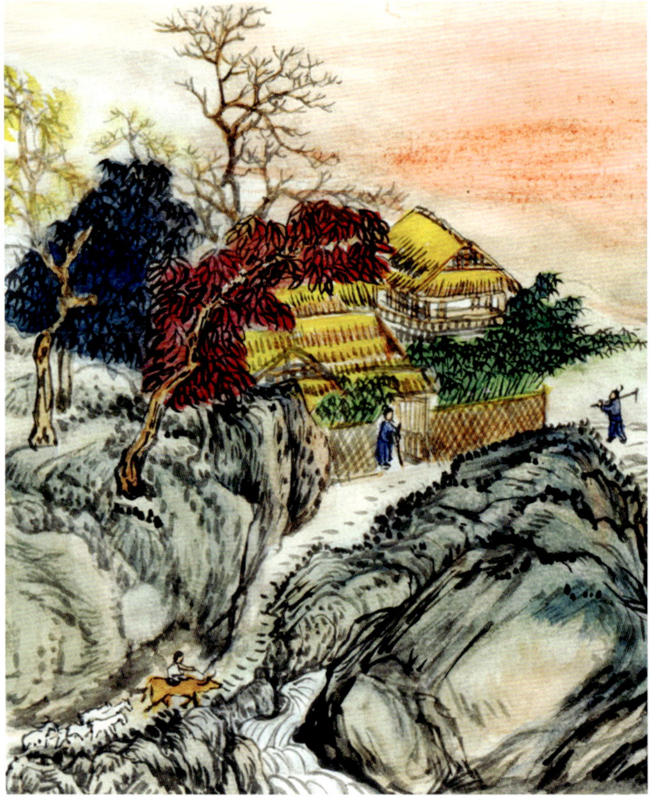

日出而作
To work at sunrise

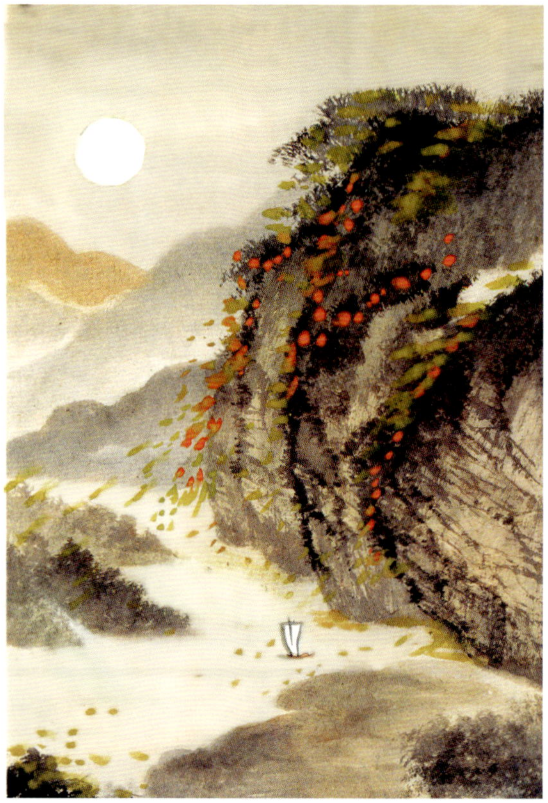

日落而息
To rest at sunset

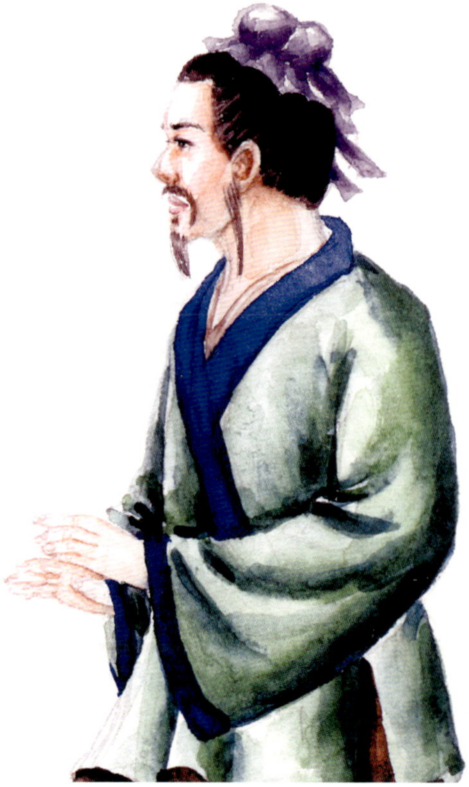

如何采吸阳气

How to absorb yang energy from nature

早晨
Morning

早上日出的时候，面向东方做深呼吸，阳气可以从鼻孔、皮肤腠理、毛孔进入人体。

At sunrise, face east, take deep breaths, and then yang energy will enter the body through the nostrils, skin and pores.

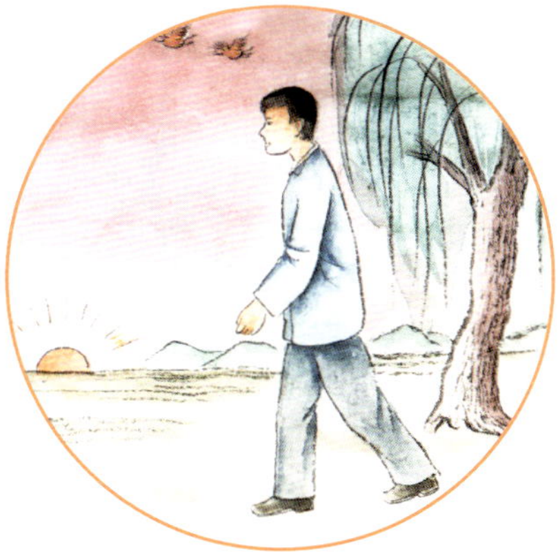

正午
Noon

正午的时候，日头当顶，人到户外后，可以让太阳的日精从位于人头顶处的百会穴进入人体。

At noon when the sun is at the zenith, go outdoors and let yang energy radiated from the sun enter the body through Baihui Point at the top of our head.

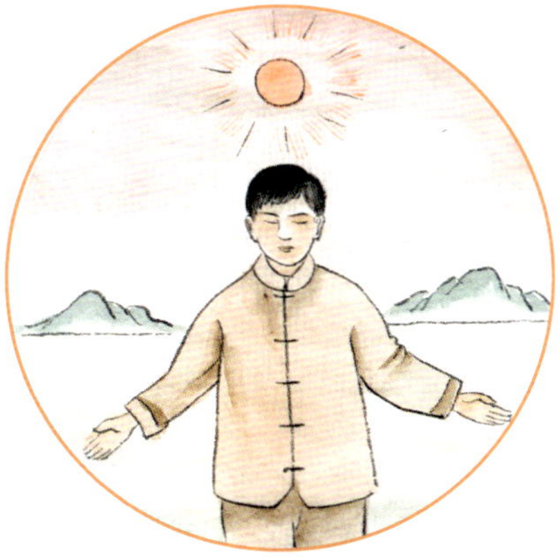

傍晚
Evening

傍晚日落红霞起的时候，可以到户外，尽可能地采吸日精。这是一天中最后一次吸取日精的机会。

At sunset or dawn, go outdoors, because it is the last chance in the day for us to absorb yang energy.

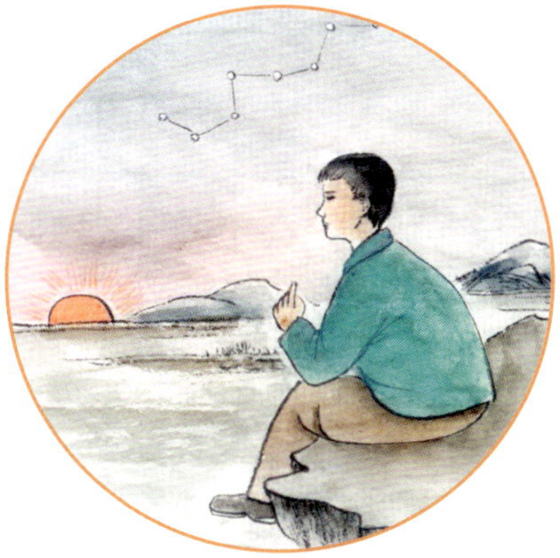

高处
Height

在山川丘陵高处，可以面向南方，使阳气更快地进入人的身体。

At a high place on a mountain or hill, face south, and it will be faster for yang energy to enter our body.

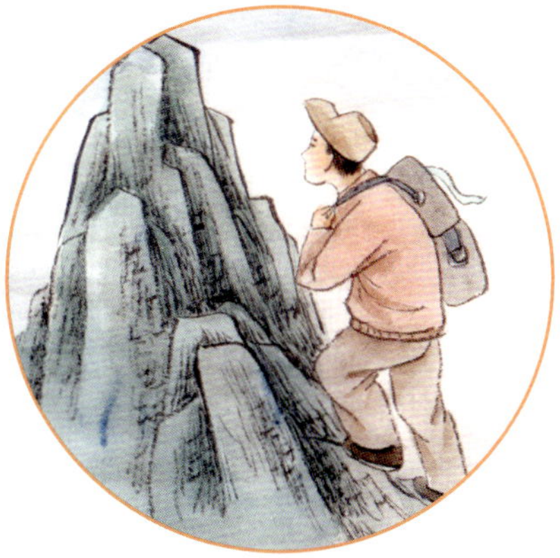

人体的生命周期

Processes of a human life

古人在长期的观察与实践中，逐渐对人体生长发育过程，有了规律性的认识。《黄帝内经》就详细地描述了人从生到死的生长周期。如女子以七八岁为基数，大多经历七个阶段，完成从生长到衰老的过程，男子以八岁为基数，大多经历八个过程。

●男子生命历程

八岁：肾气充实起来，头发茂盛起来，乳齿也更换了。

十六岁：肾气旺盛，天癸产生，精气满溢而能外泻，两性交合，就能生育子女了。

二十四岁：肾气充满，筋骨强健有力，真牙生长，这时牙齿已经长全。

三十二岁：这时筋骨丰隆盛实，肌肉丰满健壮。

四十岁：肾气衰退，头发与牙齿都开始脱落。

四十八岁：人体上部阳气逐渐衰竭，面部憔悴无华，头发和两鬓逐渐花白。

五十六岁：肝气衰弱，筋的活动不能灵活自如，身体抵抗力下降。

六十四岁：天癸枯竭，精气不再充盈，肾脏开始慢慢衰弱，牙齿头发脱落，形体衰疲。身体沉重，步伐不稳，这时已不能生育子女。

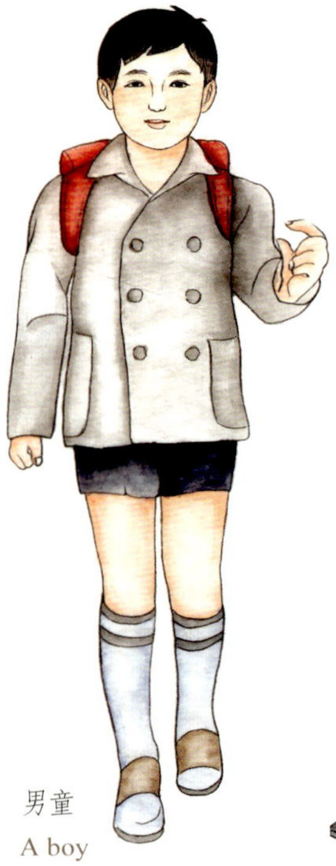
男童
A boy

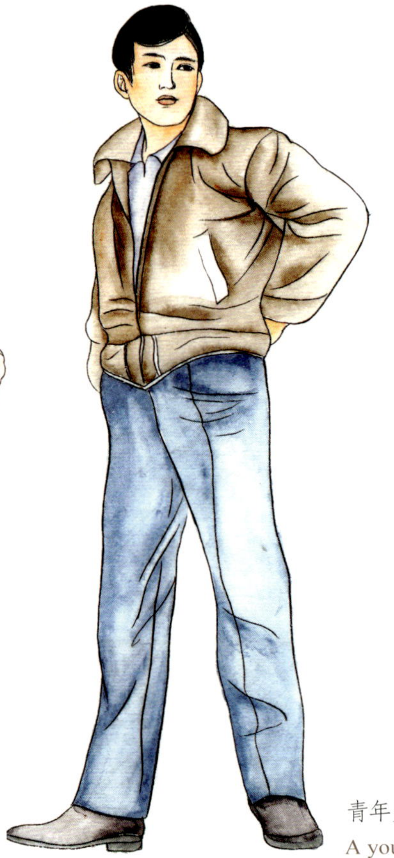
青年男子
A young man

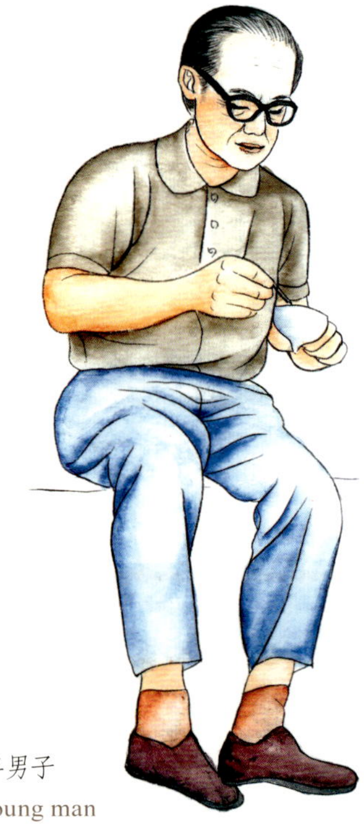
老年男子
An old man

Over years of observation and practice, ancient Chinese gradually perceived the laws of the growth of human body. The *Inner Cannon* details a life cycle from birth to death. For example, it divides a woman's life into seven -year periods, and a man's life into eight-year periods. Most women undergo seven seven-year periods; while men undergo eight eight-year periods. In this way, they complete a life cycle from birth to decrepitude.

A man's processes of life

At 8: His kidneys gain inner energy. His hair grows thick. And it is also time for them to change milk teeth.

At 16: The inner energy at the kidney abounds. Tiangui, or "kidney essence", engenders. His inner energy is so abundant that it naturally flows out. If he intercourses with a woman, he can make her pregnant with his baby.

At 24: His kidneys are full of inner energy. His tendons and bones become strong. His molar teeth grow out. By now, all his teeth have grown out.

At 32: His tendons and bones are fully developed, and his muscles rounded and robust.

At 40: His inner energy declines at the kidney. He begins to lose hair and teeth.

At 48: Yang energy in the upper part of the human body gradually declines. His complexion becomes wan and sallow, and the hair on the head and on the temples gradually turn gray.

At 56: His inner energy at the liver weakens. His tendons are no longer flexible and his immunity deteriorates.

At 64: His tiangui, or "kidney essence", drains. His inner energy is no longer abundant. His kidneys begin weakening, he starts losing hair and teeth, and he shows signs of aging. His body seems heavy, and his steps unsteady. He can no longer make women pregnant.

●女子生命历程

七岁：肾气盛旺了起来，乳齿更换，头发茂盛起来。

十四岁：天癸产生，任脉通畅，太冲脉旺盛，月经按时来潮，具备了生育子女的能力。

二十一岁：肾气充满，真牙生出，这时牙齿就长全了。

二十八岁：筋骨强健有力，头发的生长达到最茂盛的阶段，此时身体最为强壮。

三十五岁：阳明经脉气血渐衰弱，面部开始憔悴，头发也开始有脱落的现象。

四十二岁：三阳经脉气血衰弱，面部憔悴无华，此时头发开始由黑变白。

四十九岁：任脉气血虚弱，太冲脉的气血也衰弱了，天癸枯竭，月经断绝，形体渐渐衰老，因此失去生育能力。

A woman's processes of life

At 7: Her kidneys gain inner energy. Her milk teeth are being replaced, and her hair growing thick.

At 14: Her tiangui, or "kidney essence", engenders. Inner energy moves along the Ren Channel in an unobstructed manner, and inner energy in the Taichong Channel abounds. She begins menstruating and acquires the ability of conceiving babies.

At 21: Her kidneys are full of inner energy. Her molar teeth grow out. By now, all her teeth have grown out.

At 28: Her tendons and bones are robust and strong. She has the thickest hair and the strongest body in her life.

At 35: Her qi and blood in the Yangming Channel gradually decline; her complexion is turning sallow and she begins loosing her hair.

At 42: Her qi and blood in the Sanyang Channel decline; her complexion turns sallow and her hair begins turning gray.

At 49: The qi and blood in the Ren Channel decline, and so do those in the Taichong Channel. Her Tiangui, or "kidney essence", drains. She no longer menstruates. Her body shows signs of old age. Therefore, she has lost her fertility.

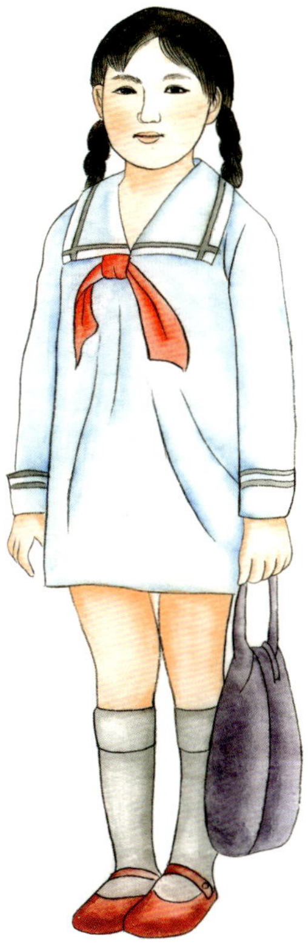

女童
A girl

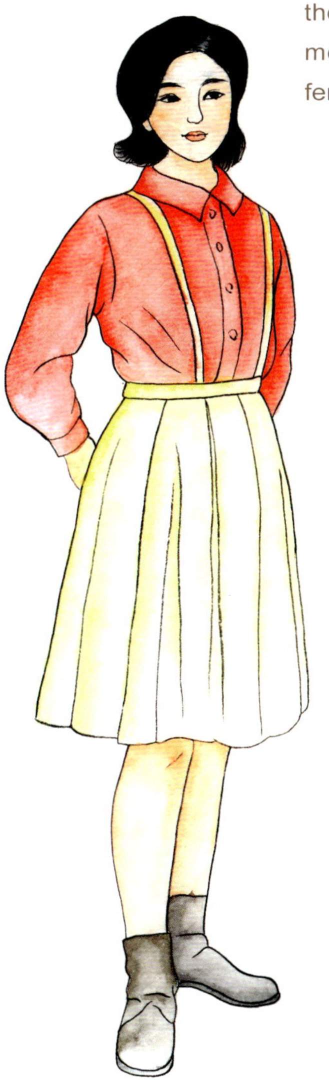

青年女子
A young woman

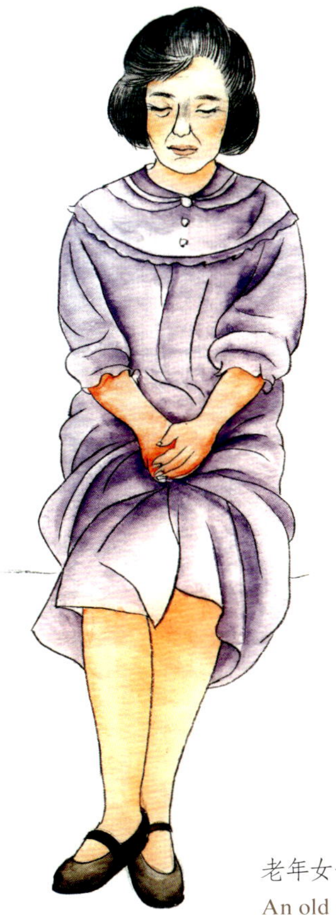

老年女子
An old woman

剖析衰老的奥秘

Analysis of the mystery of aging

衰老带来的机体改变

Physical changes caused by aging

人的生理机能是逐渐衰退的，最早表现在形体、外貌——如皮肤、毛发的细微变化上，随着年龄的增长，人的容颜、牙齿、形体都会发生较大的变化。

The deterioration of human's physiological functions is a gradual process. The earliest slight changes mostly take place in one's shape and appearance. The commonest are the changes of the skin and hair. As one ages, changes begin to take place in his/her appearance, teeth and shape.

皮肤 Skin

30岁 30 | 37岁 37 | 40岁 40 | 50岁 50 | 58岁 58 | 60岁 60

皱纹在眼角、耳前及口角两边相继出现。

Wrinkles appear first at the corners of the eyes, in front of the ears, and at the corners of the mouth.

皮肤由于脂肪和弹力纤维的消失而松弛，眼睑、耳部的皮肤下垂。

Skin becomes slack because the gradual disappearance of fat and elastic fibers. The skin at the eyelids and ears start to droop.

皮肤会出现褐色的色素斑，也被称为老年斑、老年疣。

Brown pigmented spots, known as senile plaques and senile warts, begin to appear at the skin.

毛发 Hair

30岁 30 | 36岁 36 | 40岁 40 | 50岁 50 | 60岁 60 | 75岁 75

鼻毛开始变白，这时鼻毛比头发更快开始老化。

Hair in the nose turns gray, earlier than hair on the head.

40岁头发开始变白。到60岁一般会全部变白。

At the age of 40, hair begins the graying process. Generally at the age of 60, all hair will turn gray.

60岁以后，约有80%的老人出现脱发，75岁时则多达90%。

After 60, about 80% old people start loosing hair. The percentage rises to 90% at the age of 75.

视力 Vision

30岁 30 | 40岁 40 | 50岁 50 | 60岁 60

晶状体的弹性变差，其屈光能力逐渐减小，因而视调节能力也就逐渐降低，便发生了"老花眼"。

When the elasticity of the crystalline lens deteriorates, their dioptric capacity becomes poor and they begin to have presbyopia.

晶状体的衰老还会使其透明性降低或丧失，这时便会形成白内障。

Aging also makes crystalline lens less or no longer transparent. At this point, the old will suffer from cataract.

听力 Hearing

30岁 30 | 40岁 40 | 50岁 50 | 60岁 60 | 65岁 65

听力开始逐渐减退。

Hearing begins deteriorating gradually.

50岁开始自感听力减退。

The deterioration of hearing starts at the age of 50.

65岁以上的老人中，听力减退的占27.4%。

Of people older than 65, 27.4% suffer from hearing deterioration.

四种生命活动基本特征的探讨

Four basic features of life

生命活动的基本特征

Basic features of life

生命的特征

Features of life

新陈代谢

Metabolism

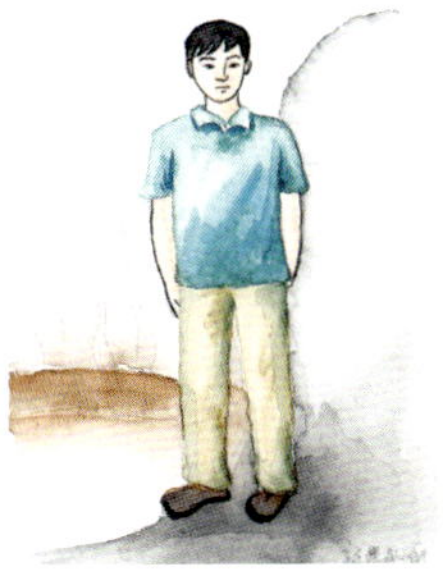

生命过程就是不断地气化（阳）与成形（阴）的过程，即有机体同外界进行不断的物质交换和能量交换的过程。

A life cycle is a process of constantly assimilating qi (yang) and taking form (yin), or in other words, a process of constant material and energy exchange.

反应性

Reactivity

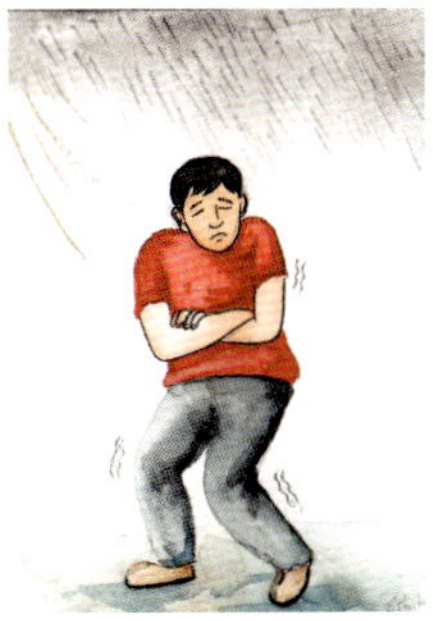

生命体在受到来自外界和内部的刺激时，会产生各种反应，如冷热刺激的反应，瞳孔对光的反应等。

When it receives stimuli from the outside or inside, a life organism will produce various reactions, for example, the reactions to coldness and heat, the reactions of pupils to light, etc.

生长与发育

Growth and development

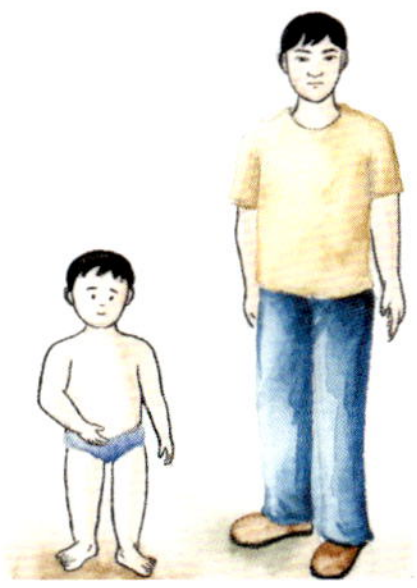

任何生命都会经历从受精卵开始，经过胚胎期、幼年期、成年期、老年期，一直到死亡的过程。

Every human life starts from a fertilized ovum, undergoes the embryonic stage, juvenile stage, adult stage and aging period, and finally dies.

生殖和遗传

Reproduction and heredity

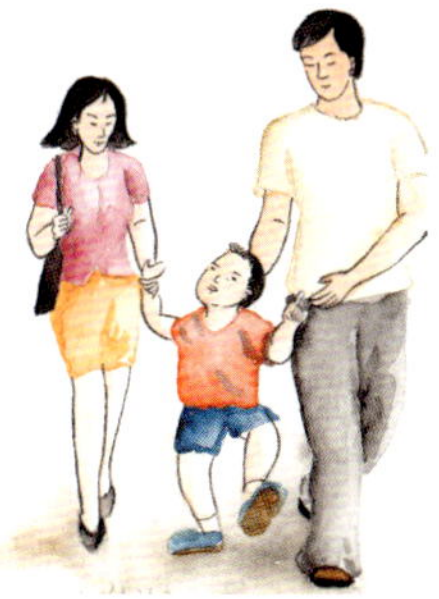

生殖与遗传，是生命得以绵延不绝的根本，同时也是生命维持稳定性的基础。

Reproduction and heredity are essential to the continuation of life and fundamental to the stability of life.

生命的运动形式

Forms of life

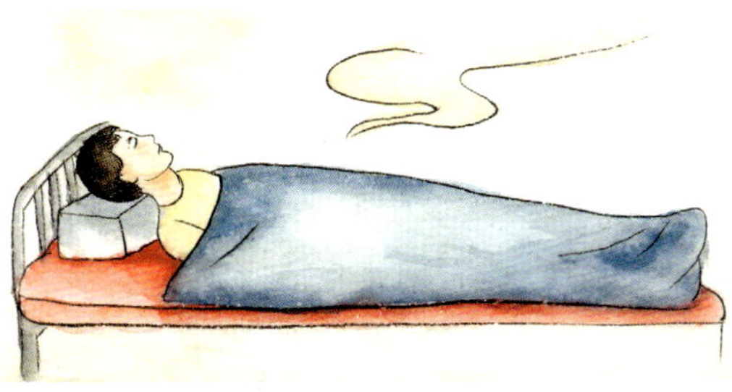

死去的人

The dead

物质的升降出入停止

Cessation of material exchange

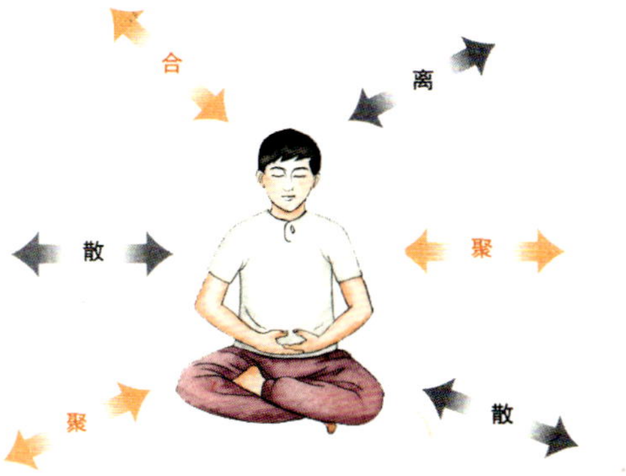

活着的人

The living

物质的升降出入活跃

Active material exchange

肆　养形健身

IV.　Fitness Keeping and Health Promotion

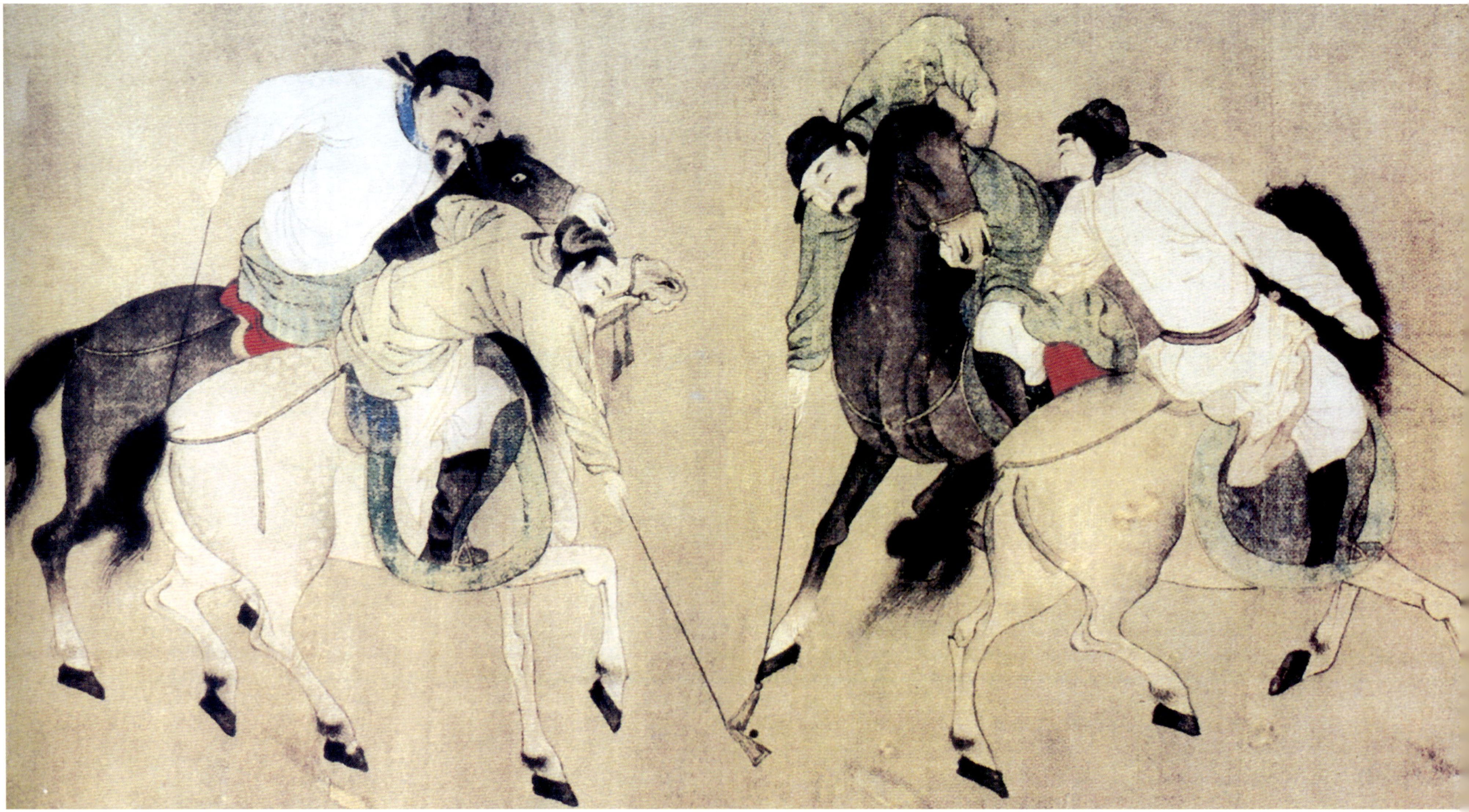

美好的生命寓于健康的身体。爱惜我们的身体发肤，是我们对于人生的热爱，对于生命的尊严的敬畏。形体是精神和生命的物质基础，保养形体要点在于严防伤害和保精养血强身。

A happy life is based on a healthy body. Efforts to preserve our body, hair and skin have sprung from our love for life and awe for the dignity of life. The body is the residence of the spirit and life. For one who wishes to preserve bodily health, it is pivotal to steer it out of harm's way and maintain the 'essence' (jing), nourish the blood and strengthen the body.

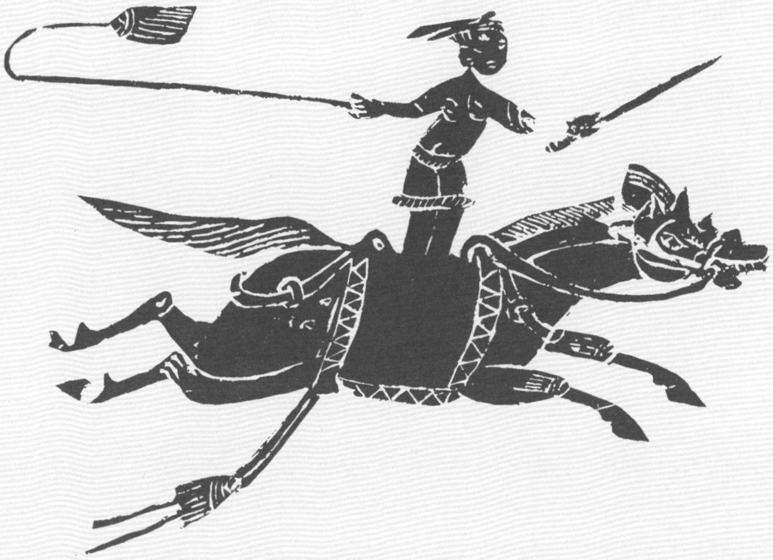

四季养生

Regimens in different seasons

司马迁说“春生、夏长、秋收、冬藏，此天地之大经也，弗顺则无以为纲纪”，《黄帝内经》也提出应“提挈天地，把握阴阳”，就是说人应该掌握、效法阴阳变化的规律，适应自然气候和外界环境的变化。“法于阴阳”在养生学上主要是指“四季气候与养生相应”。

Si Maqian said, “Life is borne in spring, growing in summer, harvested in autumn, and stored in winter, which is the world’s great law, and there would be no disciplines if it were violated.” *Inner Canon* also proposes to “guide and support the world, to grasp keep in shape “, that is, we should master and follow the changing law of yin and yang, adapt to climate and changes in the natural environment. In regimen theory, “following the law of the yin and yang” expounds the idea that the change of four seasons is consistent with the change of regimen.

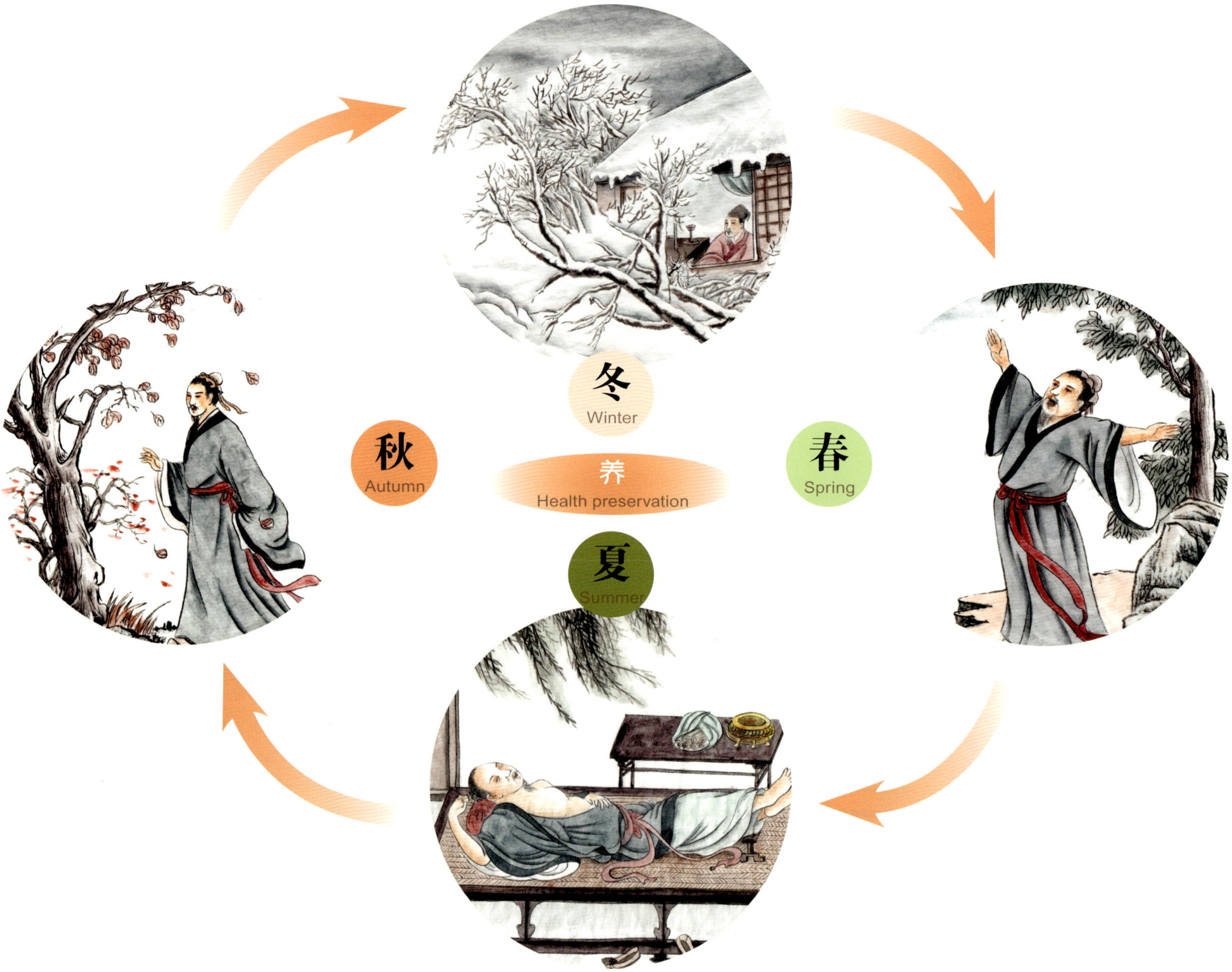

春季养生

Spring regimen

春天
Spring

立春 Spring begins → 雨水 The rains → 惊蛰 Insects awaken → 春分 Vernal equinox → 清明 Qingming → 谷雨 Grain rain

春季养生原则

Regimen of preserve health in spring

精神调养 Mental health preservation

戒怒
Avoid anger

要学会控制情绪，当你怒从心头起，要和人吵架的时候，要及时提醒自己，用理智的力量来控制怒气。

Learn to control your mood. That is, when you are about to flare up and start a quarrel with some one, admonish yourself in time and rein your anger with reason.

疏泄不良情绪
Get rid of bad mood

把积聚、抑郁在心中的不良情绪通过适当的方式宣达、发泄出去，以尽快恢复心理平衡。

Give vent to your pent-up positive feelings in appropriate ways so as to regain the equilibrium of the mind.

保持精神愉快
Maintain a happy mood

要培养开朗的性格，就要使情志有朝气，即保持精神愉快，这点特别重要。

To build a cheerful personality, you need to keep yourself happy—this is particularly important.

饮食调养 Dietary regimen

温补阳气的食物
Food that warmly invigorates yang qi

李时珍在《本草纲目》中，引用了《风土记》的内容“以葱、蒜、韭、蓼、蒿、芥等辛嫩之菜，杂和而食”。葱、蒜、韭是养阳的佳蔬良药。

In his *Compendium of Materia Medica*, Li Shizhen, Chinese herbalist, recommended that “fresh and pungent ingredients including scallion, garlic, leek, smartweed, crown daisy and mustard be mixed for food.”Scallion, garlic and leek are vegetables that nurture *yang*, or “masculine and positive strength”.

多食甜，少食酸
Eat more sweet food and less sour food

当春天来临之时，人们要少吃点酸味的食品，而要多吃些甜味的食物，这样做的好处是能补益人体的脾胃之气。

When spring arrives, people should take less sour foods and more sweet ones. In this way, the “inner energy” at the spleen and stomach may be supplemented.

春季三个月，始于立春止于立夏。春天是万物生发的季节，春归大地，万物复苏，欣欣向荣。人体阳气也顺应自然，向上向外疏发。

The three months of spring starts from the Beginning of Spring, and ends with the Beginning of Summer. Spring is the growing season of everything. Everything is reviving and thriving as soon as spring returns to the earth. In harmony with nature, yang qi of the human body at this time is growing up and flowing out.

春季起居

Circadian rhythm in spring

春季应晚睡早起。春天，睡卧时间如果太长会损害人体阳气，人应多参加室外活动，舒展形体，避免倦懒思眠。

During the spring, people should adjust their circadian rhythms by going to sleep late and getting up early. Too much sleep in spring may depress the yang qi in the body; therefore, simple exercises such as body-stretching and a few outdoor activities are recommended to help people shake off drowsiness and become invigorated.

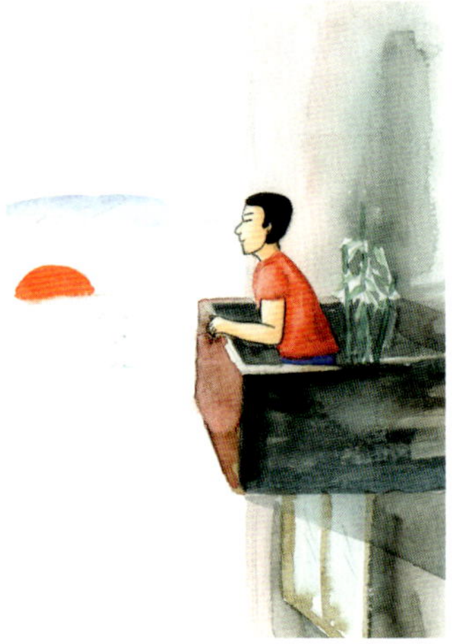

早起
Get up early

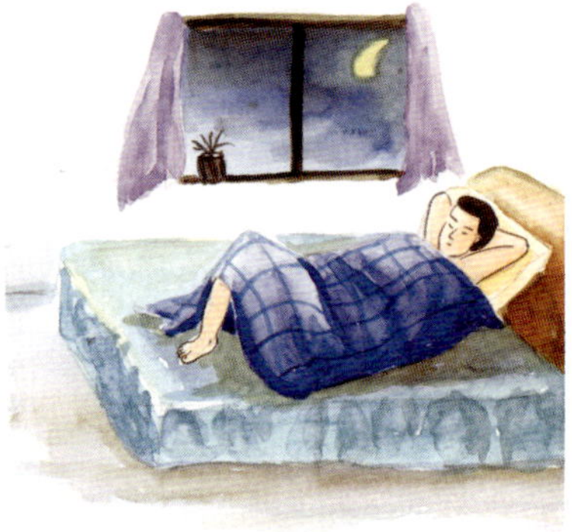

晚睡
Sleep late

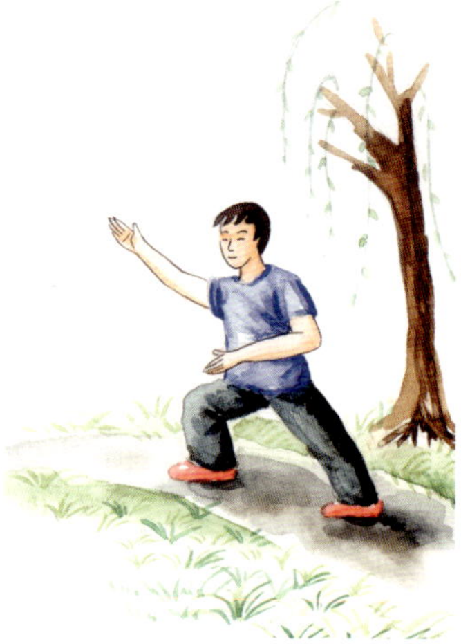

舒展形体，增加锻炼
Increase physical exercises

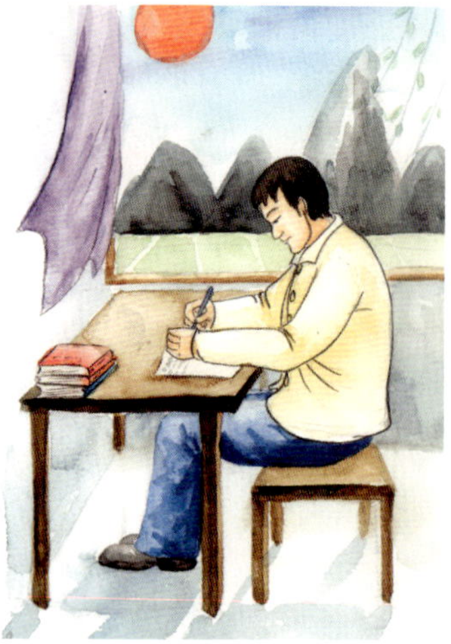

多开窗通风
Open the windows frequently for better ventilation

春季养生三重点

Three keys of health preservation in spring

1 调神务使“志生”

春天里人的志意应当顺其生发之气，精神舒畅，情志条达，宽怀戒怒，避免生恼怒和愤恨，保持乐观情绪。

2 活动以充生机

春天应抖擞精神，加强体育锻炼，主动运动、持之以恒。

3 宽身利于“发陈”

冬去春来，春阳升发，天地俱现生机，万物以荣。人体也是如此，人应顺应春气，舒展形体，使气血流通，精神活跃。

1. Balance the mind so as to nourish the spirit

In spring, a season that nurtures growth, one should be free from worries, be broad-minded and tolerant, avoid anger and resentment, and stay optimistic.

2. Exercise the body so as to energize the spirit

In spring, in response to the vitality of the season, one should improve his health through more active and persistent exercise.

3. Relax the mind so as to nourish growth in spring

When spring comes, positive life-energy rises and all living beings thrive between heaven and earth. The same is true of the human body. Therefore one should exercise his limbs in order to promote the circulation of blood and vital energy and enliven his spirits.

夏季养生

Summer regimen

夏天
Summer

立夏 Summer begins → 小满 Grain buds → 芒种 Grain in ear → 夏至 Summer solstice → 小暑 Slight heat → 大暑 Great heat

夏季养生原则

Principles for health preservation in summer

精神调养 Mental health preservation

克服烦腻情绪，振作精神
Overcome boredom and cheer up

夏天昼长暑酷，人容易疲劳，易产生烦腻情绪，因此要注意宣泄郁结之气，振作精神，克服倦怠。

In the long days and sweltering heat of summer, people are prone to get tired and fretful. As a result, it is necessary for people to find an outlet for pent-up negative emotions so that they can enliven their spirit and shake off the fatigue.

克服烦躁易怒情绪
Overcome agitation and irritability

夏天要注意克服因心绪烦腻而产生的焦躁易怒情绪。

In summer people are inclined to become irritable and restless because of the boredom and upset brought by the weather. So it is worth people's special attention to take control of their emotions.

夏天之主"湿"
Dampness is the main feature of summer

饮食调养 Dietary regimen

湿
Dampness

- 伤阳气 Hurt yang qi. → 饮食上 In diet → 忌油腻 Avoid greasy food；宜温热 Warm drinks and food are preferred
- 伤脾阳 Hurt the yang qi of spleen. → 饮食上 In diet → 宜清淡 Mild food is advisable

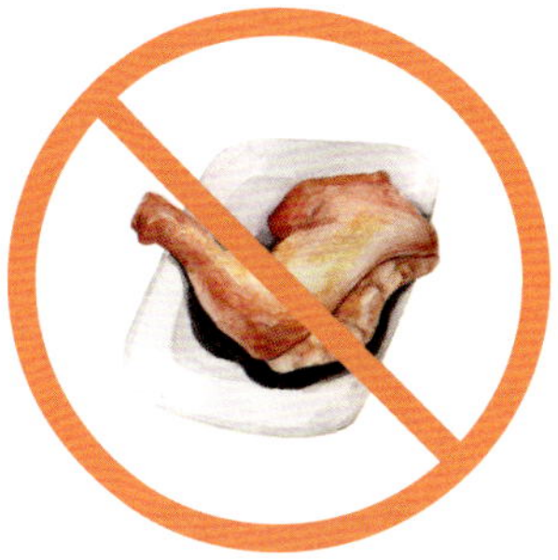

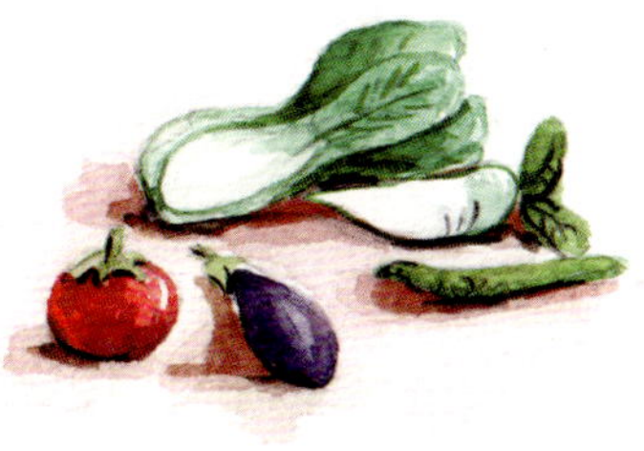

长夏的湿邪之气最易侵犯脾胃，导致消化吸收功能低下。因此长夏的饮食应清淡、少油腻，并以温食为主。

The functions of the spleen and stomach are prone to disruption by unhealthy factors of a long summer. Consequently, the digestive function will malfunction. Therefore, the dietary principles of long summer favor light foods and disfavors oily foods. And the diet should consist mainly of lukewarm foods.

夏季三个月，始于立夏止于立秋。夏季是万物繁荣茂盛的季节，天地阴阳之气上下交合，人体阳气亦旺盛。

The three months of summer starts from the Beginning of Summer and ends with the Beginning of Autumn. Summer is the season of lush prosperity of all things, when yin qi and yang qi of nature intercourse from up and down. Yang qi of the human body also grows strongest.

夏季起居

Circadian rhythm in summer

夏季昼长夜短，气温较高，应晚睡早起。夜晚不可露天睡觉，以免受凉。夏季应午休补充睡眠，确保精力充沛。

In summer when days are longer than nights, due to the hot weather, people should go to sleep late and get up early. Open-air sleeping is not recommended for it is easy to cause a cold, while taking a nap at noon is a good way to remedy insufficient sleep and refresh the spirit.

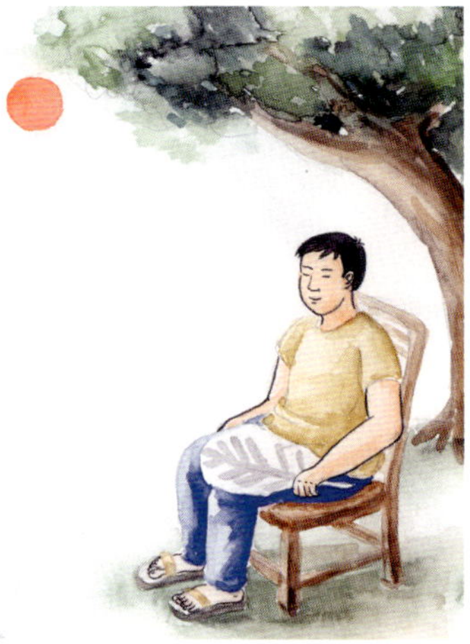

早起
Get up early

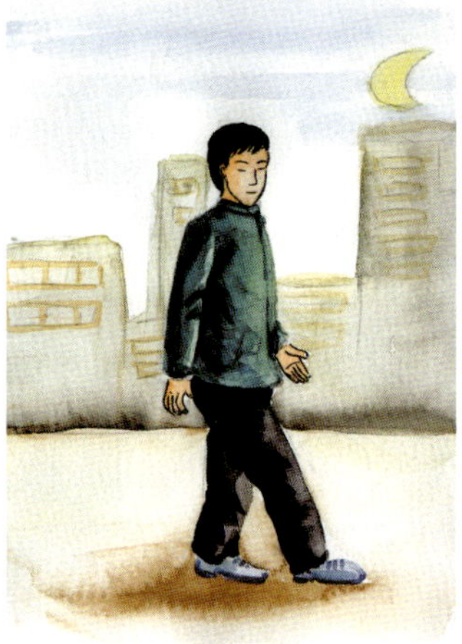

晚睡
Sleep late

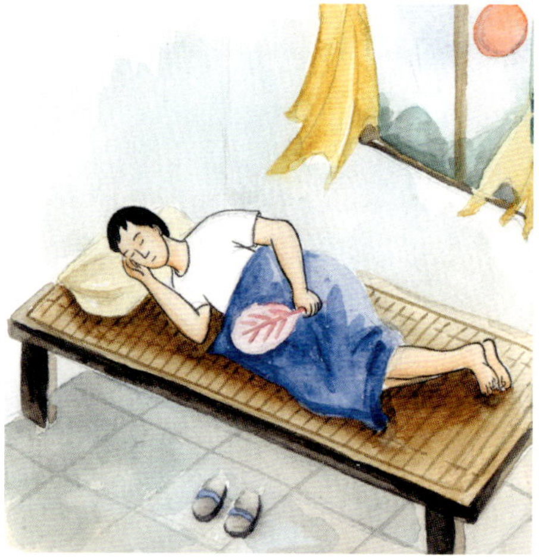

夏季应午休来补偿睡眠
A nap at noon is advisable in summer

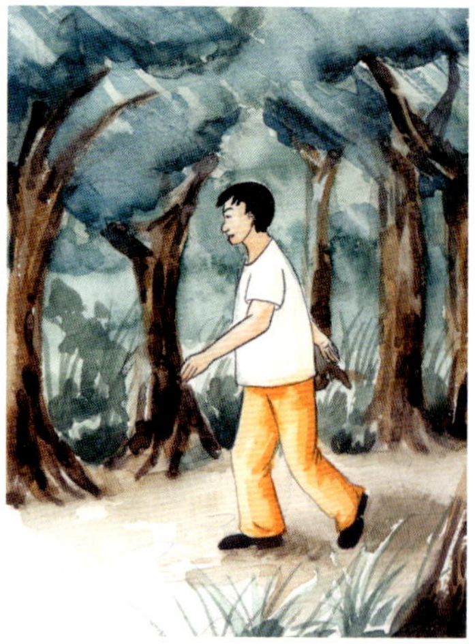

夏季适宜到大自然中健身
Better exercise in nature in summer

夏季养生三重点

Three principles for health preservation in summer

三种养生重点
Three principles for health preservation

运动保健
Physical exercises for health

夏天气温高、湿度大，因此，在夏季健身，最好到大自然中去，此外，读书习字、品茶吟诗、益友倾谈、观景纳凉，也是夏季养生的好方法。

Because of the high temperature and humidity in summer, it is the best exercise to go out into nature. Besides, reading, practicing calligraphy, having tea, organising poetry parties, chatting with friends.

冬病夏治
To cure winter diseases in summer

冬季常发的慢性病及一些阳虚阴盛的疾患，往往可以通过伏夏的调养得以好转。

Common chronic diseases and some ailments caused by yang insufficiency and excess of yin in winter may improve through recuperating efforts in the hottest days of summer.

谨防疰夏
Take precautions against the summer malady

对于此病，人们可以采取芳香悦脾，辟秽化湿的方法，减少食量，少吃油腻，清淡饮食，使脾健胃和。体质虚弱、易患疰夏之人，在秋冬季可服用一些补肺健脾，益气养精的食物。

To treat this disease, we should tonify the spleen with aromatic herbal medicines, advise the patient to abstain from dirt and try to eliminate the dampness. As for the patient, he/she should eat less, eat light foods and abstain from oily foods so as to tune up the spleen and the stomach.

秋季养生

Autumn regimen

秋天 Autumn

立秋 Autumn begins → 处暑 The limit of heat → 白露 White dews → 秋分 Autumn equinox → 寒露 Cold dews → 霜降 Hoar-frost falls

秋季养生原则

Principles of health preservation in autumn

精神调养 Mental health preservation

克服悲伤抑郁情绪
Overcome depression and sadness

秋天花木凋零，万物萧条，容易引起悲伤、凄凉、垂暮之感。因此应注重调摄精神，开放心胸，保持积极的生活状态。

Autumn is the season when all lives in nature begin to fade. The bleak scenery can easily make people feel sad and depressed. Thus it is important for people to adjust their mood and open up their mind to build up a positive attitude toward life.

注意保养精神
Avoid exhaustion and store up energy

秋天阳气开始收敛，应注重保养精神，避免大幅消耗精力。

Autumn is a time for people to preserve yang qi, the vital energy in the human body, so people should attach great importance to not consuming much of their physical strength in order to maintain their energy.

饮食调养 Dietary regimen

秋天应多吃清热生津、养阴润肺的食物
In autumn, eat more food that can clear away heat, help to generate saliva, nourish yin, and moisten the lungs

秋天津液易耗，易出现口干舌燥、咽喉疼痛、肺热咳嗽等症状，人应多吃清热生津、养阴润肺的食物。

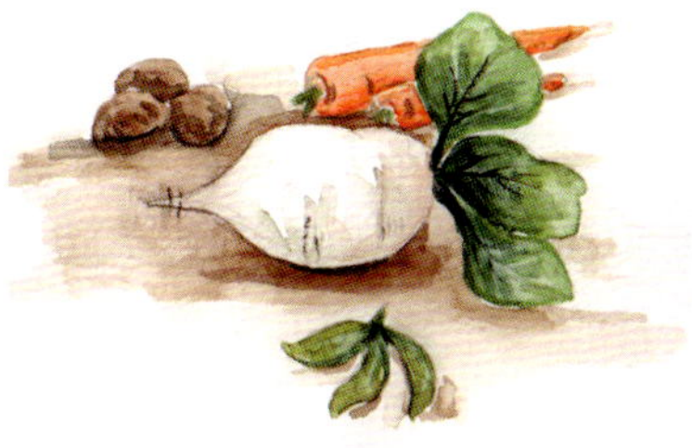

The dry weather in autumn can easily cause a loss of the body fluid and lead to a series of physical discomfort such as feeling parched and thirsty, coughing due to the lung heat, and having sore throats. Thus people should eat more heat-clearing food that can stimulate the production of body fluid, thereby nourishing the yin energy and moistening the lungs.

多食甘咸补阳的食物
Eat more sour food and less pungent food

秋季养生，气血宜收不宜散。应少吃寒凉之品，宜食用甘咸补益性食物来补充津液。

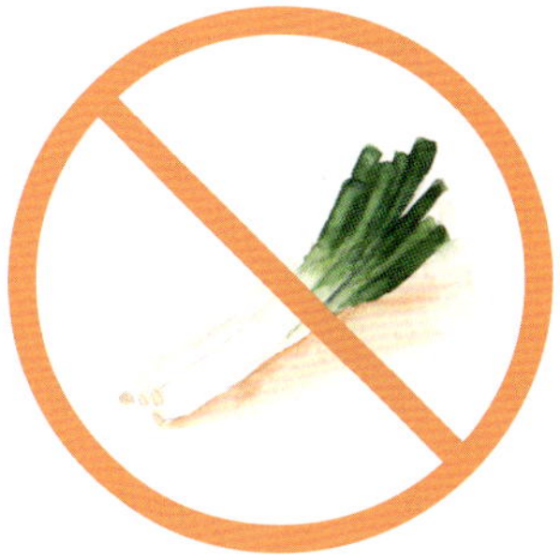

In autumn, you should preserve your blood and vital energy rather than disperse them. Eat less pungent food like scallion and ginger, and consume more acidic food.

秋季起居

Circadian rhythm in autumn

立秋之季已是天高气爽之时，应“早卧早起，与鸡俱兴”。早卧是为了顺应阳气的收敛，早起则为舒展肺气，防止肺气收敛太过。

秋季三个月，始于立秋止于立冬。秋天是万物成熟的收获季节，天地间阳气日退，阴寒渐生，人体阳气也随之内收。

Since the autumn days are crisp and invigorating, people should follow the rule of “going to sleep early and rising up upon hearing the crow of the roosters”. Going to sleep early can help to preserve yang qi while rising up early can promote the flow of qi in the lungs and also help revive the energy in the bodies.

The three months of autumn starts from the Beginning of Autumn and ends with the Beginning of Winter. Autumn is the harvest season with maturity of all things, when yang qi between heaven and earth is fading day by day and yin qi is gradually increasing. So yang qi of the human body begins to decline.

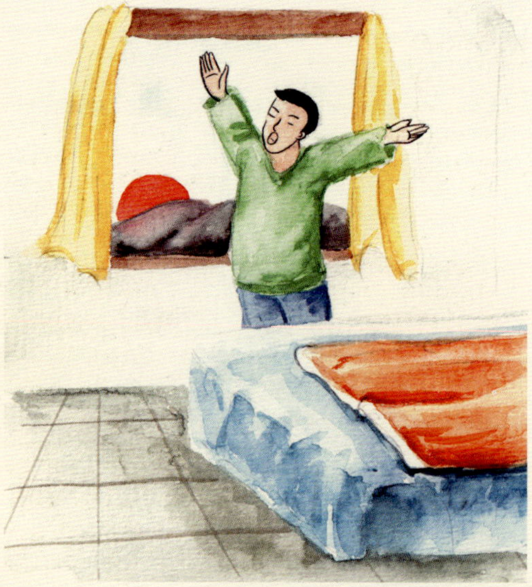

早起

Get up early

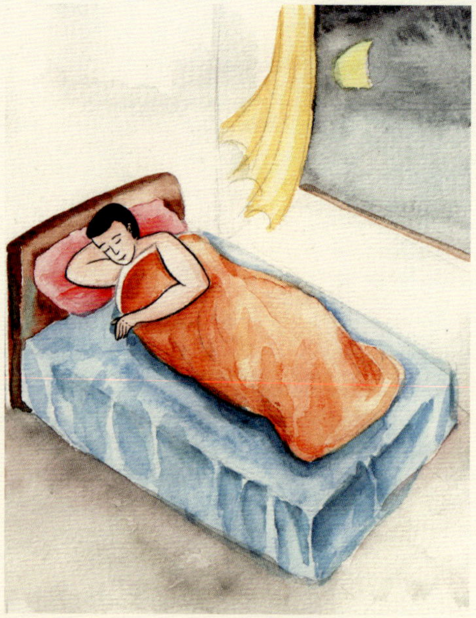

早睡

Go to bed early

秋天是开展各种运动锻炼的大好时机，每人可根据自己的具体情况选择不同的锻炼方式。

Autumn is a good time to participate in various kinds of sports and exercises. Individuals can choose different way to exercise according to their physical conditions.

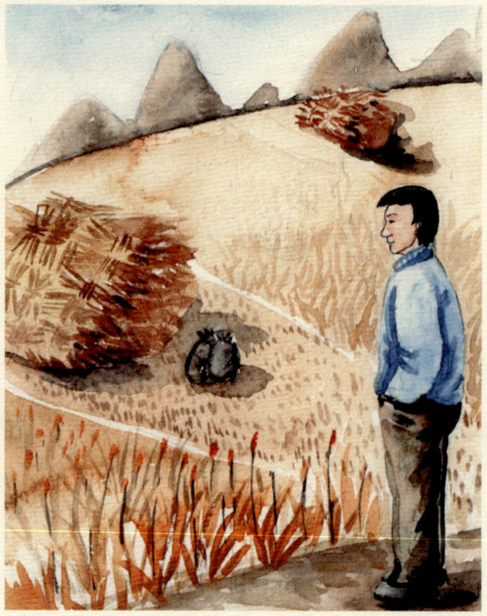

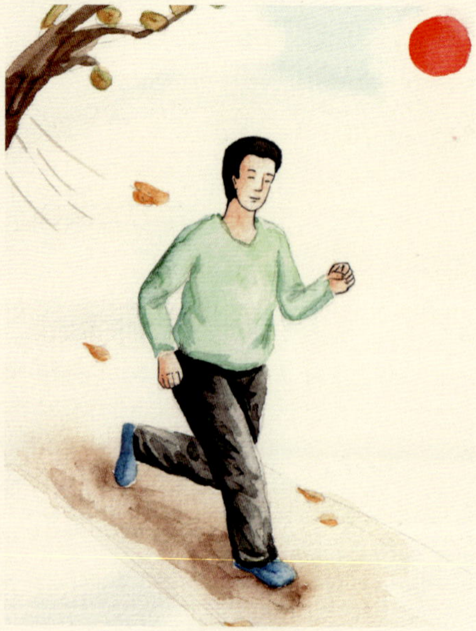

秋季应注意保养精神，不要大量消耗精力。

Store up energy and avoid over exhaustion.

冬季养生

Winter regimen

冬天 Winter

立冬 Winter begins → 小雪 Light snow → 大雪 Heavy snow → 冬至 Winter solstice → 小寒 Slight cold → 大寒 Great cold

冬季养生原则

Principles of health preservation in winter

精神调养 Mental health preservation

保持心神宁静 Stay calm

冬季养生，重在精神的调摄，要保持精神情绪的宁静，切勿烦扰妄动。

In winter, to nurture your mind, you should stay calm and avoid disturbance and improper excitement.

养精蓄锐 Conserve your energy

冬季要养精蓄锐，调心养神，保证有充足的睡眠时间，要注意运动适量，为春机勃发做好准备。

In winter, to take care of your mind and spirit, you should have enough sleep and maintain a proper amount of exercise. Thus you can preserve and nurture your spirit in preparation for the burst of vitality in spring.

饮食调养 Dietary regimen

少食生冷 Eat less raw and cold food

冬季应少吃生冷食物，避免损伤脾胃阳气。

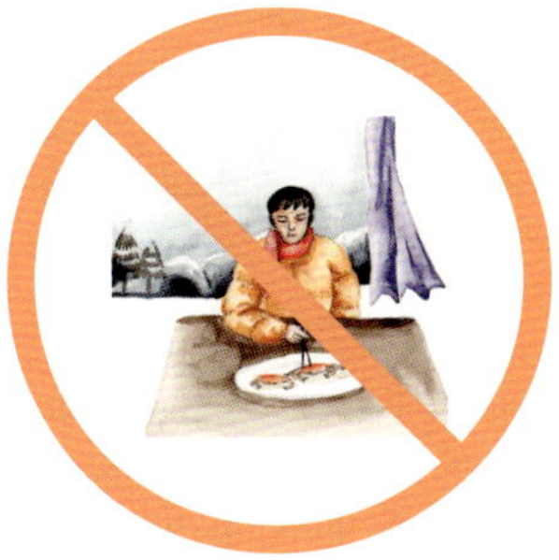

Raw or cold food should be excluded from daily meal in winter in case that it will injure the vital energy in the spleen and stomach.

多食滋阴潜阳的食物 Eat more food that nourishes yin for suppressing hyperactive yang

冬季养生，气血宜收不宜散。应少吃葱、姜等辛辣发散之品，食用酸性食物来补偿。

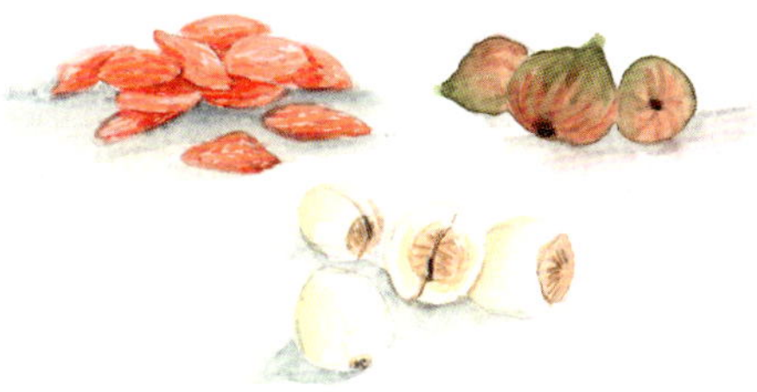

The regimen in winter focuses on preserving qi flow and blood circulation rather than dispersing them. Thus pungent food with the effect of dispersing such as shallot and ginger should be avoided, while more acid food should be taken in.

冬季起居

Circadian rhythm in winter

冬季三个月，始于立冬止于立春。冬季是万物闭藏的季节，阴气盛极，阳气潜伏，草木凋零，昆虫蛰伏，人体阳气潜藏。

冬季天气寒冷，万物蛰伏，应早睡晚起。

The three months of winter starts from the Beginning of Winter and ends with the Beginning of Spring. Winter is the season of storage of all things, when yin qi is booming and yang qi is lying low with the withered vegetation and dormant insects, and yang qi of the human body is lurking.

In the cold weather of winter, all lives lie dormant, so human beings should also rest early and get up late.

冬天是万木凋零、生机潜伏闭藏的季节，人体的阳气也随着自然的变化潜藏于内。因此，冬季养生应以敛阴护阳为根本。

Winter is the season when numerous plants wither and the vital force lies dormant. The yang energy in the human body withdraws back into the body, in correspondence with the cycle of nature. Therefore, in terms of health preservation, we should astringe yin energy and conserve yang energy in line with the laws of nature in winter. To nourish the mind, it is advised that we should "...keep your ambitions and resolutions to yourself and do not reveal them to others; if you have made a decision, keep it as a secret joy." Try to stay calm, regulate your sentiments, maintain the tranquility of the mind, keep your private thoughts to your self, and free yourself from cares and worries, thereby conserving your yang energy in the body.

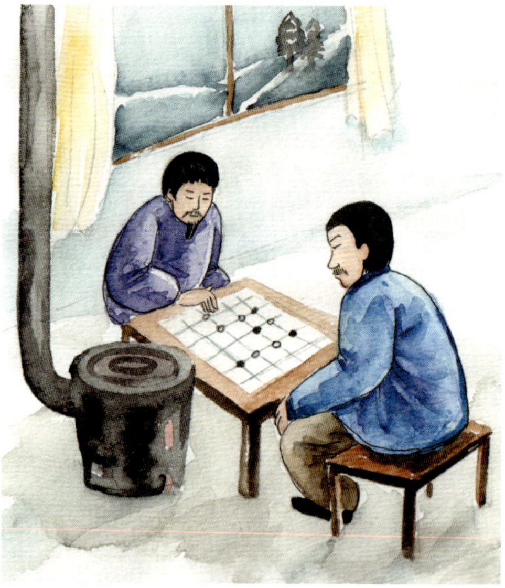

在生机潜伏、万物闭藏的冬季里，要养精蓄锐，使阳气内藏。

During winter when most lives lie dormant and inactive, it is important for people to store up and nourish the vital energy.

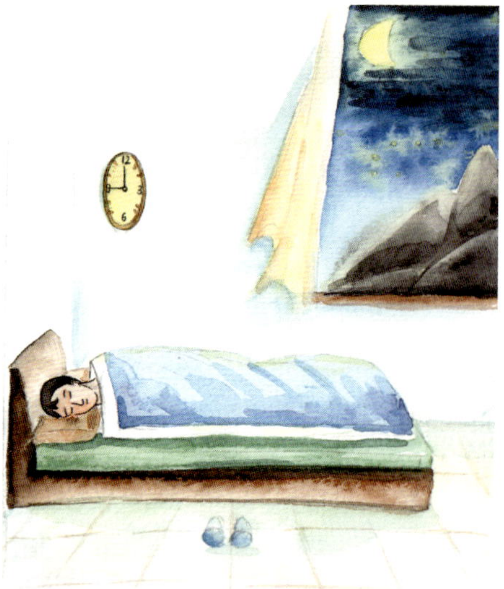

冬季气候寒冷，万物蛰伏，应早睡晚起。

In the cold weather of winter, all lives lie dormant, so human beings should also rest early and get up late.

冬季养生三重点

Three principles for health preservation in winter

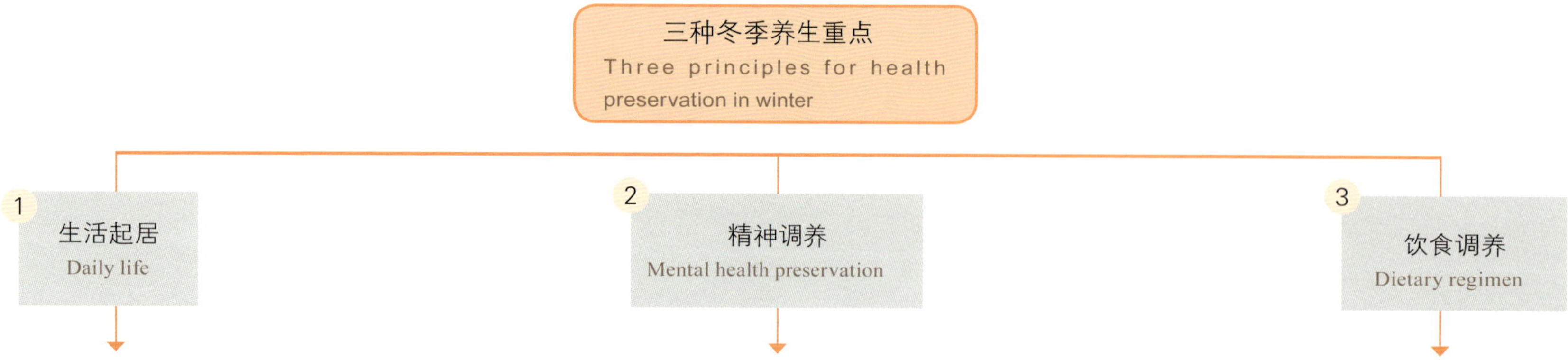

在生机潜伏、万物闭藏的冬季里，要养精蓄锐，使阳气内藏。

In winter, when life is latent and all creatures go into hiding, you should preserve your energy so as to store up your yang qi.

保持精神情绪的宁静，避免烦扰妄动，使体内阳气得以潜藏。

Maintain the tranquility of the mental and emotional states and avoid mental disturbance so as to conserve yang energy in the body.

冬季天气严寒，万物伏藏，易感受寒邪，应少吃生冷食物，以免损伤脾胃的阳气。

Maintain the tranquility of the mental and emotional states and avoid mental disturbance so as to conserve yang energy in the body.

调节四季情志

To regulate emotions in the four seasons

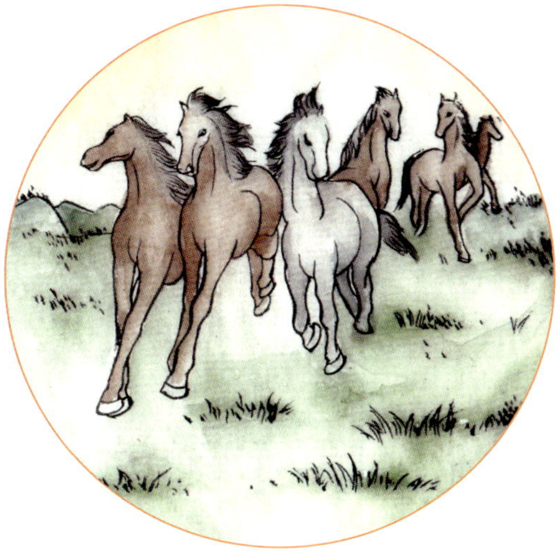

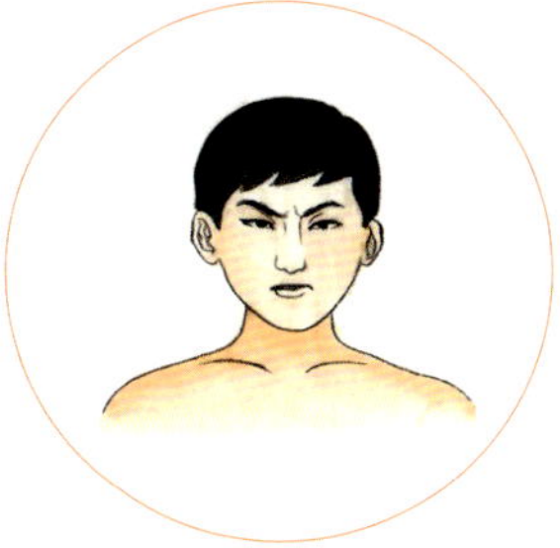

春在志为怒

In spring, one is emotionally susceptible to anger

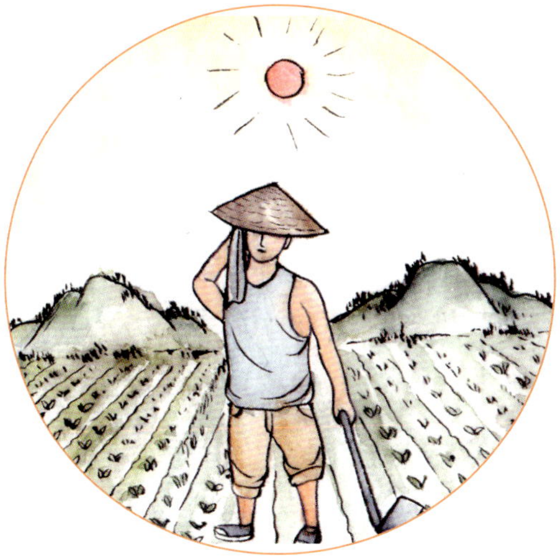

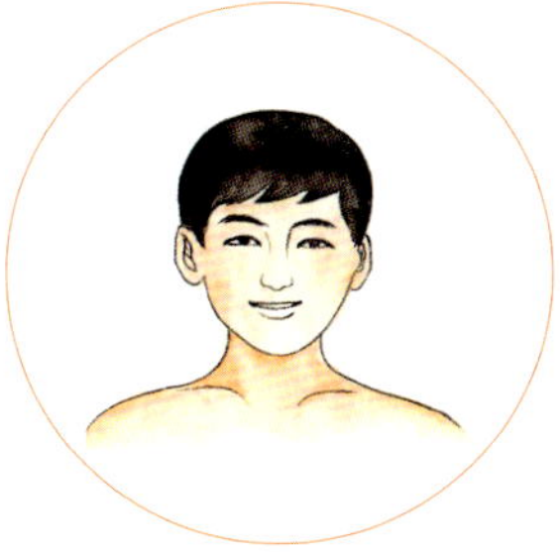

夏在志为喜

In summer, one is emotionally susceptible to joy

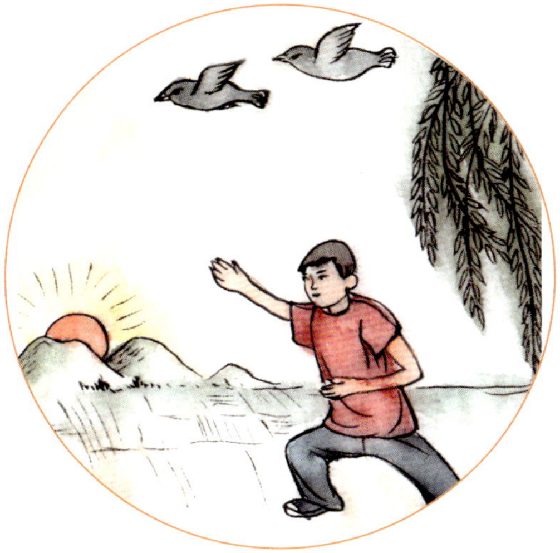

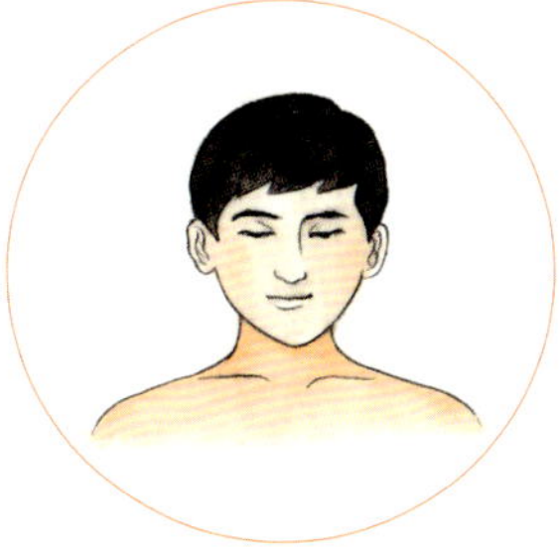

长夏在志为思

In a prolonged summer, one is emotionally susceptible to too much thought

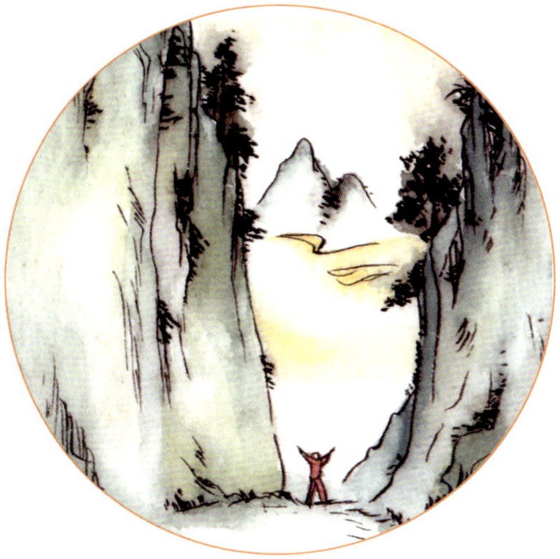

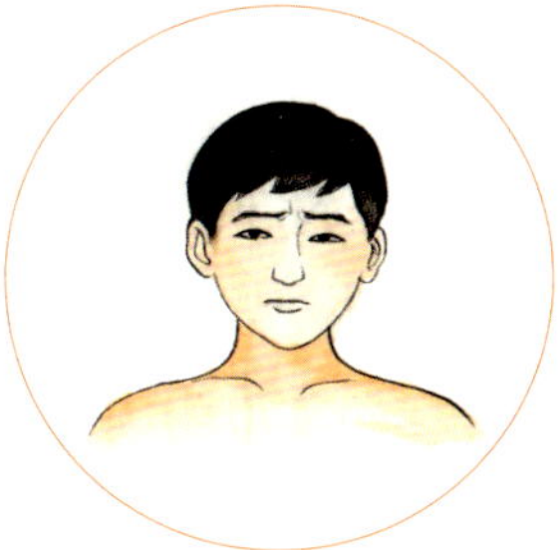

秋在志为忧

In autumn, one is emotionally susceptible to anxiety

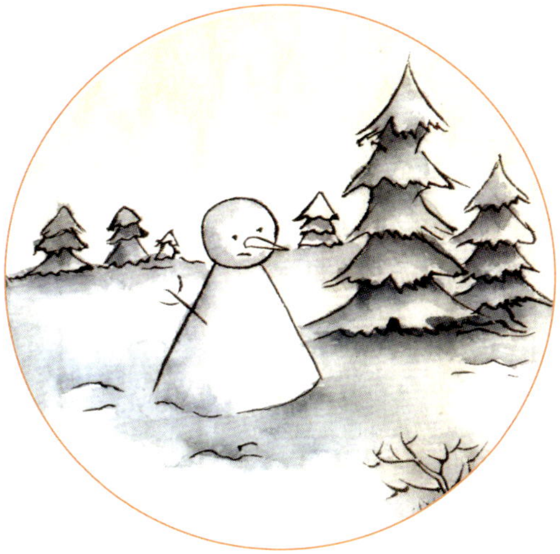

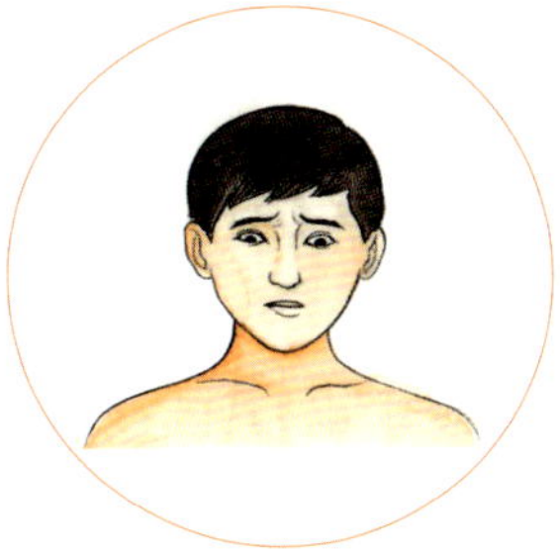

冬在志为恐

In winter, one is emotionally susceptible to fear

养生要随自然变化调节情志。

Health preservation requires the adjustment of moods according to the change of nature.

五官调护

The nursing of facial features

每日早、中、晚梳头，由前到后，再由后至前；由左向右，再由右向左，如此循环往复，梳头数十次至五十次。头部按摩可疏通经络，流畅气血。面部按摩可在每天早晨起床或临睡前进行，两手并拢，从鼻翼两侧开始上推至前额，然后两手分开沿面颊推下，反复进行，以使面部感到温热为度。此法简便易行，持之以恒，既可美容又能延寿。

We can comb our hair in the morning, at noon and at night, first from front to rear, from back to front, and then from left to right, from right to left, repeating again and again for dozens of times. Head massage can make blood flow smoothly. Face massage can be conducted in the morning while getting up, or before going to sleep. The method is as follows: put hands together, starting from both sides of the nose, push upwards to the forehead, and then push along the cheeks with separate hands, repeat until the face feels warm. The method is simple and easy, if persisted, it can make us beautiful and prolong our life.

口：要讲究口腔卫生，“津宜常咽”、“齿宜常叩”。

We should pay attention to oral hygiene, “salvia should always be swallowed,” and “it is healthy to practice often upper teeth knocking lower teeth.”

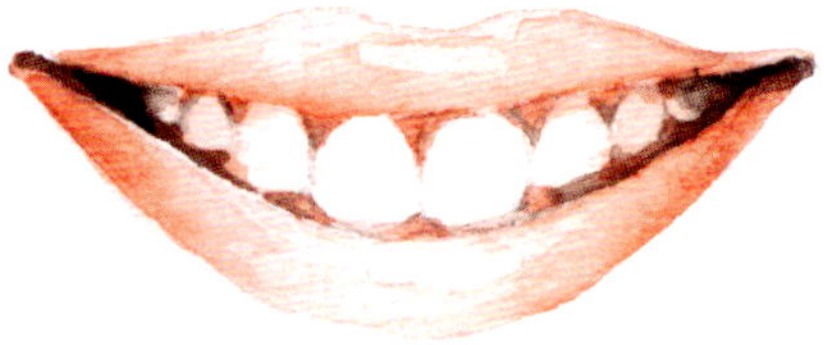

健康的口齿

Healthy mouth and teech

目：“养目力者，常瞑。”此外，“运睛”也是养目的方法，双目之珠从左转向右，再从右转到左。转睛要慢，转结应紧闭少时，再突然大睁。如此数次，能去内障外翳，纠正近视、远视。

To protect the eyesight, we should often close the eyes. “Moving the eyeballs” is also recommended, that is, to move the eyeball from the left to the right, and then from the right to the left. Eyeball movement should be conducted slowly and when finished, close eyes for a while, and then suddenly open eyes wide, which, if repeatedly conducted, can remove cataract and correct myopia and hyperopia.

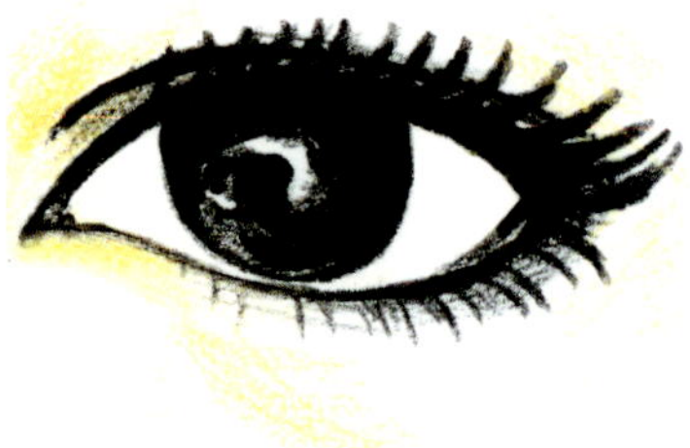

健康的眼目

Healthy eyes

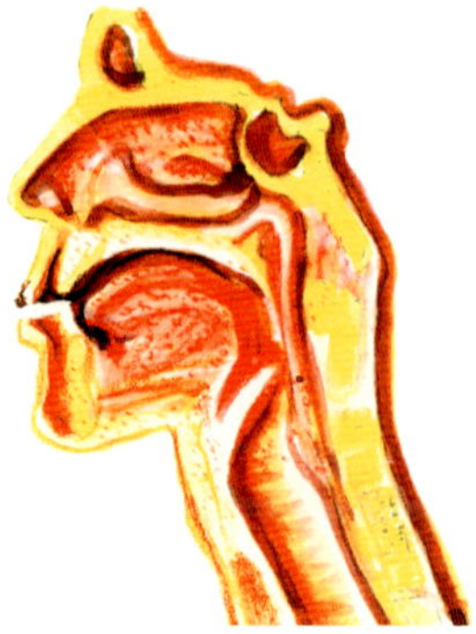

人的鼻腔与口腔、咽喉、呼吸道相通

Human’s nasal cavity is connected with oral cavity, the pharynx and larynx, and the respiratory tract.

耳：《遵生八笺》中有言“两手掩耳，即以第二指压中指上，用第二指弹脑后两骨作响声，谓之鸣天鼓”。

Eight Notes on How to Have a Healthy Life introduces a method to protect one’s hearing: “put your hands over your ears, with the second fingers pressed on the middle fingers, and then flips the back of the head with the second fingers,and you will hear your head bones sound, which is called ‘knock the bell of heaven’.”

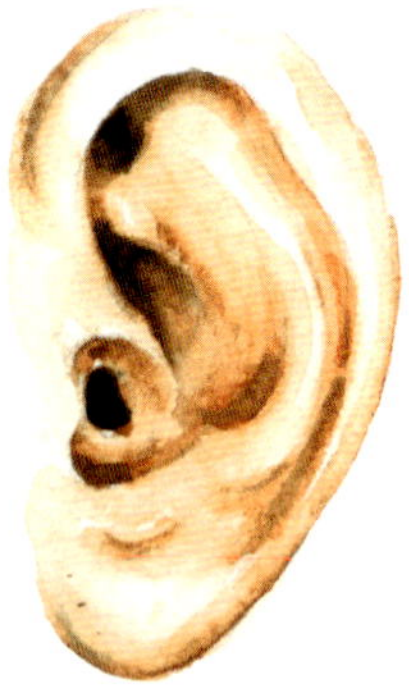

要保持耳部的清洁

Keep the ears clean

鼻：肺气通于鼻，鼻是呼吸道的门户，故中医学强调对鼻进行保健按摩，即用冷水冲洗鼻子，以预防感冒。

Nose: nose is the channel through which the qi in lungs travels. It also serves as an important gateway to the respiratory tract, so Chinese traditional medicine attaches great importance to the daily care and massage of the nose by cleaning nose with cold water so as to prevent colds.

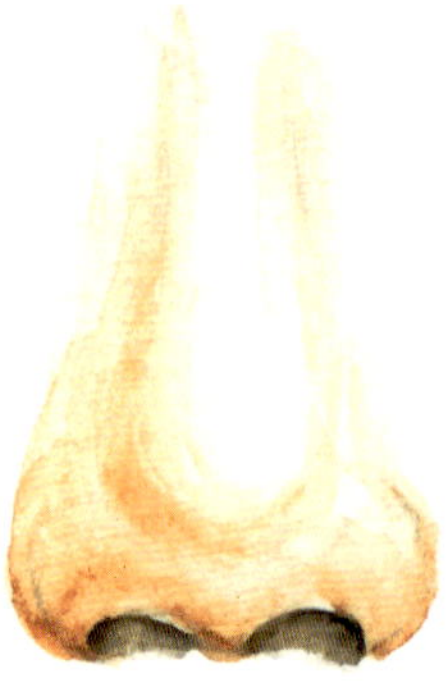

要保持鼻部的清洁

Keep the nose clean

五官保健功法

Exercises for the health of facial features

面部保健功法

Exercise for face health

1. 将两手掌互相摩擦生热，从下颏部起向上推摩面肌（图 1）。

2. 将两手食、中、无名指并拢，以两手中指按于唇下正中（即承浆穴），沿下唇向两口角（即地仓穴）推摩，再向唇上正中（即人中穴）推摩，反复 7 次（图 2）。

3. 以两手中指从鼻下、鼻翼旁向上推摩至两眉头，然后两手的食、中、无名指并拢，从额头正中线向外分抹，反复 21 次（图 3）。

4. 以两手食指揉按目内角的睛明穴 20 次后，沿下眼皮向外推抹至目外角，再从睛明穴沿上眼皮向外推抹至太阳穴，反复 14 次（图 3）。

1. Rub your palms against each other till they are warm, and rub them against your face from the chin upward (Fig. 1) .

2. Bring together the index finger, the middle finger and the fourth finger of each hand. Press your middle fingers on the middle point right beneath your lower lip (Chengjiang Point). Rub them along the lower lip toward the corners of your month (Dicang Point) and then toward the middle point right above your upper lip (Renzhong Point) for 7 times (Fig. 2).

3. Rub your middle fingers from the parts right beneath or beside your nose upward to the tips of your eyebrows. Then bring together the index finger, the middle finger and the fourth finger of each hand, and rub them from the central line of your forehead outward Do this 21 times (Fig. 3).

4. Rub Jingming Point on the inside of your eye sockets with your index fingers 20 times. Then rub them along the lower eyelids outward toward the outside of your eye sockets. Then rub them along the upper eyelids from Jingming Point outward to your temples for 14 times (Fig. 3).

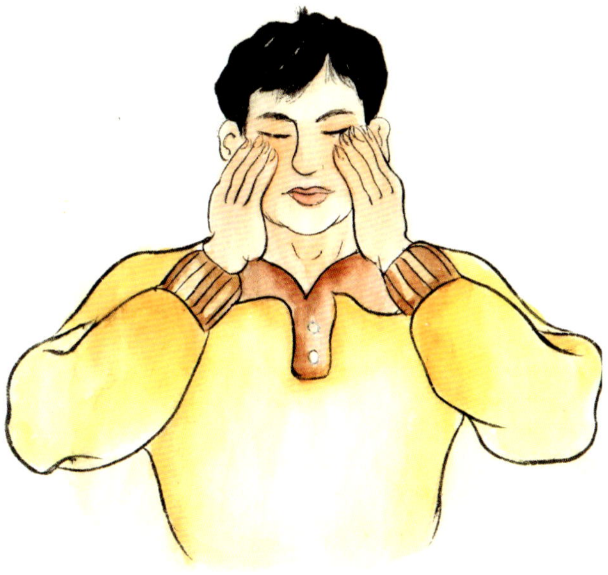

1

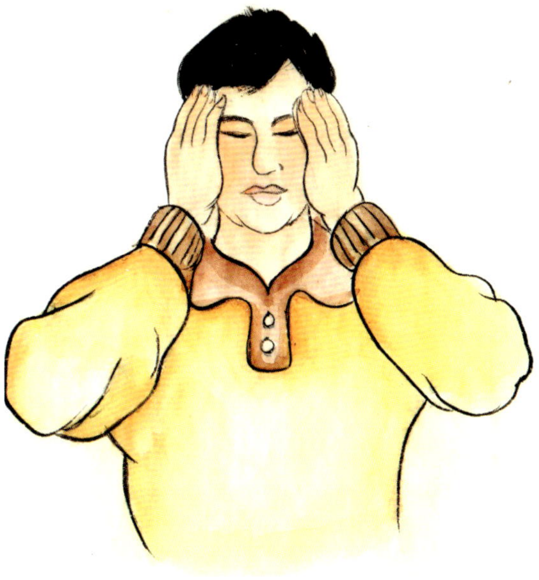

2

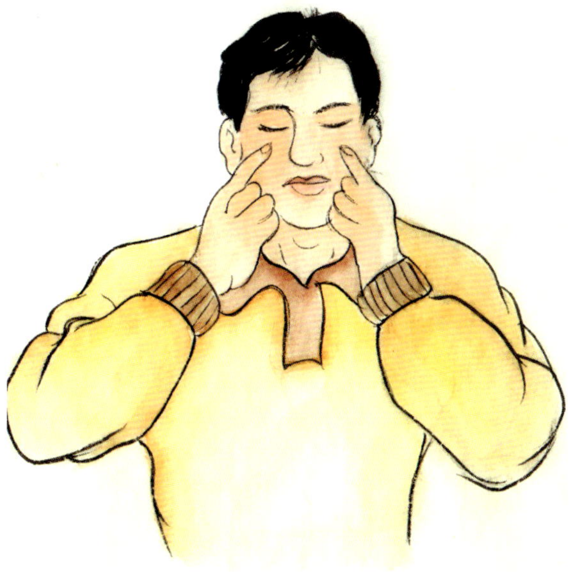

3

眼部保健功法

Exercise for eye health

1. 每天睡醒，先不睁眼，两手握拳，将两拇指背靠拢、擦热，或将一拇指背在另一掌心上擦热。之后，于目内眦慢慢揉按 14 次，再从目内眦向下，沿眼睛四周抹摩 14 圈。眼仍微闭，眼球向左暗转 7 次，再向右暗转 7 次，然后紧闭约一分钟，再突然猛睁双眼（图 1）。

2. 以拇指关节突起部揉按眉头外开 5 分处之小孔部，各 27 次。再以拇指背从目内角下沿眼眶下缘向外分抹 30 次（图 2）。

3. 拇指在前，食指在后，反复捏、旋两耳各 30 次。五指并拢，搓热，从眉心向外推抹至脑后，反复 27 次（图 3）。

4. 用舌舔唇、牙，待唾液多时，分数口咽下。

5. 以两拇指关节突起部同时按压两目内角，此时呼气并松手，直至自觉气运通畅时为止。

6. 跪下，臀部坐于足跟，两手按地，头先左后右徐徐后转，目视后下方，左右各 5 次。要求心神集中后转至最大限度（图 4）。

1. When you wake up every day, keep your eyes closed for a while. Make a fist with each hand. Put the back of your thumbs together and rub them against each other till them are warm, or rub the back of the thumb against the other palm till it is warm. Press your thumbs on the inner side of the eye sockets and rub gently for 14 times. Move them down and rub around your eyes for 14 times. Eyes still half-closed, turn your eyeballs to the left 7 times and to the right 7 times. Keep your eyes tightly shut for about a minute, and open them suddenly (Fig. 1).

2. Rub with the joints of your thumbs the point 5 centimeters from the tips of your eyebrows 27 times. Then rub the back of your thumbs along the lower edge of your eye sockets from the inner canthi outward for 30 times (Fig. 2).

3. Knead and twist both ears 30 times, with the thumbs at the front and the index fingers at back. Bring the fingers of each hand together and rub them till they are warm. Rub them from the point between your eyebrows outward to the back of your head for 27 times (Fig. 3).

4. Lick the lips and teeth with the tongue. When the saliva builds up, swallow it in several batches.

5. Press and rub the inner canthus with the joints of two thumbs. Exhale at the meantime. Let loose your hands until your breath flows smoothly and freely.

6. Kneel down and rest the buttocks on the heels. Put both hands on the ground, then turn the head slowly to the left and right while looking back and downward. Do this 5 times, turning in both directions to the maximum extent while keeping the thoughts focused (Fig. 4).

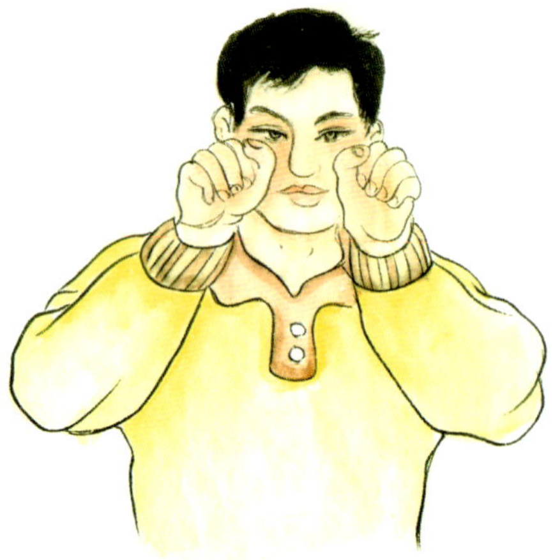

2

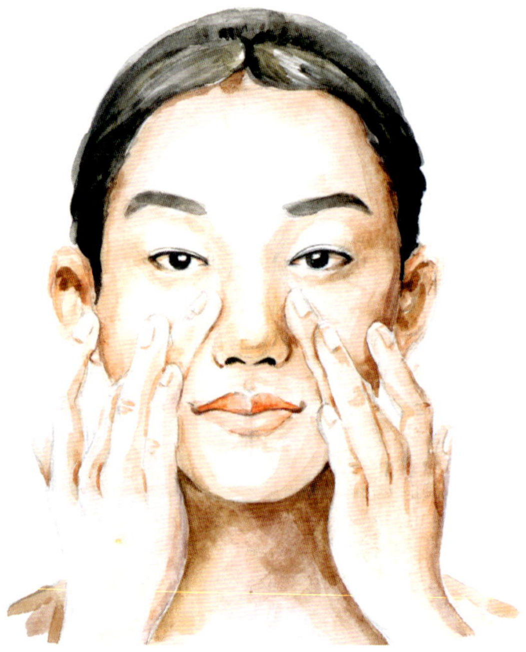

1

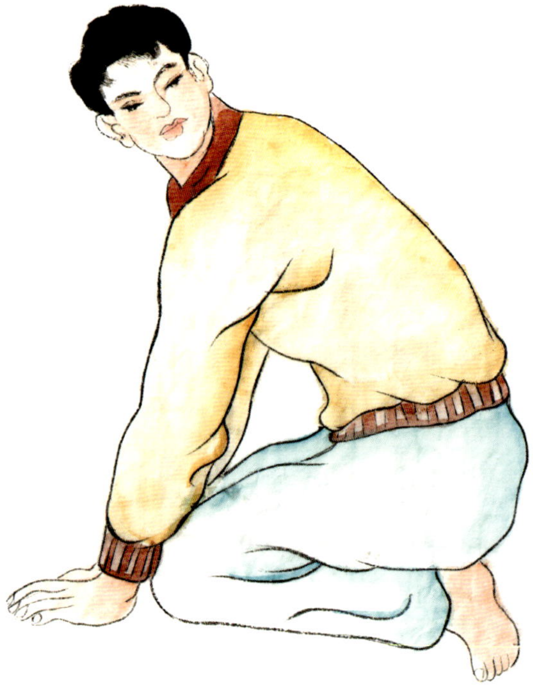

4

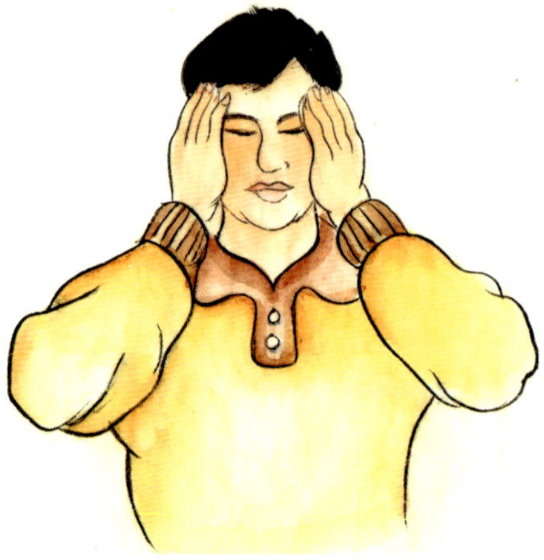

3

耳部保健功法

Exercise for ear health

1. 以两手分别按揉两侧耳轮，从下向上、再从上向下反复各 21 遍（图 1）。

2. 平坐于地，伸一足，屈一足，两臂向前伸直，两腕背曲，掌心朝前，如推门状，然后头向左，再向右缓缓转动，左右各 7 次（图 2）。

1. With both the hands, rub the exteriors of the ear helixes 21 times first from bottom to up and then from top to bottom (Fig. 1).

2. Sit on the ground, with one leg reaching out and the other bent. Stretch the arms forward horizontally, with the palms facing forward as if you are pushing a gate open with your hands. Then slowly turn your head leftward 7 times and then rightward 7 times (Fig. 2).

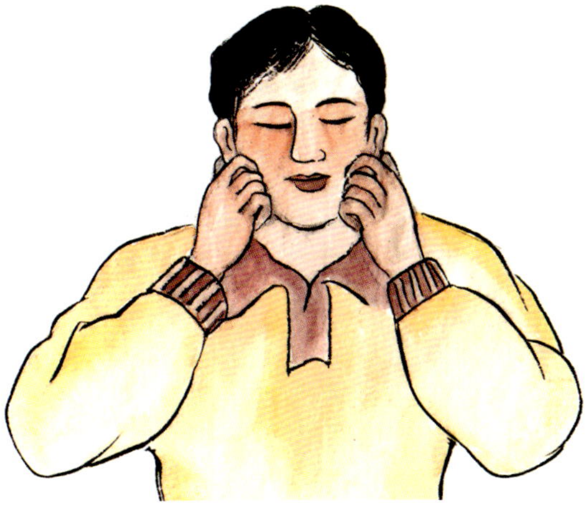

1

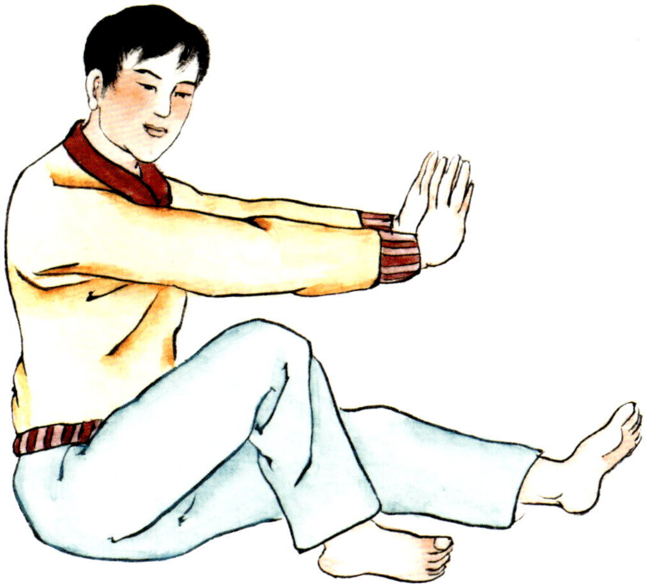

2

鼻部保健功法

Exercise for nose health

1. 将双手食指互相擦热，沿鼻两侧作上下揩擦 36 次（图 3）。

2. 每晚睡前伏卧去枕，两小腿成直角上竖，足掌朝天，用鼻缓缓深吸气，再徐徐呼出，反复 14 次（图 4）。

1. Rub your forefingers until it heats up. Then rub the two sides of your nose up and down with them 36 times (Fig. 3).

2. Every night, before going to bed, remove the pillow, lie on the stomach with the two calves upright and the soles upwards , inhale deeply with nose and exhale slowly. Repeat this 14 times (Fig. 4).

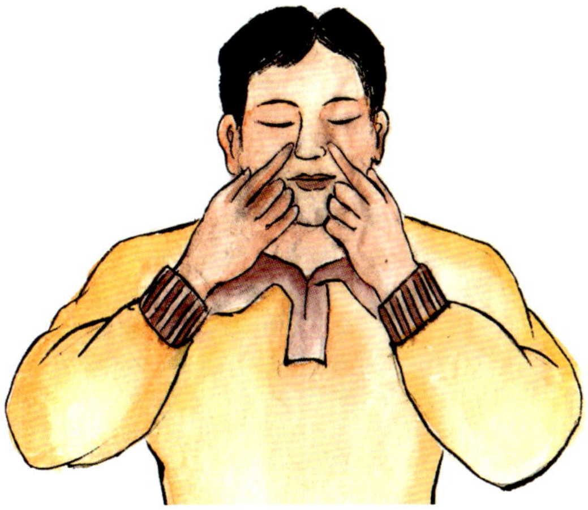

3

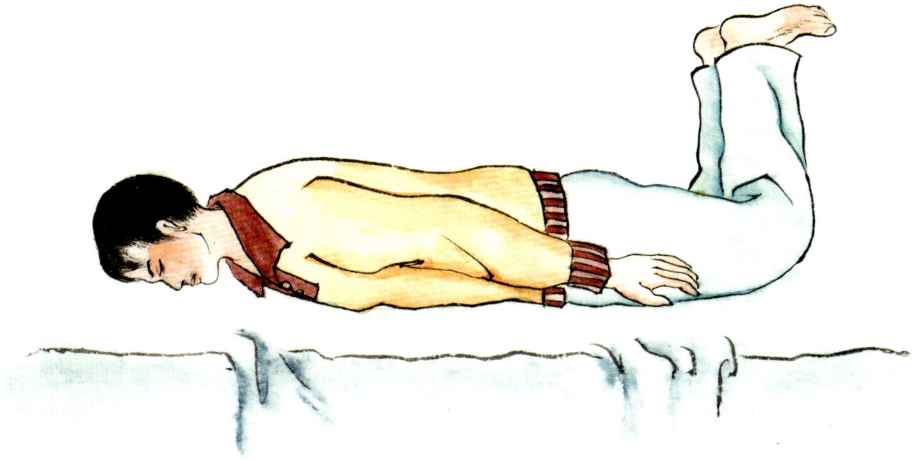

4

腿、足及身体调护

Caring for legs and feet

俗话说“人老先老腿”。调护腿足的有效方法有：

濯足法：即用热水泡脚。濯足可以使腿部血脉通畅，改善局部营养，可调畅周身之气血，消除疲劳，有助于睡眠。

腿足导引：干洗腿即揉腿肚活动。搓足心，“足心宜常搓”。中医认为摩擦涌泉，可滋肾水，降虚火，有镇静安神之功。

背宜常暖；胸宜常护；谷道宜常提。

腿部功法

Leg exercise

双脚并拢，伸直手臂前推，不屈膝直腰下摸脚面，双手前推起身，直推至双手掌心朝向天空，如此往复 3 次 (下图)。

Stand with feet together. Stretch forward the arms, and then bent straight down until your fingers reach the feet. After that, stretch your arms upward to the sky. Repeat this for 3 times (See picture below).

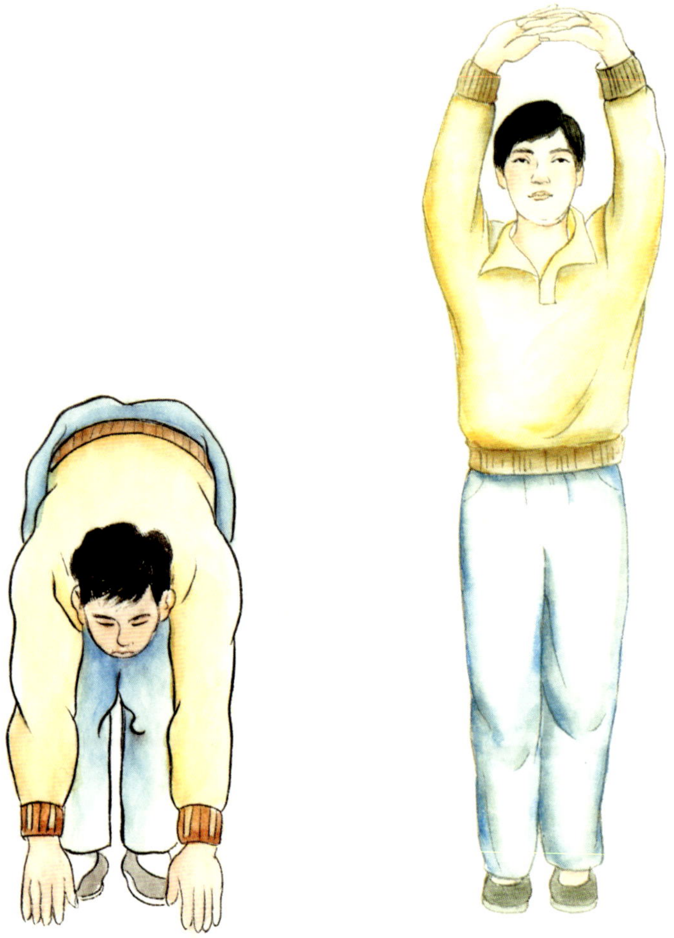

As the saying goes, "The legs are first old when persons are getting old."

Foot bath: a hot water foot bath may improve blood circulation at the legs, even all over the body; relieve fatigue, and help with sleep.

Leg-and-foot Tao Yin exercises: rub the legs; rub the calves; “The centre of the sole should be rubbed often”. Chinese medicine believes that rubbing Yongquan Point can nourish the kidney, subdue the excessive heat caused by a deficiency in Yin energy, and calm the mind.

Keep your back warm and the chest protected; often exercise the levator muscle of anus.

足部保健功法

Exercise for feet health

1. 正坐挺膝，伸直两足，上身尽力前俯，两手用力抓握足心 (图 1)。反复 12 次 (图 2)。

2. 坐于椅、凳上，垂足；两足跟相对，将足尖向外扭，再将足尖向内扭，使足尖相对。交替各做 24 次 (图 3)。

3. 盘坐，一手抓住同侧足趾，另一手反复揩擦同侧脚的足心涌泉穴 (图 4)，直至足心发热为止。之后，该脚趾上下左右动转数次。调手后如法反向练习。

4. 一足下跪，臀部坐于跪足跟上，两手向后撑地，另一脚用力伸、曲，连做 24 次再换腿如法练习 (图 5)。

1. Sit upright with the legs and feet stretched straight, then bend forward as hard as possible, and grasp the middles of the soles with strength(Fig. 1). Repeat the process 12 times (Fig. 2).

2. Sit on a chair or stool and let your legs dangle; put and keep the heels together, separate the toes of the two feet as far apart as possible, and then bring them back together. Repeat this process 24 times (Fig. 3).

3. Sit cross-legged with one hand grasping the toes of the foot of the same side; with the other hand, rub Yongyuan Point on the sole of the corresponding foot (Fig. 4) until the rubbed part gets warm. After that, bend the toes of the rubbed foot up and down, left and right, several times. Do the same exercise with the other foot.

4. Get down on one knee with the bottom on the heel of the bent leg. Support the body with the arms and then stretch and bend the other leg 24 times. Then do the exercise again after the two legs switch their roles (Fig. 5).

腿、足按摩法

Massage for legs and feet

屈膝而坐，两手从两腿弯外伸入按于地上，把两脚压在手背上，抬起臀部，也可同时行气（即臀部抬起时吸气并尽力屏气，臀部下落时呼气，反复做之）（图6）。

Bent your knees into a crouch, and then put your hands under your feet. Raise the hip and at the same time inhale; exhale when dropping the hip. Repeat the action (Fig. 6).

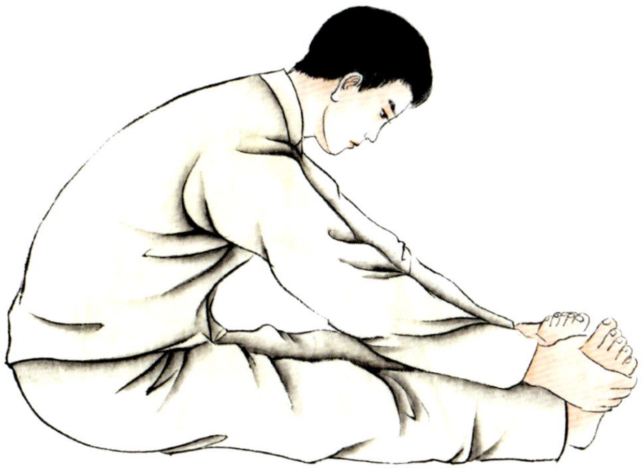

1

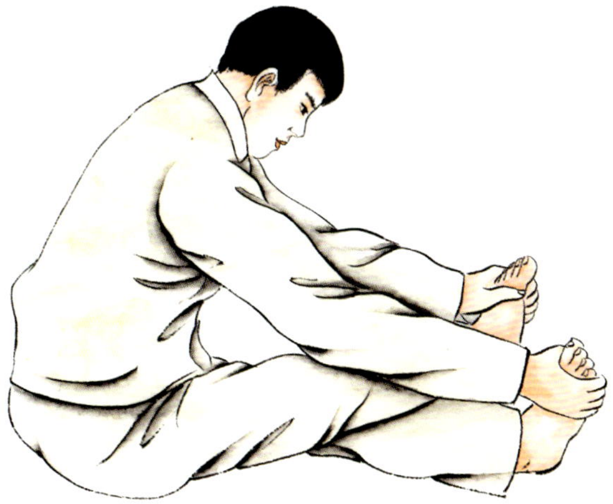

2

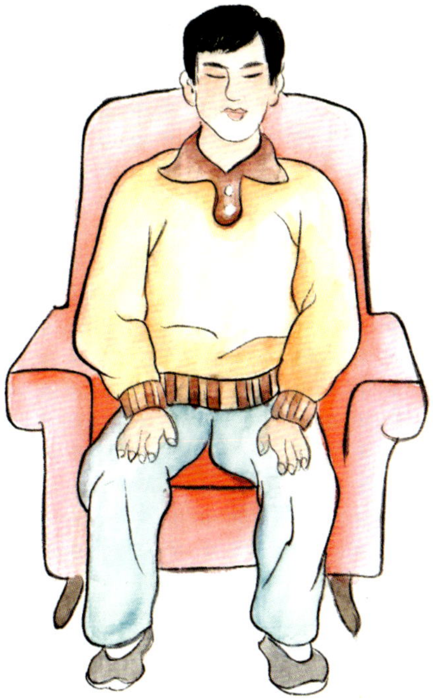

3

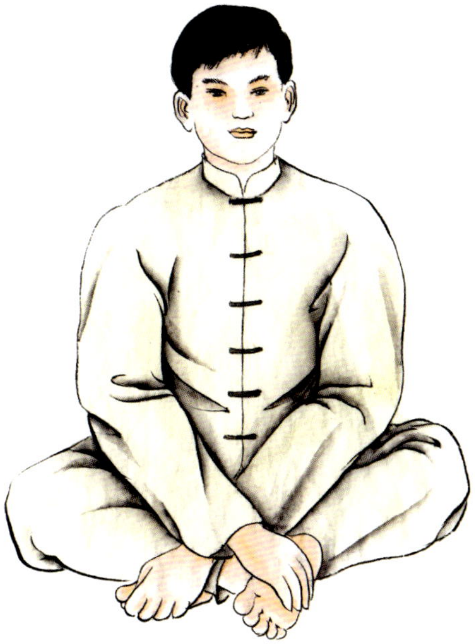

4

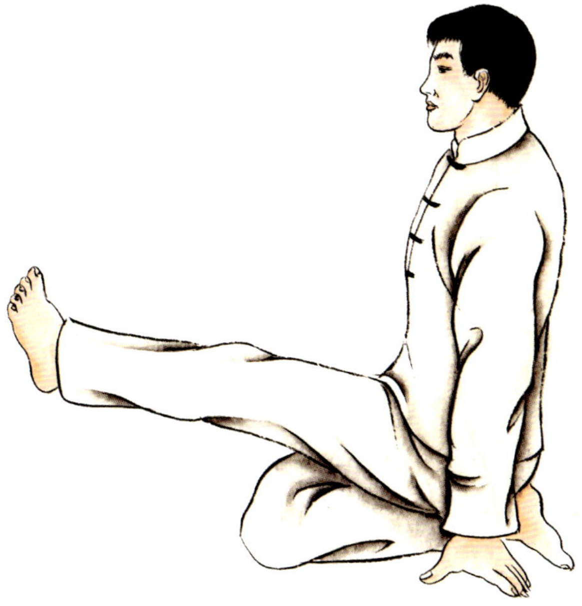

5

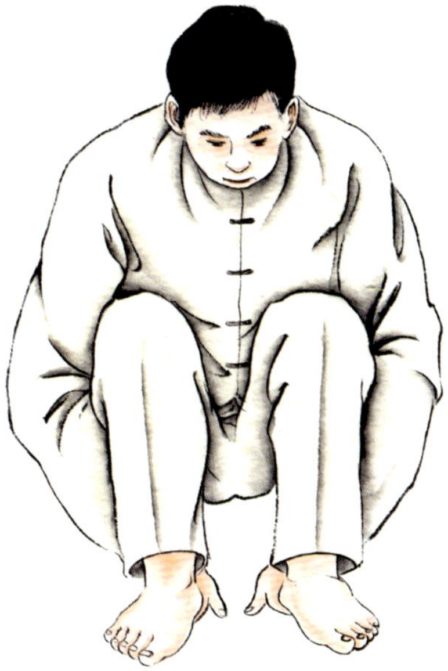

6

脏与腑

Zang organs and fu organs

五　脏

Five zang organs

“五脏“就是心、肝、脾、肺、肾五个脏器。“脏”在古代写作“藏”，有深藏在内和蕴藏之义。《黄帝内经》上称五脏“藏精气而不泻，故满而不能实”。

The “five zang organs” are the heart, liver, spleen, lungs and kidneys. In classical Chinese, zang, the character for “viscera”, has another meaning, i.e. “to hide inside or hold in store”. The *Inner Cannon* says that the five viscera “hold inner energy in store and keep it from flowing out; therefore, they can be full but not stuffed.”

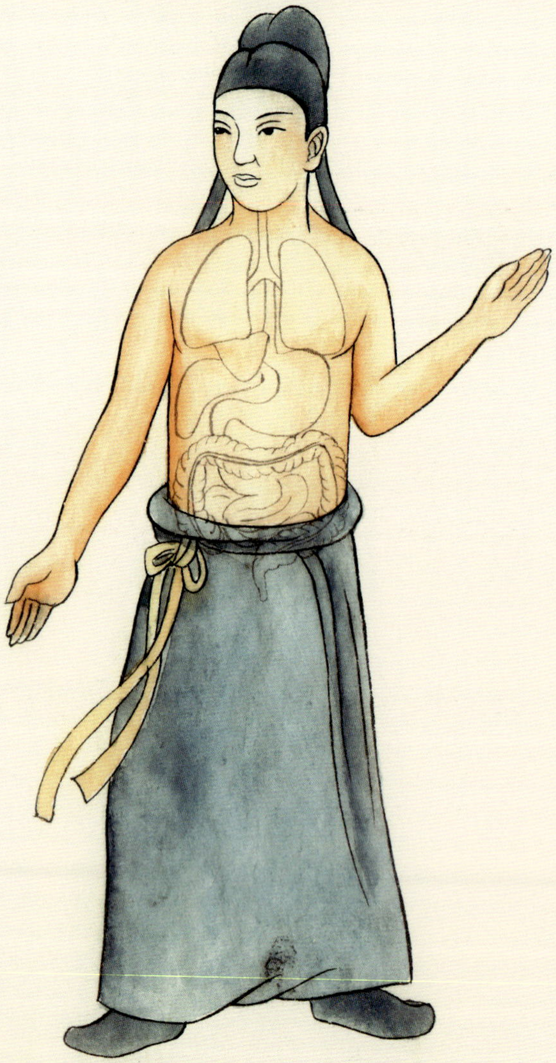

脏贮藏精气，如肝藏血，肺主气，肾藏精。五脏必须保持“藏而不泻”、“满而不实”的状态，才能充分发挥生理效能。

The zang organs are places to store blood and qi, for example, the liver stores blood, the lungs store qi and the kidneys store essence.The zang organs must be kept in a state of “full but not over flowing” so that they can fulfill their physiological functions to the full.

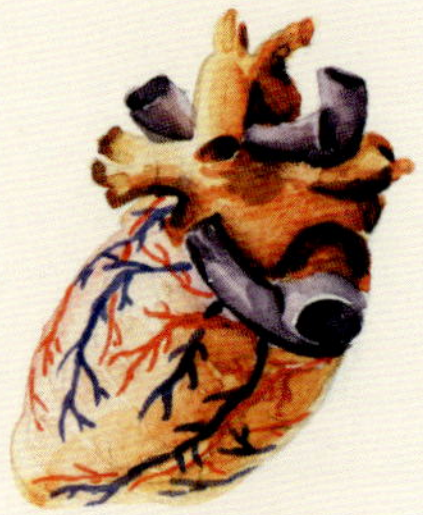

心
Heart

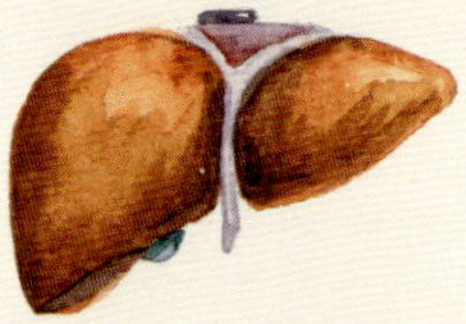

肝
Liver

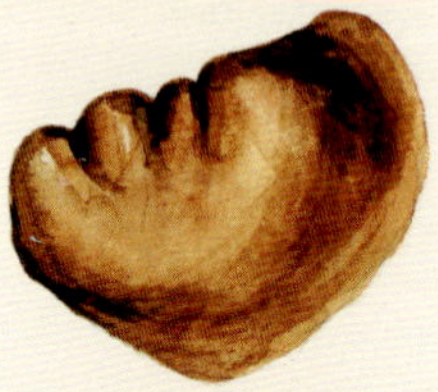

脾
Spleen

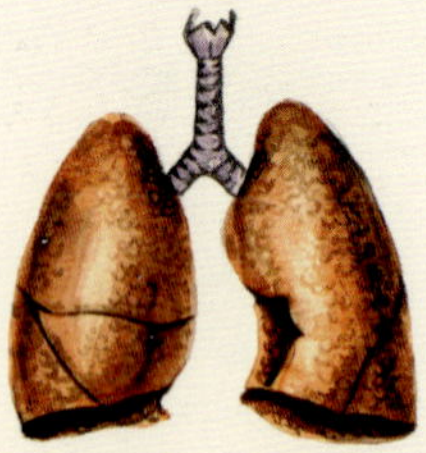

肺
Lung

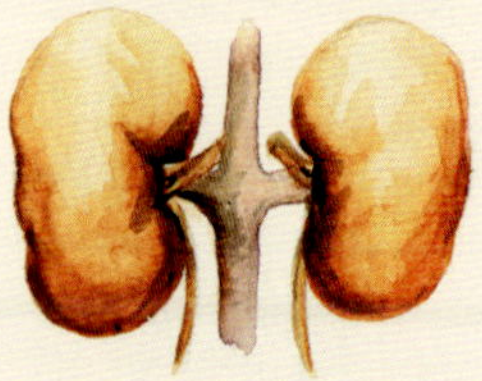

肾
Kidney

六　腑

Six fu organs

“六腑”是胆、胃、小肠、大肠、膀胱、三焦这六个脏器的总称。“腑”是以“肉月”为形旁，以“府”为声旁，指肉体房间，是储物之义。六腑容饮食。

The “six fu organs” are the gall bladder, stomach, small intestine, large intestine, urine bladder, and San Jiao. In classical Chinese, fu, the character for “bowel”, has a part which means “flesh”, with the other part meaning “room”. When the two parts are combined together, we can see that the character initially means “flesh room”. Thus the six fu organs are “flesh rooms” where drink and food are kept.

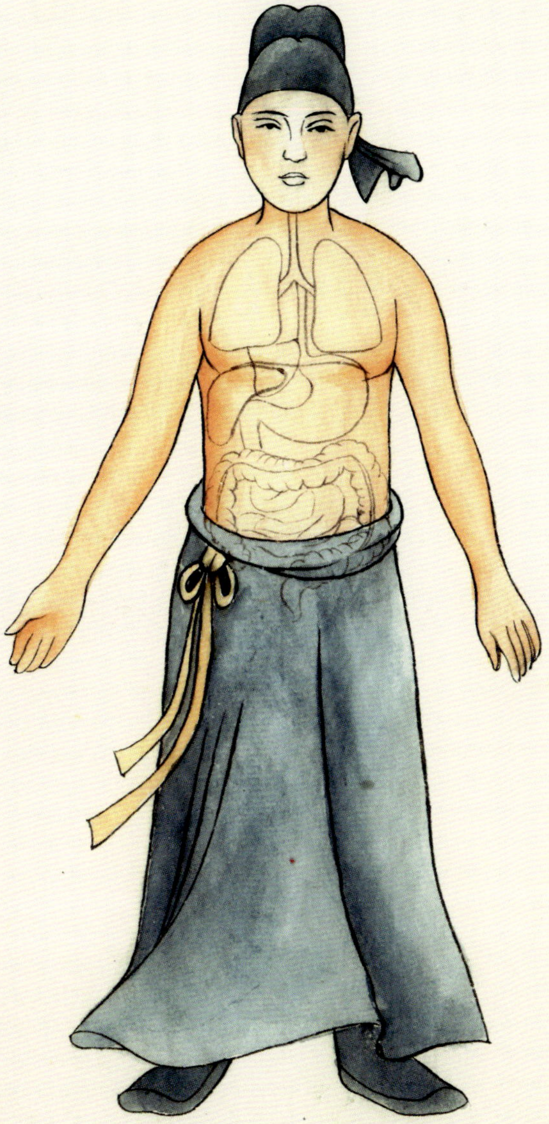

腑，传化水谷。如，胃受纳水谷，在对水谷进行初步消化后，下传入小肠；小肠接受胃下传的水谷，对其进行彻底消化，在吸收其精微后，将糟粕下注入大肠；大肠接受糟粕，吸收其中的残余水分，再将其传导至肛门排出。因此，腑除了有消化饮食水谷的功能外，还有及时将受益容纳的饮食水谷向下排送、为下一次受纳作准备的功能。

The fu organs are places to digest food.For example, the stomach receives food and digests it crudely, and then sends it to the small intestine; the small intestine receives what comes from the stomach and digests it thoroughly,absorbing the nutritional food essence and sending the waste to the large intestine; the large intestine receives the waste and absorbs the remaining water in it, then sending it to the anus to defecate. Therefore, the functions of the fu organs are not only food digestion but also timely transmission of digested food so as to prepare for the next reception.

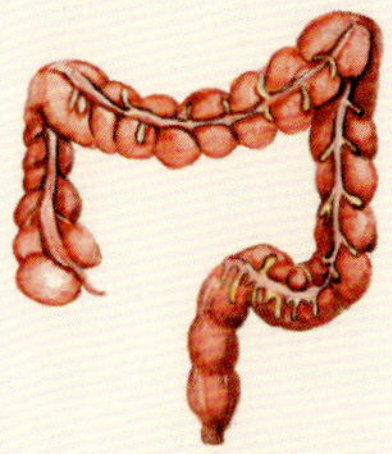

大肠
Large intestine

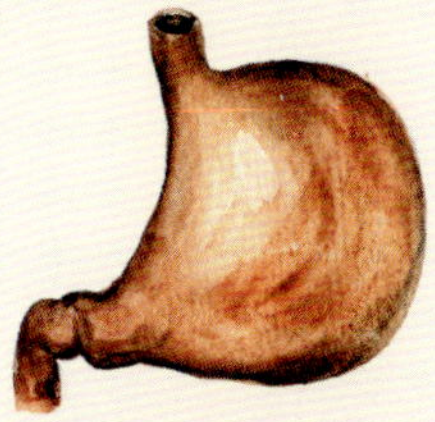

胃
Stomach

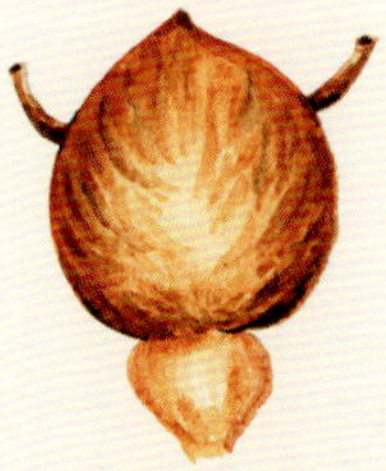

膀胱
Urine bladder

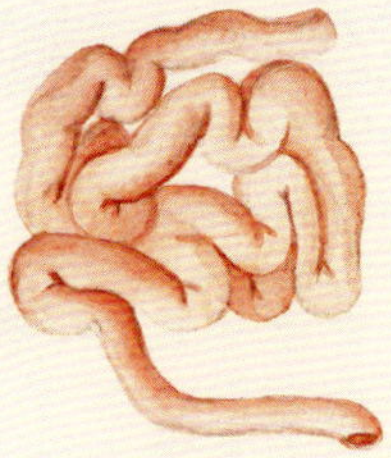

小肠
Small intestine

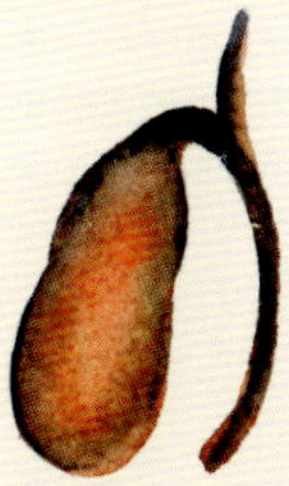

胆
Gall bladder

“七情”五志

Seven emotional states and five emotional activities

中医将喜、怒、忧、思、悲、恐、惊称为“七情”。
七情归纳合并之后为喜、怒、忧、思、恐，即“五志”。

In Traditional Chinese Medicine, there are “seven emotional states”: joy, anger, anxiety, contemplation, grief, fear and fright.

They are also reduced to the “five emotional activities” (of the five viscera): joy, anger, anxiety, contemplation and fear.

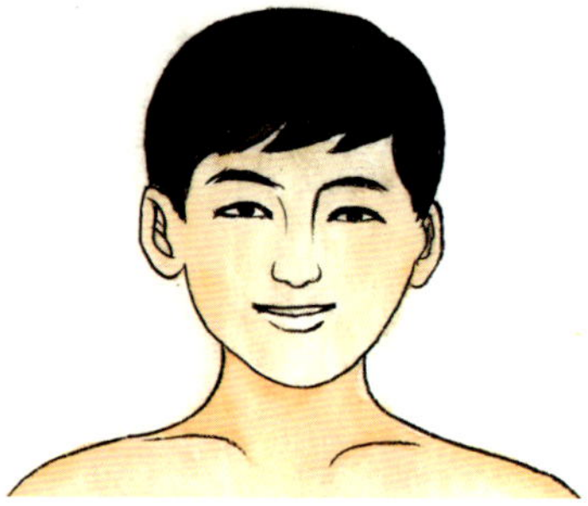

喜

joy

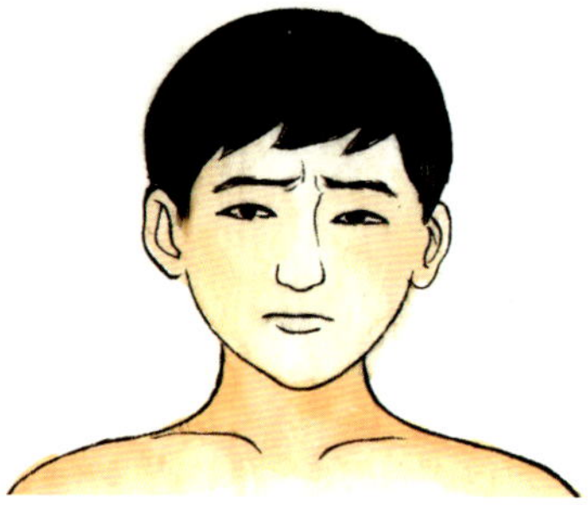

忧

anxiety

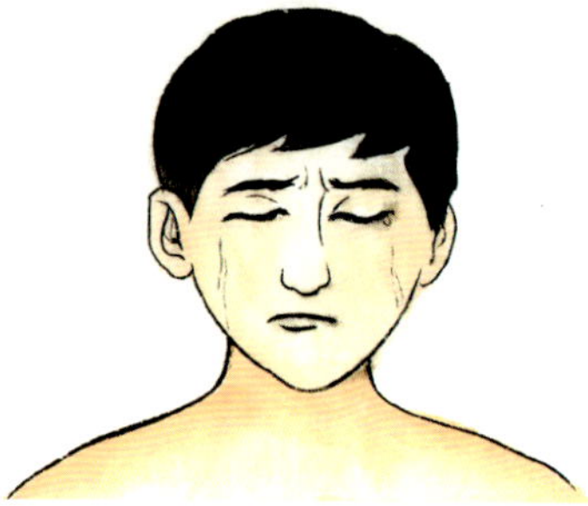

悲

grief

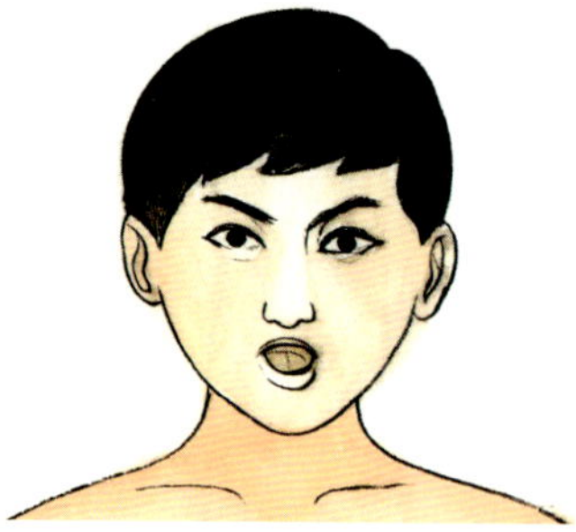

惊

fright

心志为喜

The heart corresponds to the emotion of joy.

脾志为忧

The spleen corresponds to the emotion of anxiety.

肺志为悲

The lungs correspond to the emotion of grief.

肾志为惊

The liver corresponds to the emotion of fright.

肝志为怒

The liver corresponds to the emotion of anger.

脾志为思

The spleen corresponds to the emotion of contemplation.

肾志为恐

The kidneys correspond to the emotion of fear.

怒

anger

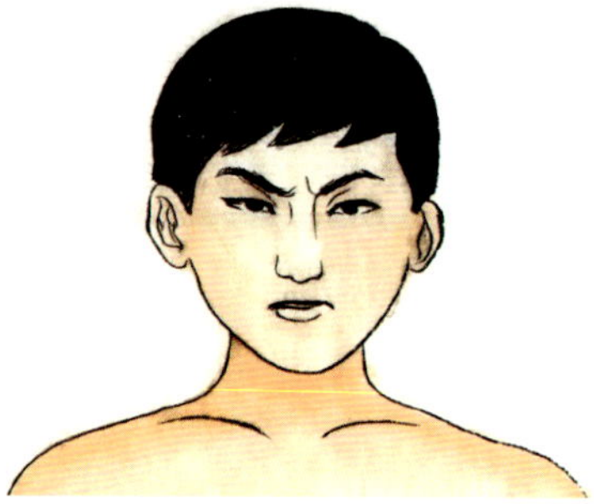

思

contemplation

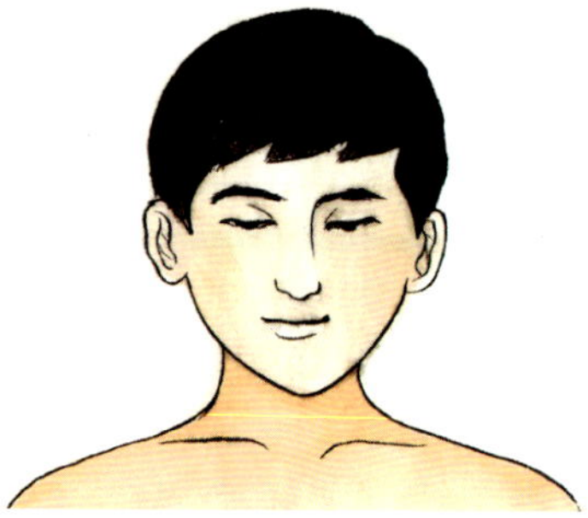

恐

fear

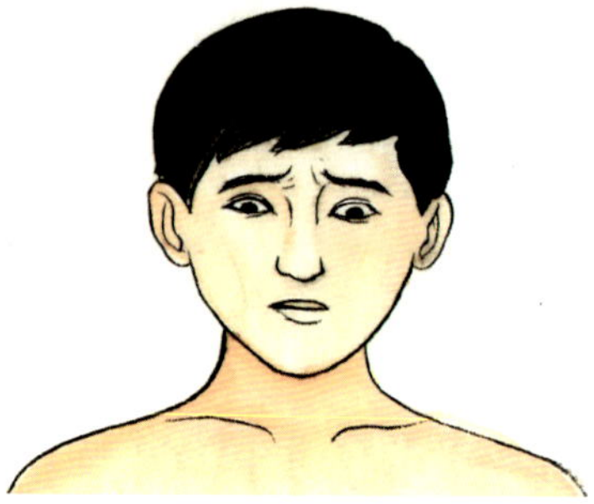

动静结合

The combination of the dynamic and the static

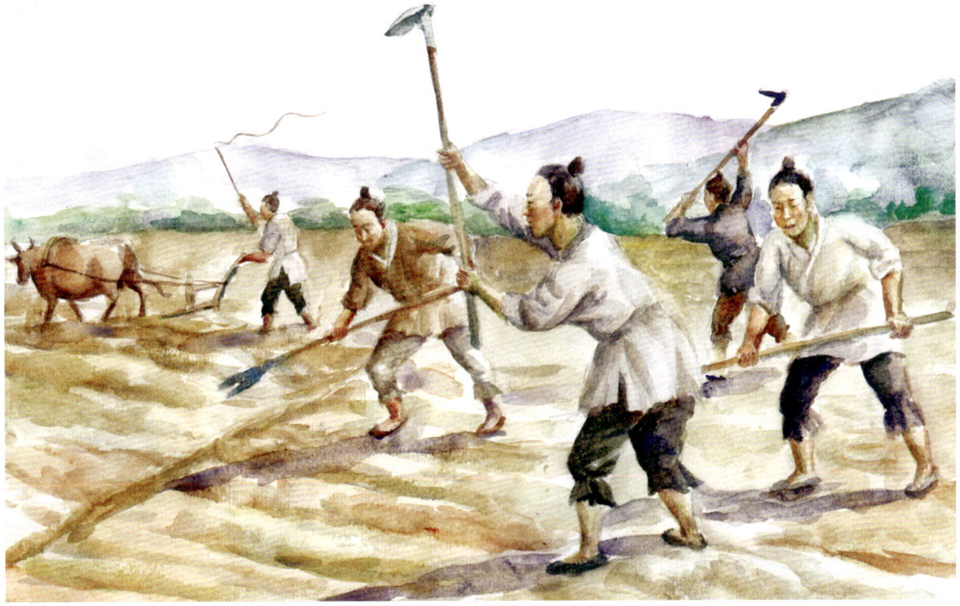

体力劳动可以延寿："服劳自动手"；"人欲劳于形，百病不能成"。我国东汉时名医华佗就指出，"人体欲得劳动，但不当使极耳"（《后汉书·华佗传》）；孙思邈亦提出"养生之道，常欲小劳，但莫大疲及强所不能堪耳"。

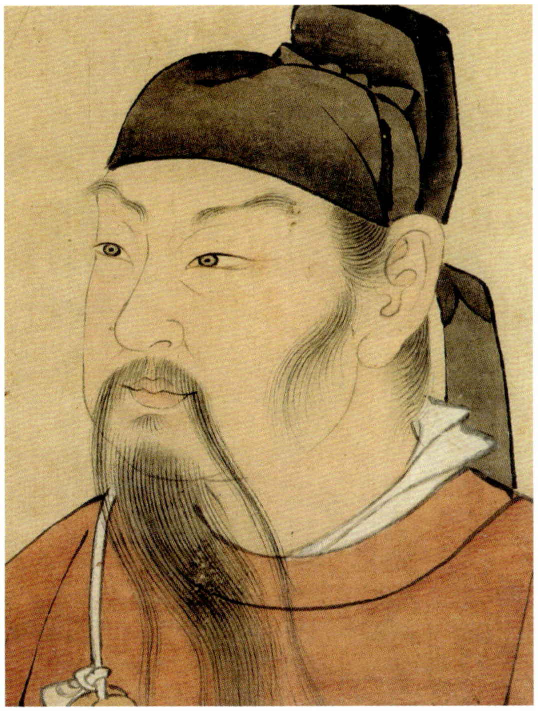

孙思邈像

Sun Simiao

生命在于运动

Life lies in movement

《吕氏春秋》说"流水不腐，户枢不蠹，形气亦然，形不动则精不流，精不流则气郁"；华佗更提出"人体欲得劳动……动摇则谷气得消，血脉流通，病不得生，譬如户枢，终不朽也"。

Spring and Autumn of Lv Family says that "Running water is never stale and the door hinge is never worm-eaten. So are the human body and qi. If the body is not moving, its fluid is not flowing. If the fluid is not flowing, the qi is pressed. "Hua Tuo also proposed that "one has to work... when the body moves the cluttered qi disappears, the blood circulates, and diseases are prevented, just as the door hinge never becomes worm-eaten."

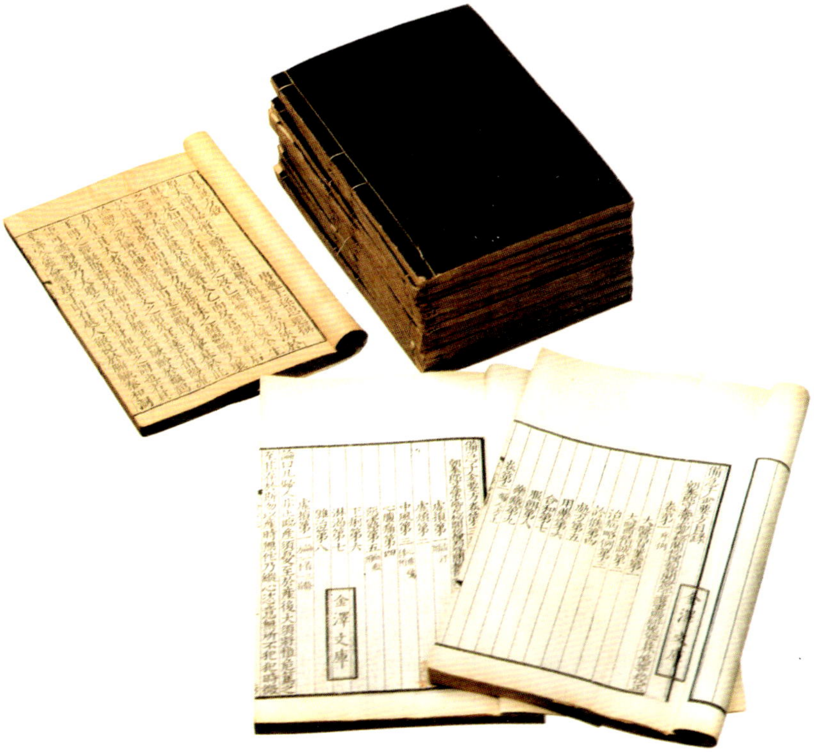

《备急千金方》、《千金翼方》书影

The Thousand (Taels of Gold) Formulas for Emergency and *Supplement to the Thousand [Taels of Gold] Formulas*

Laboring can prolong life: "Labor means do it yourself", "If one keeps laboring, he will be free from any diseases."

Hua Tuo, the famous doctor of Han dynasty in China, pointed out that "human beings should work but not beyond his limit." (*History of Later Han Dynasty: Life of Hua Tuo*) Sun Simiao also proposed that "regimen often requires small work, but great fatigue and work beyond one's limit should be avoided."

运动原则

Principles of physical exercise

生命在于运动。运动是人保持健康的最主要方式，是否有运动习惯在很大程度上决定了人能否拥有健康的身体。总结大多数健康人的养生经验，运动应注意以下几点：

1. 持之以恒：体育锻炼应持之以恒，坚持到底，特别要克服“三天打鱼，两天晒网”，才能收到良好的效果。

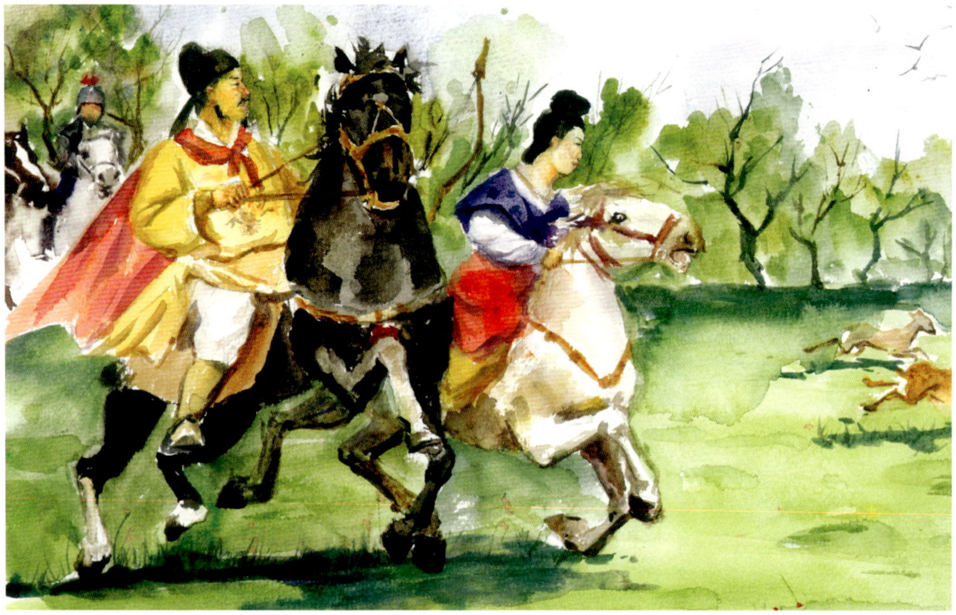

2. 循序渐进：体育锻炼应遵循循序渐进的原则，应以不产生疲劳感为度，逐步增大运动量。人的内脏器官、功能活动需要一个适应的过程，不能急于求成。

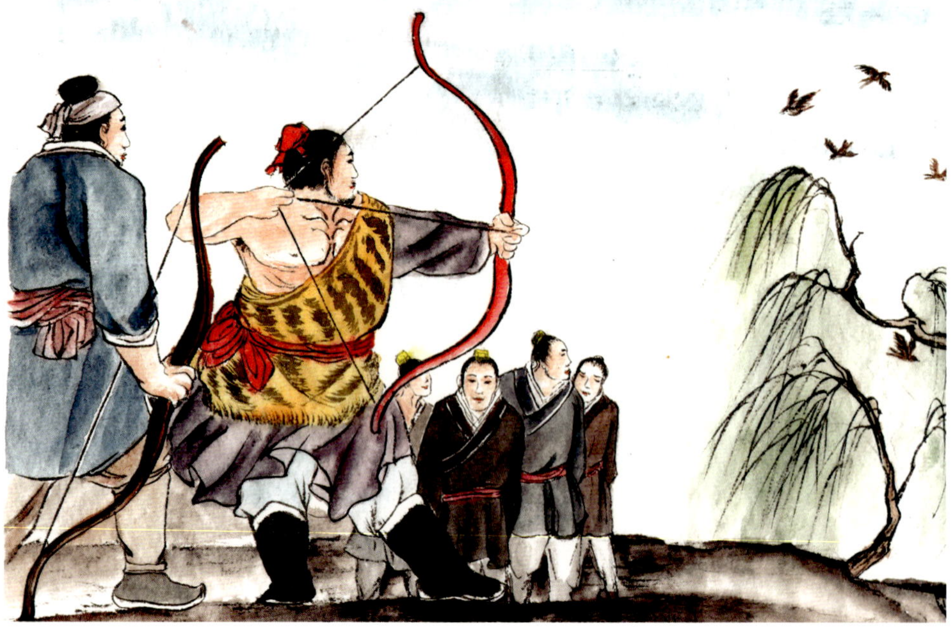

Life lies in movement. Physical exercise is essential to life, for it is the most important way to stay healthy. To have or not to have a habit of exercising is a major cause of good or poor health. Based on the experience of most healthy people, there are several points of advice to follow in exercise:

1. Persistence. One should exercise constantly and persistently. No good effect can be achieved without perseverance.

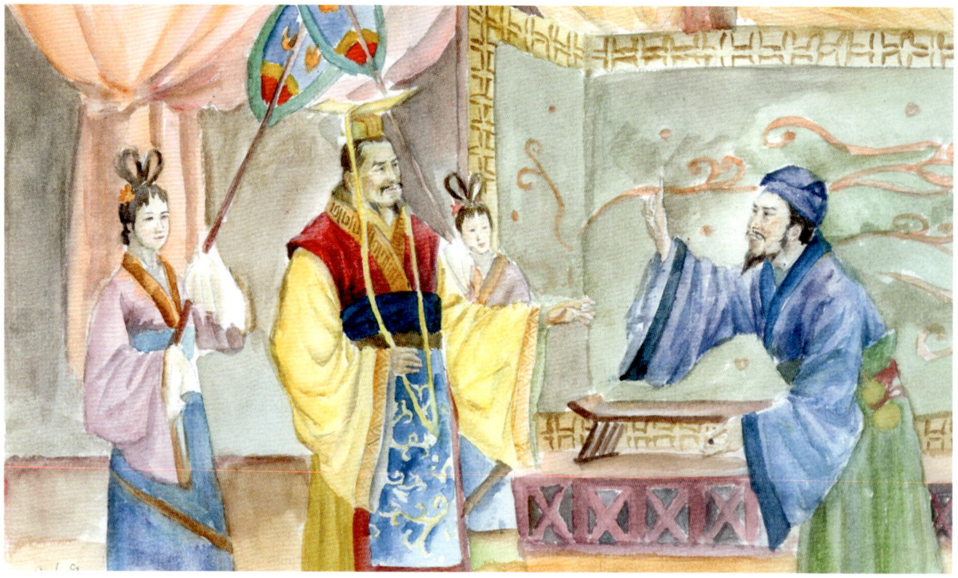

2. Step-by-step progress. Increase the amount of exercise gradually to allow your internal organs to adapt to it. Do not be impatient for results. Proper exercise is not supposed to cause fatigue.

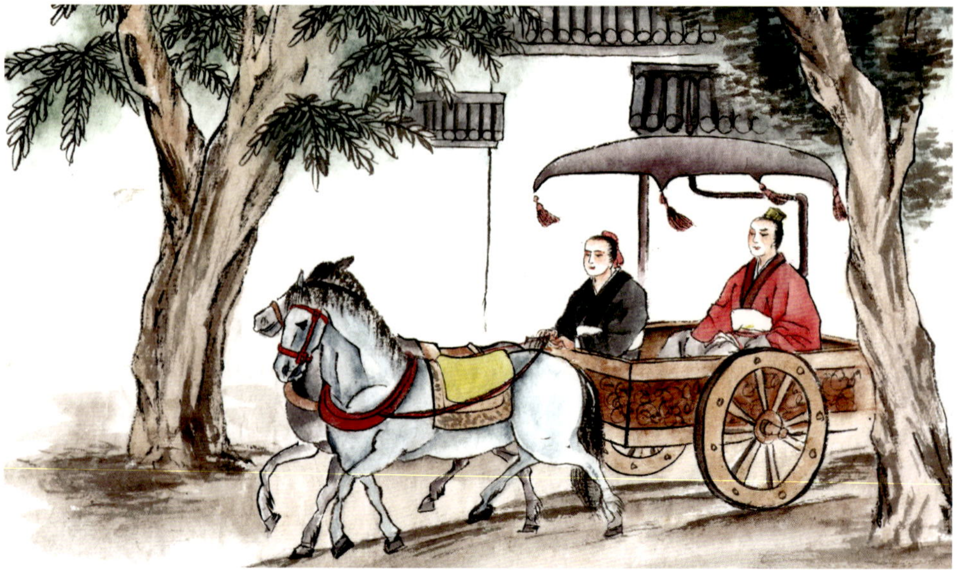

3. 动静适度：所谓动静适度，是动作应以“轻、柔、稳”为原则。在体育锻炼初期，宁少勿多，宁慢勿快，运动量要逐渐增加。

3. Proper intensity. Your movements should be soft, gentle and stable. If you have just started to exercise, don't do it too much or too fast. Intensify your exercise step by step.

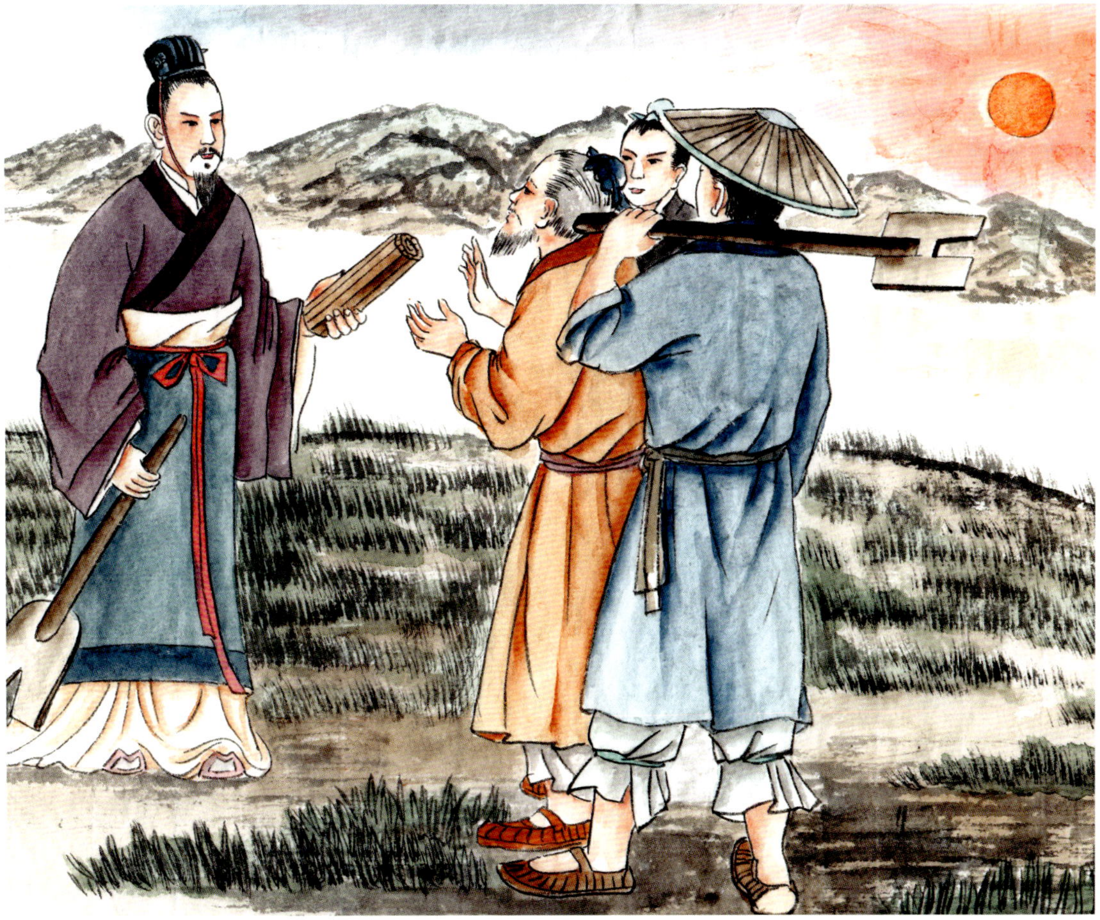

4. 运动时间：早晨空气新鲜，精神饱满，是锻炼身体的最好时间。饭后不宜马上进行活动，应休息 1 至 2 小时再进行锻炼。

4. Proper time. Early morning is the best time for exercise because the air is fresh and you are likely to be full of energy. Do not exercise after meal until you have rested one or two hours.

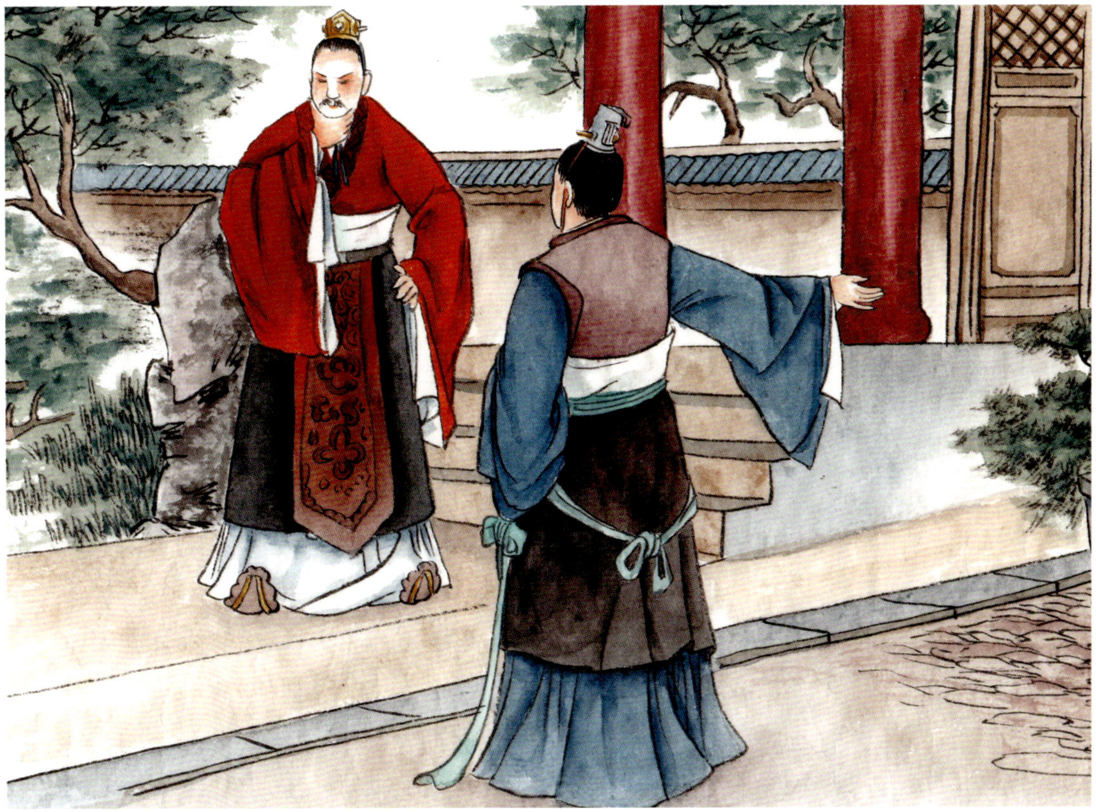

中国古代体育

Ancient Chinese sports

中国古代体育充分体现了中国文化注重人与自然和谐相处的特点。其形式丰富多彩，有蹴鞠、击鞠、捶丸、田径、摔跤、放风筝、荡秋千等，充满了中国文化的智慧。

Ancient Chinese sports are a convincing example of Chinese culture's love for life, inclination for nature and pursuit of harmony. Ancient Chinese sports are various: Cuju (which is regarded as the origin of ancient football), Jiju (like today's polo), Chuiwan (like today's hockey), track and field games, wrestling, kite playing, swing playing, etc. Ancient Chinese games, too, are replete with wisdom of Chinese culture.

一、骑马

1. Riding

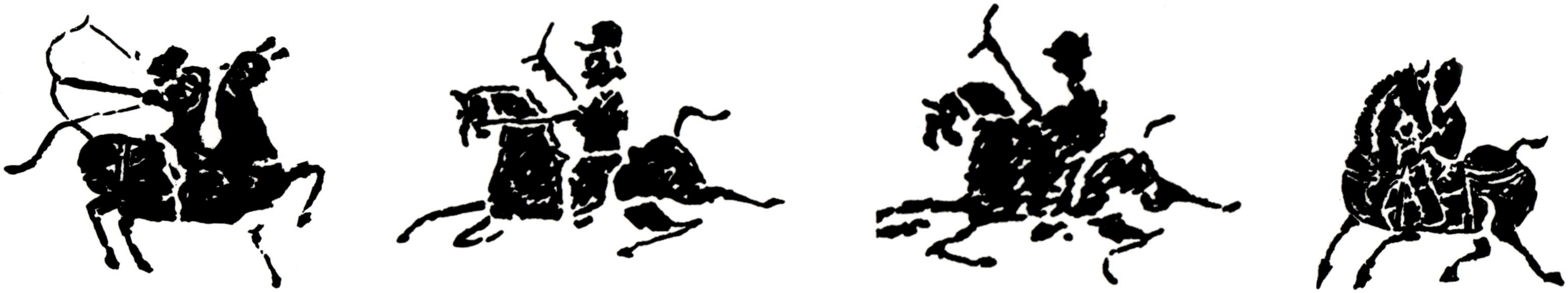

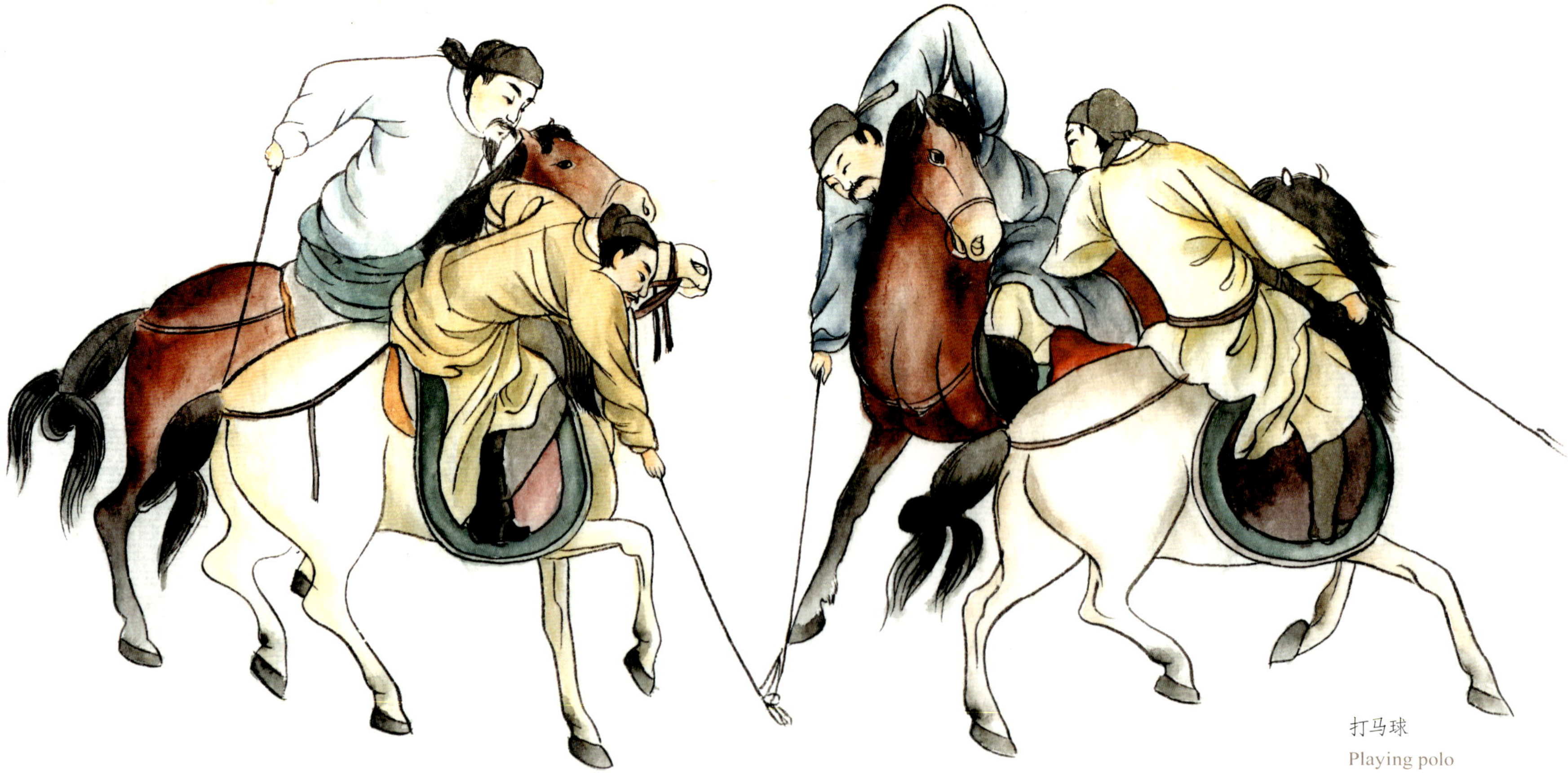

打马球

Playing polo

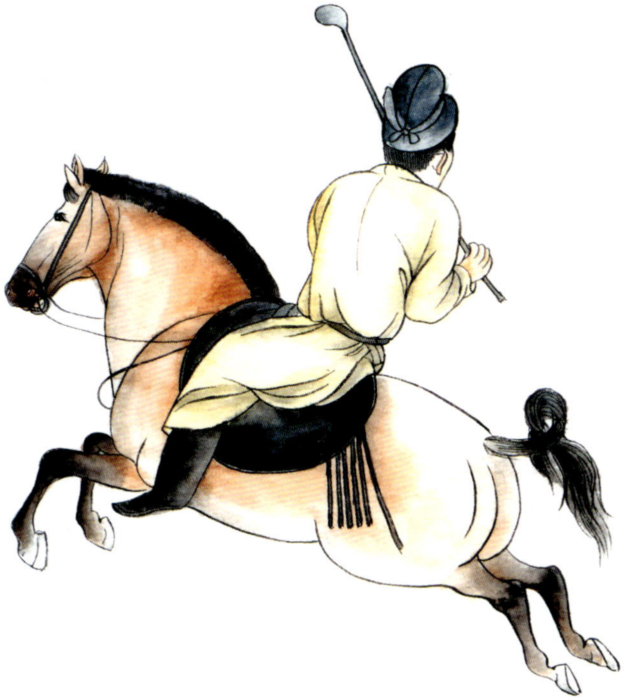

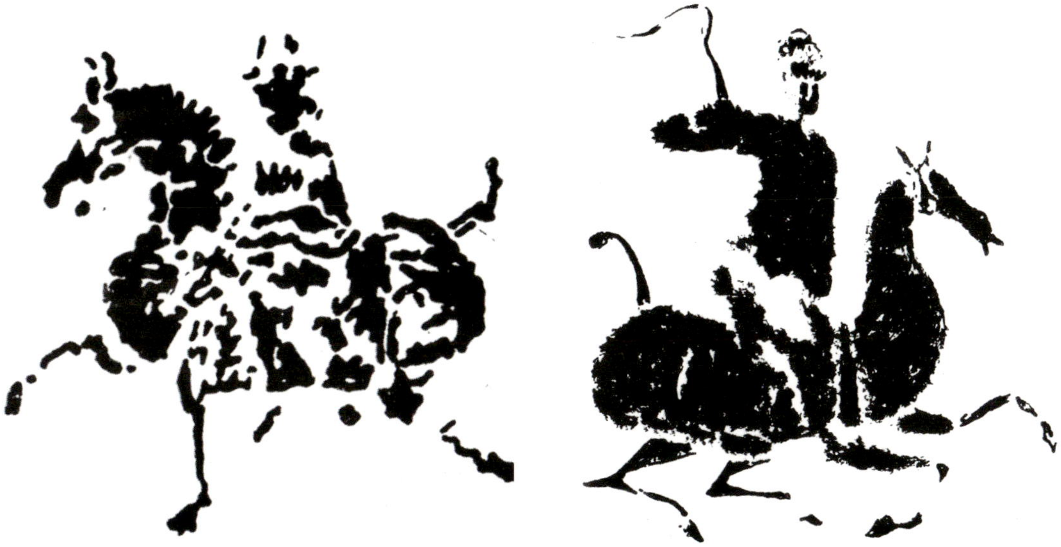

打马球

Playing polo

二、双陆、蹴鞠

2. Shuanglu and Cuju

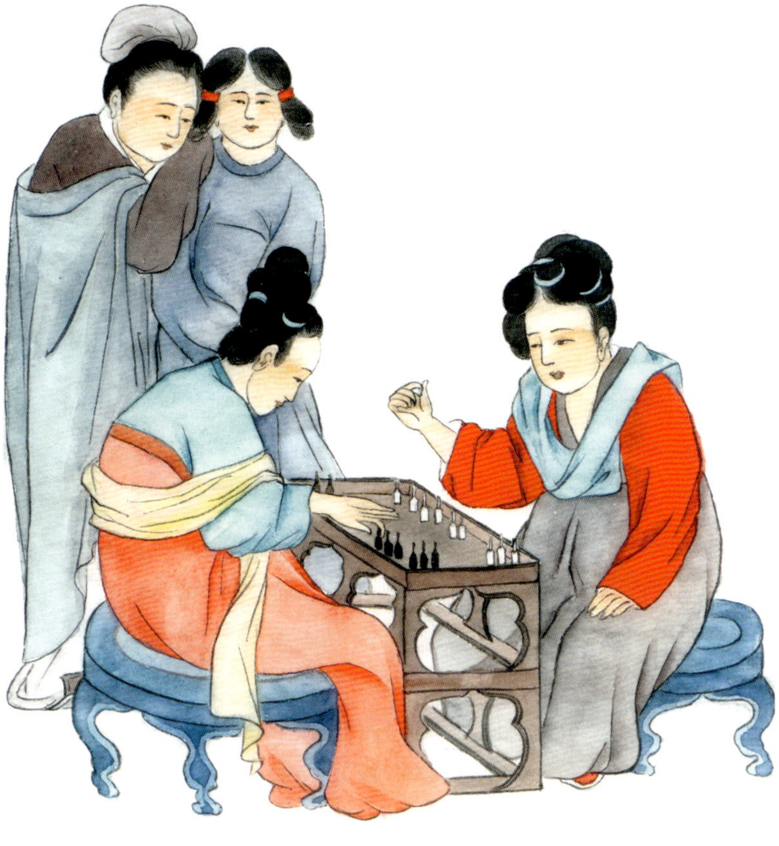

双陆

Shuanglu

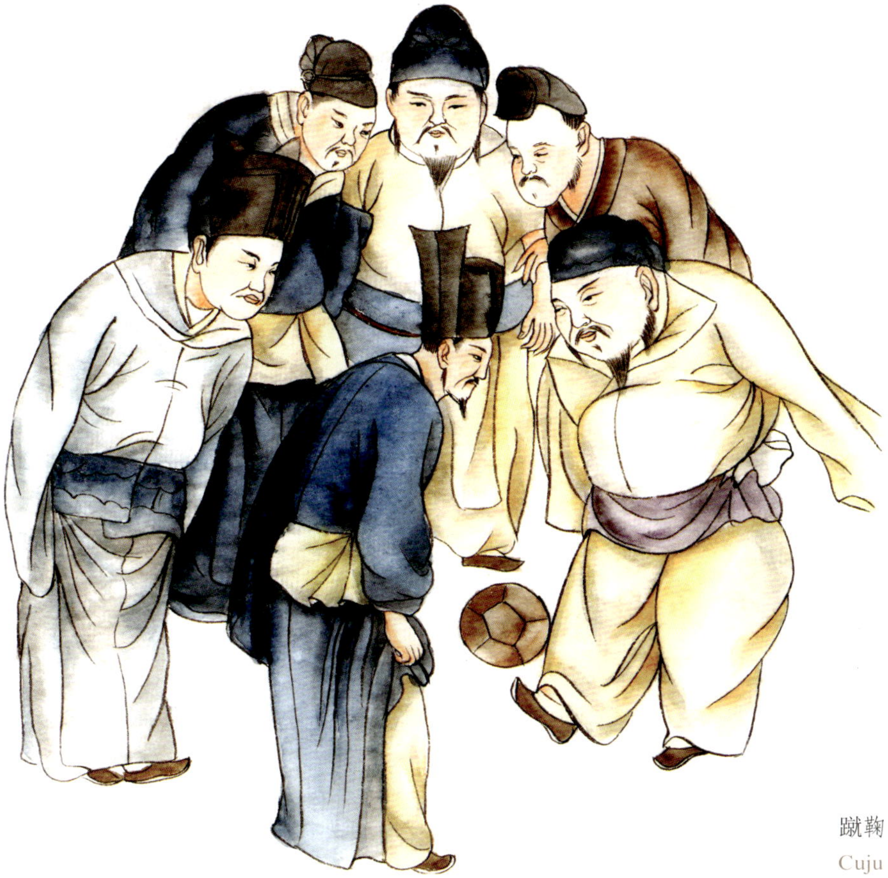

蹴鞠

Cuju

三、武术

3. Wushu

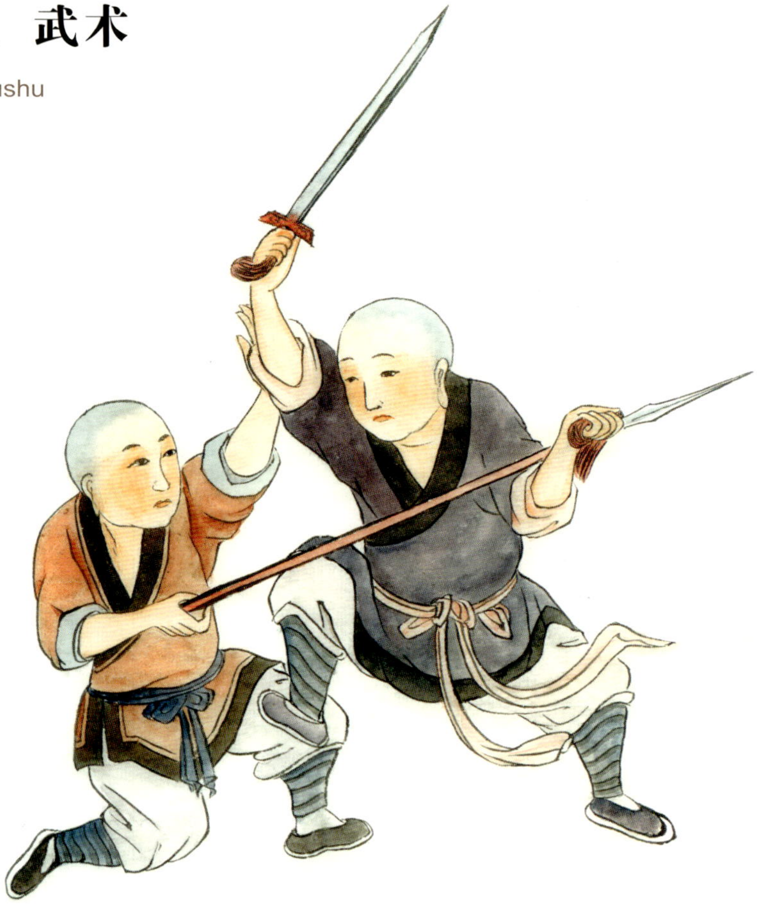

刀枪对练

Sword and spear exercise

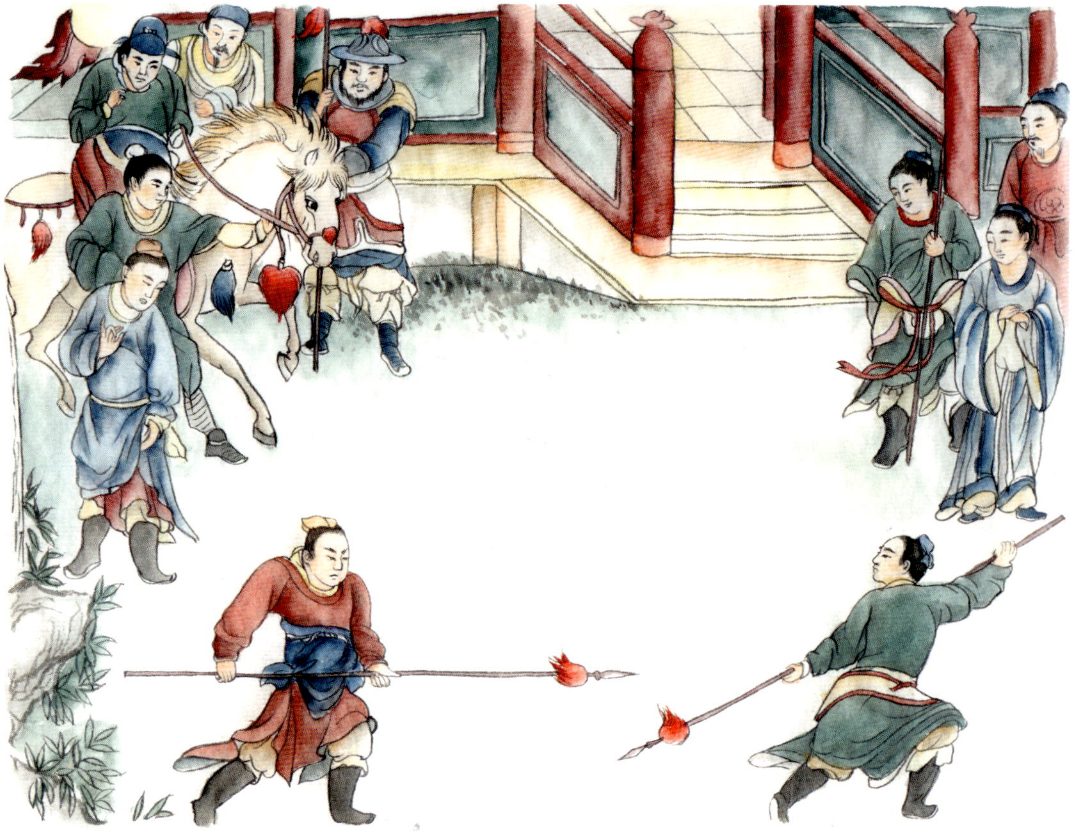

枪术

Spear exercise

四、摔跤

4. Wrestling

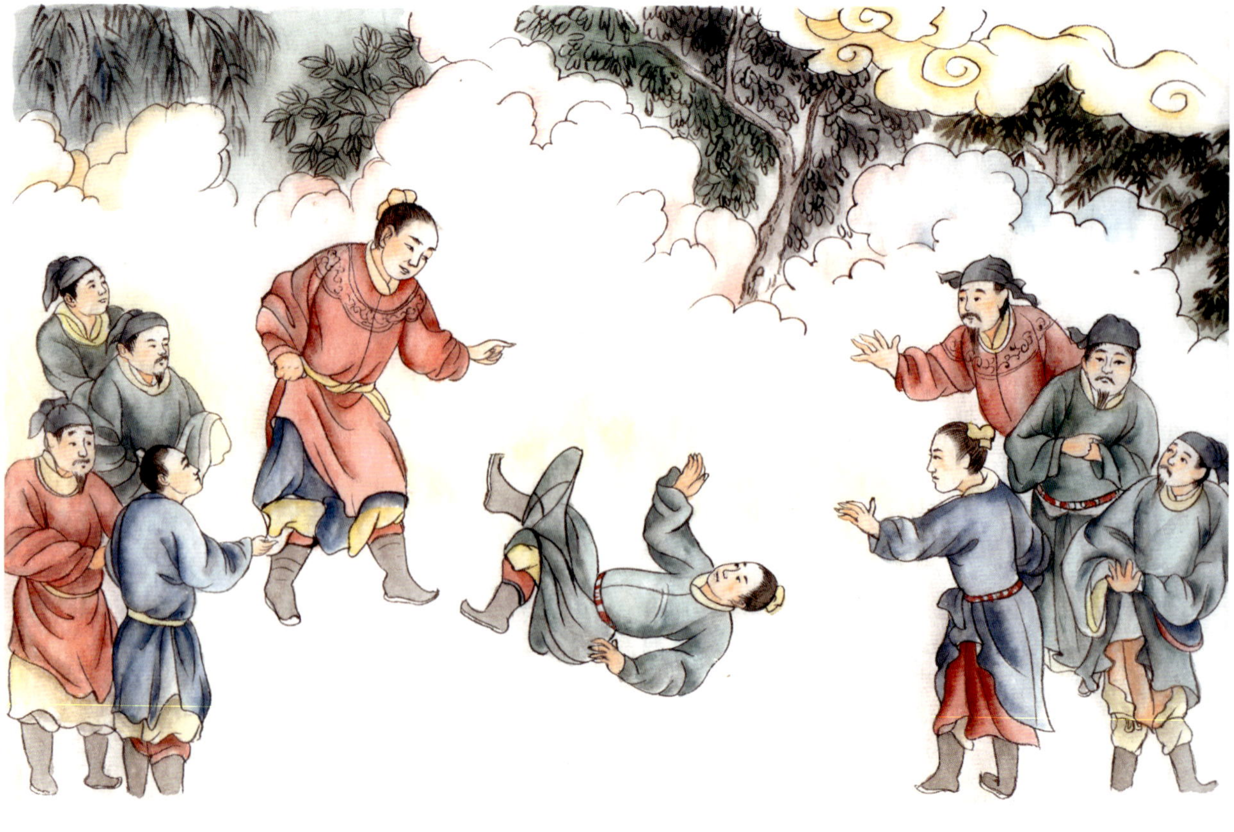

五、打球、荡秋千

5. Ball playing and swing playing

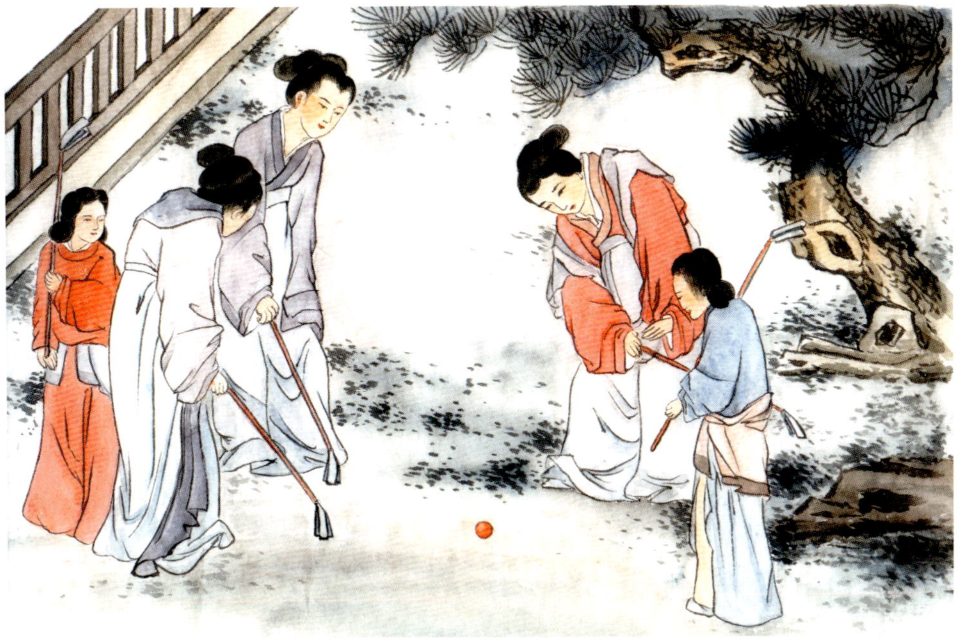

打球

Ball playing

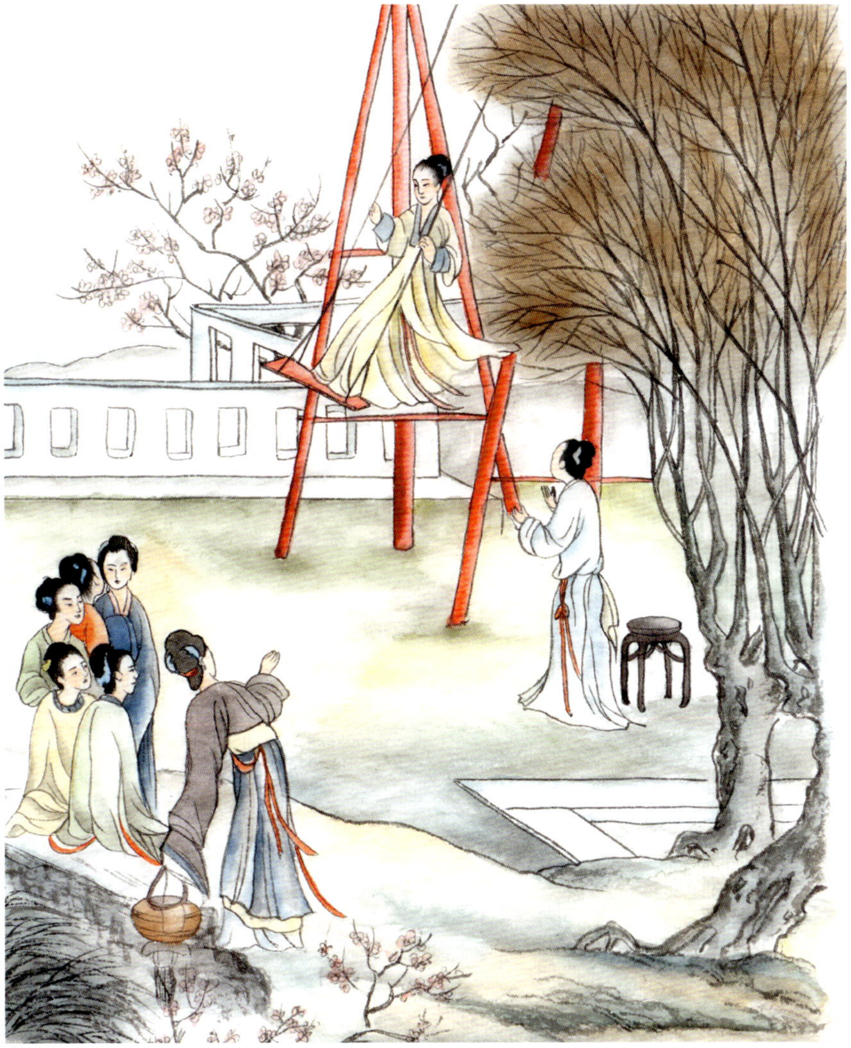

荡秋千

Swing playing

六、射箭、导引

6. Archery and Tao Yin

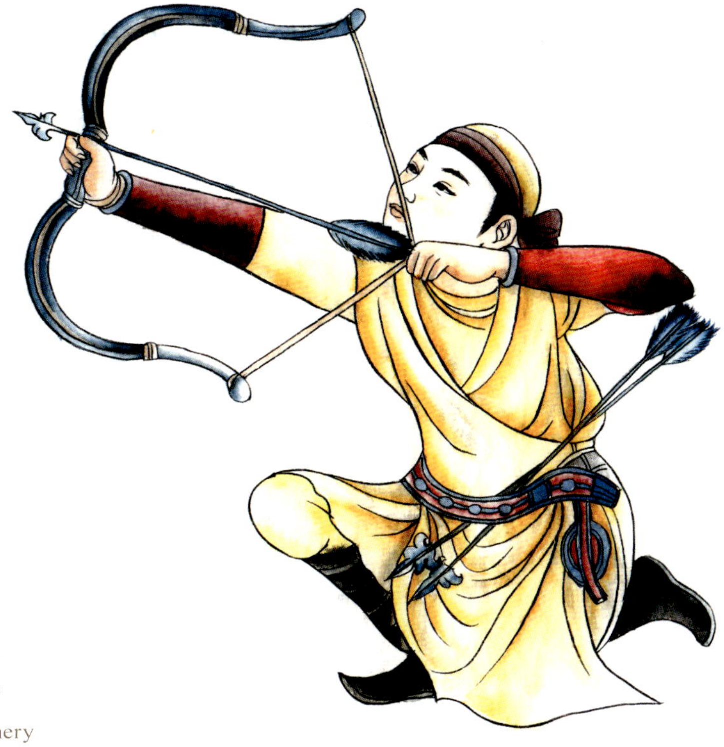

射箭

Archery

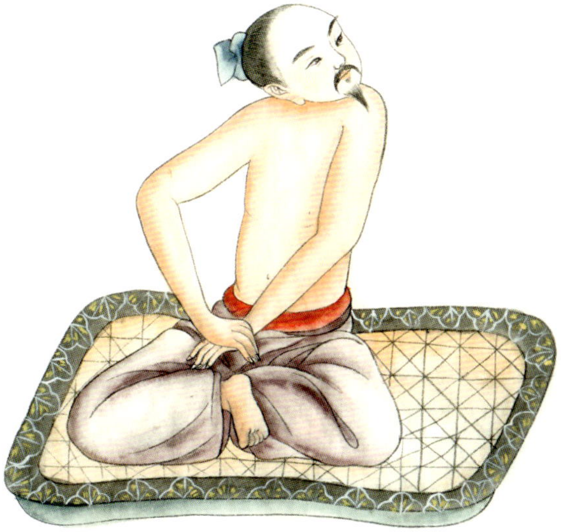

导引

Tao Yin

七、对弈、百戏

7. Chess and acrobatics

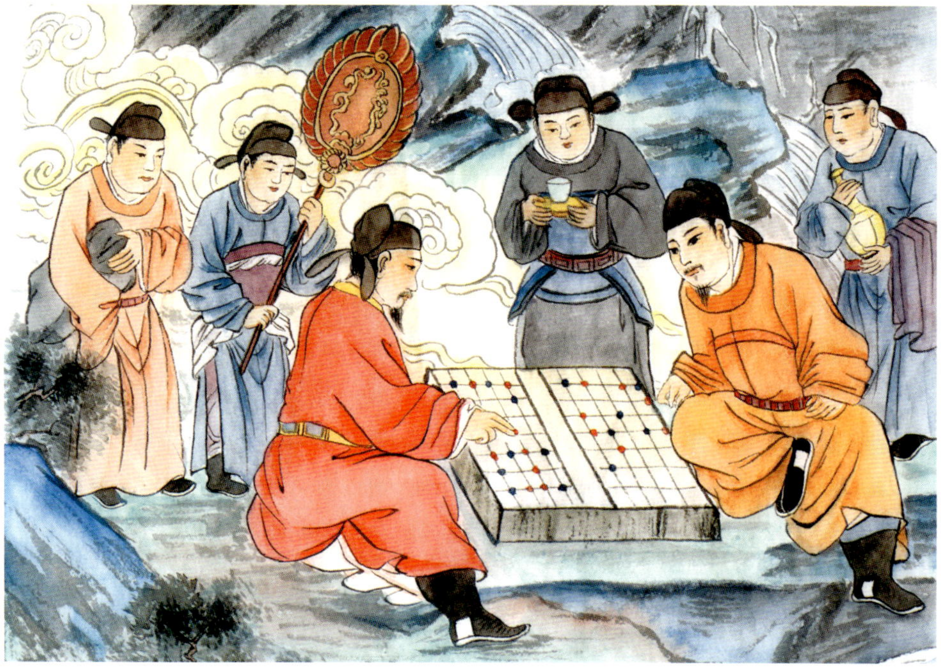

对弈

Chess

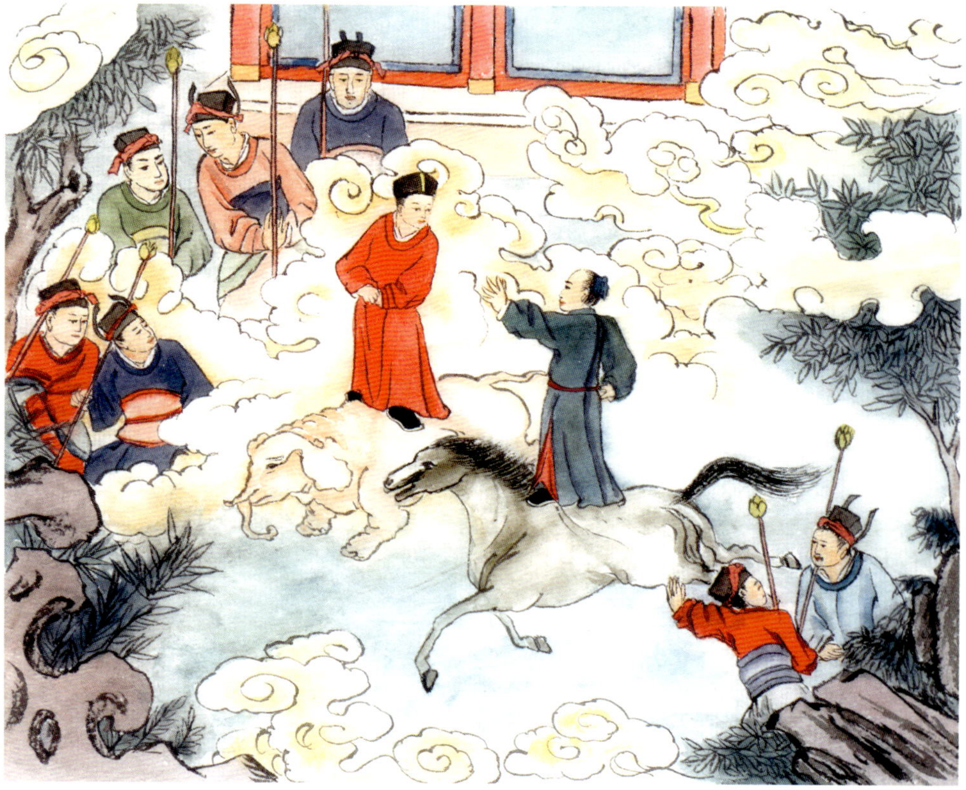

百戏

Acrobatics

八、赛龙舟、走冰船

8. Dragon boat racing and walking on the ice

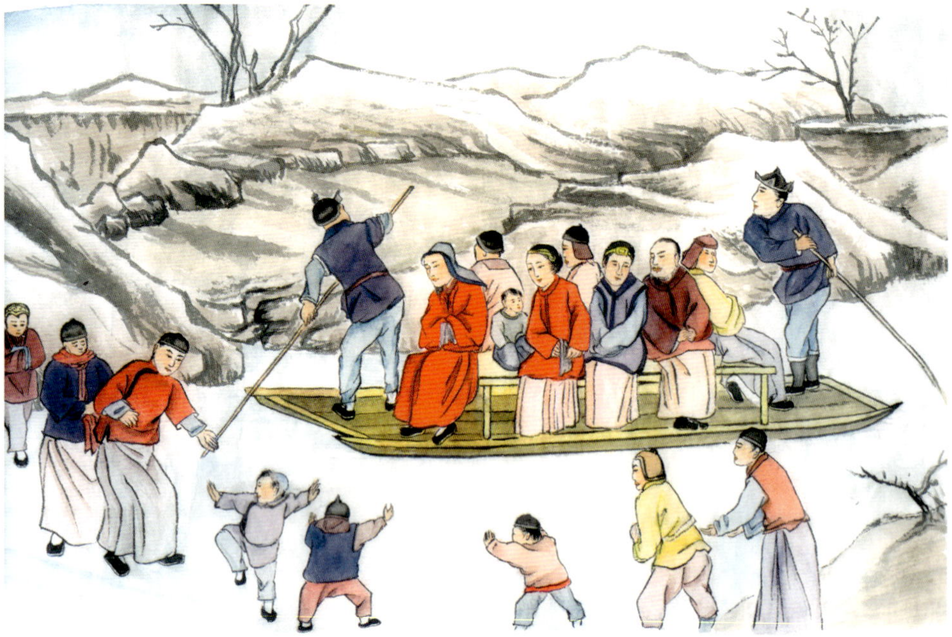

走冰船

Walking on the ice

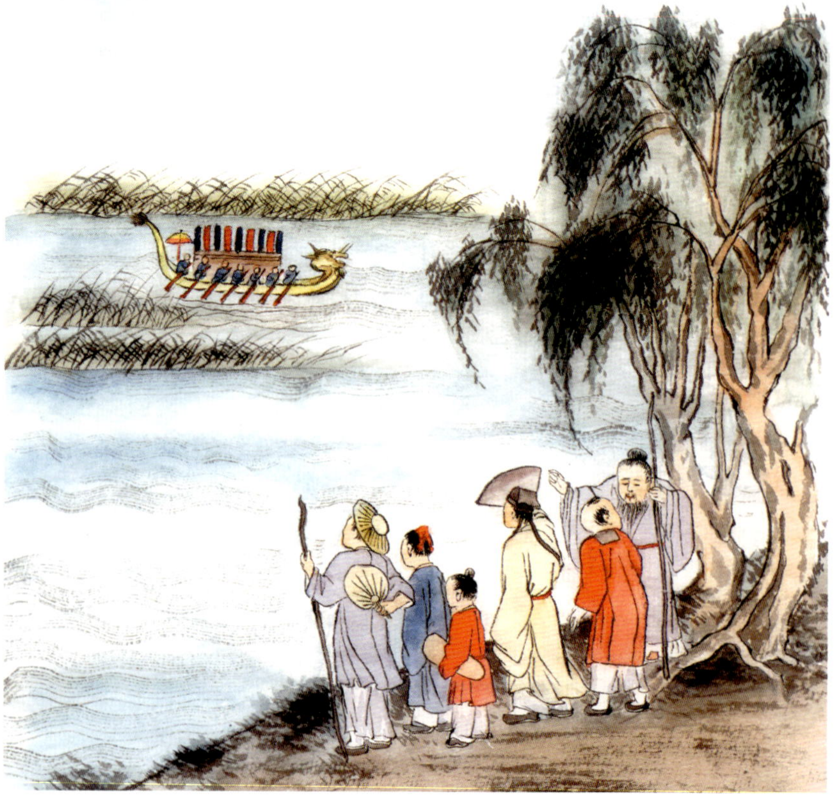

赛龙舟

Dragon boat racing

历代流传的养生强身功法选录

A selection of exercises for preserving and improving health handed down from past ages

凡以练“静”为主的功均称为内功，也可称为静功，如放松功、静养功、养生站桩功、小周天祛病益寿功等。凡以练“动”为主的功均称为外功，也可称为动功，如易筋经、五禽戏、八段锦、祛病延年功等。马王堆益寿延年导引功、十二段锦等则为内外结合功。外功和内功均能单练，也可同时练。体弱者应先练内功，待病情好转，体质增强后，再增练外功。为保健强身、益寿延年，可单练外功或内、外功结合练。一旦选练某种功法，就应坚持下去。本书选录的《内功图说》是气功养生非常有名的著作，流传很广，原名《卫生要术》，为清代潘霨所辑撰。内收十二段锦、分为内外功、易筋经、祛病延年法等功法，图文并茂，易于摹仿学习。

All exercises that focus on keeping still are called neigong (exercises to benefit internal organs) or “still exercises”. These include the Relaxing Exercise, the Tranquil Nurture Exercise, the Health-Preserving Exercise of Standing on Stakes, and the Small Universe Exercise for Resisting Diseases and Prolonging Life. All exercises that mainly consist of movements are called waigong (exercises to benefit the skin/muscles/bones) or “moving exercises”. These include the Muscle-Bone Strengthening Exercise, the Five Animal Frolics, the Eight Pieces of Brocade, and the Exercise for Resisting Disease and Prolonging Life. The Mawangdui Life-Prolonging Tao Yin Exercise and the Twelve Pieces of Brocade are combinations of the two kinds of exercise. One can practice either waigong or neigong alone, or practice a combination of them. A weak person should start from neigong, which can be supplemented with waigong when he or she has got better and stronger. To preserve and improve health and prolong life, you may practice waigong alone or combine it with neigong. Once you have decided on a particular kind of exercise, you should practice it swith perseverance. *Illustrated Explanation of Neigong Exercises*, which is excerpted in this book, is a well-known and widespread treatise on health preservation through qigong (deep-breathing exercises). Originally entitled *Essential Techniques for Health*, it was compiled by Pan Wei of the Qing Dynasty. It contains the methods of the Twelve Pieces of Brocade, Fenxing Neirong and Waigong, the Muscle-bone Strengthening Exercise, and the Exercise for Resisting Disease and Prolonging Life. These are made easy to imitate and learn by the combination of texts and pictures.

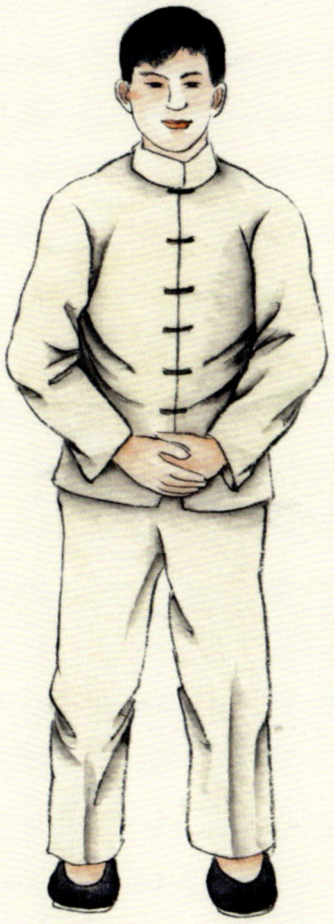

自然站桩式　两脚平行分开，间距约与两肩等宽，右手在外，左手在里，掌心向后，叠放在小腹上，两眼平视。

Natural zhanzhuang (a method of training in Chinese martial arts) posture: stand with your feet apart and parallel to each other at a distance equal to the length of your shoulders. Cover your lower abdomen with your hands, right hand over left hand, palm facing backward. Look straight ahead.

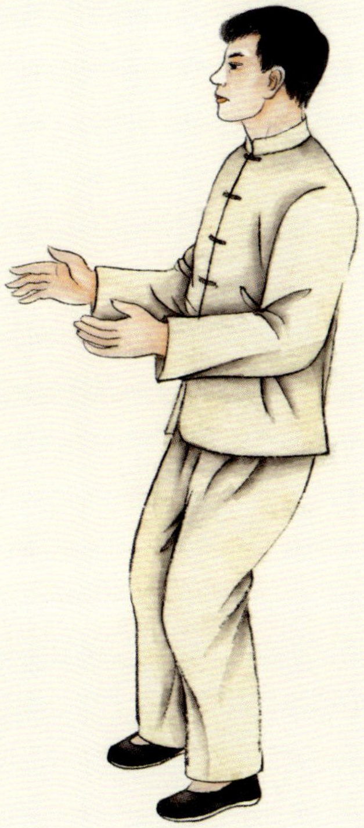

自然站立式　两脚平行分开站立。十指相对，环抱于腹前(两拇指间距8、9寸，拇指距腹2、3寸)，全身放松，心无杂念。

Natural standing posture: stand with your feet apart and parallel to each other. Hold your hands in front your belly, the fingers facing each other (26-30 centimeters between the thumbs and 6-10 centimeters from the thumbs to the belly). Relax your whole body and rid your mind of distracting thoughts.

易筋经

The Muscle-bone Strengthening Exercise

易筋经是古人强健身体，锻炼筋骨的一套行之有效的健身法，包括内功和外功两种锻炼方法，各有 12 势。其中内功采用站式，以一定的姿势，借呼吸诱导，逐步加强筋脉和脏腑的功能。

The Muscle-bone Strengthening Exercise (yi jin jing) is an effective method developed in ancient China to improve one's health and exercise one's muscles and bones. It can be practiced in the 'inner' way or the 'outer' way, each having 12 moves. When practicing the 'inner type' of the exercise, one assumes required postures while standing and uses respiration to gradually strengthen his muscles and internal organs.

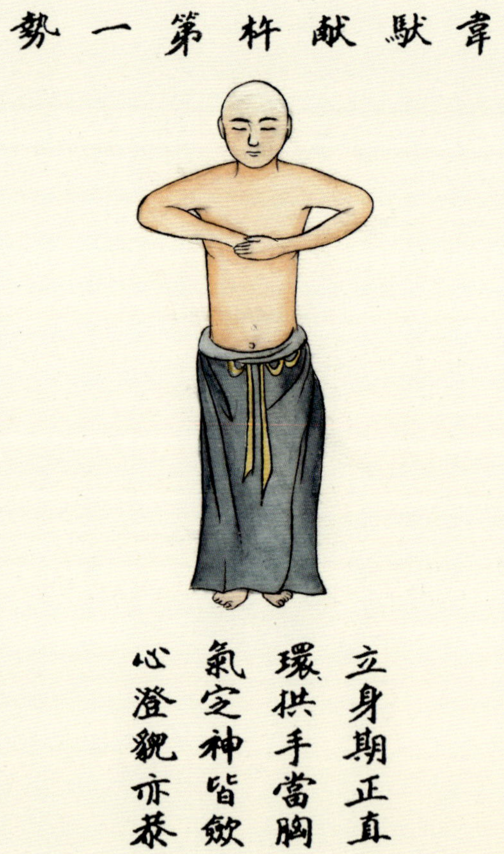

第一势：韦驮献杵第一势

两臂曲肘，徐徐平举至胸前成抱球势，屈腕立掌，掌心相对。配合呼吸做 8 – 20 次。

First movement: Wei Tuo offers his pestle (1)

Bend your arms and raise them slowly to your chest as if holding a ball. Bend your wrists and hold your hands upward, palms facing each other. Do this 8 to 20 times while breathing properly.

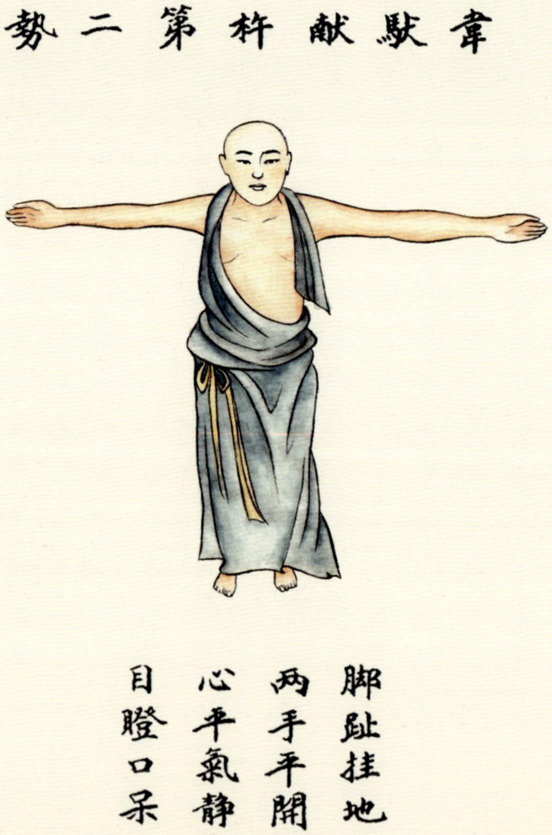

第二势：韦驮献杵第二势

两足分开，与肩同宽，两手自胸前徐徐外展；立掌，掌心向外；两目前视。配合呼吸做 8 – 20 次。

Second movement: Wei Tuo offers his pestle (2)

Stand with your feet apart at a distance equal to the length of your shoulders. Slowly spread your arms from the chest outward. Hold your hands upward, palms facing forward. Look straight ahead. Do this 8 to 20 times while breathing properly.

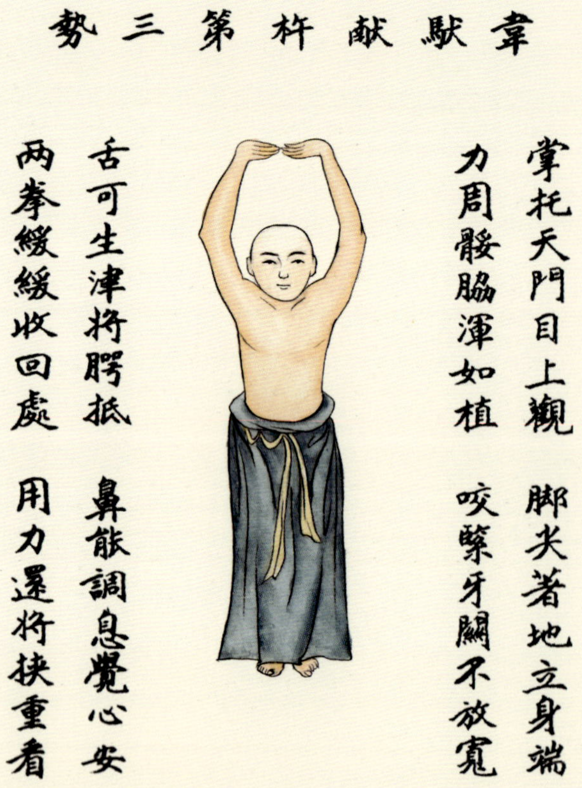

第三势：韦驮献杵第三势

两脚开立，足尖着地，足跟提起；双手上举高过头顶，掌心向上；沉肩曲肘，仰头。反复 8 – 20 次。

Third movement: Wei Tuo offers his pestle (3)

Stand on tiptoe with your feet apart and heels off the floor. Raise your hands over your head, palms facing upward. Lower your shoulders, bend your arms, and look up. Do this 8 to 20 times.

摘星換斗勢

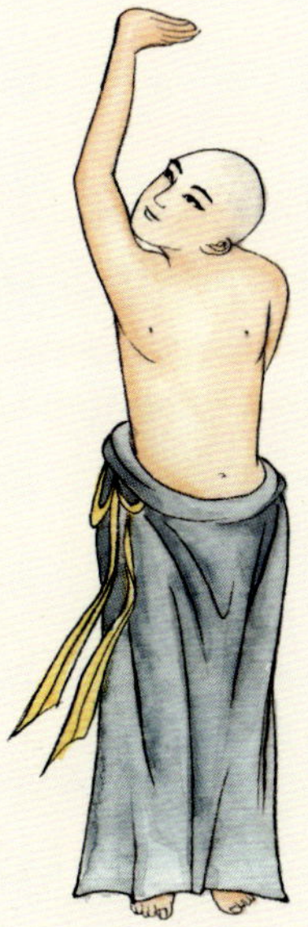

第四势：摘星换斗势

右脚稍向右前方移步，与左脚形成斜八字，右虚步。吸气时，头往上顶；呼气时，全身放松。连续 5 – 10 次。

Fourth movement: pluck a star to replace the Big Dipper

Move your right foot slightly forward to the right to form an angle with the left foot, the right foot standing on tiptoe. Move your head up when inhaling, and relax the whole body when exhaling. Do this 5 to 10 times continuously.

倒拽九牛尾勢

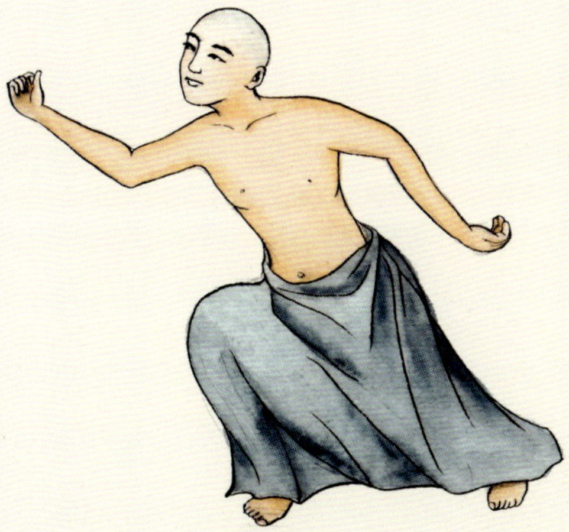

第五势：倒拽九牛尾势

右脚前跨一步，屈膝成右弓步。右手握拳，举至前上方，双目观拳。反复 5 – 10 次。

Fifth movement: pulling nine oxen by the tail

Take a step forward with your right foot and bend your right knee. Make a fist with your right hand and raise it upward in front of you, fixing your eyes on it. Do this 5 to 10 times.

出爪亮翅勢

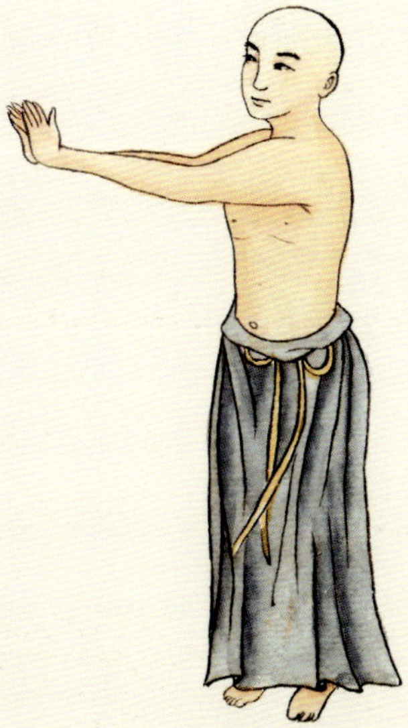

第六势：出爪亮翅势

两脚开立，两臂前平举，立掌。配合呼吸 8 – 12 次。

Sixth movement: show the claws and spread wings

Stand with your feet apart and hold your arms level and forward, hands upward. Do this 8 to 12 times while breathing properly.

九鬼扳馬刀勢

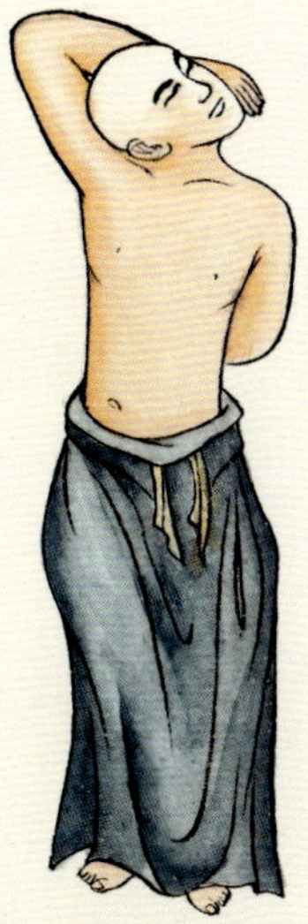

第七势：九鬼拔马刀势

脚尖相衔，足跟分离成八字形；两臂向前成叉掌立于胸前。右手成抱颈状，足趾抓地。配合呼吸吸反复 5 – 10 次。

Seventh movement: nine demons drawing sabers

Bring the tiptoes of your feet together, with heels apart. Cross your arms in front your chest, with your right hand appearing to hold your neck. Grasp the floor with your toes. Do this 5 to ten 10 while breathing properly.

三盤落地勢

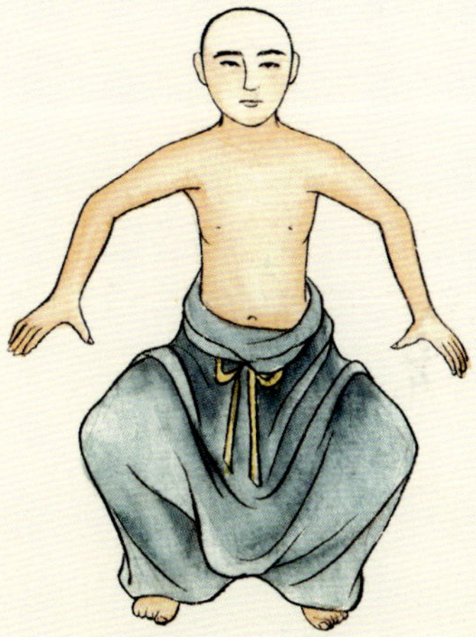

第八势：三盘落地势

两足分开，下蹲，双手下按；然后两掌翻起，起立时脚步要正。

Eighth movement: separate the feet and squat

Pushing the two hands downward; then upturn the palms and stand up, keeping the feet straight to the front.

青龍探爪勢

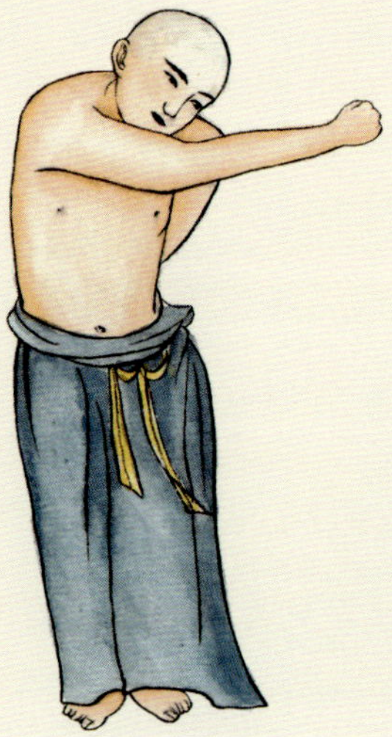

青龍探爪
左從右出
修士效之
掌平氣實
力周肩背
圍收過膝
兩目注平
息調心謐

第九势：青龙探爪势

两脚开立，两手成仰拳护腰。右手向左前方伸探，五指捏成勾手，上体左转。配合呼吸连续 5 – 10 次。

Ninth movement: black dragon reaches out its claw

Stand with your feet apart and make fists with both hands, fingers upward, at your waist. Reach out your right hand forward to the left, bending the fingers, and turn your torso left. Do this 5 to 10 times while breathing properly.

卧虎撲食勢

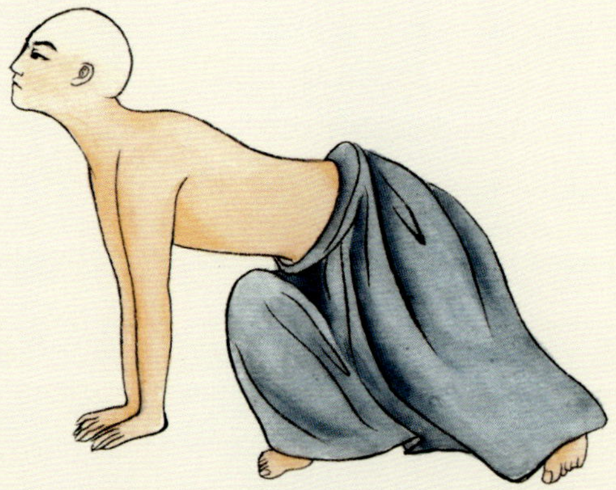

兩脚分蹲身似傾
屈伸左右腿相更
昂頭胸作探前勢
偃背腰還似砥平
鼻息調元均出入
指尖著地賴支撑
降龍伏虎神仙事
學得真形也衛生

第十势：卧虎扑食势

右脚向右跨一大步，屈右膝下蹲，成右弓左仆腿势；上体起伏，前探后收，如猛虎扑食。动作连续 5 – 10 次。

Tenth movement: crouching tiger pounces on its prey

Take a big step to the right and bend your right knee while keeping your left leg straight. Bend your torso forward and retract your back as if you were a tiger ready to pounce on your prey. Do this 5 to 10 times continuously.

折躬勢

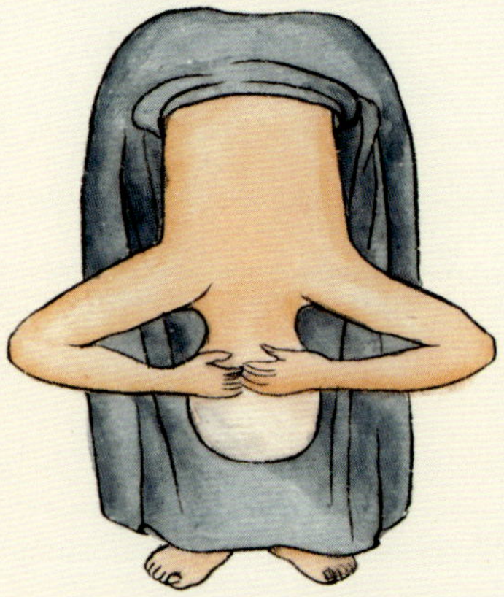

兩手齊持腦
垂腰至膝間
頭惟探胯下
口更齧牙關
掩耳聰教塞
調元氣自閑
舌尖還抵腭
力在肘雙彎

第十一势：折躬势

两脚开立，脚尖内扣。双手仰掌缓缓向左右而上，用力合抱头后部，手指弹敲小脑后片刻。配合呼吸体力反复 8 – 20 次。

Eleventh movement: bend your body

Stand with your feet apart, with the tiptoes pointing inward. Raise both hands slowly with the palms facing upward. Hold the back of your head with force, tapping your fingers on your head for a while. Do this 8 to 20 times while breathing properly.

掉尾勢

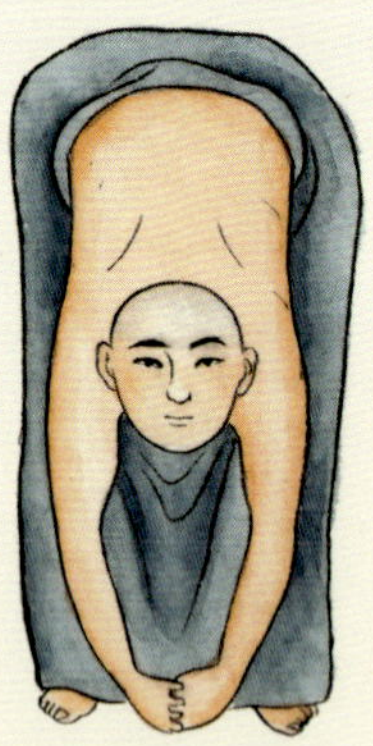

膝直膀伸　推手自地
起而頓足　二十一次
瞪目昂頭　凝神壹志
左右伸肱　以七為誌
更作坐功　盤膝垂眥
口注於心　息調於鼻
定靜乃起　厥功維備
總攷其法　圖成十二
達摩西来　傳少林寺
却病延年　功無與類
誰實貽諸　五代之季
有宋岳侯　更為鑒識

第十二势：掉尾势

两腿开立，双手仰掌由胸前徐徐上举至头顶，目视掌而移，身立正直，十指交叉，旋腕反掌上托；如此反复 21 次。收功：直立，两臂左右侧举，屈伸 7 次。

Twelfth movement: turn the tail

Stand with your feet apart. Keep your eyes on your hands as you raise them to the top of your head, palms facing upward. While standing upright, interlace your fingers, turn your wrists, and push your palms upward. Do this 21 times. Then stop and stand upright. Raise your arms sideways, and bend and straighten them 7 times.

五禽戏

Five Animal Frolics

我国古代名医华佗精心研究虎、鹿、熊、猿、鸟的运动特点，创造“五禽戏”，既能健身，又能治病。华佗习此，活到九十多岁时，还耳聪目明，身体健康。

The Five Animal Frolics (Wu Qin Xi) was invented by Hua Tuo, an eminent physician of ancient China, who had made a careful study of the movements of tigers, deer, bears, monkeys and birds. The exercise can improve one's health and cure diseases. By practicing it regularly, Hua Tuo remained in good health in his nineties, with good sight and acute hearing.

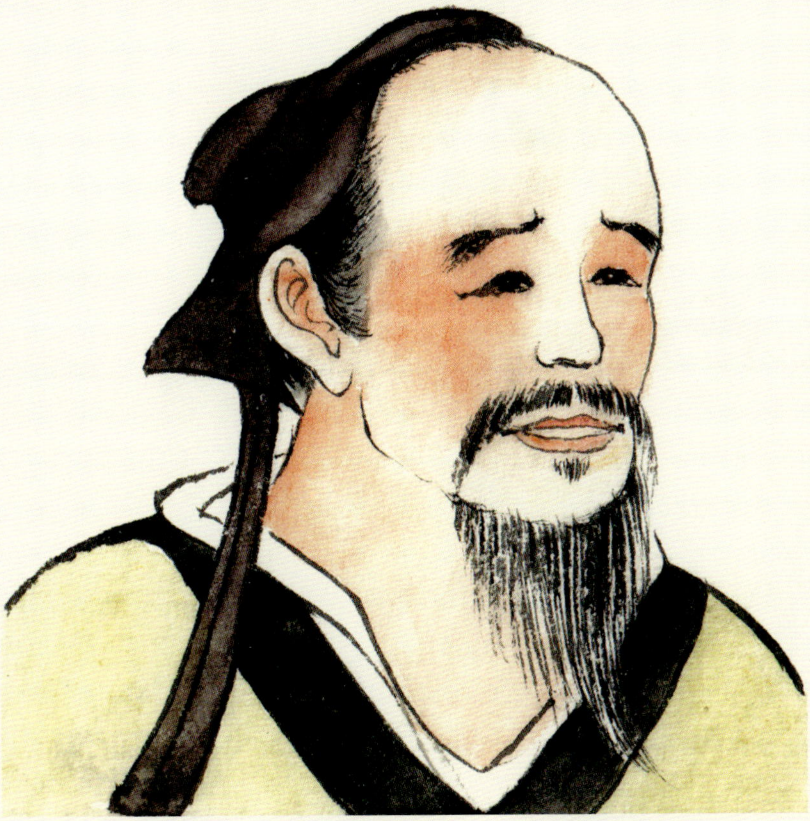

华佗像

Hua Tuo

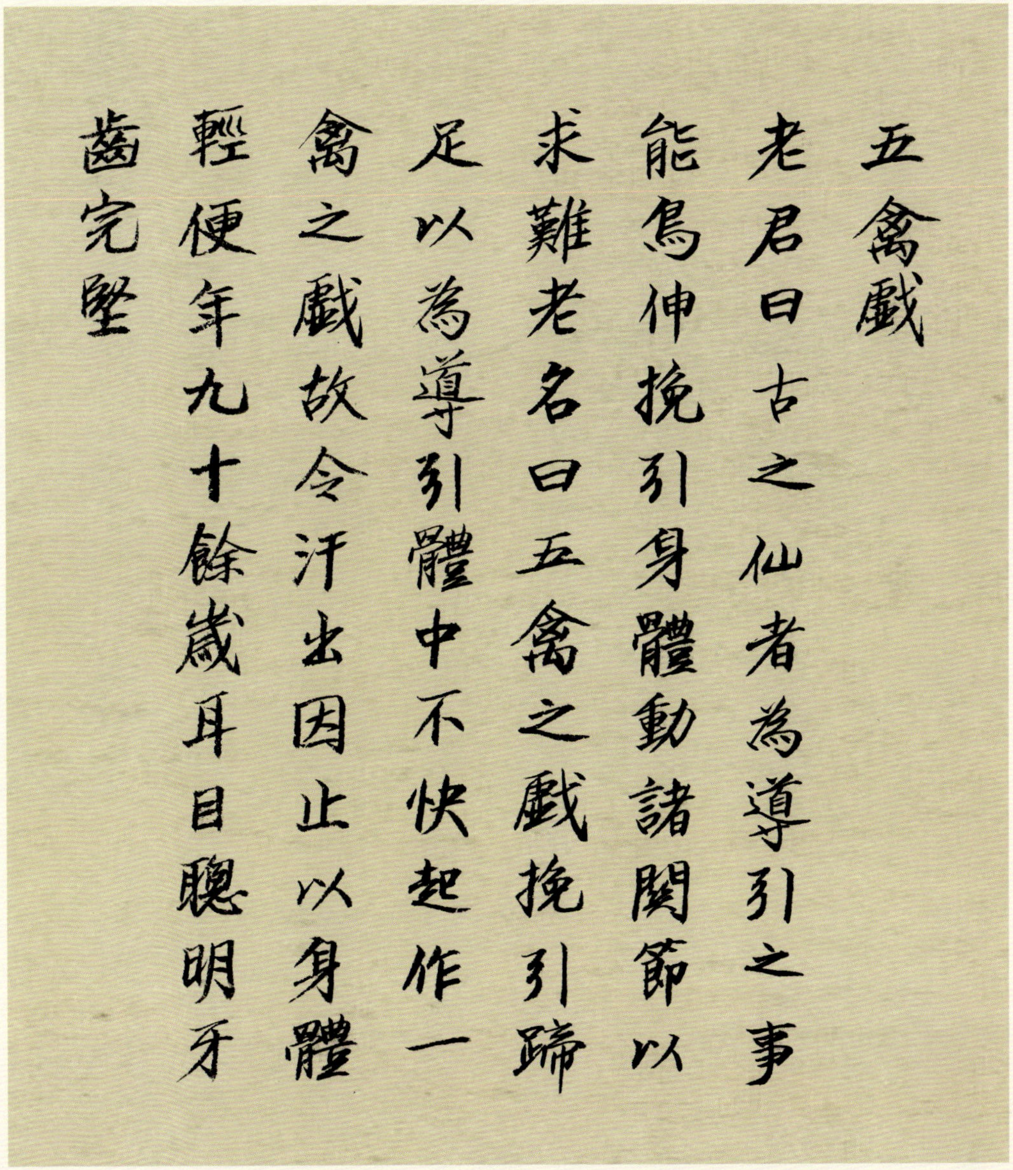

一、虎戏

1. Tiger movement

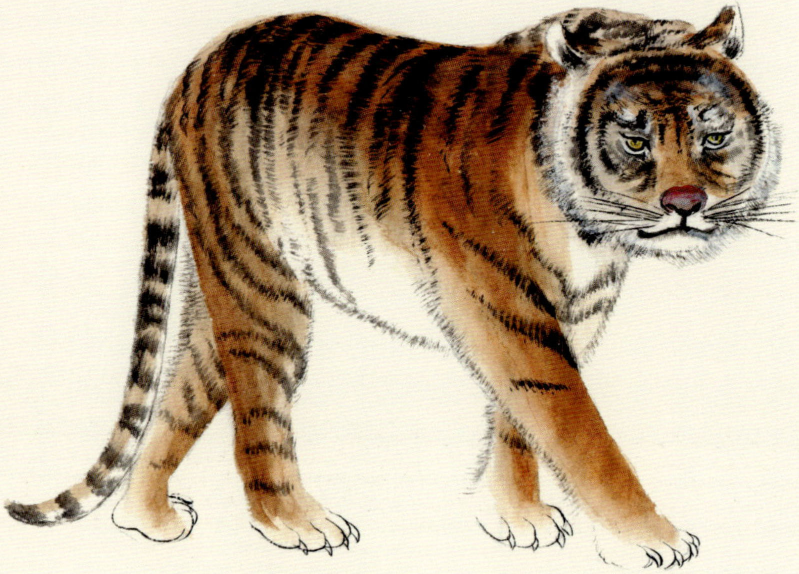

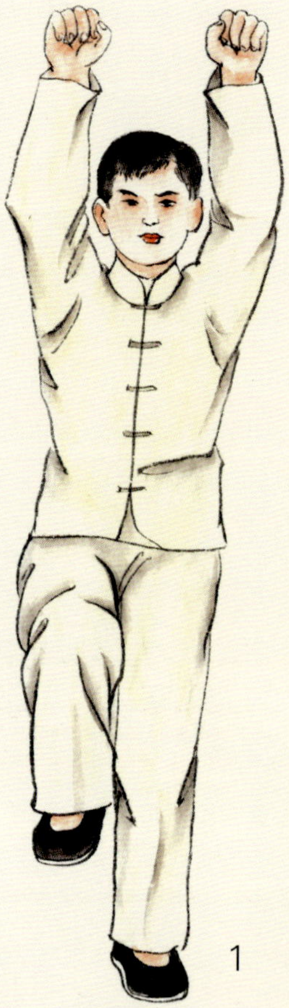

1

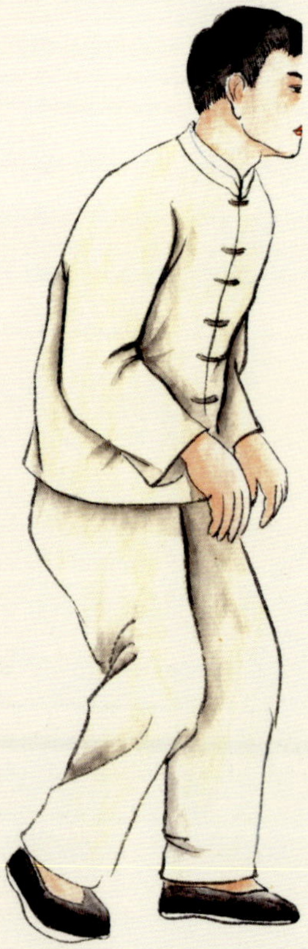

2

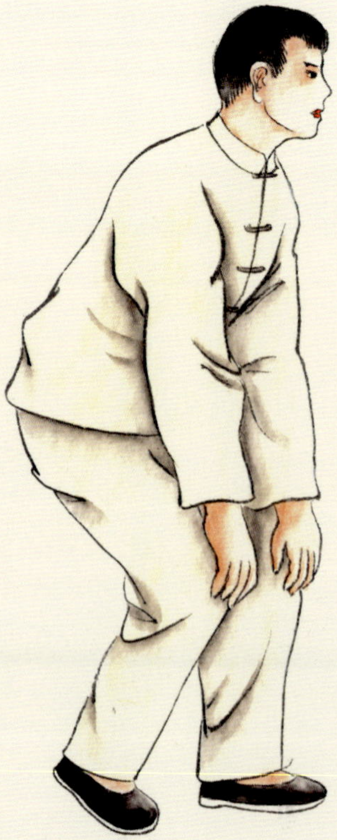

3

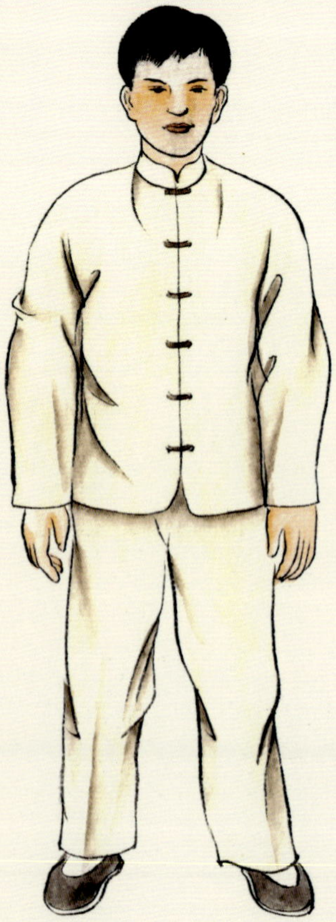

4

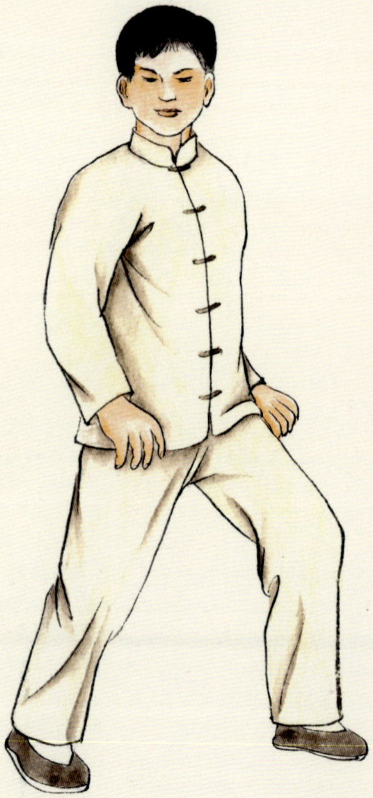

5

二、鹿戏

2. Deer movement

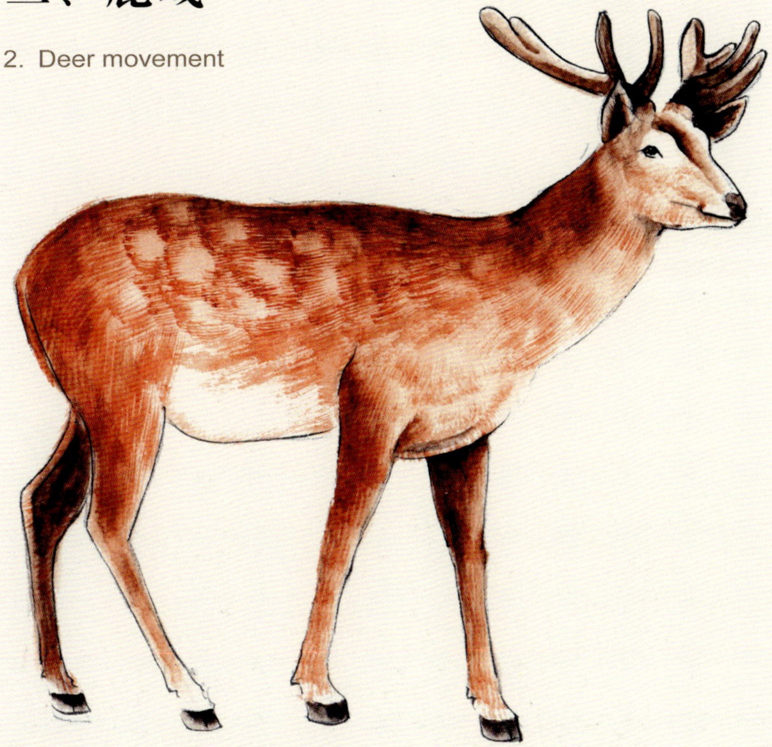

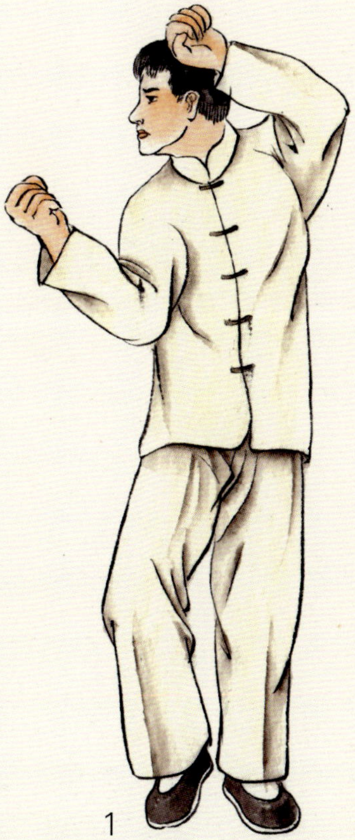

1

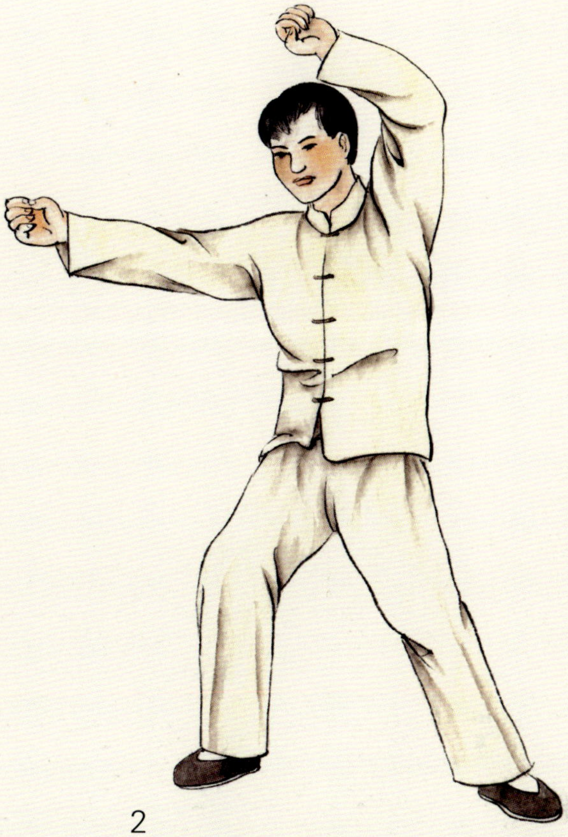

2

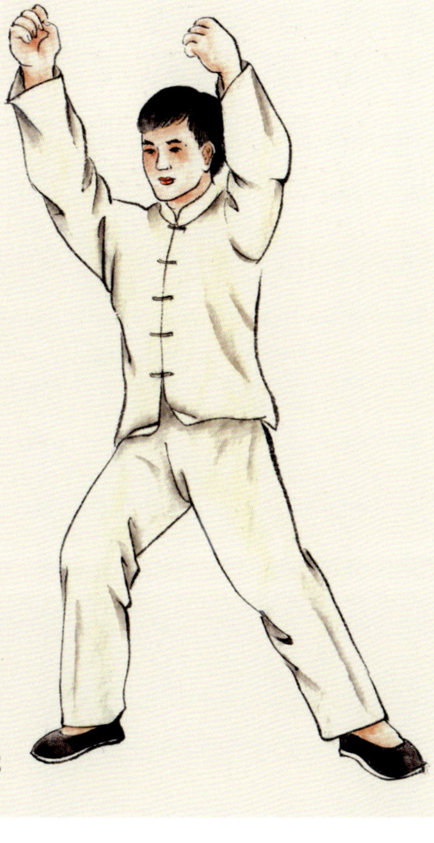

3

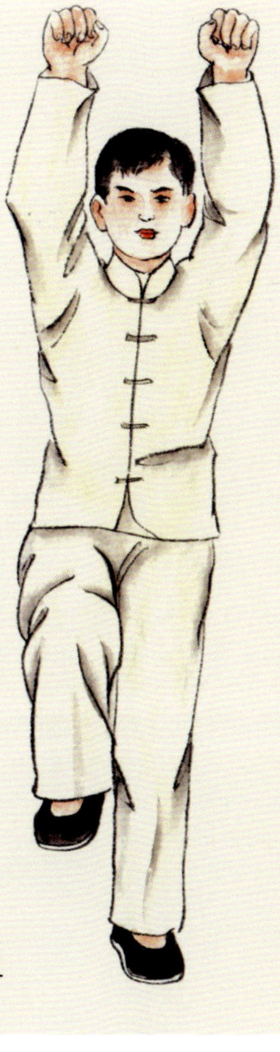

4

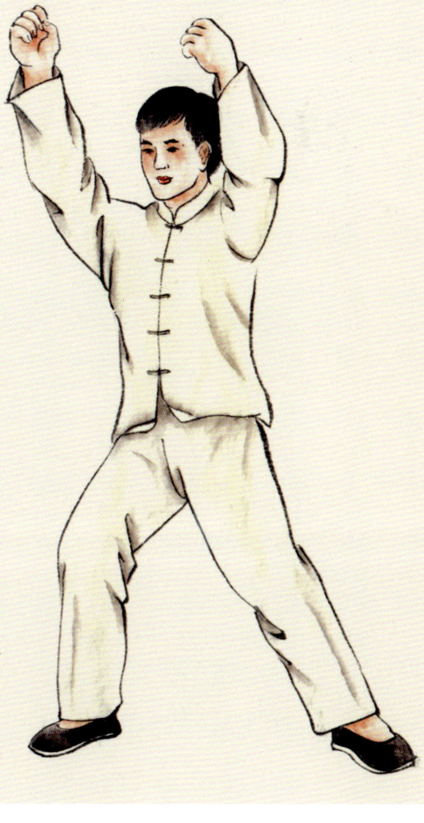

5

三、熊戏

3. Bear movement

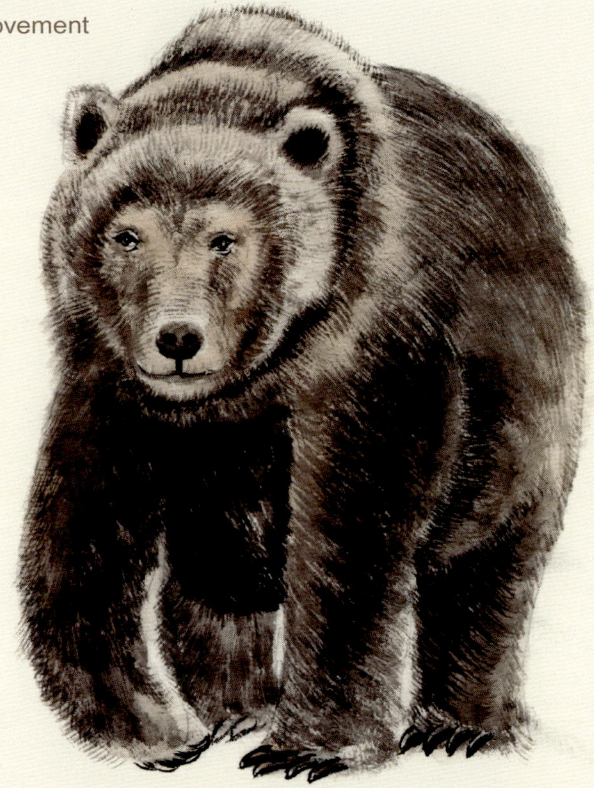

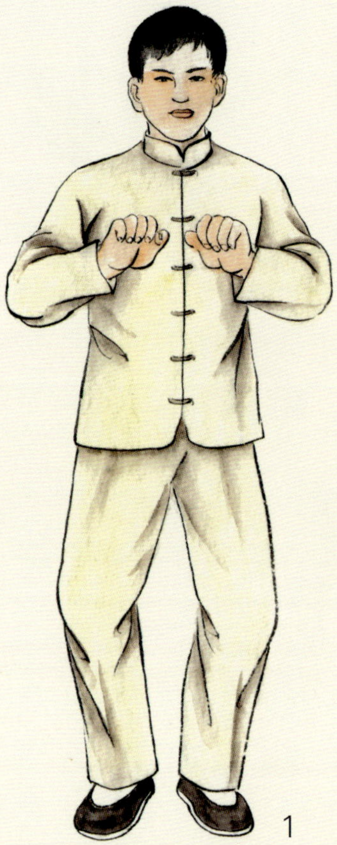

1

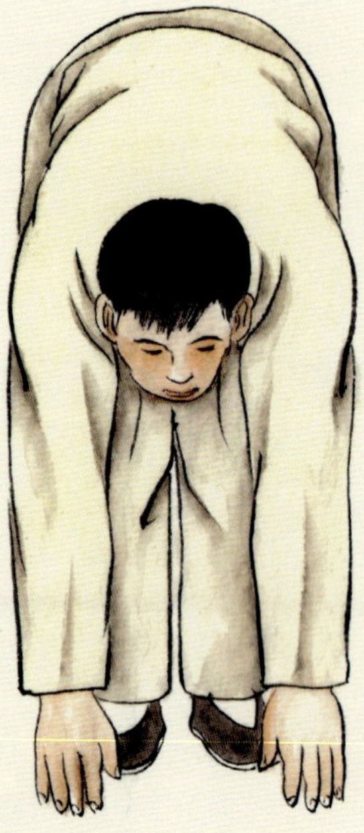

2

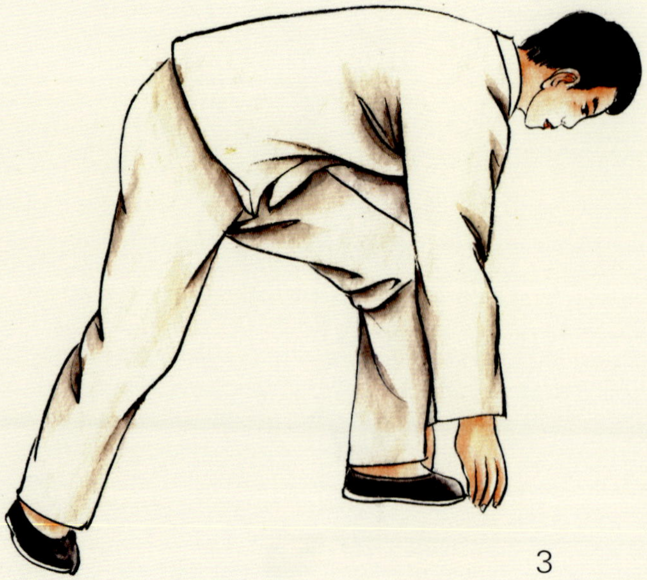

3

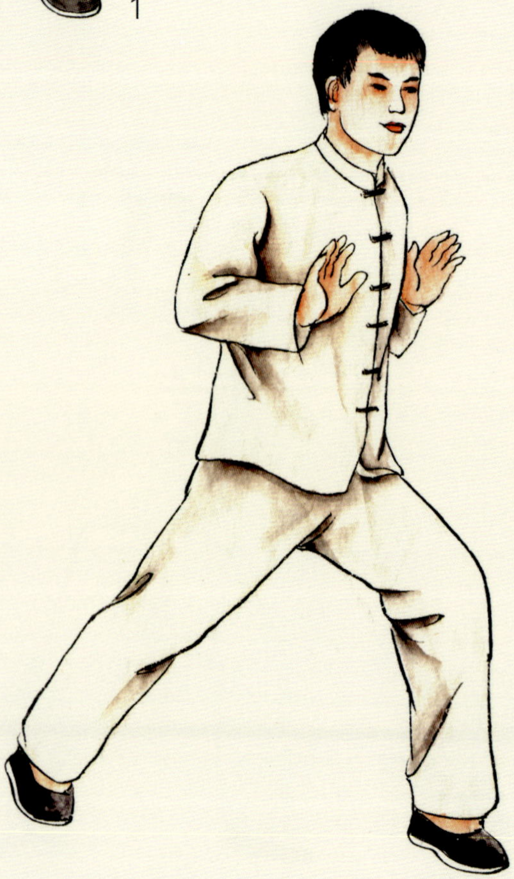

4

四、猴戏

4. Monkey movement

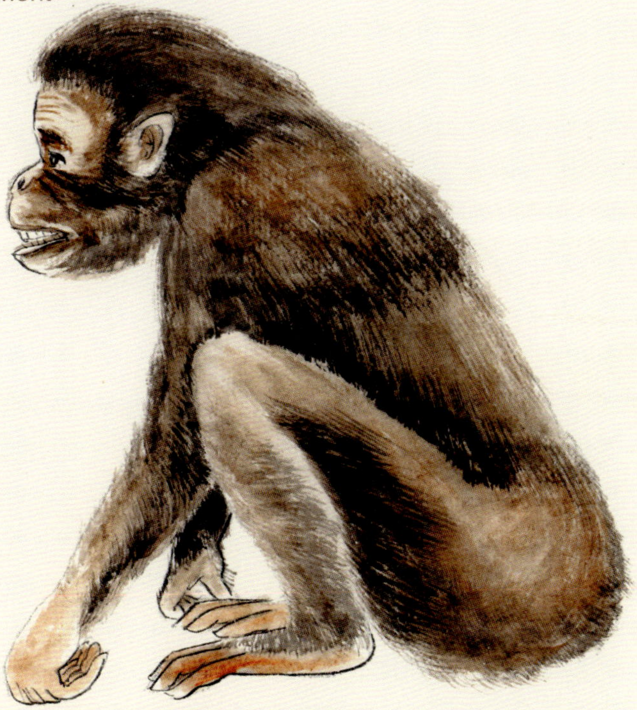

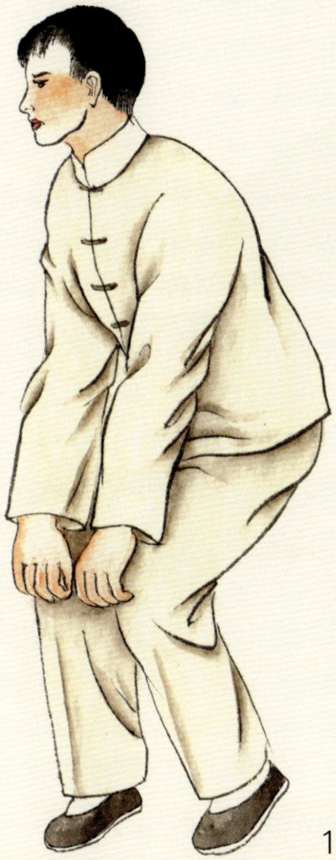

1

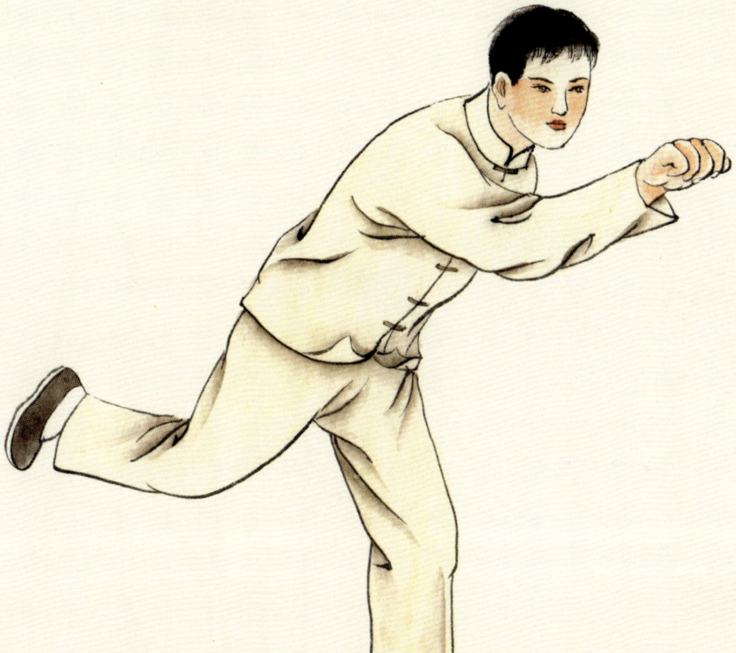

2

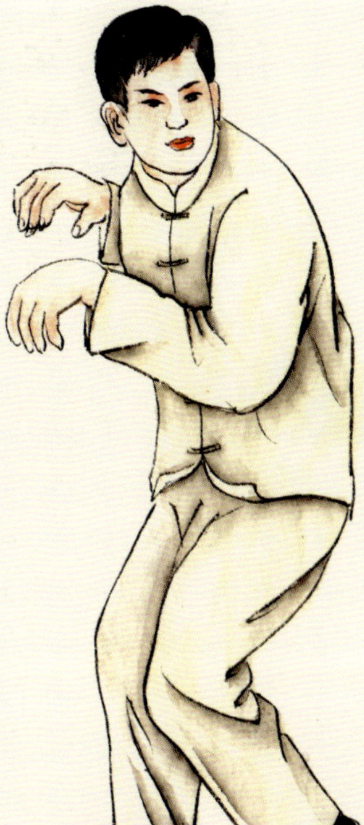

3

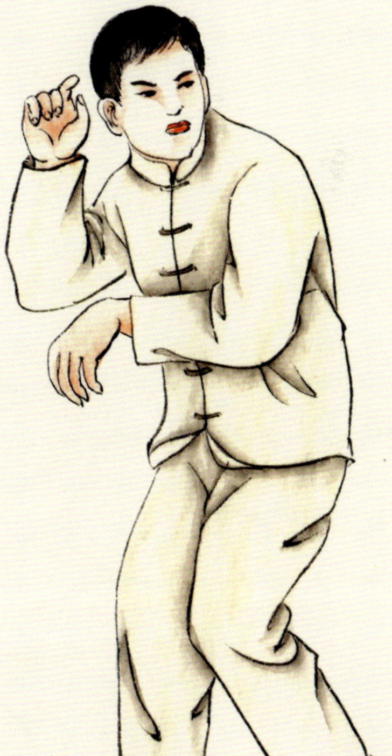

4

五、鸟戏

5. Bird movement

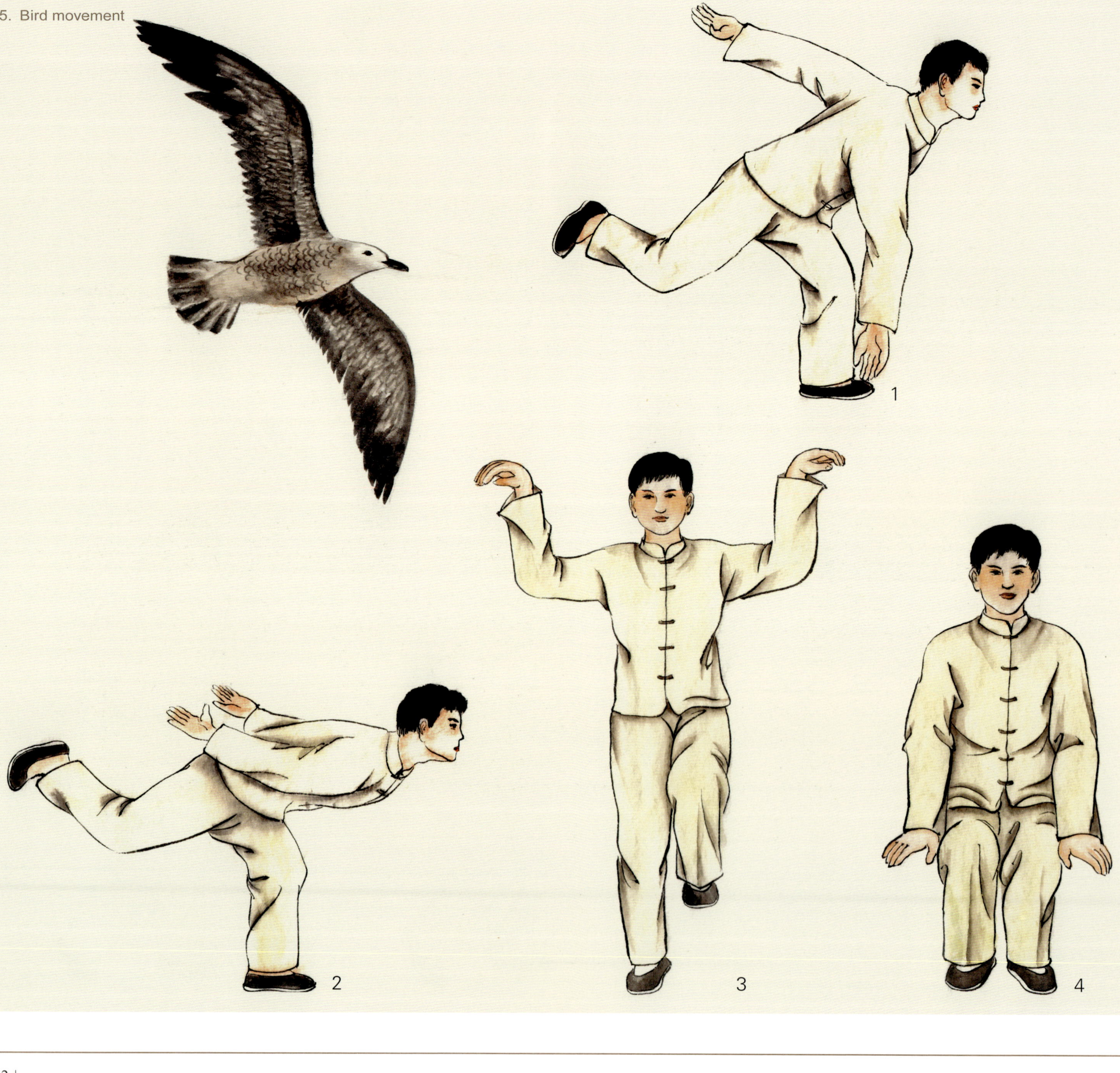

十二段锦

The Twelve Pieces of Brocade

十二段锦是由十二节动作组合而成，其全部动作进行时均取坐势。“十二段锦”功法虽然简单，但健身益寿、抗老防衰的功效显著，适合患慢性、虚弱性疾病者的调理。

The Twelve Pieces of Brocade consists of twelve movements, all executed in a sitting posture. Simple as it is, it is highly effective for improving one's health, delaying aging, and prolonging life. It is suitable for the recuperation of those afflicted with chronic or weakening diseases.

闭目冥心坐，握固静思神。

Sit with closed eyes, clasped hands, and a calm and concentrated mind.

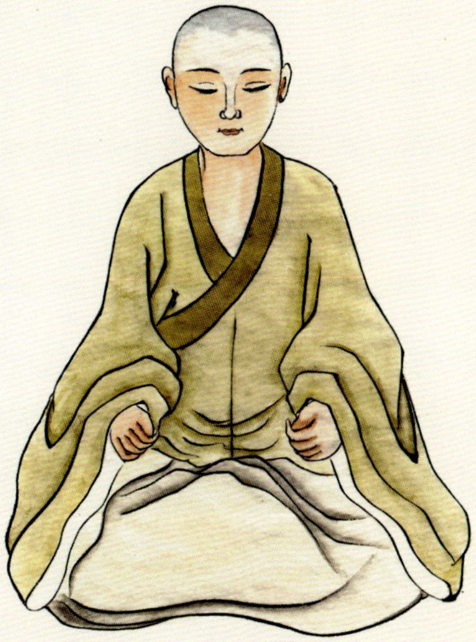

盘腿而坐，紧闭两目，排除心中杂念。握固就是握手牢固。

Sit cross-legged with your eyes tightly shut and no distracting thoughts on your mind. Clasp your hands tightly together.

叩齿三十六，两手抱昆仑。

Click your teeth thirty-six times and embrace Mount Kunlun with both hands.

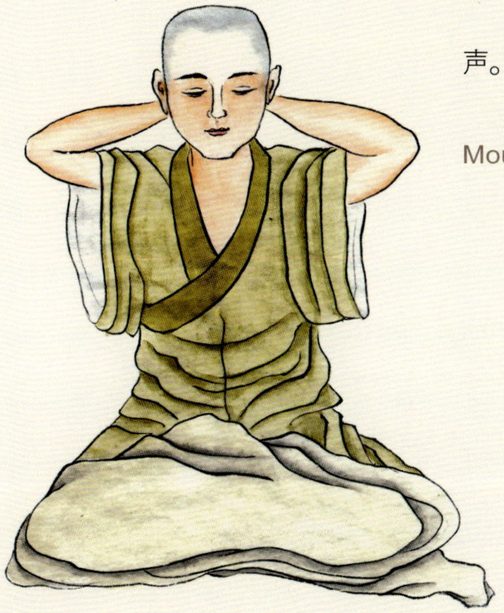

上下牙齿，相叩作响，宜三十六声。昆仑就是头部。

Click your teeth thirty-six times. Mount Kunlun means your head.

左右鸣天鼓，二十四度闻。

Beat the heavenly drum twenty-four times.

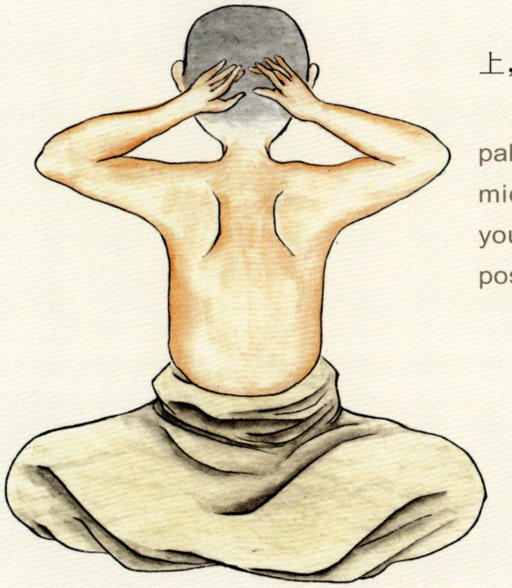

两手掌按耳，以第二指叠在中指上，用力重弹脑后，要如击鼓之声。

Cover your ears with your palms. Put the index finger over the middle finger and tap the back of your head with force. You are supposed to hear a drum-like sound.

微摆撼天柱。

Gently sway the heavenly pillar.

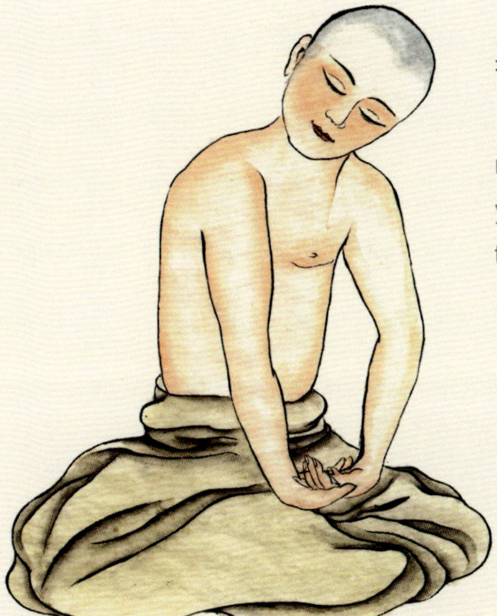

天柱即后颈，低头扭颈向左右侧视，各二十四次。

The heavenly pillar refers to the nape. Lower your head and move your neck to look at the left and then the right. Do this twenty-four times.

赤龙搅水津，鼓漱三十六。

The red dragon stirs the pool, filling your mouth with divine water. Rinse your mouth with it thirty-six times.

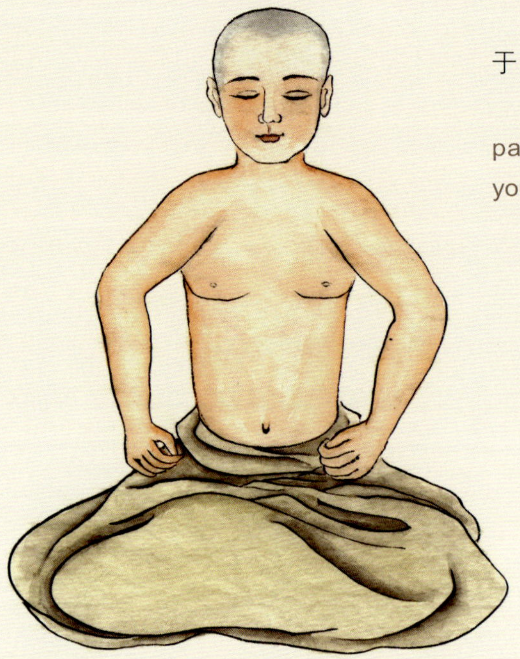

以舌顶上腭，使水津自生，鼓漱于口中三十六次。

Press the tongue against the palate to bring forth saliva. Rinse your mouth thirty-six times.

闭气搓手热，背摩后精门。

Hold your breath, rub your hands, and massage the 'essence gate' on your back.

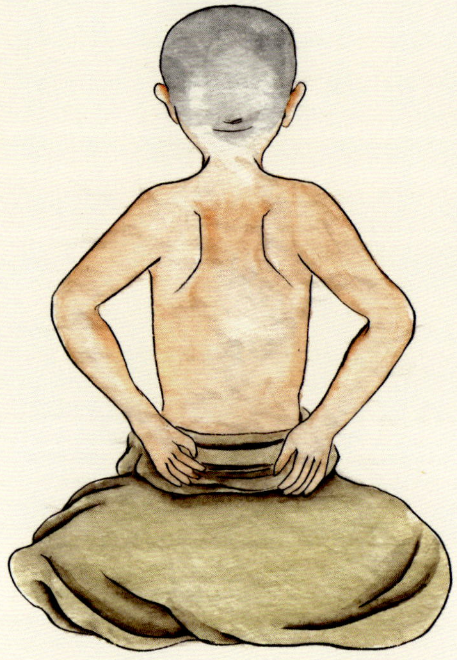

用两掌相搓擦极热，急分两手磨后腰上两边。

Rub your palms till they are very hot; then immediately part them and rub your low back.

尽此一口气，想火烧脐轮。

Use up the breath and imagine a fire burning your qilun.

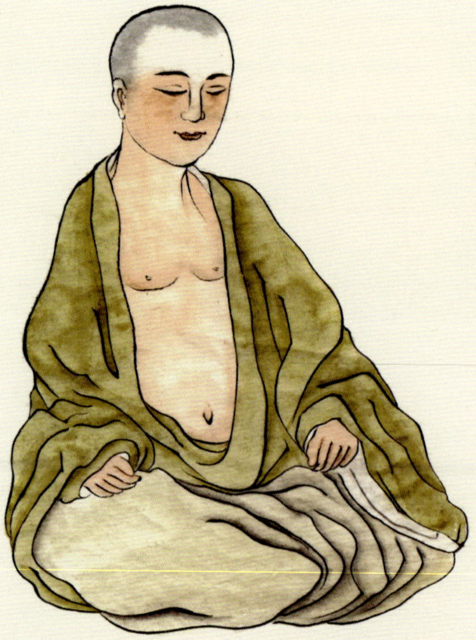

闭口鼻之气，以心暗想，运心头之火，下烧丹田。脐轮即脐丹田。

Hold your breath in your mouth and nose. Use your mind to move the fire at your heart downward to your dantian (the point two inches below the navel where one's qi resides). Qilun refers to dantian.

左右辘轳转。

Turn the windlass left and right.

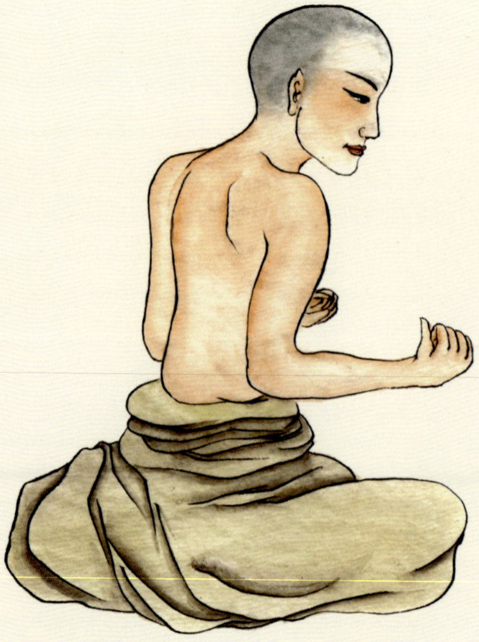

曲弯两手，先以左手连肩，圆转三十六次，右手亦如之。

Bend your arms. First touch your left hand on your shoulder and rotate your left arm thirty-six times. Repeat this with your right arm.

两脚放舒伸，叉手双虚托。

Stretch your legs, interlace your fingers, and push up.

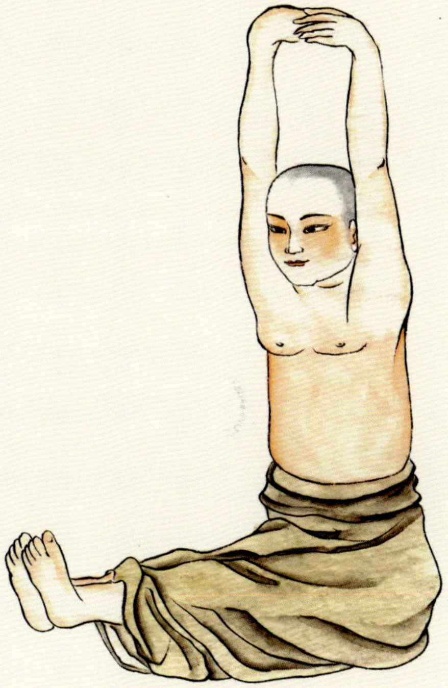

两脚平伸向前，两手指相叉，反掌向上，作力上托。

Reach your feet straight forward. Interlace your fingers, turn your palms upward, and push them up with force.

低头攀足频。

Lower your head and pull your feet repeatedly.

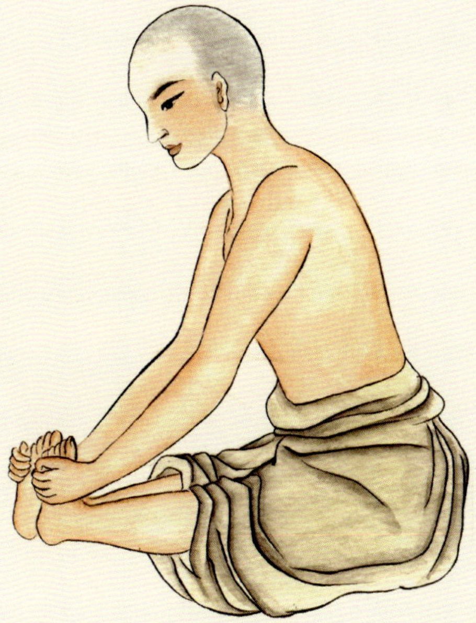

以两手向所伸两脚底作力扳之，十二次。

Reach your hands to your soles and pull your feet with force. Do this twelve times.

再漱再吞津，如此三度毕，咽下汩汩响，百脉自调匀。

Rinse your mouth again, and swallow it. Repeat this, so that it is done thrice. With the gurgling sound, all your energy channels are well-regulated.

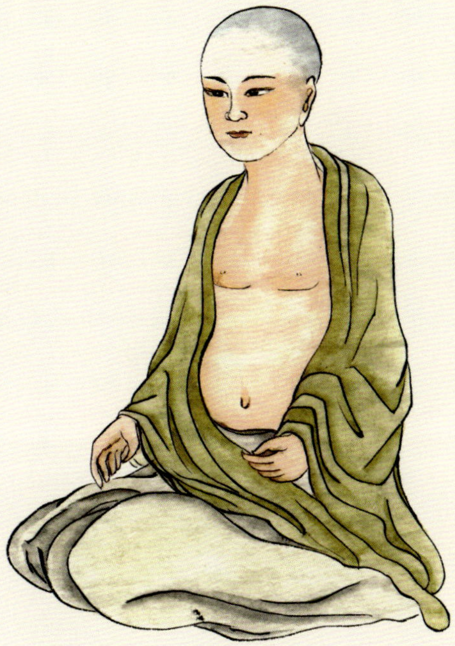

再用舌搅口内，再鼓漱三十六。连前一度，此再两度，共三度，毕。

Move your tongue about your mouth again. Then rinse your mouth again thirty-six times. Repeat the procedure, which has been executed before, so that this is done three times in all.

河车搬运毕，想发火烧身，旧名八段锦。子后午前行，勤行无间断，万病化为尘。

When the 'river cart' has been loaded, imagine a fire that burns your body. The old name for this exercise is Eight Pieces of Brocade.

Practice it between midnight and midday every day, and all diseases will turn to dust.

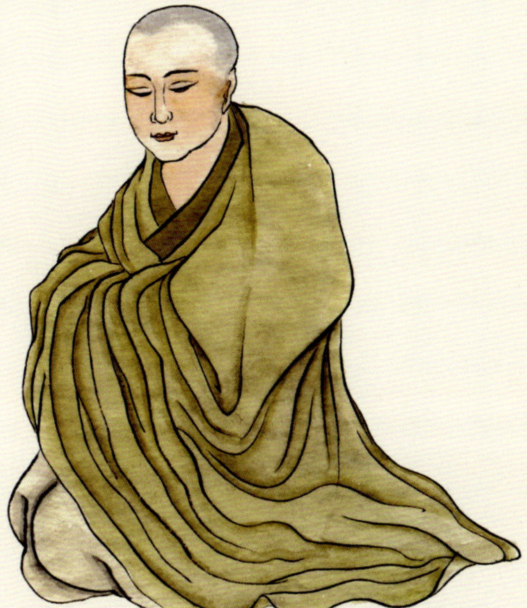

延年九转法

The Nine Movements for Prolonging Life

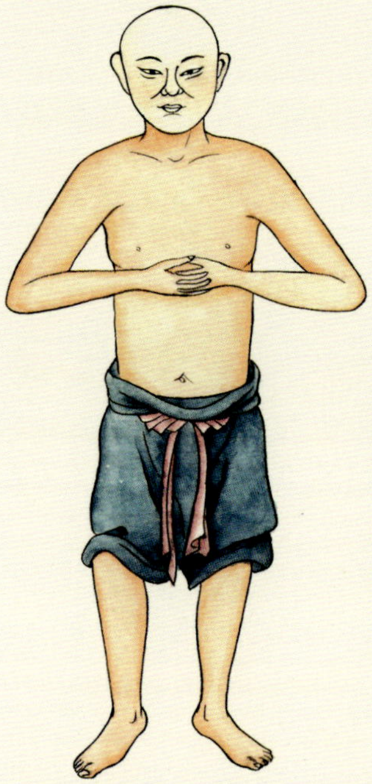

以两手中三指按心窝，由左顺摩圆转二十一次。

Press the three middle fingers of both hands on the pit of your stomach and rub it clockwise twenty-one times.

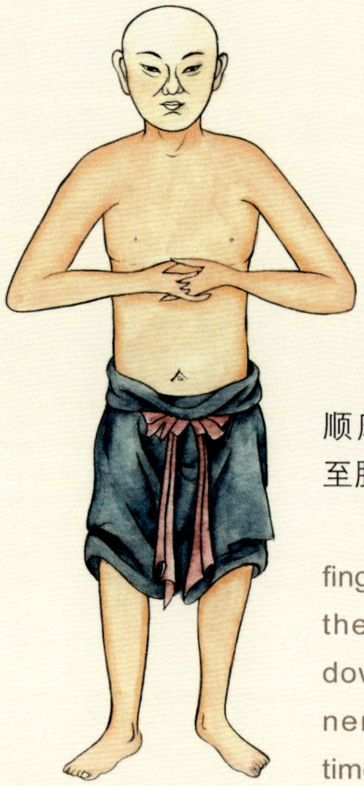

以两手中三指，由心窝顺摩而下，且摩且走，摩至脐下高骨为度。

Push the three middle fingers of both hands from the pit of your stomach downward till the prominent bones twenty-one times.

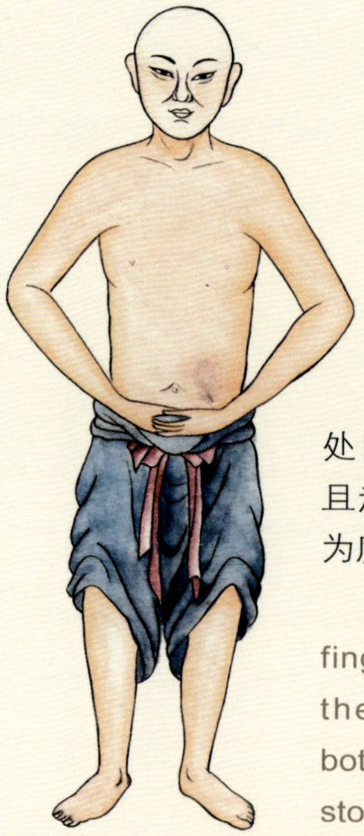

以两手中三指，由高骨处向两边分摩而上，且摩且走，摩至心窝，两手交接为度。

Rub the three middle fingers of both hands from the prominent bones up both sides till the pit of your stomach, where your hands should touch each other.

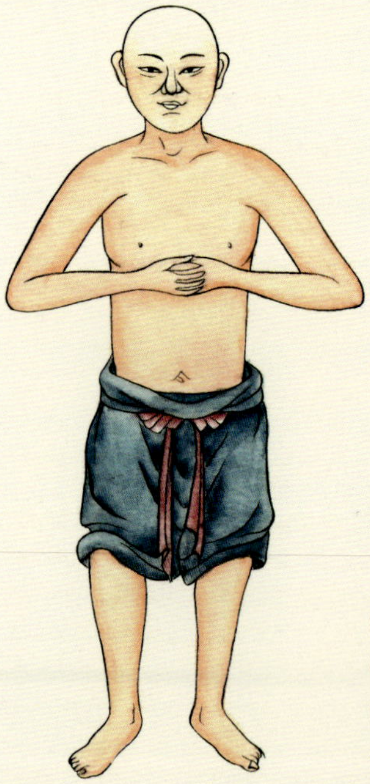

以两手中三指，由心窝向下，直推至高骨二十一次。

Push the three middle fingers of both hands from the pit of your stomach downward till the prominent bones twenty-one times.

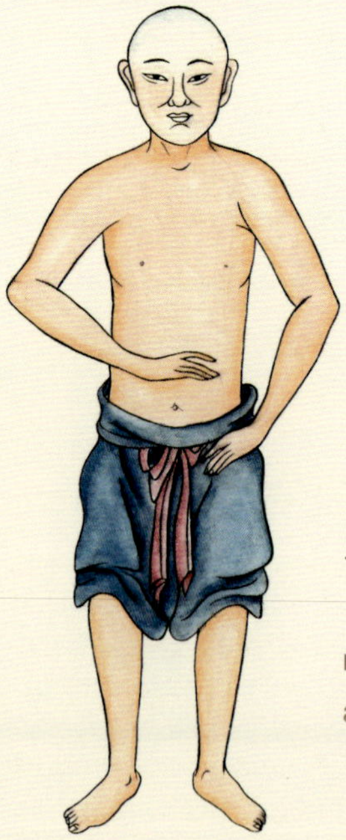

以右手由左绕摩脐腹二十一次。

Put your right hand to the right of your navel and rub around it twenty-one times.

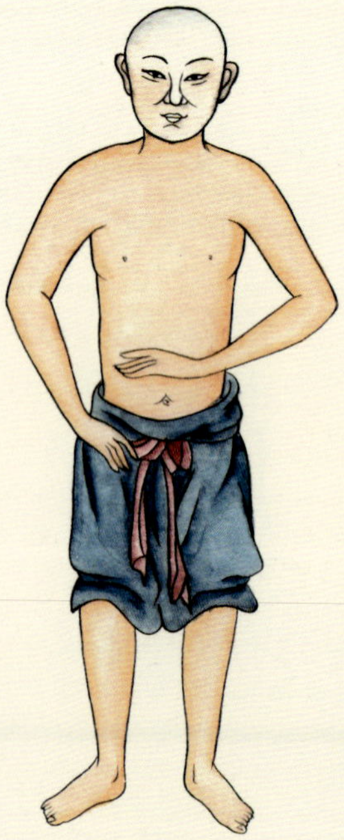

以左手由右绕摩脐腹二十一次。

Put your left hand to the left of your navel and rub around it twenty-one times.

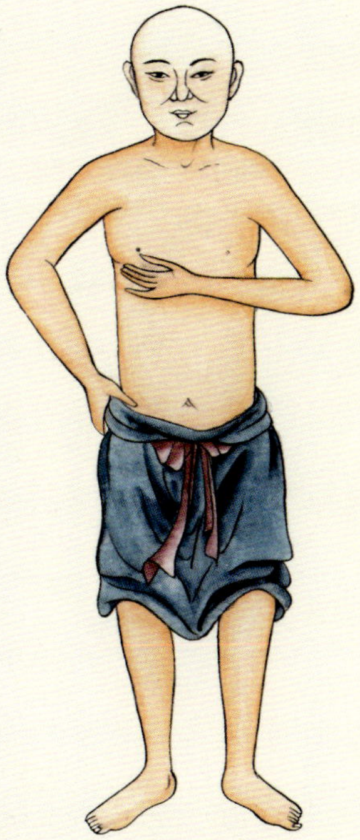

以左手将左边软肋下腰肾处，自左乳下直推至腿夹二十一次。

Hold the left side of your waist where your kidney is with your left hand. Push the three middle fingers of your right hand from the part below your left breast to your crotch twenty-one times.

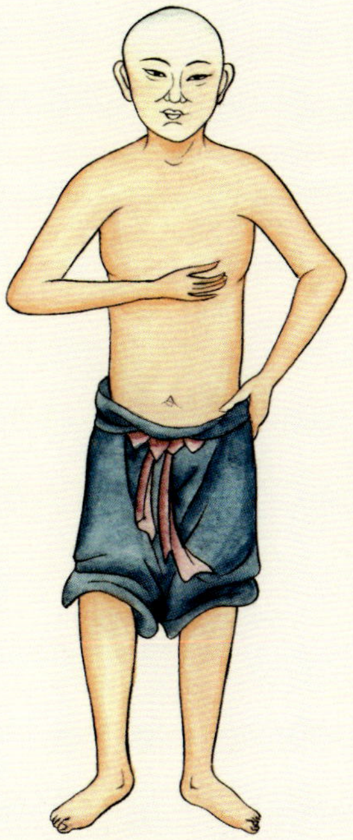

以右手将右边软肋下腰肾处，自右乳下直推至腿夹二十一次。

Hold the right side of your waist where your kidney is with your right hand. Push the three middle fingers of your left hand from the part below your right breast to your crotch twenty-one times.

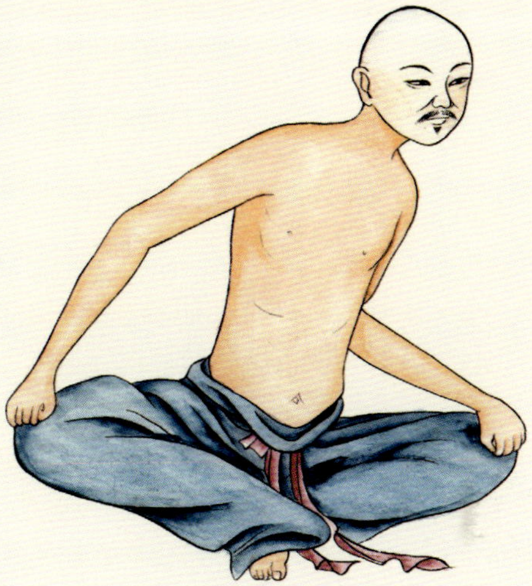

推毕遂趺坐，以两手分按两膝上。将胸自左转前，由右归后摇转。毕。

When this is over, sit cross-legged. Put both hands on your knees. Turn your chest clockwise. This is the end of the exercise.

太极拳

Tai Chi Chuan

“太极”一词源出《周易》,《周易·系辞上》说 :“是故易有太极，始生两仪。两仪生四象，四象生八卦，八卦定吉凶。”太极即为天地未开、混沌未分阴阳之前的状态，两仪即为太极的阴、阳二仪，或说为天地。中国古代哲学用阴阳、乾坤、刚柔的对立统一来解释宇宙万物和人类社会的一切变化，指出了它们之间既互相对立斗争又相互滋生依存的关系，这是非常伟大的智慧，也是太极拳的理论基础。

The word Taiji (the Supreme Ultimate, or the Great Primal Beginning) originates from *Book of Changes* (*I Ching*). The First Part of the Appended Judgments ('Xi Ci') in this book says, 'Therefore there is in the Changes the Great Primal Beginning. This generates the two primary forces. The two primary forces generate the four images. The four images generate the eight trigrams. The eight trigrams determine good fortune and misfortune.' Taiji refers to the state of chaos prior to the separation of heaven from earth, and that of yin from yang. The 'two primary forces' are yin and yang, or heaven and earth. In ancient Chinese philosophy, the unity of opposites, such as yin and yang, heaven and earth, and firmness and softness, serves to explain all changes in the universe and human society in terms of their opposition to each other and inter-dependence. Such extraordinary wisdom forms the theoretical basis of Tai Chi Chuan.

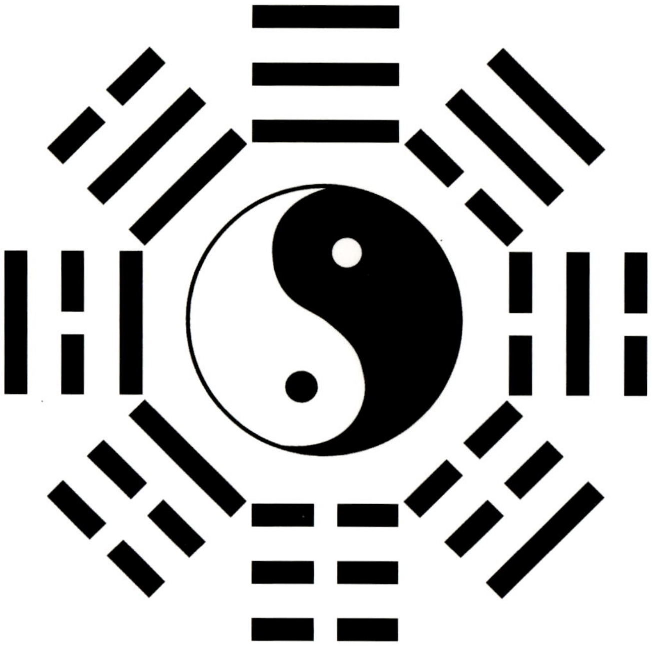

中国武术中流传范围最广，影响力最大，练习者最多的拳种，非太极拳莫属。特有的养生健身功能和蕴含的深刻哲理，让太极拳受到了全世界的关注，越来越多的人喜欢上这项运动。如今，太极拳已传播到 150 多个国家和地区，成为世界上参与人数最多的运动项目，大约有一亿三千万人正在习练太极拳。

Tai Chi Chuan has surpassed any other kind of Chinese martial arts in circulation, influence, and the number of practitioners. It has spread to over 150 countries and regions, arousing worldwide interest for its unique health-preserving effects and profound philosophy. Practiced by some 130 million people, it has become the sport with the largest number of participants in the world.

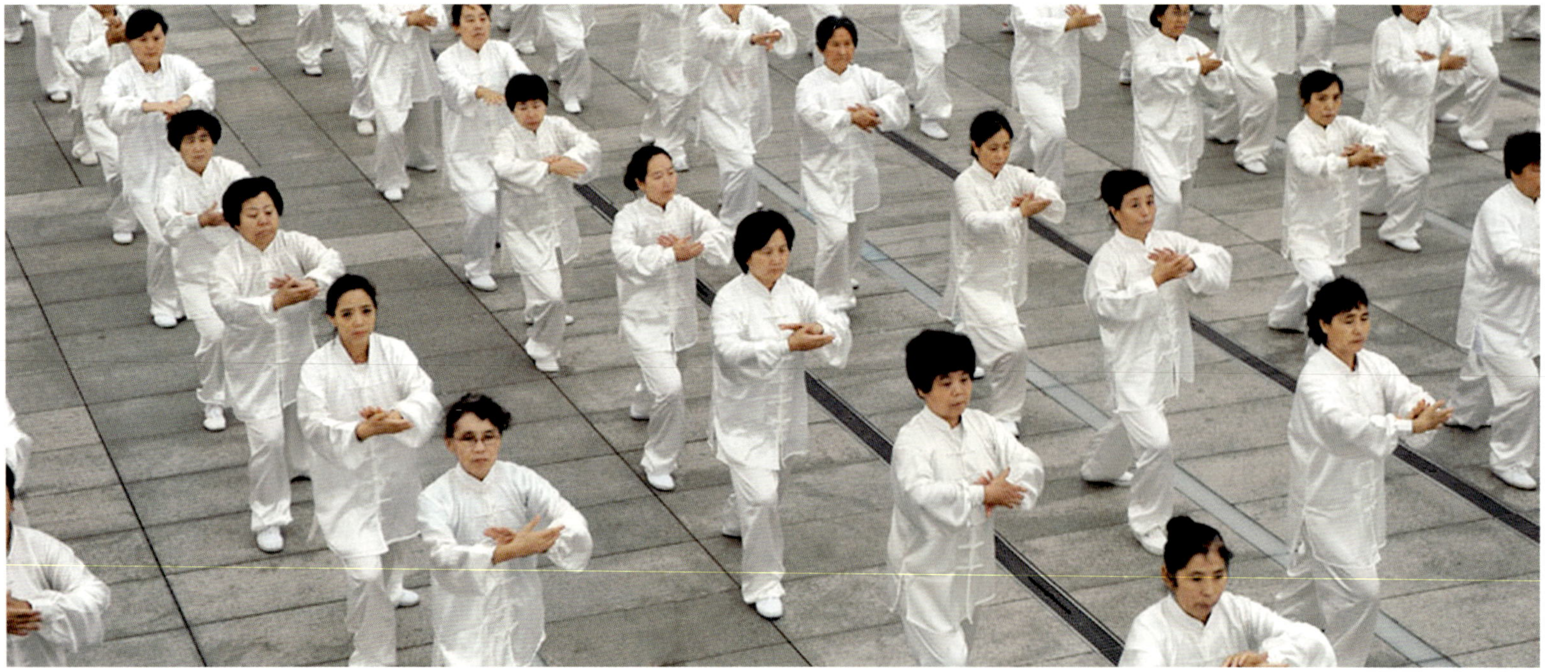

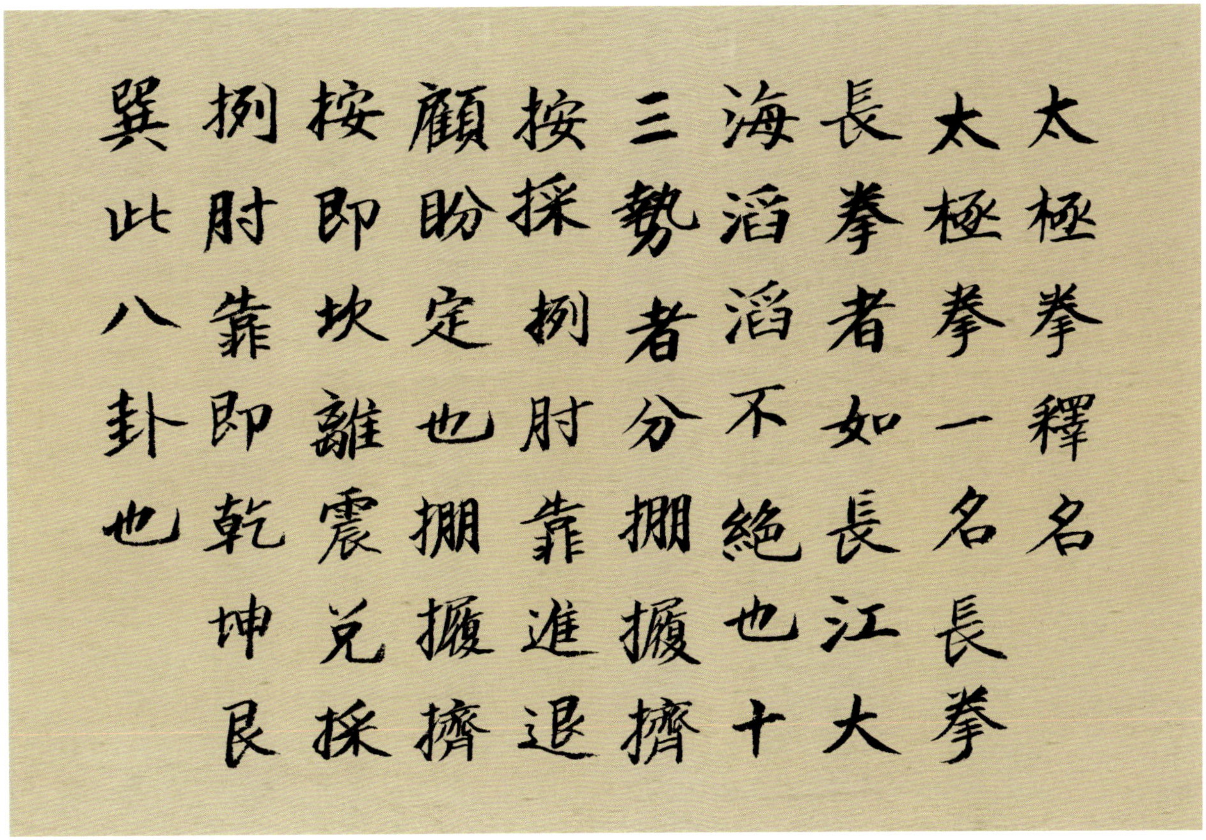

传统体育的很多技击技术都是以损害人体机能为代价的，太极拳则不然，它是人充实生活，修炼人格，获得全面发展的极佳方式。太极拳在创立的过程中，以武术动作为核心，吸收了中国传统医学、养生学的精髓。习练太极拳对调理人的身体、修炼人的精神、完善人的性格、提升人的涵养都有非常大的好处，能够让人保持身心健康，祛病延年。有研究表明，练习太极拳可以改善人体的呼吸系统、微循环系统和消化系统，提高人的肌体平衡力和控制力，促进血液循环，预防骨质疏松，增强免疫力。太极拳，这一古老的拳术正在为造福人们的生活作出越来越大的贡献。

During its creation and development, Tai Chi Chuan, which was based on movements in martial arts, incorporated the essence of traditional Chinese medicine and health-preserving methods. It is highly beneficial to the regulation, cultivation and improvement of one's physical and mental health, character and self-restraint. It can resist diseases, prolong life, and ensure mental and physical health. For example, research has shown that practicing Tai Chi Chuan can improve the respiratory system and the digestive system, enhance immunity, and aid blood circulation and psychological balance. In particular, it is clearly effective for improving the microcirculatory system, preventing osteoporosis and enhancing balance control.

It is universally acknowledged that practicing Tai Chi Chuan is good for the preservation of psychological and moral health. It can help to cultivate the virtues of generosity, tranquility, composure and prudence. In many of the numerous arts of attack and defense, various effects are achieved at the expense of physical health. In comparison, Tai Chi Chuan, which integrates boxing, the preservation and improvement of health, and mental cultivation, is an excellent approach to self-fulfillment and all-around development. This ancient boxing art is giving more and more benefit to our life.

王宗岳的《太极拳论》是太极拳界公认的经典著作，全文如下：

太极拳论

Treatise on Tai Chi Chuan

太极者，无极而生，动静之机，阴阳之母也。动之则分，静之则合。无过不及，随曲就伸。人刚我柔谓之走，我顺人背谓之粘。动急则急应，动缓则缓随。虽变化万端，而理唯一贯。由着熟而渐悟懂劲，由懂劲而阶及神明。然非用力日久，不能豁然贯通焉。虚领顶劲，气沉丹田，不偏不倚，忽隐忽现。左重则左虚，右重则右杳。仰之则弥高，俯之则弥深，进之则愈长，退之则愈促。一羽不能加，蝇虫不能落，人不知我，我独知人。英雄所向无敌，盖皆由此而及也。斯技旁门甚多，虽势有区别，概不外壮欺弱，慢让快耳。有力打无力，手慢让手快，是皆先天自然之能，非关学力而有为也。察四两拨千斤之句，显非力胜；观耄耋能御众之形，快何能为。立如平准，活似车轮，偏沉则随，双重则滞。每见数年纯功，不能运化者，率皆自为人制，双重之病未悟耳。欲避此病，须知阴阳；粘即是走，走即是粘，阴不离阳，阳不离阴；阴阳相济，方为懂劲。懂劲后，愈练愈精，默识揣摩，渐至从心所欲。本是舍己从人，多误舍近求远。所谓差之毫厘，谬之千里，学者不可不详辨焉。是为论。

《太极拳论》在太极拳界里的地位就相当于《论语》之于儒家，《老子》之于道家，它面世以后，所有讲解太极拳的论著可以说都是对它的阐释和发挥。

Taiji is born of *wuji* and is the mother of *yin* and *yang*.
In motion it separates. In stillness it combines.
Without excess, no urgency, follow while bending, engage while extending.
When the opponent is hard, I am yielding; it is called *zou*.
When I adhere to the opponent, it is called *nian*.
If the opponent's movement is quick, then I am quick.
If the opponent's movement is slow, then I follow slowly.
Though transformation produces ten thousand outcomes, the principle is unchanging.
By martial proficiency, one gradually awakens *dong jin*.
From dong jin, one progresses toward *shen ming*.
Without long, persistent and arduous practice, one cannot pass through to deeper knowledge.
Empty the neck to lead energy to the head-top.

Wang Zongyue's *Tai Ji Quan Lun* (Treatise on Tai Chi Chuan) is universally acknowledged as a classic by the Tai Chi Chuan community. The full text goes as follows:

Sink *qi* to the *dantian*.
No leaning or leaning-on.
Suddenly hide, now appear.
If the left-side is weighted upon, the left-side empties.
If there is pressure on the right-side, the right-side disappears.
Facing up, it becomes even higher. Looking down, it becomes even deeper.
Advancing, it further lengthens. Retreating, it becomes increasingly urgent.
One feather cannot be added, and a fly cannot alight.
The opponent does not know me—only I know him.
A hero moving toward invincibility—thus prevailing over all.
There are many paths to skillfulness but although they use different powers,
for the most part they don't go beyond the strong bullying the weak, and the slow resigning to the swift.
The powerful hitting the weak and slow hands submitting to swift hands:
theses are all the results of natural advantages and not of well-trained power.
Consider the saying, 'Four ounces turns a thousand pounds.'
Obviously this cannot be a victory through strength.
Witness an old person resisting numerous people: how can it be due to swiftness?
Stand precisely balanced. Resemble a cart-wheel.
Sinking to one side allows following. Symmetrical force is stagnant.
If one has spent years practicing skills but still cannot neutralize,
and is rather, always governed by the opponent,
one has not apprehended the fault of symmetrical weightedness.
If one desires to avoid this defect, one must know yin and yang.
To adhere means to receive. To yield means to adhere.
Yin cannot leave yang; yang cannot leave yin.
Yin and yang mutually aid and change each other.
Grasping this aspect, one can arrive at dong jin.
After dong jin is acquired, more practice will improve the essence.
Silently memorize and deeply ponder and gradually one can accomplish anything one pleases.
Fundamentally, 'give up self-centeredness and accept others'.
Many mistakenly 'give up the near to seek the far'.
It is said, 'A slight deviation will lead one thousands of paces astray.'
The pupil must clearly distinguish, hence this treatise. (Translated by Sam Masich)

Tai Ji Quan Lun is as important to the Tai Chi Chuan community as *The Analects* is to Confucianism, or *Lao Tzu* to Taoism. All books on Tai Chi Chuan published since its appearance can be regarded as commentaries on it.

太極拳論

太極者無極而生動靜之機陰陽之母也動之則分靜之則合無過不及隨曲就伸人剛我柔謂之走我順人背謂之黏動急則急應動緩則緩隨雖變化萬端而理唯一貫由着熟而漸悟懂勁由懂勁而階及神明然非用力日久不能豁然貫通焉虛領頂勁氣沉丹田不偏不倚忽隱忽現左重則左虛右重則右杳仰之則彌高俯之則彌深進之則愈長退之則愈促一羽不能加蠅蟲不能落人不知我我獨知人英雄所向無敵蓋皆由此而及也斯技旁門甚多雖勢有區別概不外壯欺弱慢讓快耳有力打無力手慢讓手快是皆先天自然之能非關學力而有為也察四兩撥千斤之句顯非力勝觀耄耋能禦眾之形快何能為立如平準活似車輪偏沉則隨雙重則滯每見數年純功不能運化者率皆自為人制雙重之病未悟耳欲避此病須知陰陽黏即是走走即是黏陰不離陽陽不離陰陰陽相濟方為懂勁懂勁後愈練愈精默識揣摩漸至從心所欲本是捨己從人多誤捨近求遠所謂差之毫釐謬之千里學者不可不詳辨焉是為論

太极八法

The Eight Methods of Tai Chi Chuan

掤、捋、挤、按、采、挒、肘、靠，是太极拳中最基本的手法，又称“太极八法”。它是太极拳所有拳式的基础，八法的劲别各不相同。吴氏太极拳揽雀尾一势八法俱备，下面我们就用图示展示其动作和用法。

揽雀尾，此动作有象形之意。有将对方向我击来之手臂比喻为鸟雀的尾巴，把自己的手臂比喻为绳索，有随着对方手臂的屈伸、上下、左右的动向而缠绕不使其逃脱的意思。

There are the Eight Methods of Tai Chi Chuan: ward off, roll back, press/squeeze, push/press, pluck, split, elbow strike, and body strike/bump [peng, lu, ji, an, cai, lie, zhou, kao]. These form the foundation for all the maneuvers, and they differ in the degree of energy (jin). In Wu's Tai Chi Chuan, the maneuver called Roping the Bird's Tail is an epitome of all the eight methods. Its movements and techniques are shown in the following pictures.

Grasp bird's tail In this maneuver, your opponent's arm coming at you is likened to a bird's tail, and your own arm to a rope, which follows the movements of your opponent's arm, 'twisting' around it and preventing the 'bird' from escaping.

第一动 左抱七星(掤)

First move: embracing seven stars on the left (peng, or warding off)

用意想“会阴穴”向右后下方移动，使尾骶骨与右脚跟上下对正。然后松左肩、坠左肘，左掌会自动地向前上方抬起，到掌心向后上方，拇指与鼻尖前后对正为度，同时右掌也自动地向胸前移动至中指尖贴近左臂弯处为止，掌心朝前下方。然后坠右肘，松右肩，这时左脚会自动地朝正前方把腿舒直，脚跟着地，脚尖翘起（成坐步式）。两眼从左掌拇指上方平远视，重心在右腿，意在右肩（图 1）。

用法：如对方击来右拳，我则以左肘粘其右肘，并以右腕粘其右腕，使其右臂伸直不叫它弯曲，此时对方即被拿起来了（图 2）。

Thinking of your perineum, move downward to the right so that the sacrum is right above the right heel. Relax the left shoulder and lower the left elbow so that the left hand automatically raises forward until the palm faces up backward, with the thumb directly in front of the tip of your nose. Meanwhile, you right hand moves toward the chest until the tip of the middle finger is close to the bend of your left arm, with the palm facing down and forward. Lower your right elbow and relax your right shoulder so that your left foot automatically moves right ahead, straightening the left leg, with the heel on the ground and the toes raised. Look straight ahead into the distance over your left thumb. Rest the center of gravity on your right leg, and think of your right shoulder (Fig. 1).

How to use it: If the rival strikes you with his right fist, 'adhere' your left elbow to his right elbow and 'adhere' your right wrist to his right wrist in order to keep his right arm straight so that he would be warded off (Fig. 2).

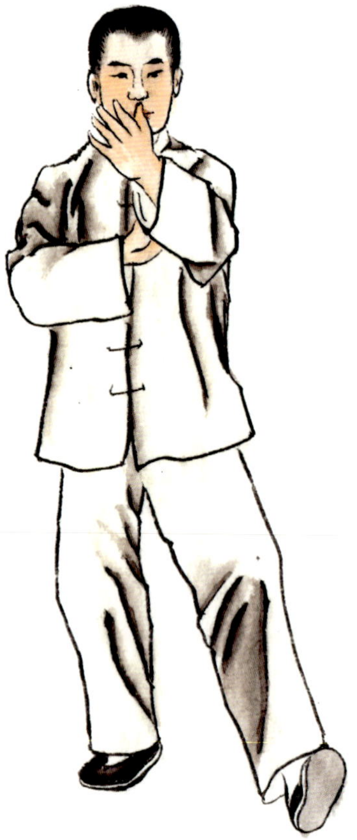

1

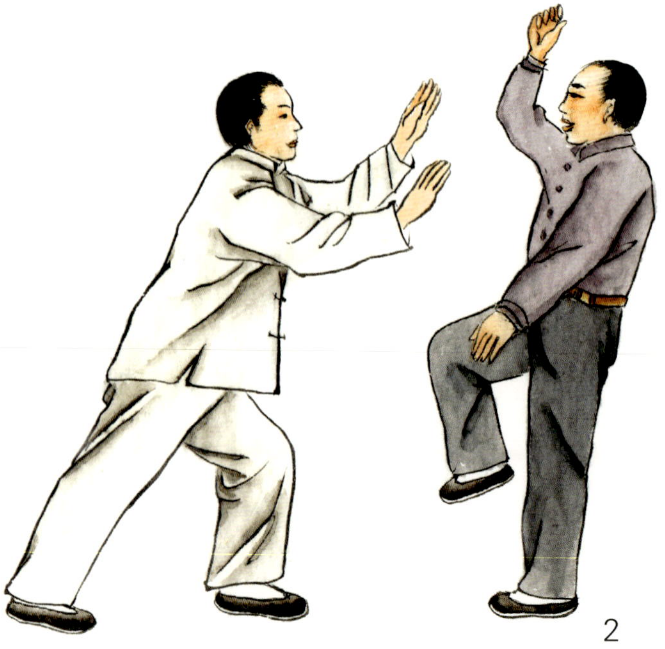

2

第二动 右掌打挤

Second move: pressing/squeezing (ji) with the right hand

用意想松右肩，坠右肘，右掌会自动地向前移至掌心与左掌脉门相贴时为止。这时左臂自动形成平曲横于胸前，左掌掌心向后，指尖朝右，右掌掌心向前，指尖朝天，以食指尖与鼻尖前后对正。与此同时，左脚逐渐落平，左膝前弓，右腿在后伸直（成左弓箭步）。重心在左腿，两眼从右食指上方向前平远视，意在脊背（图3）。

用法：接上动随之，用“挤劲”发之，我以左小臂横于对方之胸部前方，复以右掌向前推至左脉门处，同时脊背微向后倚。这时对方则应手踉踉跄跄跌出或仰面摔倒（图4）。

Relax the right shoulder and lower the right elbow so that the right hand automatically moves forward until the palm touches the maimen (location near the wrist for feeling the pulse) of the left hand. Now that left arm is bent and held level in front of the chest, with the palm facing backward and the fingertips pointing right; the right palm faces forward, with the fingertips pointing upward and the tip of the index finger right in front of the tip of your nose. Meanwhile, level the left food gradually, bend the left knee, and straighten the right leg in a left bow-and-arrow stance (gongjian bu). Rest the center of gravity on your left leg and look straight ahead into the distance over the right index finger while thinking of your back (Fig. 3).

How to use it: Following the previous move, execute this one with 'pressing/squeezing force'. Level your left front arm before your rival's chest, and move your right hand forward until the left maimen. Meanwhile, lean your back slightly backward. Your rival will stumble backward or fall on his back(Fig. 4).

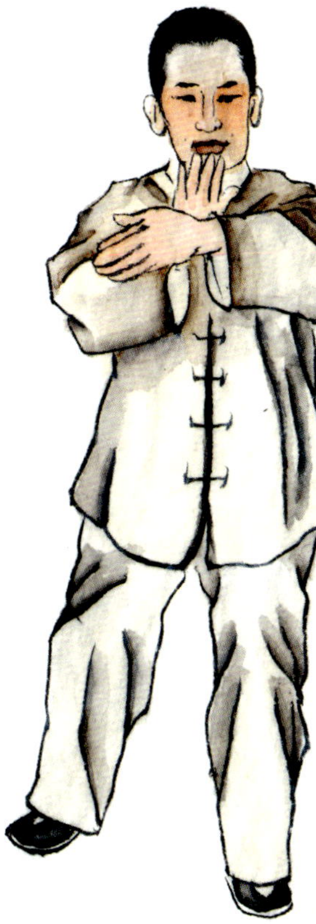

3

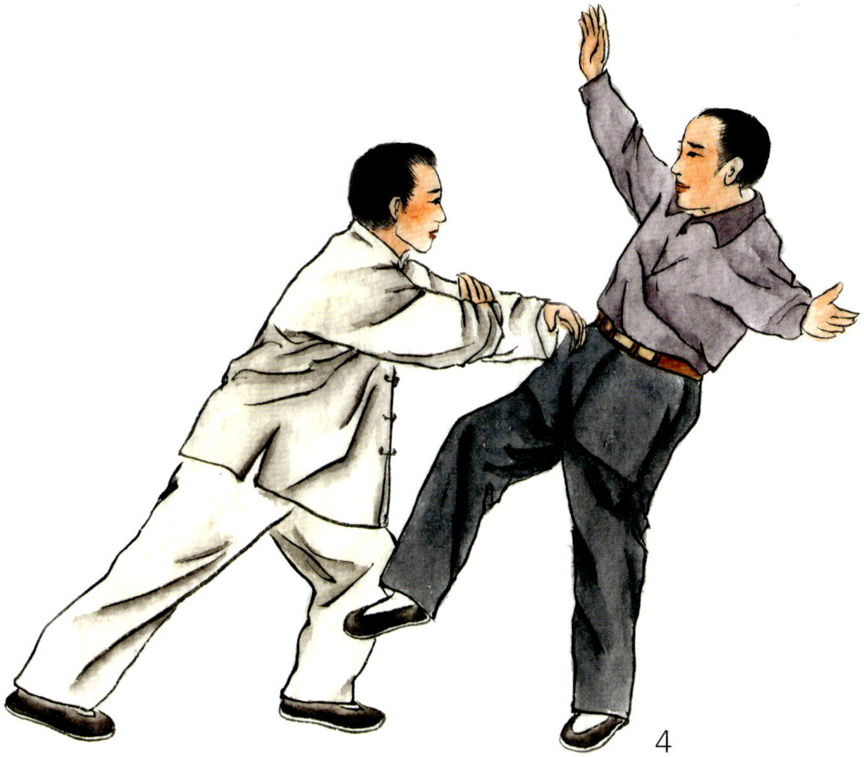

4

第三动 左掌沉采

Third move: 'plucking' (cai) with your left hand

用意想左掌使掌心与右肘相触后，掌心转向下，坠左肘、松左肩。右手上起至中指尖朝天与右肘垂直，左手虎口贴在右肘尖下。同时右脚跟回收，使膝盖与踝骨垂直，左脚不动，两脚形成 90°，重心三七开，身体自动右转，成半马裆步，重心偏在左脚，两眼注视左食指尖。意在左肩（图5、图6）。

Having touched the left palm to the right elbow, turn the palm downward, lower the left elbow, and relax the left shoulder. Raise the right hand until the tip of the middle finger points upward and is perpendicular to the right elbow, with the hukou (part of the hand between the thumb and the index finger) under the tip of the right elbow. Draw back the right heel so that the knee is perpendicular to the ankle while keeping the left foot still, so that the two feet form a right angle. Turn your body to the right to form a madang squat, resting 70% of your weight on the left foot. Fix you eyes on the tip of the left index finger and think of the left shoulder (Fig. 5, Fig. 6).

用法：对方以左肘向我右肋顶来，我则以左掌腕部粘其左腕，同时向右转身并以小臂竖直粘其左肘，然后向左后上方微微移动，即可将对方采起（拿起来）了（图7、图8）。

How to use it: When the rival strikes at my right flank with his left elbow, 'adhere' your left wrist to his left wrist and, meanwhile, turn right, raise your front arm upright and 'adhere' it to his left elbow. Move slightly back upward to the left and 'pluck' your rival (Fig. 7, Fig. 8).

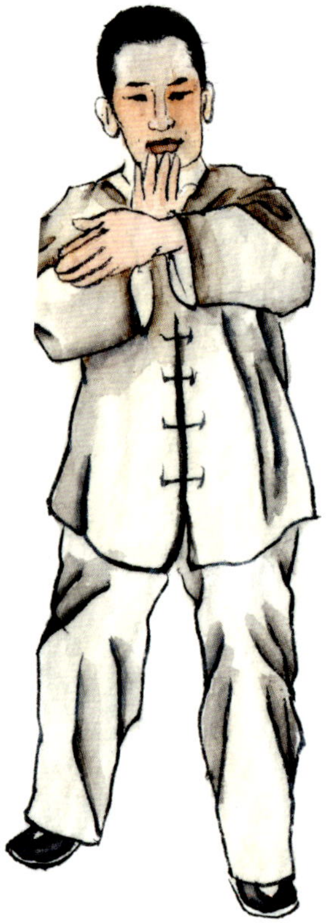

5

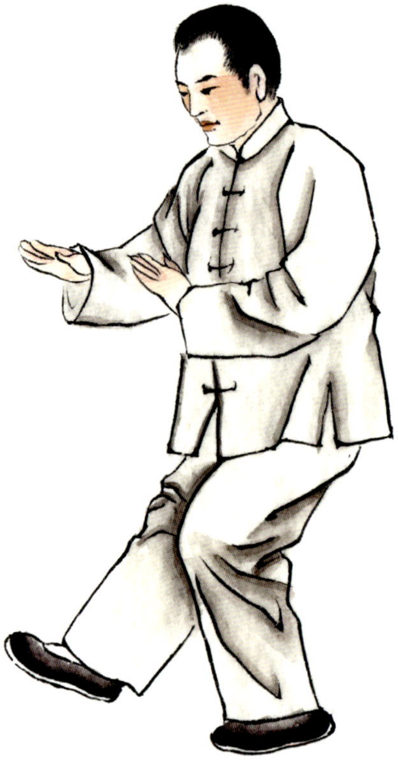

6

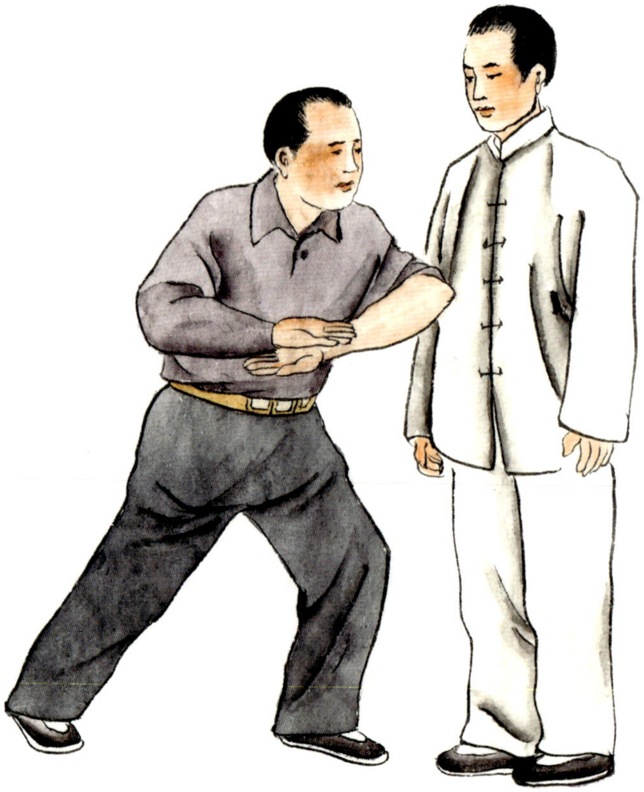

7

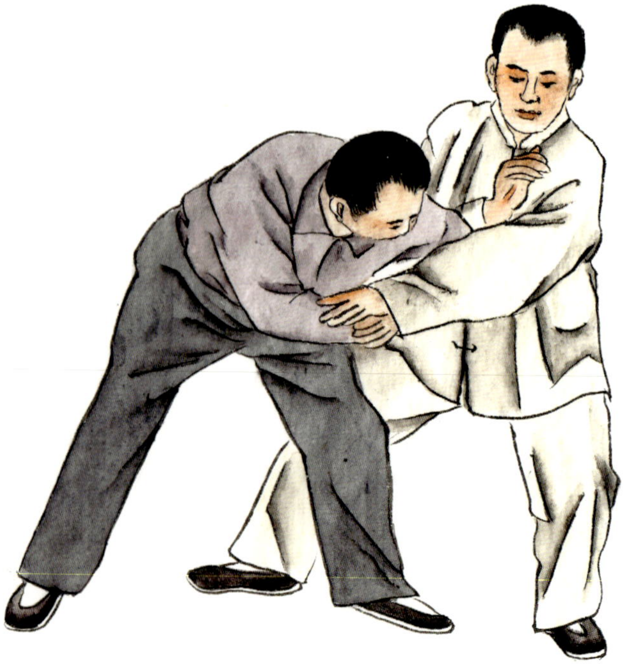

8

第四动 弓步顶肘

Fourth move: elbowing (zhou) in a bow-and-arrow stance

用意想松左肩、坠左肘，这时，右脚脚尖自动地略微抬起，左掌便自动地向前移动至掌心与右臂弯相贴时为止。这时右臂自动形成平曲横于胸前，右掌掌心向右和右肩相对，指尖朝后，左掌指尖朝前，拇指尖朝天。与此同时，右脚逐步落平，右膝弓出，左腿在后伸直（成右弓箭步）。重心在右腿，两眼从右肘尖上方向前平远视。意在右掌掌心（图 9、图 10）。

用法：我以右肘肘尖横于对方胸部前方，复以左掌向前推至右臂弯处，同时右掌掌心微向右肩靠拢。这时对方则应手跄踉跌出或立即摔倒（图 11、图 12）。

Relax the left shoulder and lower the left elbow. The toes of the right foot rise slightly, and the left hand move forward until the palm touches the bend of the right arm. Now the right arm is bent and held level before the chest, with the right palm facing the right shoulder and the fingertips pointing backward, and the fingertips of the left hand pointing forward except the tip of the thumb, which points upward. Meanwhile, level the right foot gradually, bend the right knee, and straighten the left leg to form the right bow-and-arrow stance. Rest the center of gravity on your right leg and look straight ahead into the distance over the tip of the right elbow while thinking of your right palm (Fig. 9, Fig. 10).

How to use it: Put the tip of your right elbow before your rival's chest and push your left hand forward to the bend of your right arm. Meanwhile, bring your right palm slightly closer to your right shoulder. Your rival will stumble or fall immediately (Fig. 11, Fig. 12).

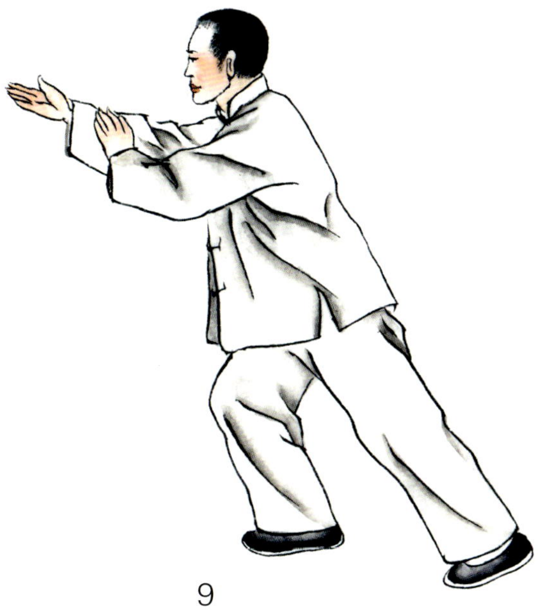

9

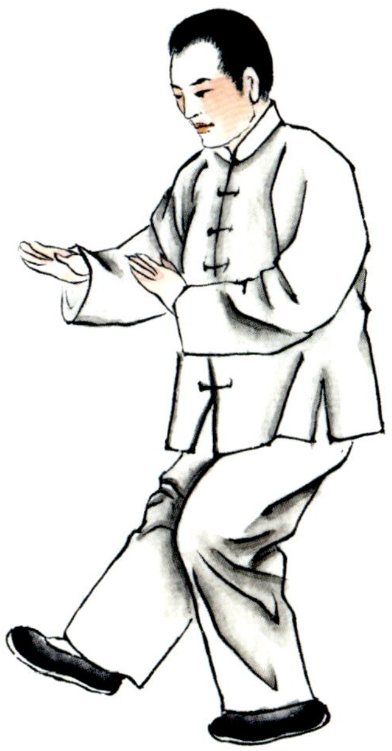

10

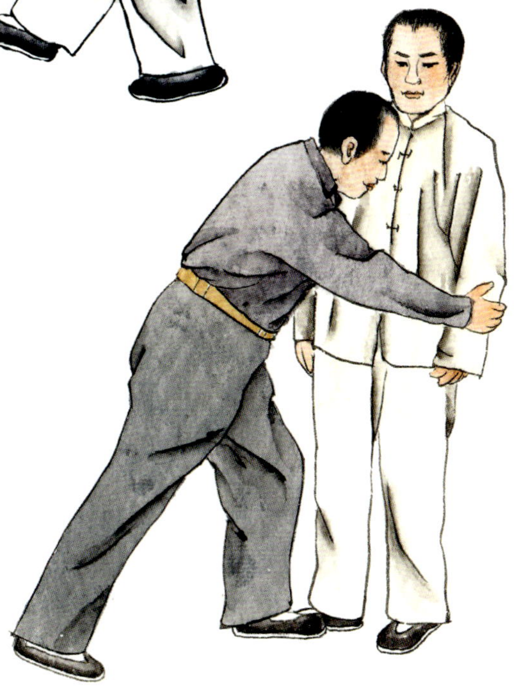

11

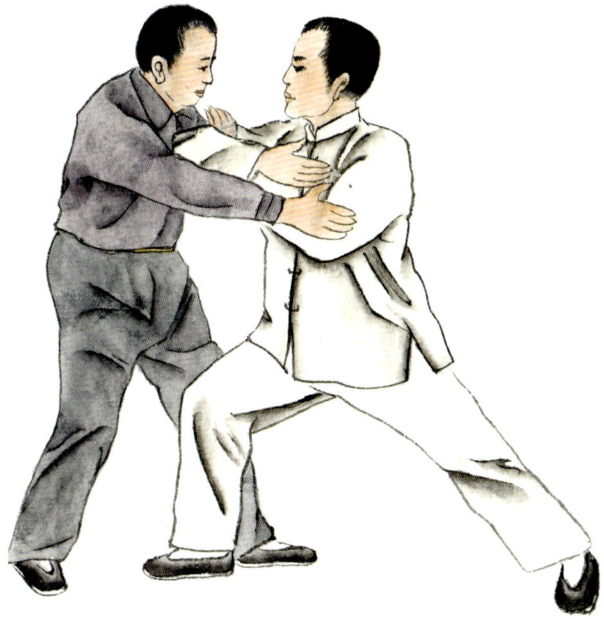

12

第五动 左肩打靠

Fifth move: bumping (kao) with the left shoulder

用意想右掌的五指指甲，从拇指开始逐递想每个指甲与空中（天）成水平，这时右臂自动伸直，掌心也随之翻转朝地面，然后使右臂从身之右前上方走弧形降落至身之右后下方。这时用意想哪里，哪里就放松。此动作是从右手的小指肚开始依次放松的，即从小指、无名、中、食、拇指指肚、手心与手腕、肘关节一直松到肩关节。此动作做完形成右弓箭步，重心仍在右腿，左肩朝正前方，上体半面转向右。左右两臂微曲、两掌掌心均朝下，虎口上下斜对成圆状。两眼注视右手食指指尖（图 13）。

用法：发靠劲，似雷霆之迅速不及掩耳。其姿势以自己身体之有关部位靠对方之身，使其不能得力，无论用肩、肘、背、胯、膝等部位，均可靠之。此式用法是接上一个动作肘打，而被对方采劲化解反攻，我即用左肩向其胸部（即原右肘所触之位置）猛击（图 14）。

Think of the nails of the five fingers of your right hand, one by one from thumb. Make them parallel to the sky in your mind. The right arm automatically straightens and the palm turns downward, facing the ground. Lower the right arm from its position to the upper right of your body along a curve to the lower right. Think of various parts of the body and relax it accordingly. In this move, relaxation starts from the inside of the little finger of the right hand and proceed one by one to the fourth finger, the middle finger, the index finger, the inside of the thumb, the palm, the wrist, the elbow joint, and the shoulder joint. At the end of this process you assume a right bow-and-arrow stance, with the center of gravity still on the right leg, your left shoulder facing straight forward, and your torso turned halfway right. Bend your arms slightly, both palms downward, with the hukou of both hands joined into a circle. Fix your eyes on the tip of the index finger of the right hand (Fig. 13).

How to use it: Execute this move very fast and suddenly with a 'bumping force'. You may bump him with your shoulder, elbow, back, hip or knee. This move follows the previous one. If your rival has neutralized the previous move and strikes back at you, bump his chest (i.e. what was touched by your right elbow) with your left shoulder (Fig. 14).

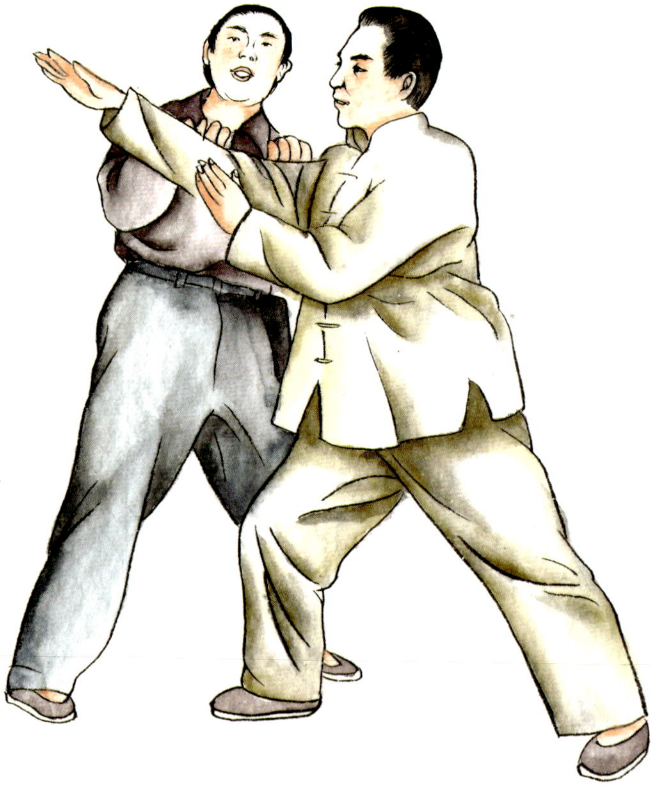

13

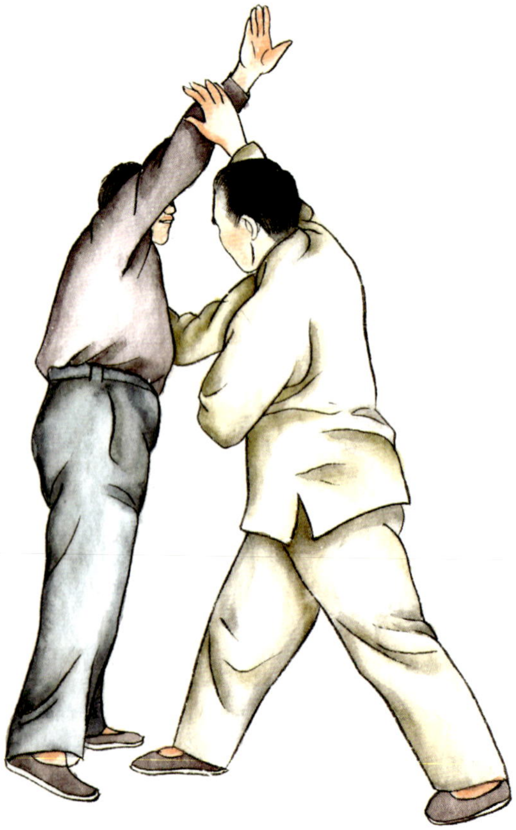

14

第六动 右掌上挒

Sixth move: splitting (lie) upward with the right hand

用意想右肩松力、右肘下坠、右掌掌心自动松转向上，从右肋开始移动经左肋、前胸、至右臂舒直与右肩前后对正略高于肩，掌心向上，指尖向前，左掌掌心向下以中指和无名指尖扶在右掌脉门。与此同时，身子要随手的动作而自动地运转（即身子怎样动都不要管它，任其自然保持正直）。重心变换了一次，系由右腿移到左腿，复由左腿又转移到右腿。两眼从右掌食指尖上方，向前平远看。意在右脚（图15）。

用法：劲之法与采劲相反。分劲为挒，其姿式抓住以后而拧为挒。主要是手与脚而产生（图16）。

Relax with right shoulder and lower the right elbow. The right palm automatically turns upward and moves from the right flank past the left flank and chest until the right arm is straight and right ahead of and slightly higher than the right shoulder, palm upward and fingertips forward. Turn your left palm downward, and touch your middle finger and fourth finger on the maimen of your right hand. Meanwhile, the body automatically moves along with the movement of your hands (i.e. keep your body naturally upright without minding how it moves). The center of gravity moves from the right leg to the left leg and then back to the right leg. Look straight ahead into the distance over the tip of the index finger of your right hand while thinking of your right foot (Fig. 15).

How to use it: 'Splitting' (lie) is opposite to 'plucking' (cai). A splitting action, which need two forces executed in opposite directions, consists of grasping and twisting. It is mainly done with one's hands and feet (Fig. 16).

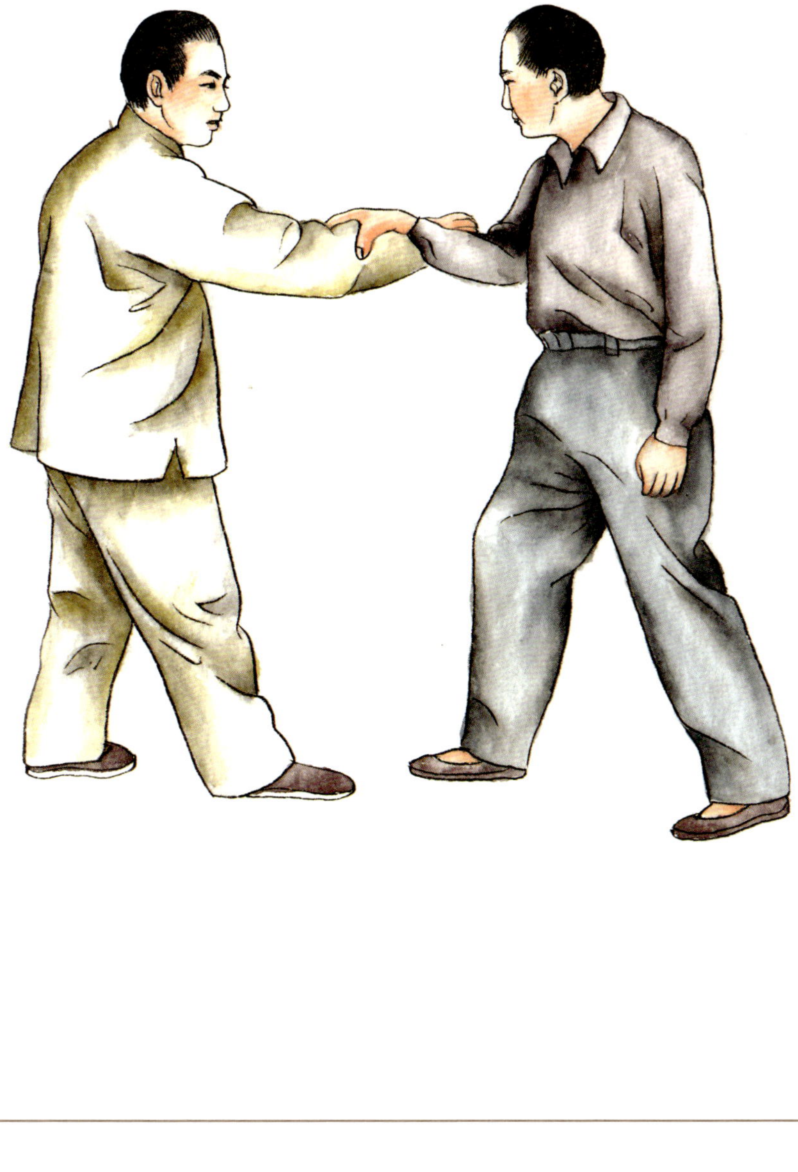

15

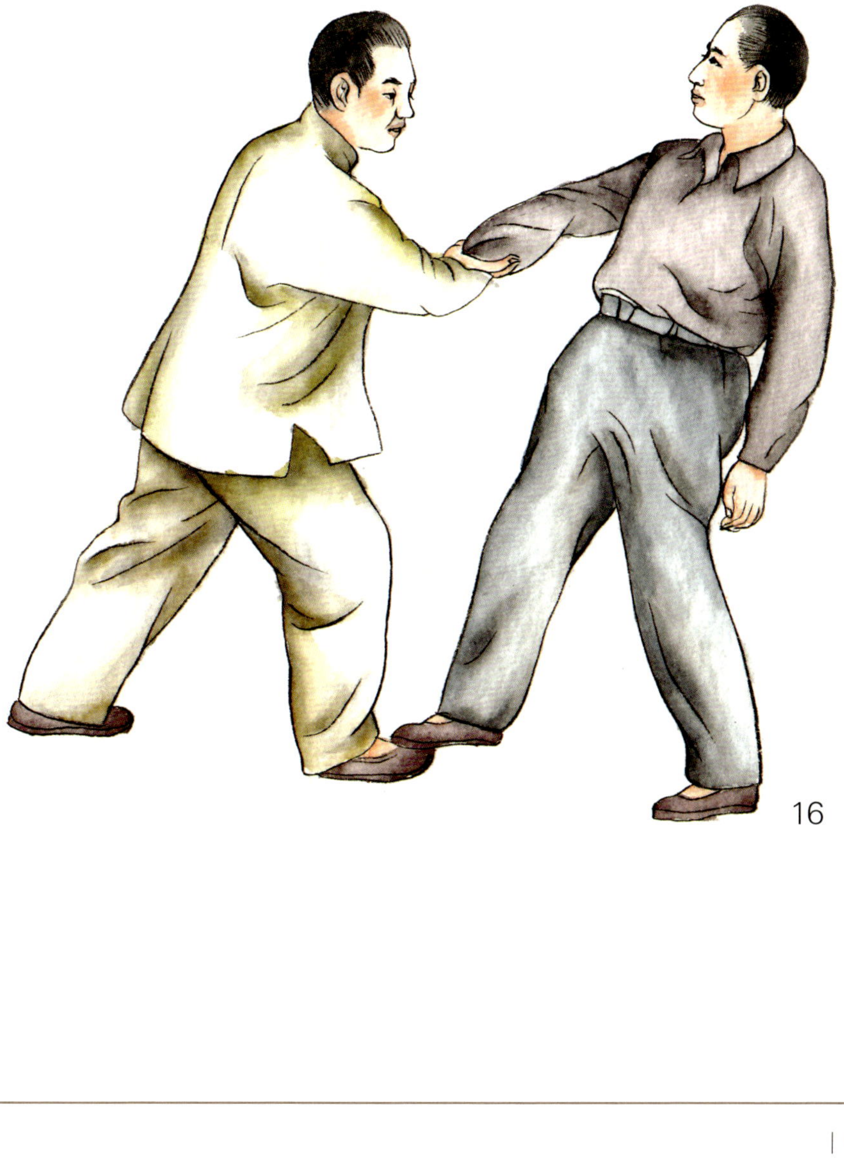

16

第七动 两掌回捋

Seventh move: rolling back (lu) with both hands

用意想右掌掌心向内，以食指指肚从左眉梢向右划至左眉攒时，掌心转向外再以食指的指甲从右眉攒划至右眉梢为止。眼神始终注视右掌食指指尖。与此同时，左腿自动地屈膝略蹲，右腿舒直，脚跟着地，脚尖翘起，重心在左腿。左掌与右掌均朝外，两掌分开距离约十五厘米，意在两眉中间（图 17）。

用法：捋劲之法是破手之法。例如对方以手来攻（即斜上方的力），刚刚接触我身时（图 18），我则以右掌粘其左腕，左掌粘其右肘，同时往右后上方捋出（图 19），与此同时，身子略微右转则使对方所发之力落空而应手跌出（图 20）。

Turn the palm of your right hand inward. Scrape the inside of the index finger from the outer tip of your left eyebrow to the right until its inner tip. Turn the palm outward, and scrape the nail of the index finger from the inner tip of the right eyebrow to its outer tip. During the process, fix your eyes on the tip of the index finger of your right hand. Meanwhile, slightly bend your left knee and straighten your right leg, with the heel on the ground and the toes raised. Rest the center of gravity on your left leg. Turn both palms outward at a distance of about 15 cm. Think of the part between your eyebrows (Fig. 17).

How to use it: 'Rolling back' serves to neutralize the 'warding off' technique. Suppose your rival attacks you with pengshou (an oblique upward force). As soon as he touches you (Fig. 18), 'adhere' your right hand to his left wrist and 'adhere' your left hand to his right elbow; meanwhile, roll backward to the upper right (Fig. 19). Turn your body slightly right so that the rival will miss his target and stumble (Fig. 20).

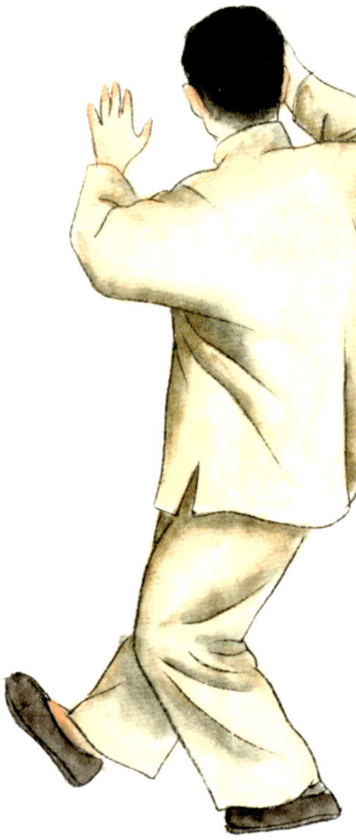

17

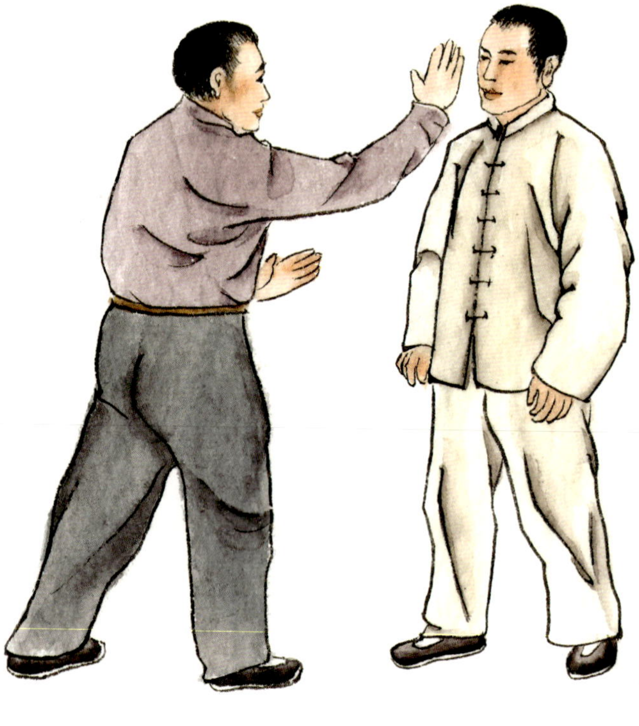

18

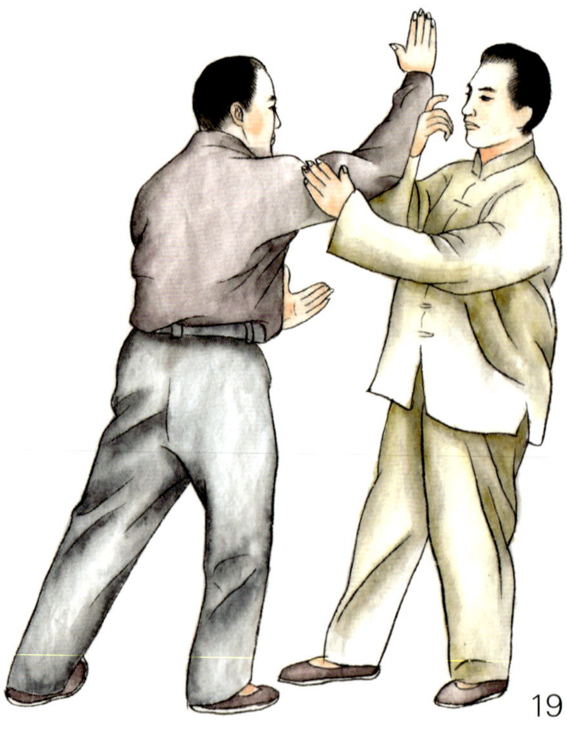

19

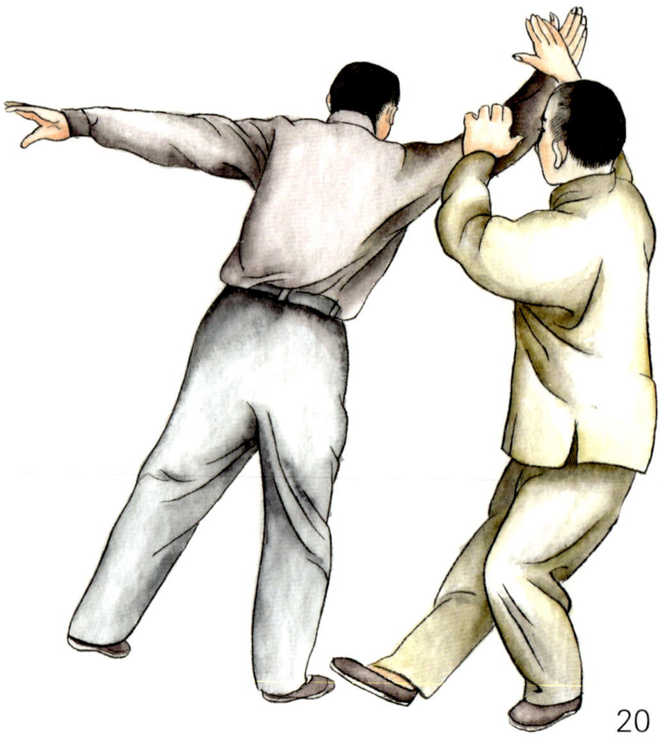

20

第八动 右掌前按

Eighth move: pressing (an) forward with the right hand

用意想左手腕，左肘逐渐放松，一直松到左肩为止。同时右脚脚尖自动地向左转（正对南方），随之，屈膝微蹲，左腿舒直，左脚位置不动，两脚形成“丁八步”。重心在右腿，这时左右两掌距离不变，只是随同身子从正北向左转到正南时为止，掌心均朝下。右掌高与乳平，左掌与心口窝平。两眼视线从右食指尖转移到左食指指尖，意在前胸（图21）。

用法：按劲之法可以破挤劲。如对方用挤手（即平行直力）击来（图22），我则以双手轻轻扶于其后臂之肘腕部的上面，不可用力，只要粘住不离开就行，但要点在于“涵胸”（即胸部略微一收敛），同时两掌微微向前舒展略带弧形即得（图23）。这时对方则应手而倒或是跌坐在地上（图24）。

Thinking of your left wrist, gradually relax your left elbow and up to your left shoulder. Meanwhile, the toes of your right foot automatically turn left to face due south. Bend your right knee slightly and straighten your left leg while keeping your left foot still so that your feet form a dingba posture. Rest the center of gravity on the right leg. Keep the distance between your hands as they move left with your torso from due north to due south, both palms downward. Hold your right hand at the height of your breast and your left hand at the height of your heart. Move the line of sight from the tip of your right index finger to that of your left index finger while thinking of your chest (Fig. 21).

How to use it: The pressing technique can be used to neutralize the squeezing technique. If your rival strikes at you with 'squeezing' (straight and level) force (Fig. 22), gently touch your hands to his upper arm above the elbow. Simply 'adhere' to it and do not apply any force. Most importantly, you must contract your chest a little bit and, meanwhile, gently extend your hands forward in a slight curve (Fig. 23). Your rival will lose balance or fall on his buttocks (Fig. 24).

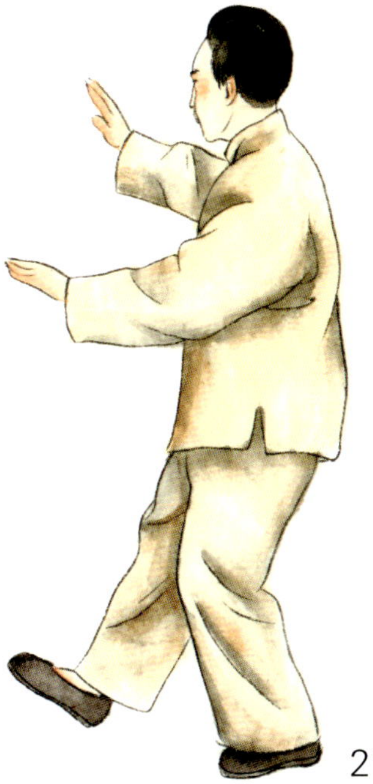

21

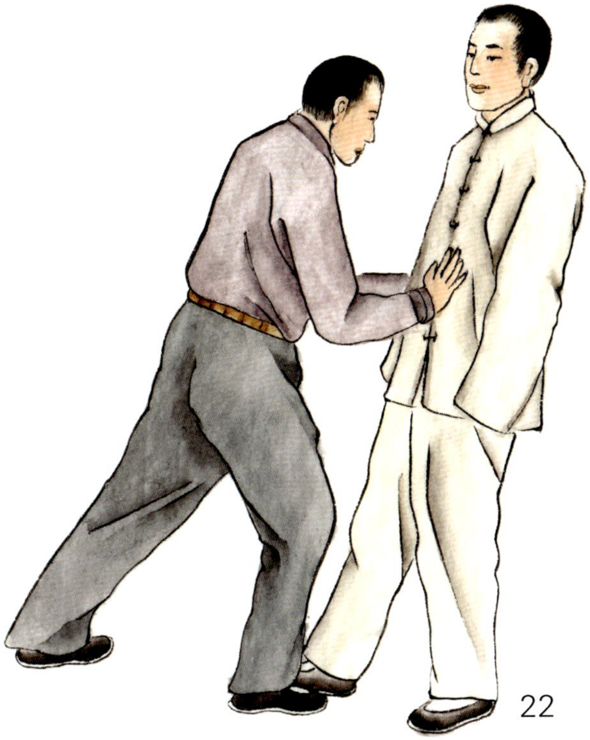

22

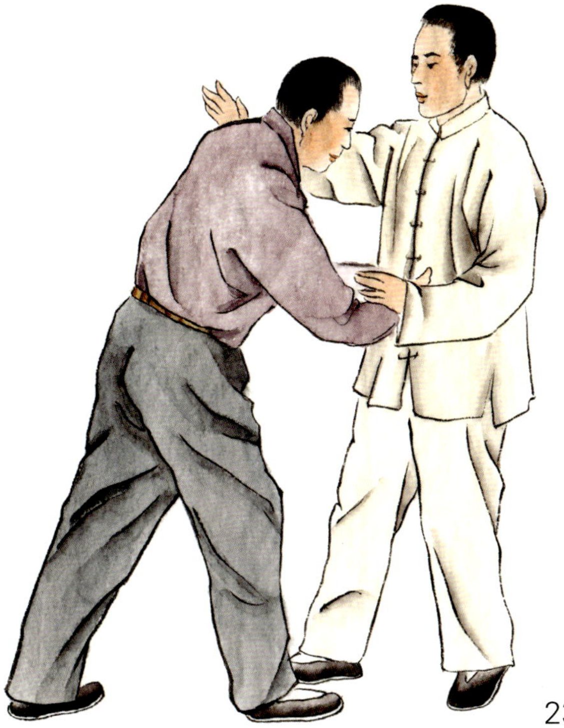

23

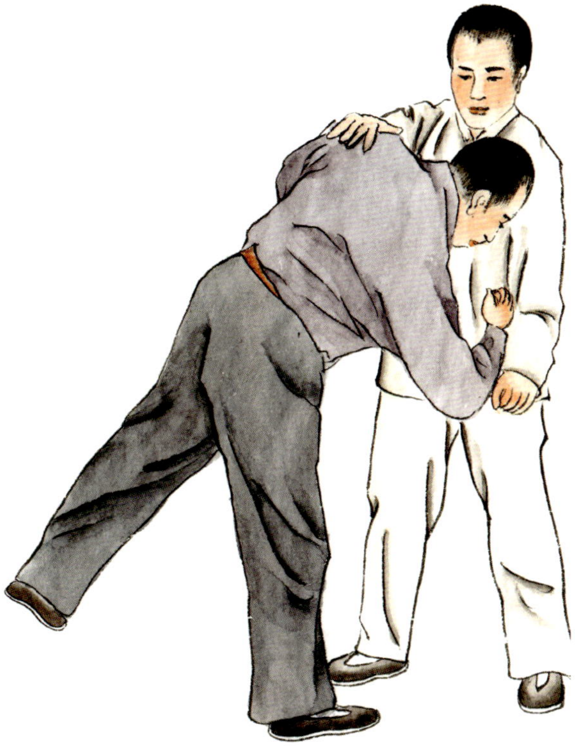

24

吴式太极拳三十七式

The Thirty-Seven Movements of Wu Style Tai Chi Chuan

太极拳，是武术项目，也是体育运动和健身项目，在中国有着悠久的历史。太极拳是我们的祖先古人依据《易经》阴阳变化的辩证哲学、中医经络学、道家导引吐纳法综合创造的一套符合人体节律和大自然运转规律的拳术。太极拳讲究运动时身体中正安舒、轻灵圆活、松柔慢匀，如“行云流水，连绵不断”，既自然又富含哲理，使人在愉悦中防病祛病，身心健康。下面是《吴式太极拳三十七式》：

Tai Chi Chuan is a type of martial art, a sport and an exercise with a long history in China. It is a kind of boxing conducive to health and in compliance with the law of nature, which was invented by ancient Chinese according to the dialectic philosophy about yin and yang in *I Ching*, or the *Book of Changes*, the theory of energy channels in traditional Chinese medicine, and the Taoist practices of Tao Yin and tuna (breathing technique for longevity). It requires the movements of the body to be relaxed, flexible, gentle, slow, even, and 'natural and smooth like clouds and streams'. Conforming to nature and highly philosophical, this is an enjoyable exercise that enables one to resist diseases and stay healthy both mentally and physically. The following are the thirty-seven movements of Wu Style Tai Chi Chuan:

预备式

Preparation

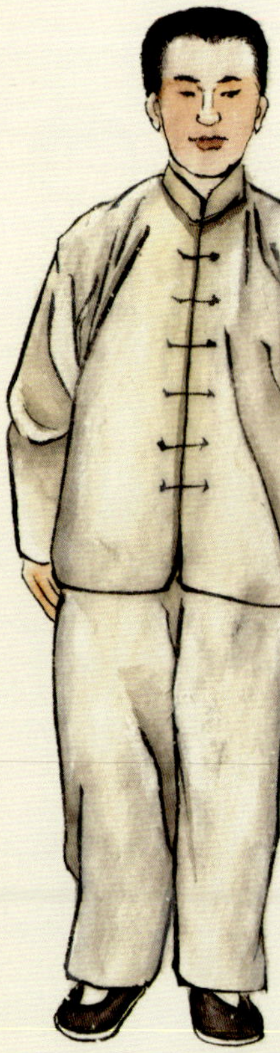

1

一、起势

1. Commencing

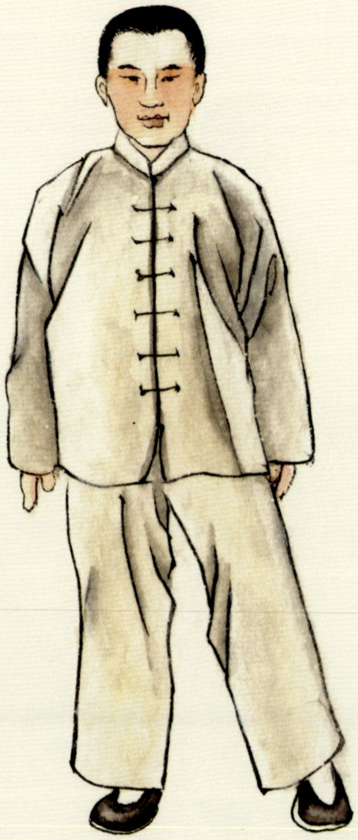

1

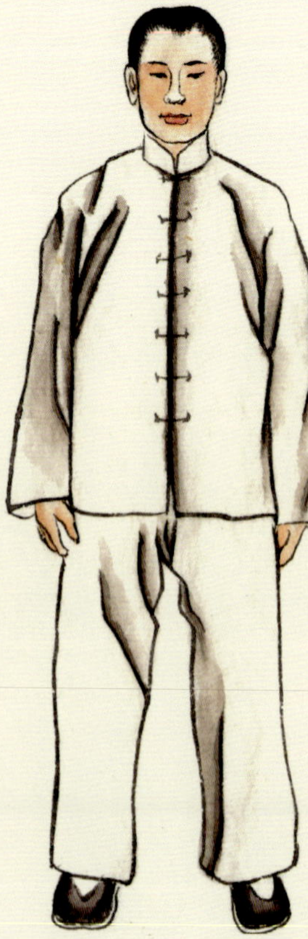

2

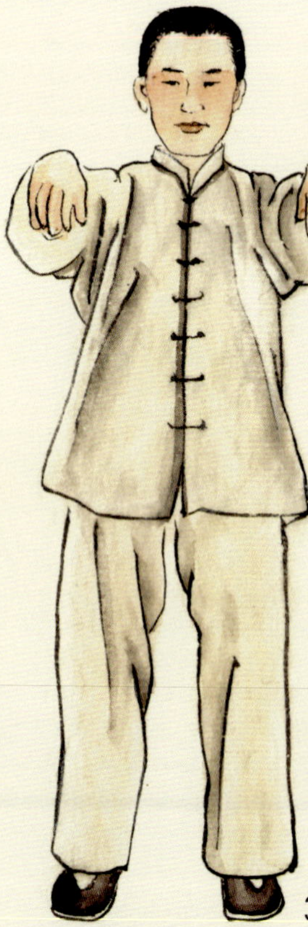

3

二、揽雀尾

2. Grasp bird's tail

双手揽住飞鸟的尾巴之意。

grasping the tail of a bird with both hands

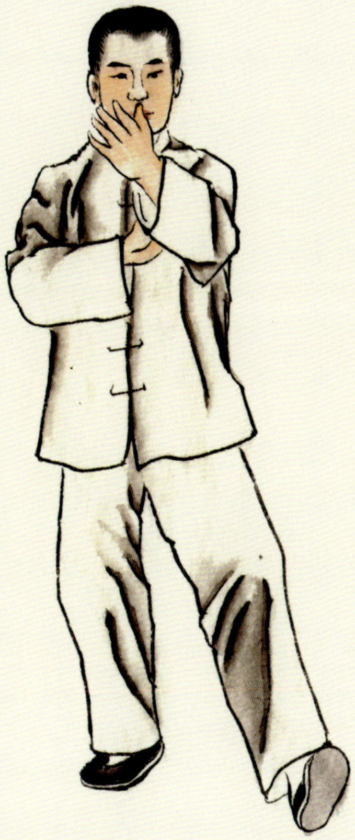

1

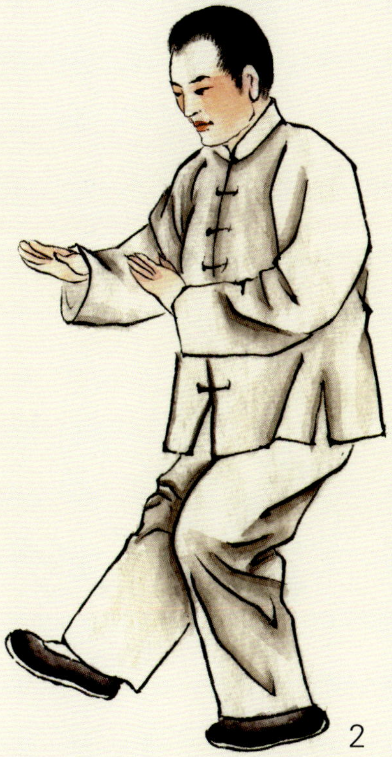

2

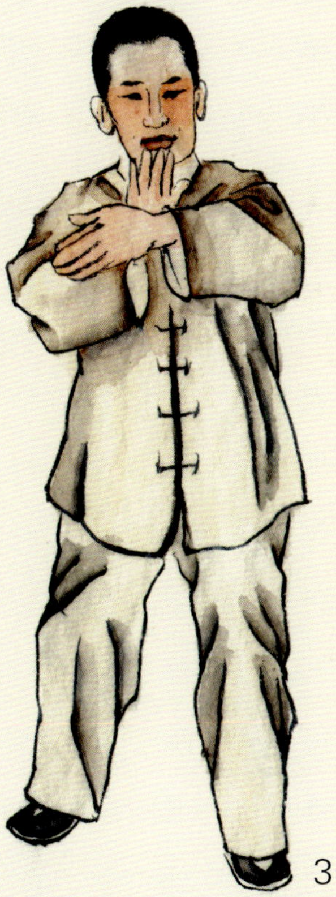

3

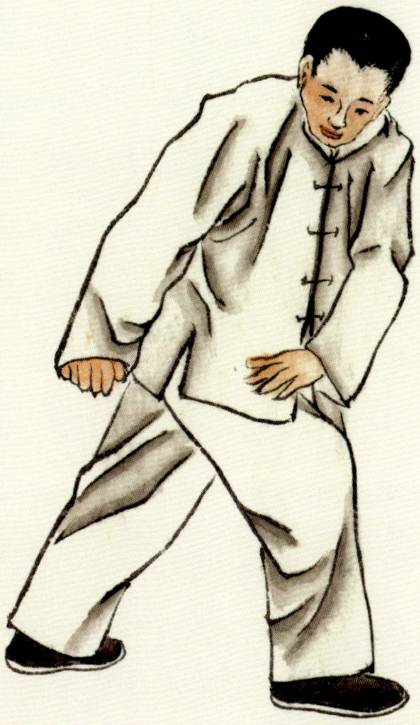

4

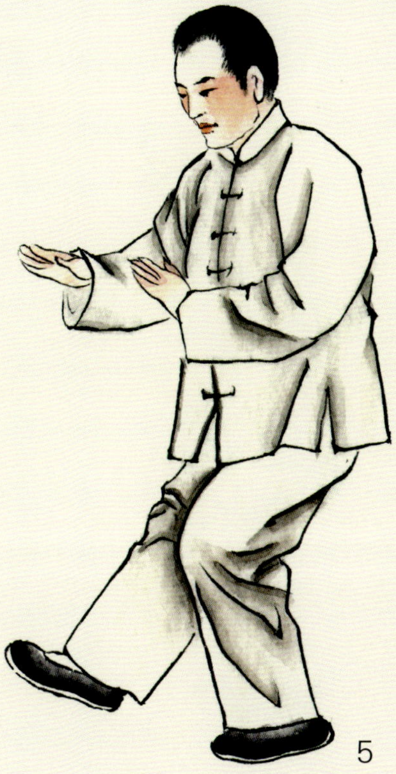

5

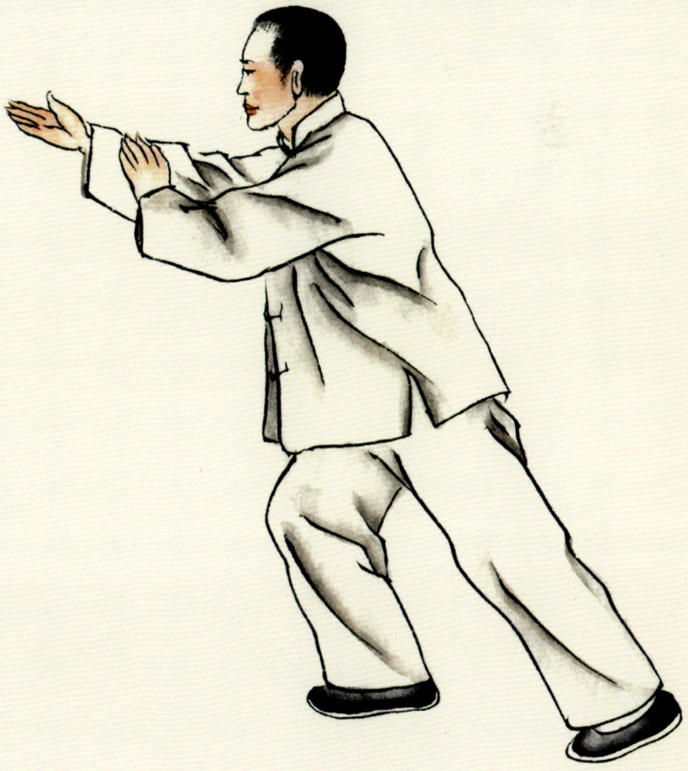

6

三、搂膝拗步

3. Brush knee and twist step

以手绕过膝盖为“搂膝”，手与脚运动的前后形成左右交叉式为“拗步”。

'Brush knee' means passing your hands across your knees, and 'twist step' means moving the hands and feet so that they cross each other.

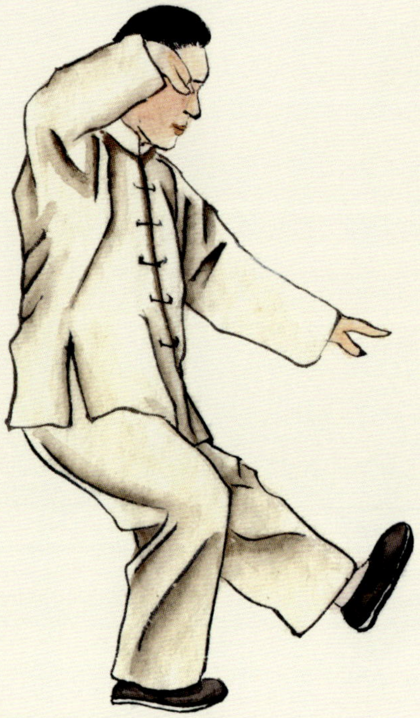

1

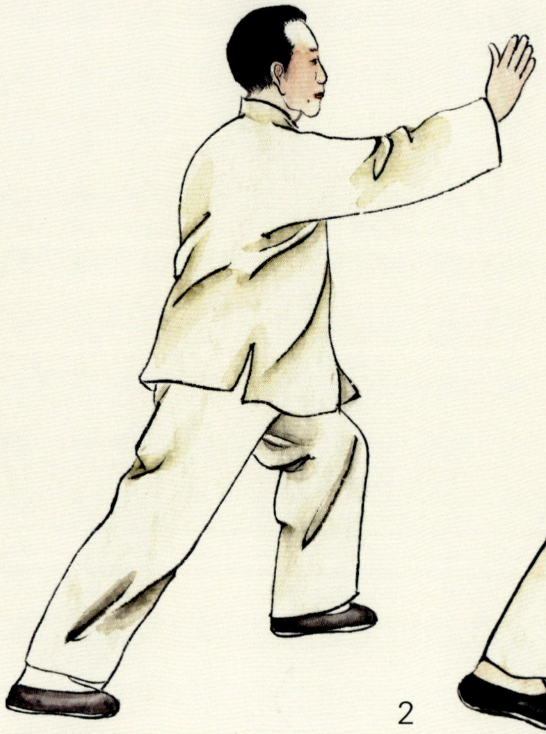

2

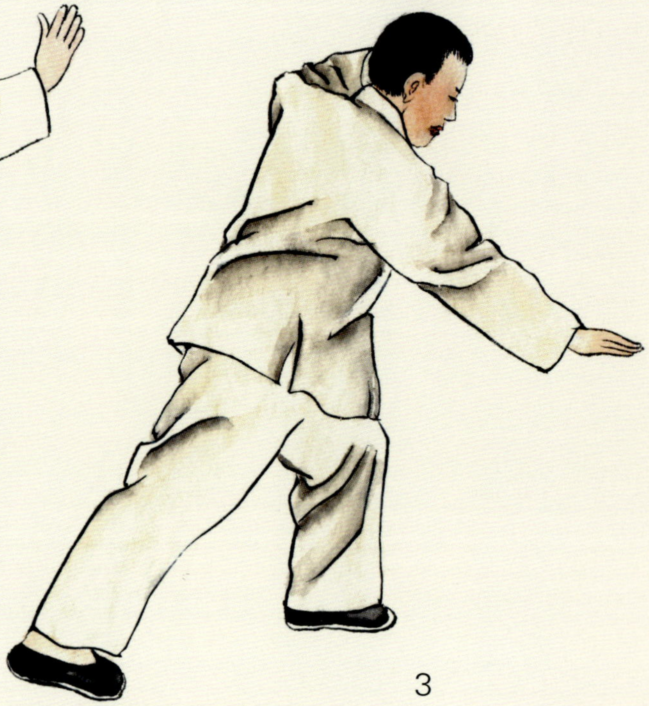

3

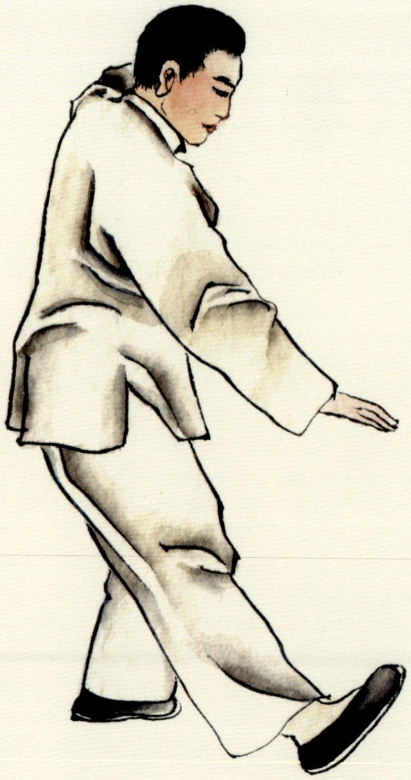

4

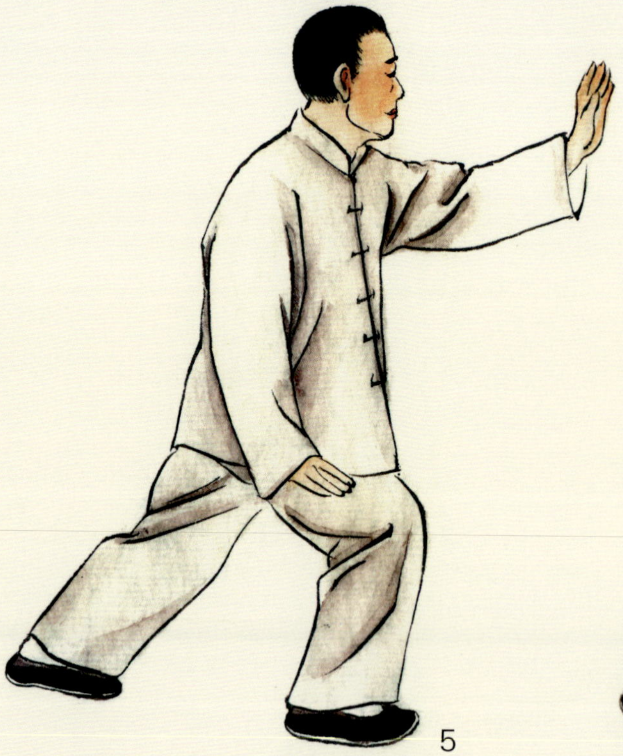

5

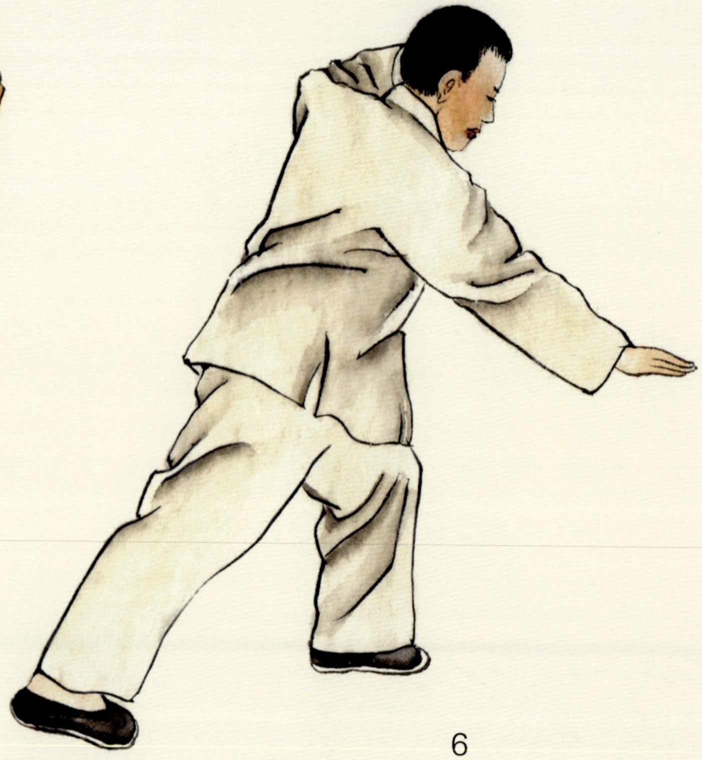

6

四、手挥琵琶

4. Play the pipa

两手好似挥弹琵琶的样子。

Move the hands as if you were playing the pipa (guitar-like Chinese instrument).

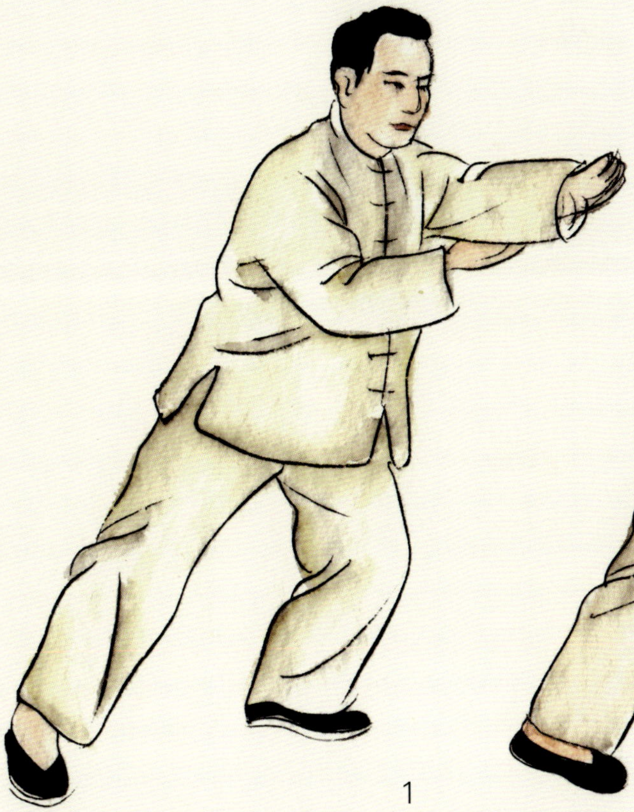

1

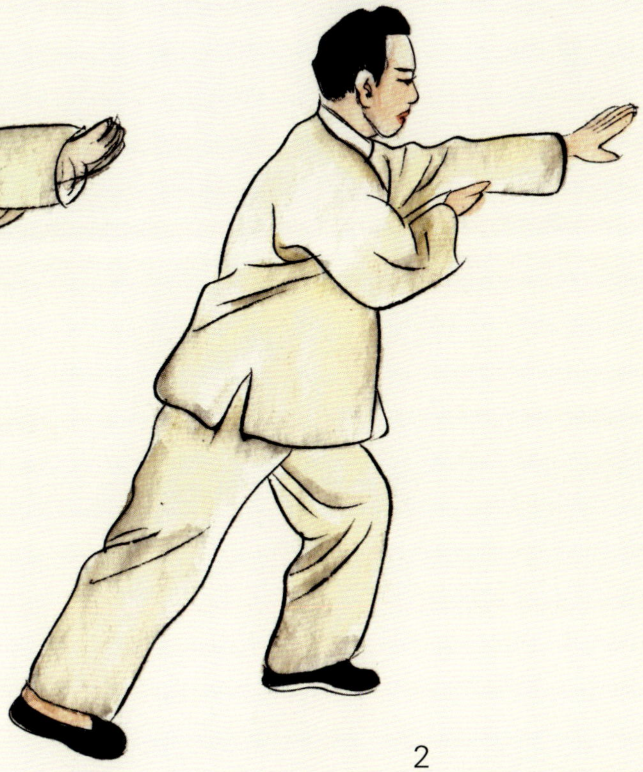

2

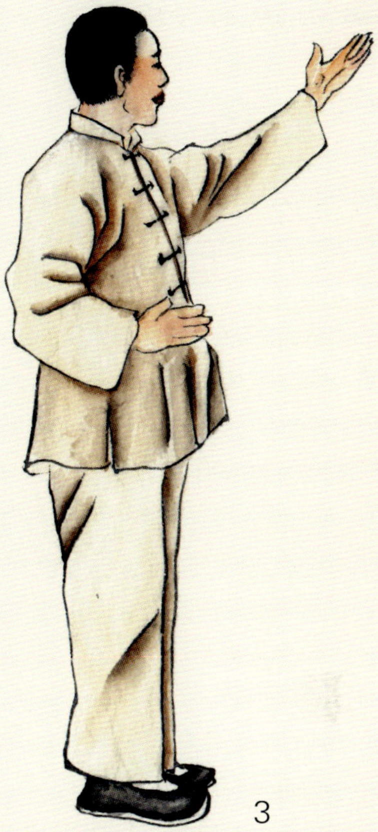

3

五、野马分鬃

5. Part the wild horse's mane

动作如骏马左右摆鬃。

The movement is like a steed shaking its mane left and right.

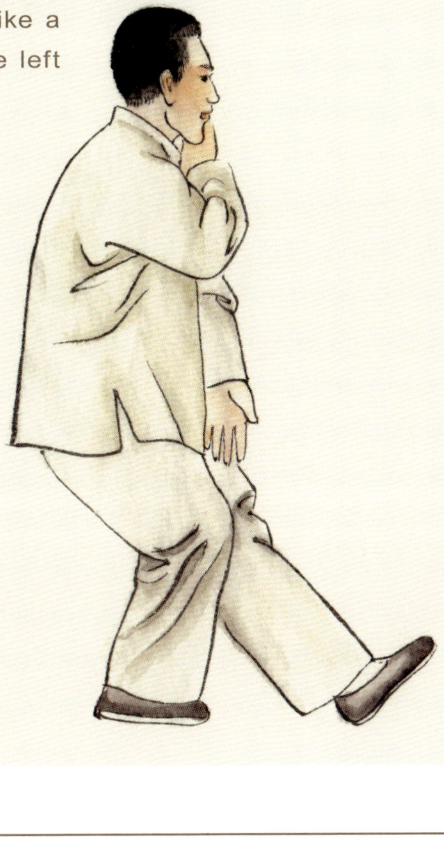

1

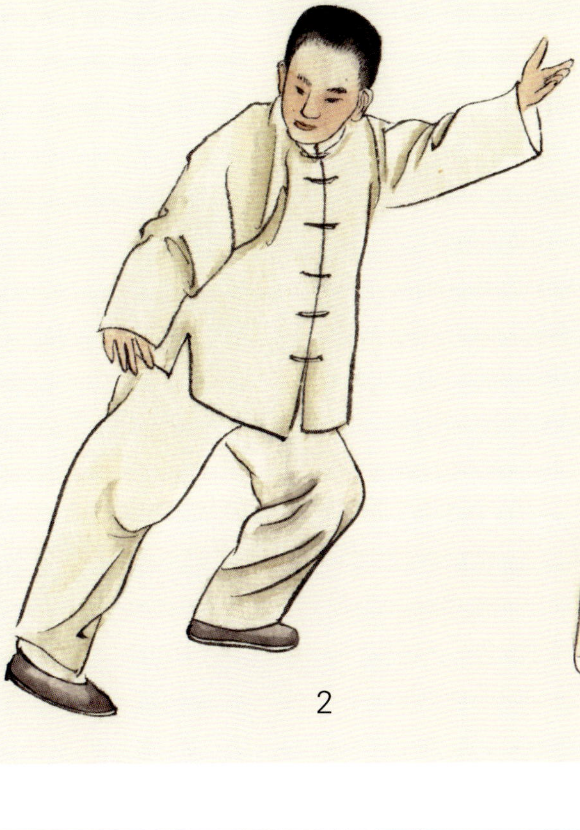

2

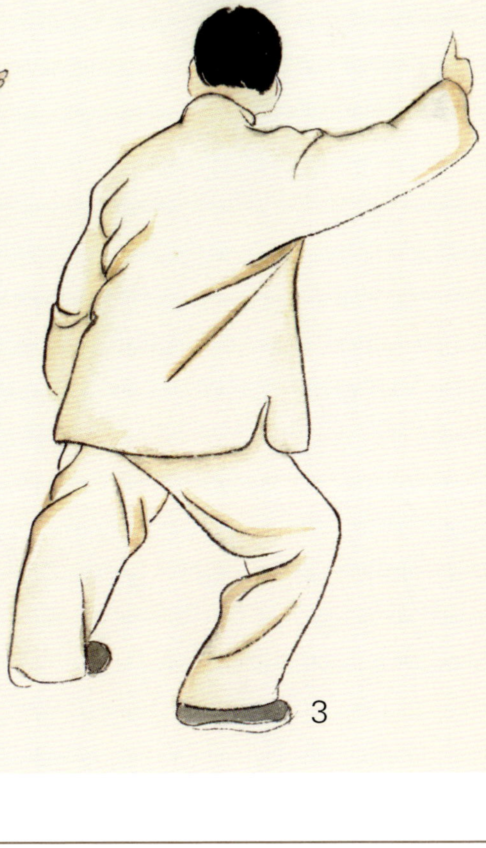

3

六、玉女穿梭

6. Fair lady works with shuttles

动作左右运转交织有如玉女在运梭织锦。

Make circular and crossing movements like a fair lady weaving brocade with shuttles.

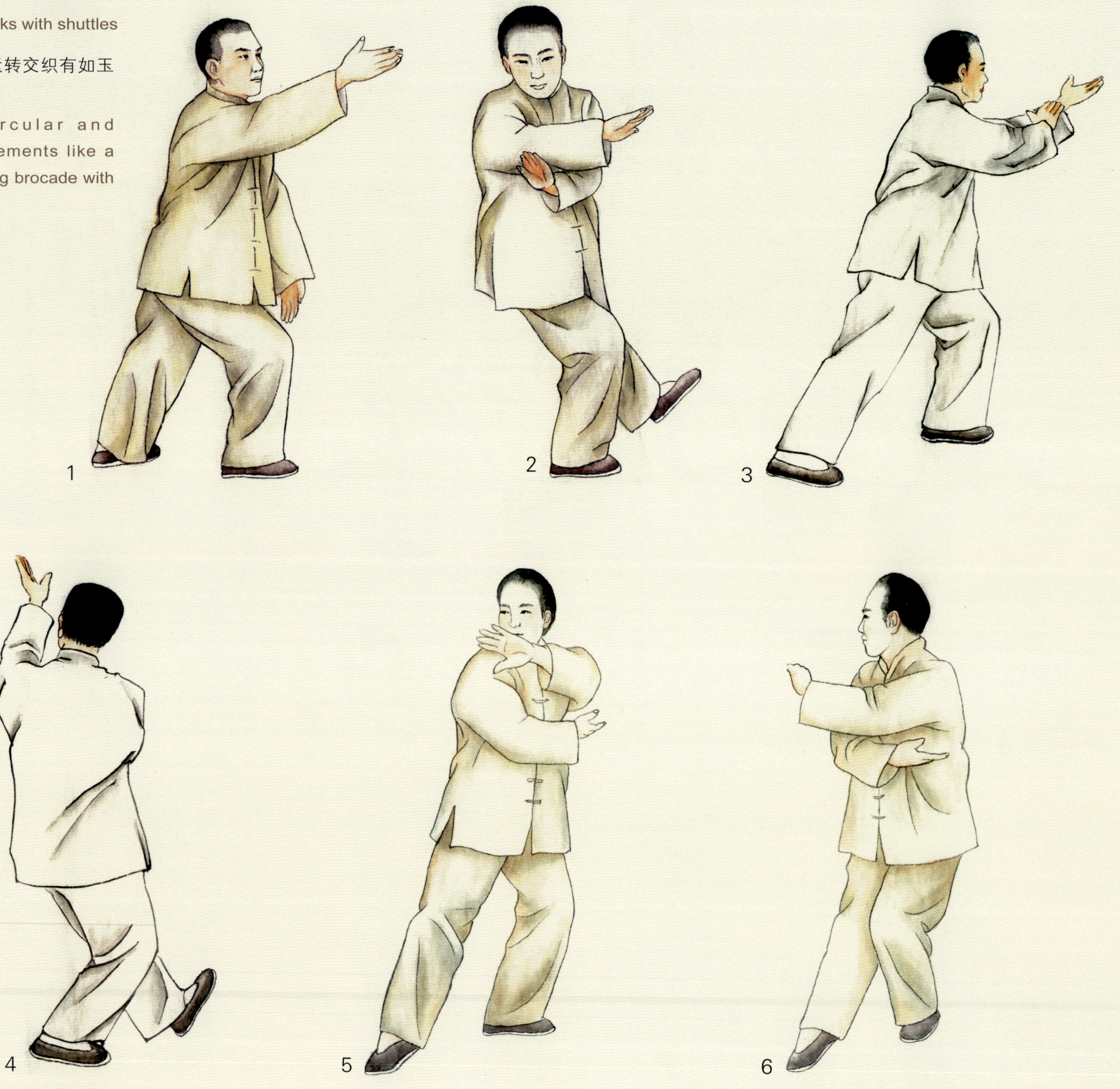

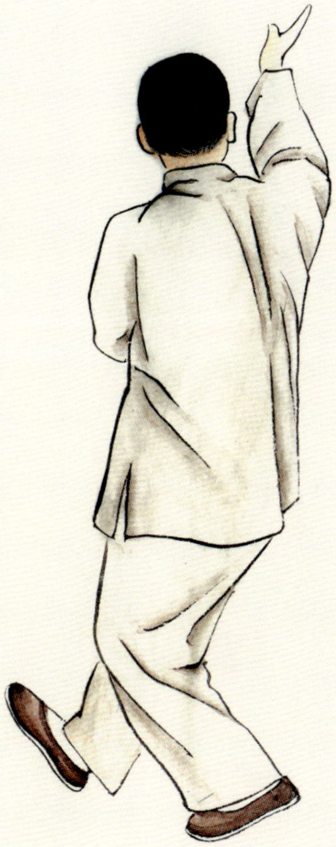
7

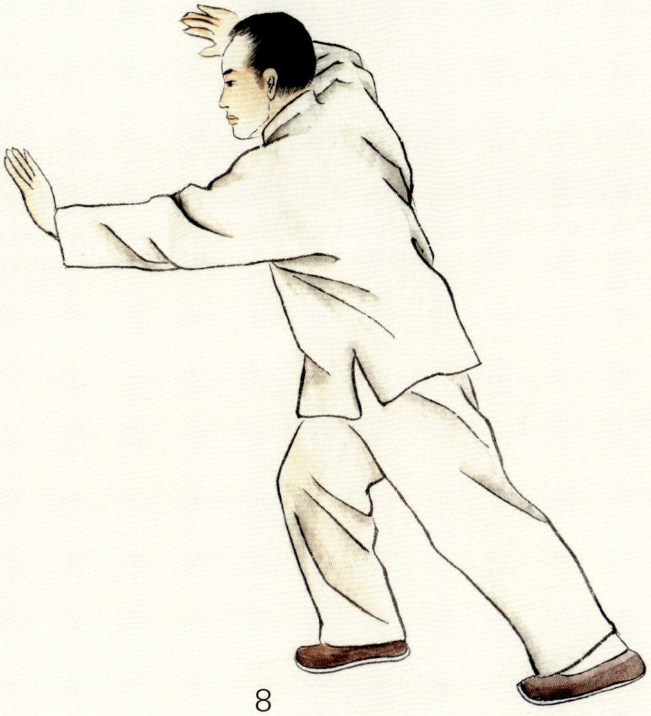
8

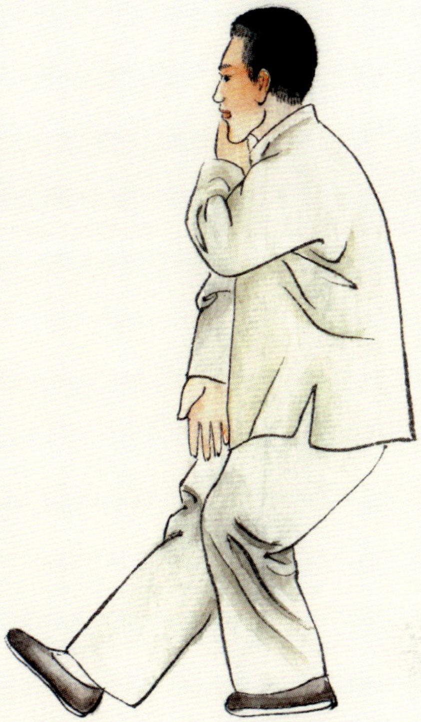
9

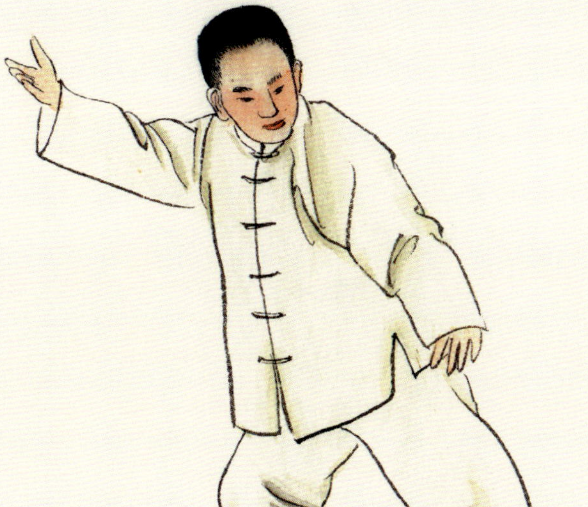
10

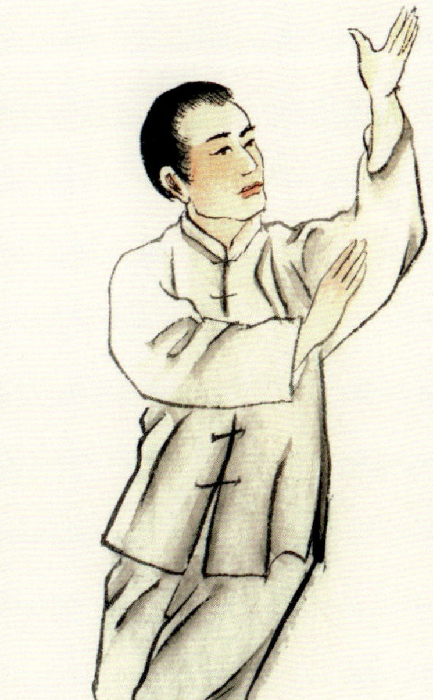
11

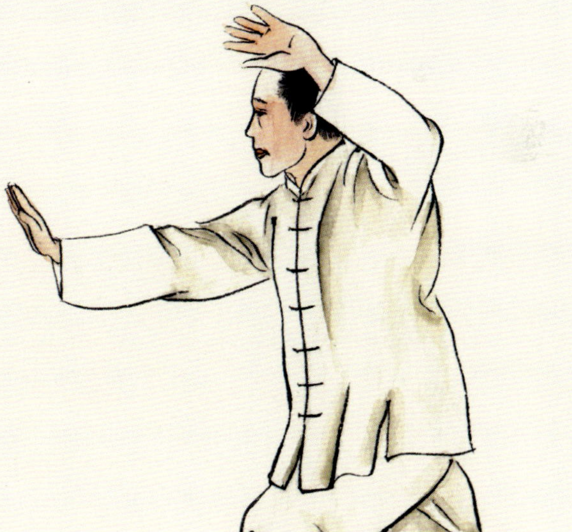
12

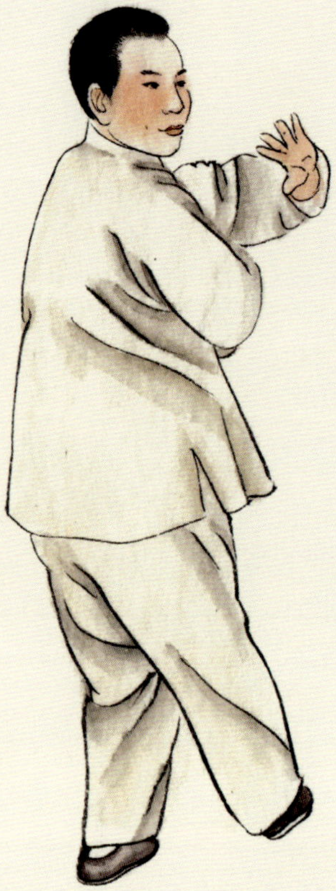

13

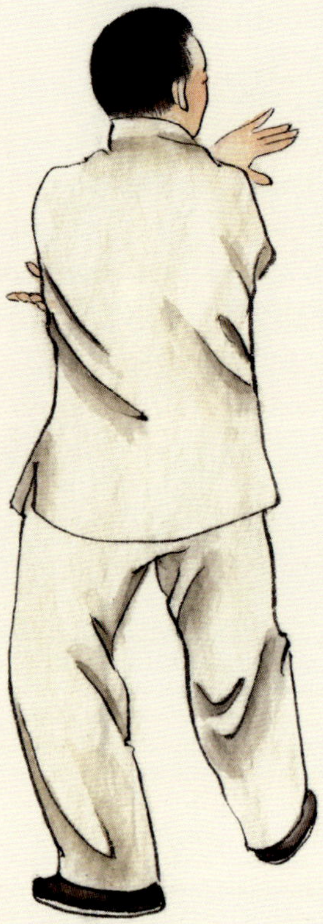

14

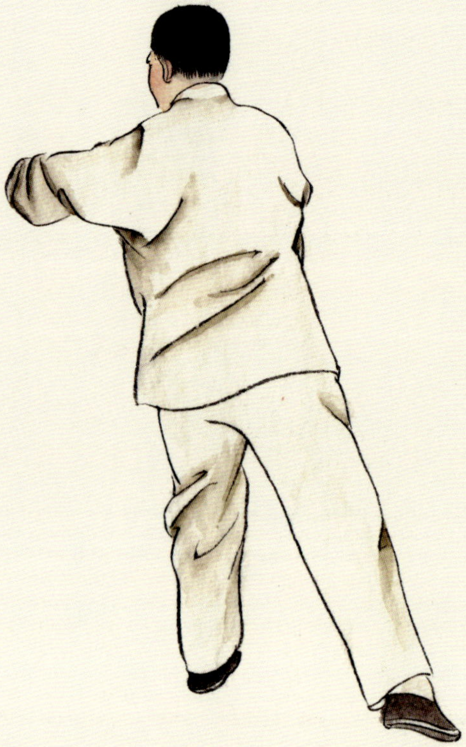

15

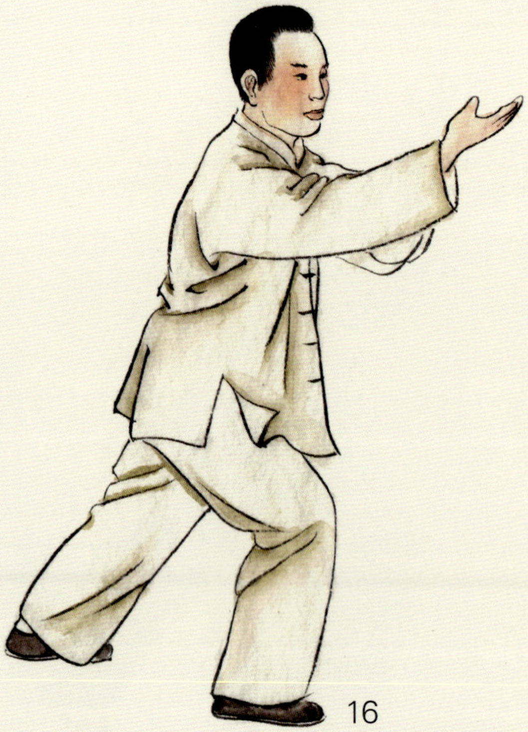

16

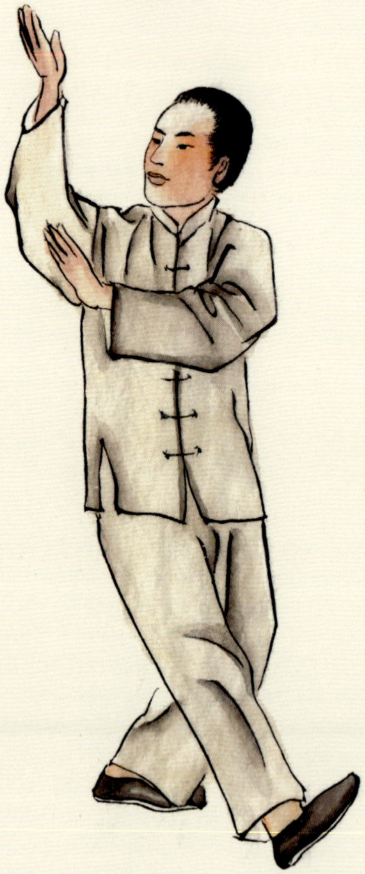

17

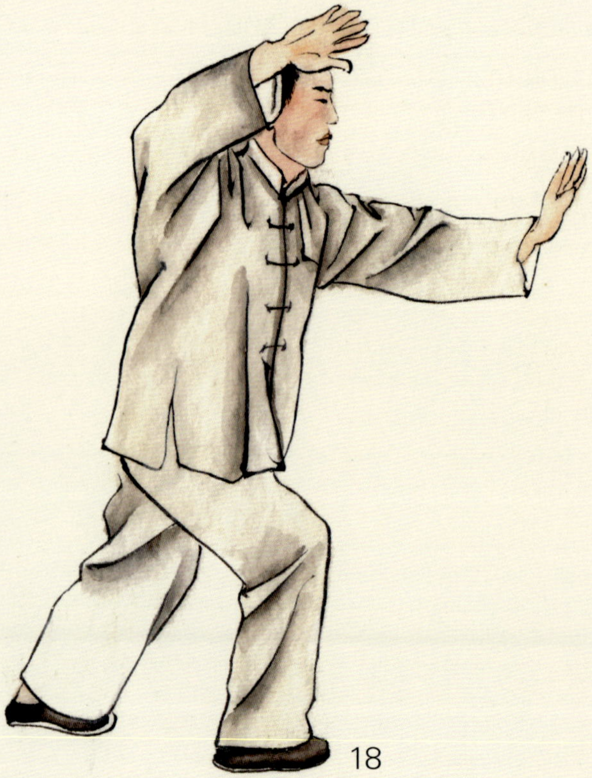

18

七、肘底看锤

7. Fist under the elbow

两掌均变为拳，以肘下拳为主，乃防守之意。

Make fists with both hands and punch from below the elbow for defense.

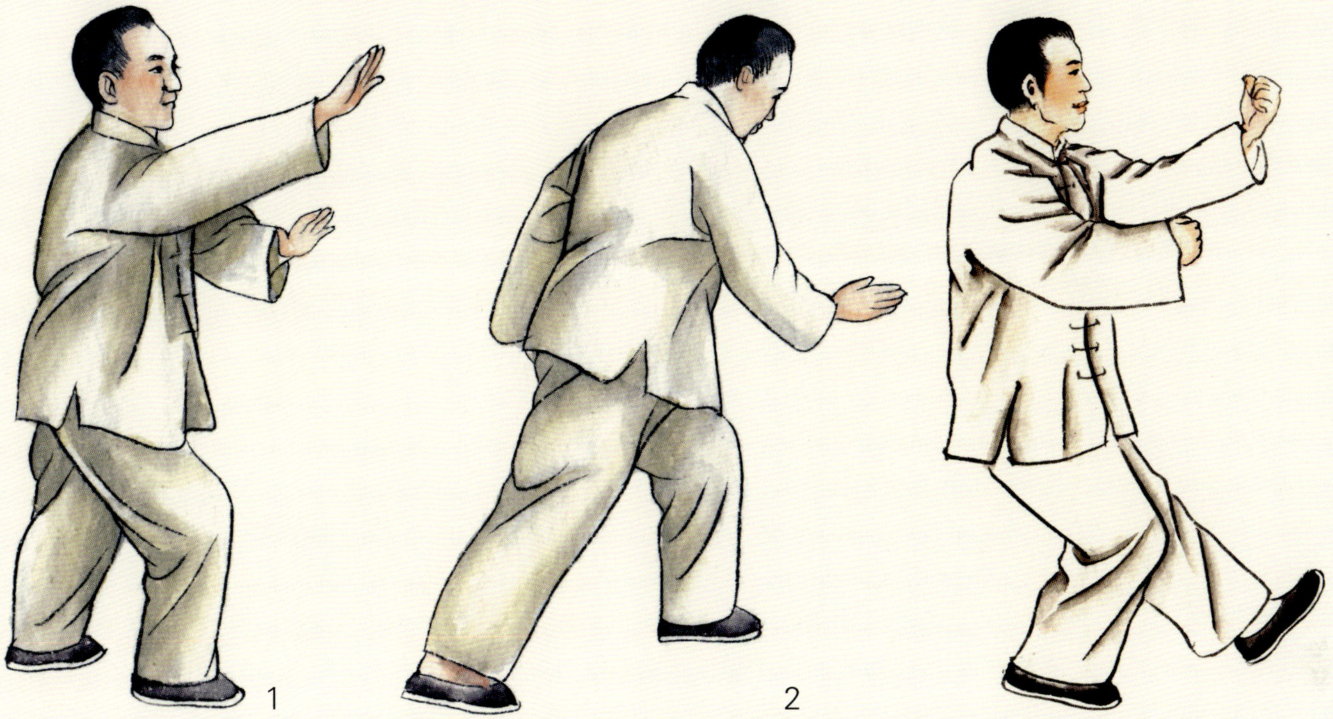

1 2 3

八、金鸡独立

8. Golden rooster standing on one foot

两拳均变为掌，右手指天，提膝，做金鸡独立状。

Unclench two fists and point the right hand at the sky, lifting one knee like a golden rooster standing on one foot.

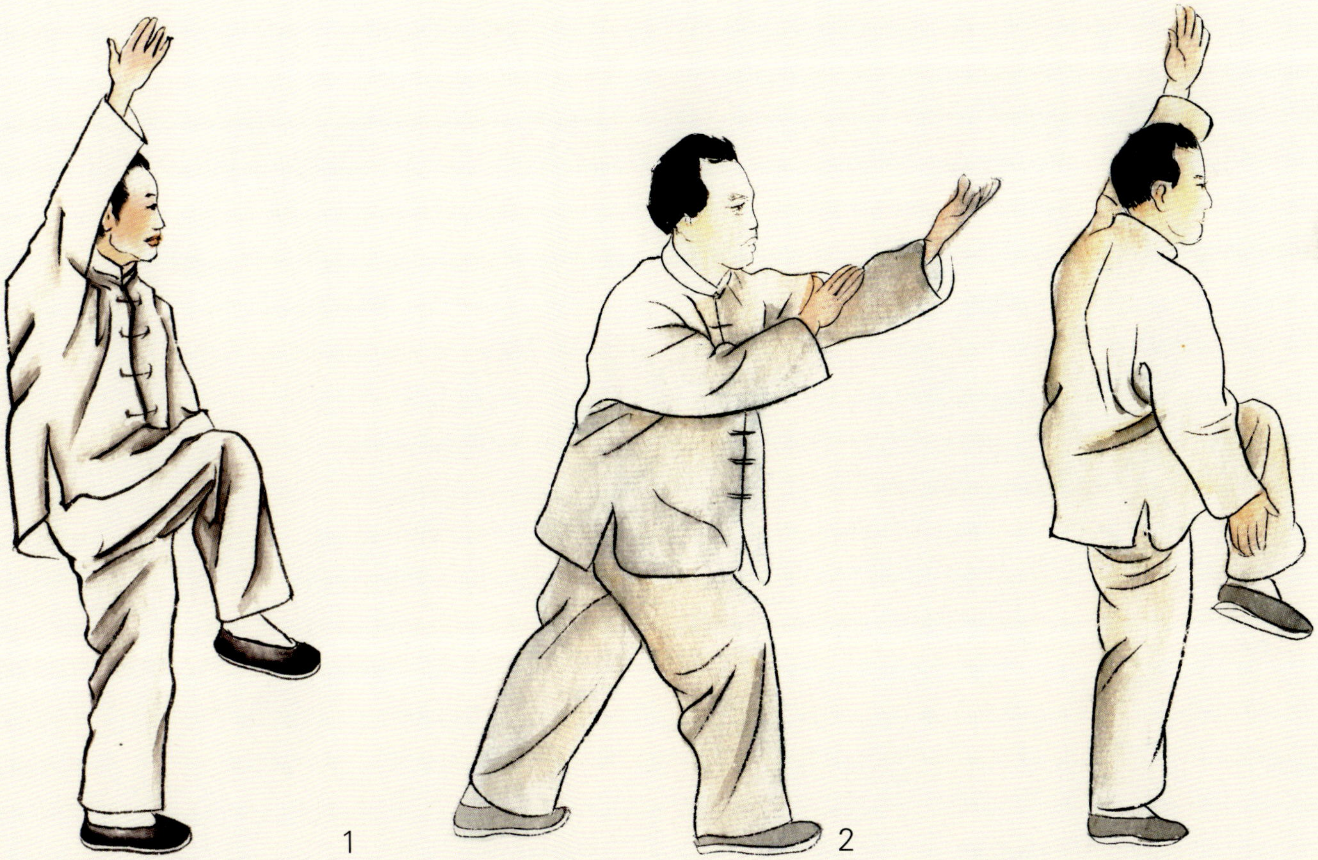

1 2 3

九、倒撵猴

9. Step back and repulse the monkey

此动作以退为进，如倒撵猿猴。

Retreat in order to advance as if you were repulsing a monkey.

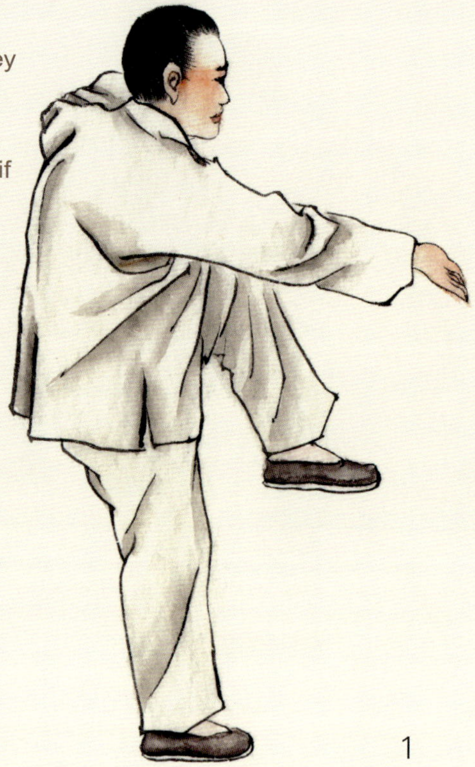

1

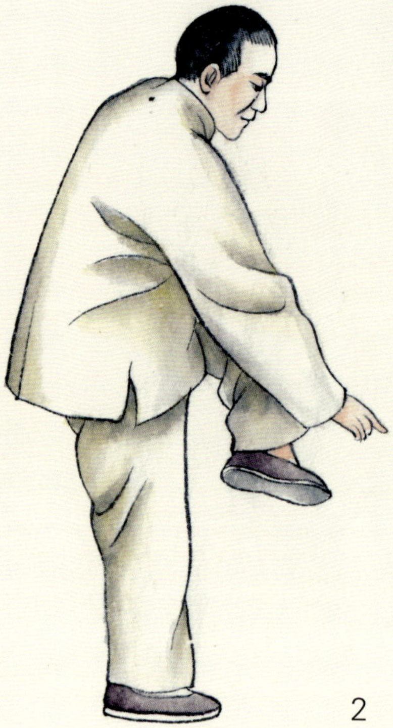

2

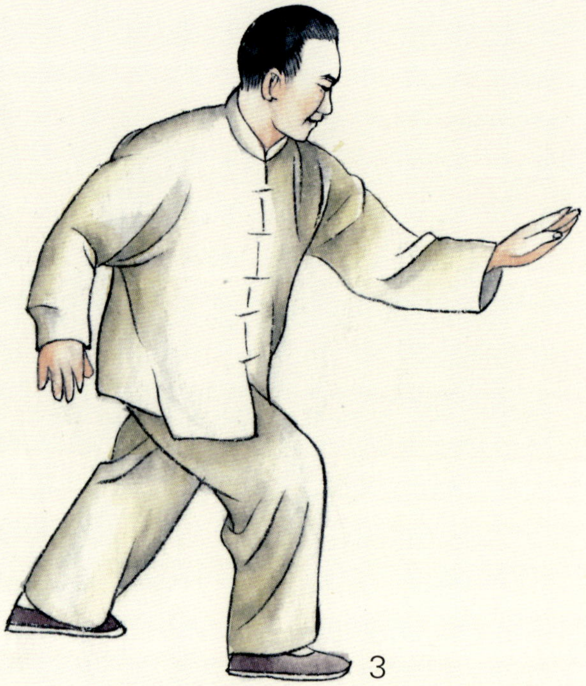

3

十、斜飞式

10. Fly diagonally

此式两臂分合闭张的动作，如大鹏展翅，斜行飞翔于上空。

Bring the arms together and apart as if you were a roc flying diagonally.

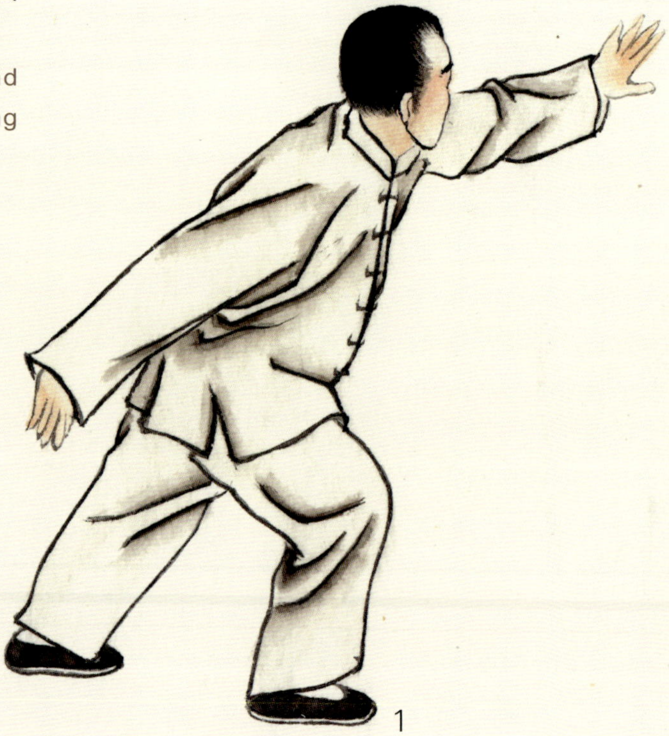

1

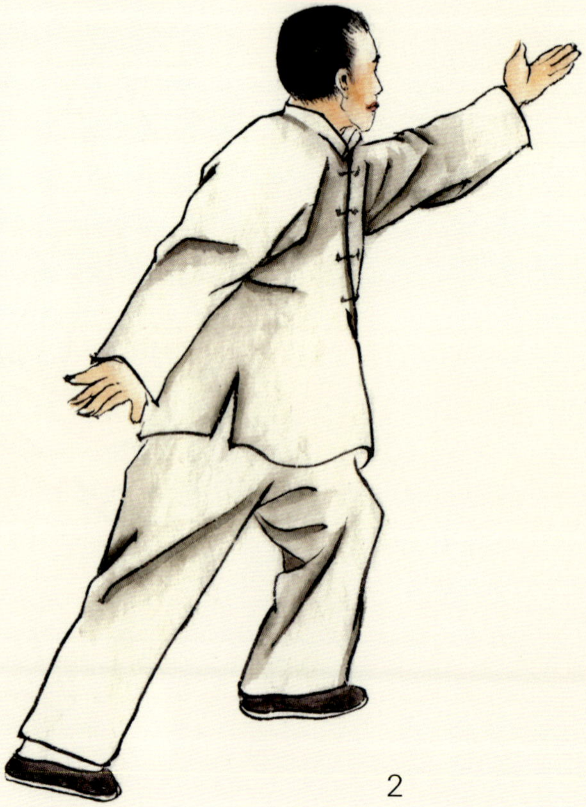

2

十一、提手上式

11. Lift arms

　　此式动作是以手臂上起如提重物状。

　　Raise your arms as if you were lifting something heavy.

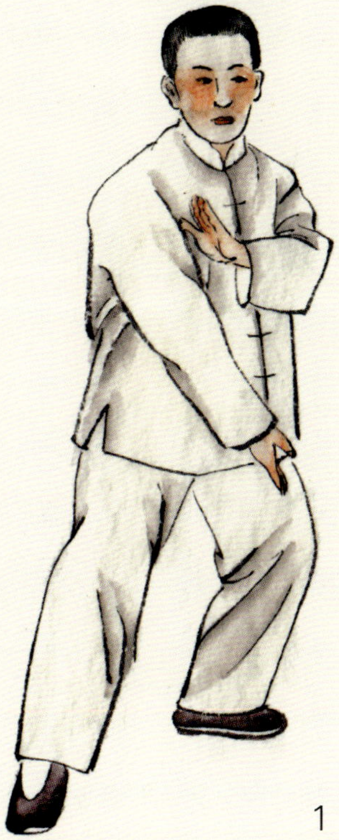

1

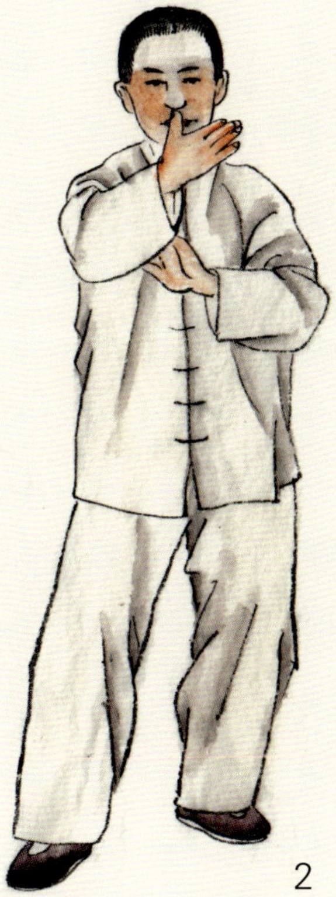

2

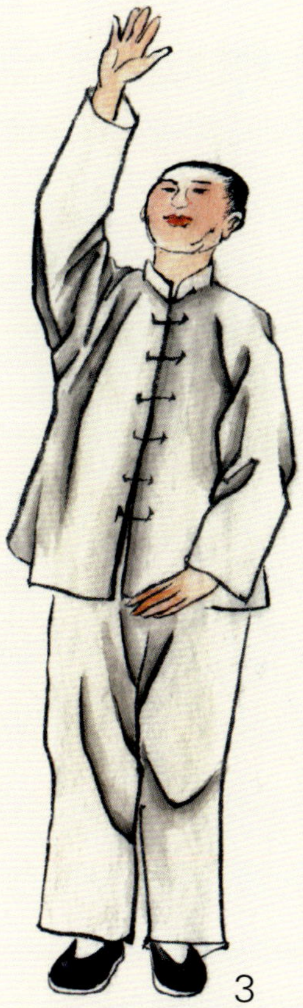

3

十二、白鹤亮翅

12. White crane spreads its wings

　　此式动作之运转形势，有如鹤之展翅。

　　This movement resembles a crane spreading its wings.

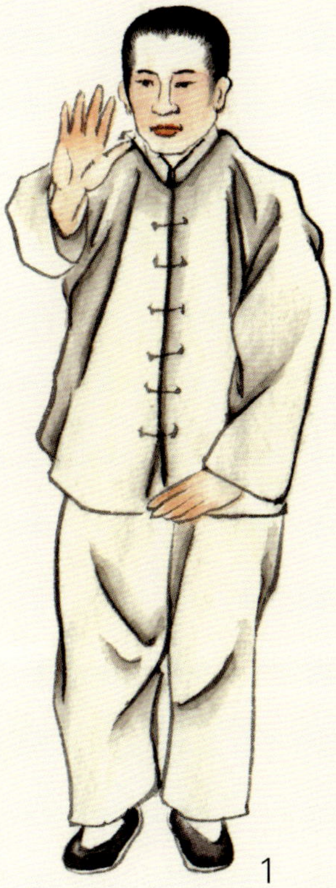

1

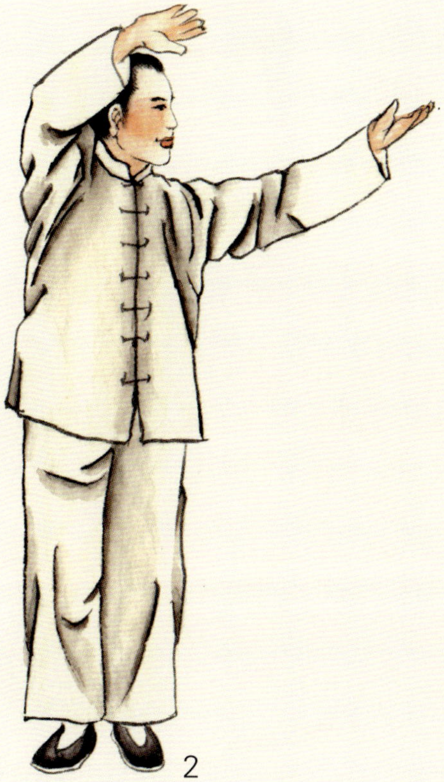

2

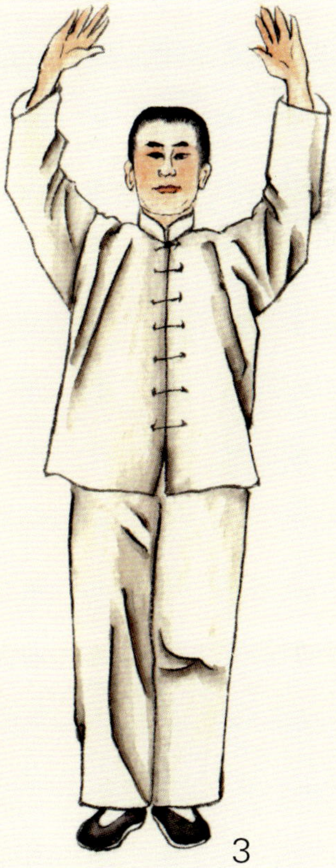

3

十三、海底针

13. Needle at sea bottom

此式以手指喻为金针下指海底。

In this movement, the fingers are compared to gold needles pointing to the bottom of the sea.

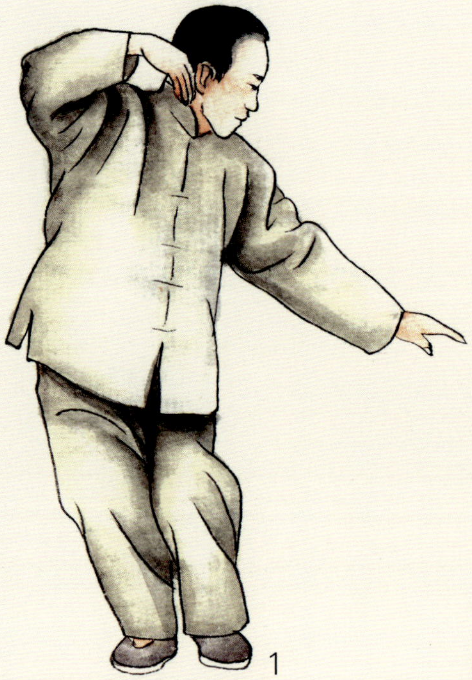

1

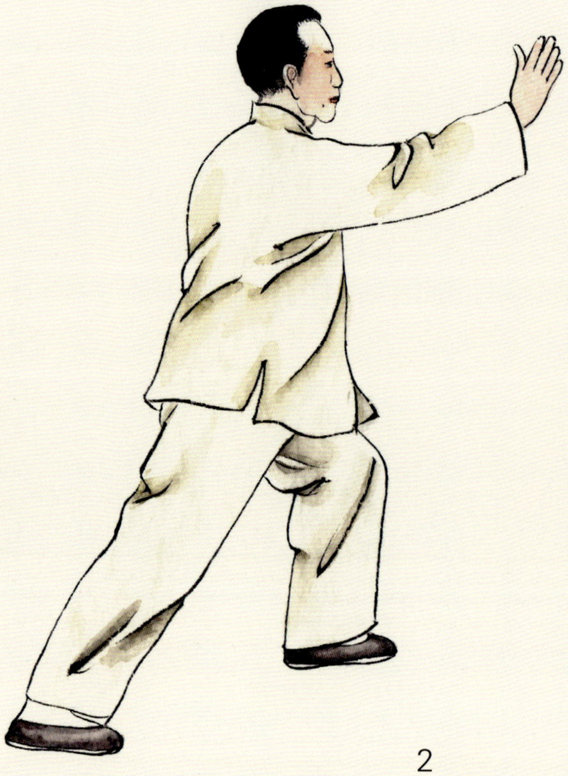

2

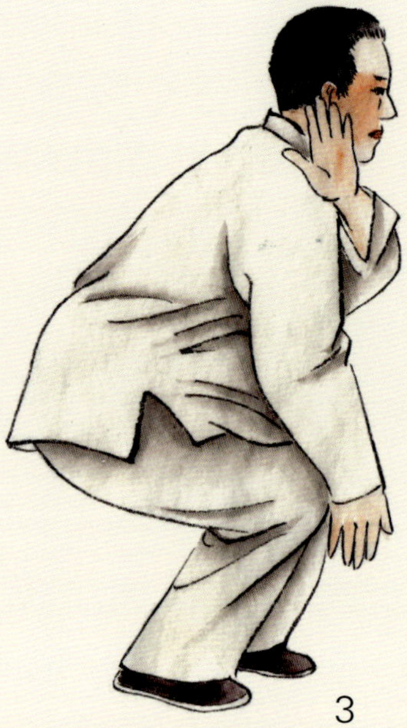

3

十四、扇通背

14. Fan through back

此式是以腰为轴，两臂展开如扇。

In this movement, turn the body and stretch out two arms like a fan.

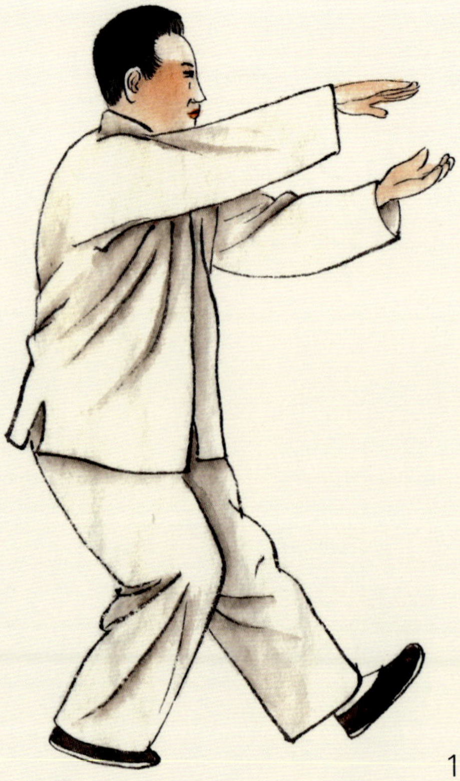

1

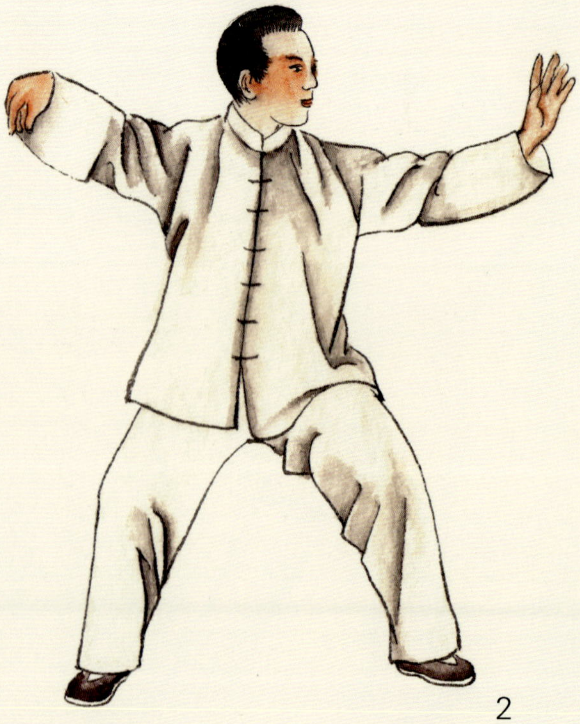

2

十五、左右分脚

15. Separation kick

此式所谓分脚，即指脚踢出时，要求脚背绷脚尖挑起而左右分踢之意。

Bend the top of your feet and kick to the left and right.

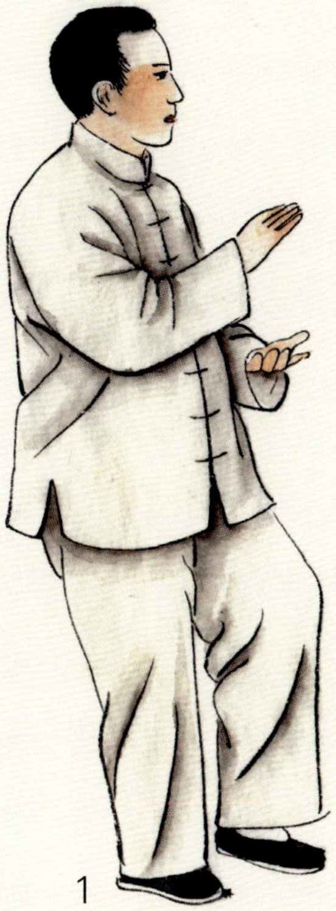

1

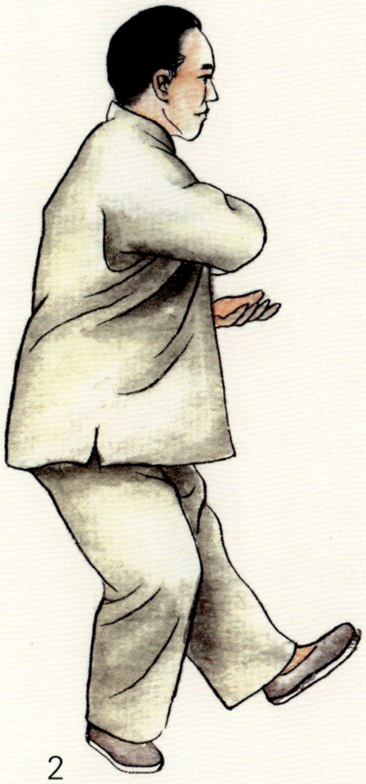

2

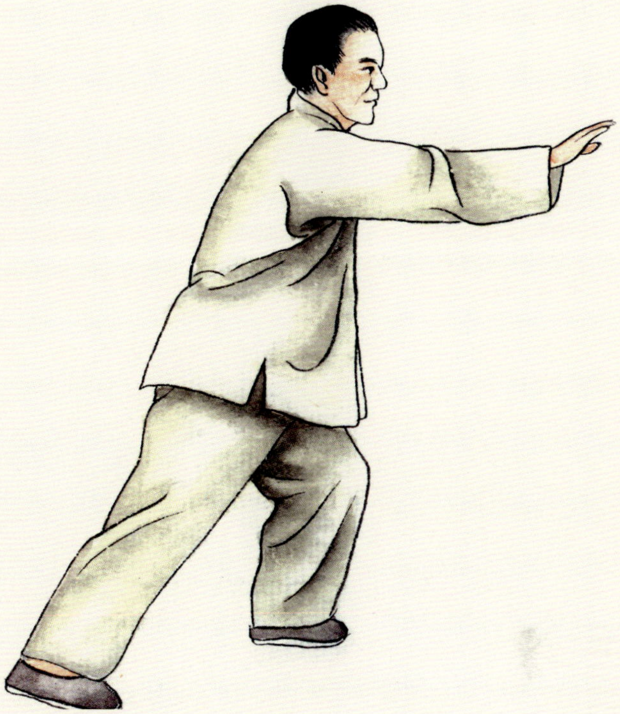

3

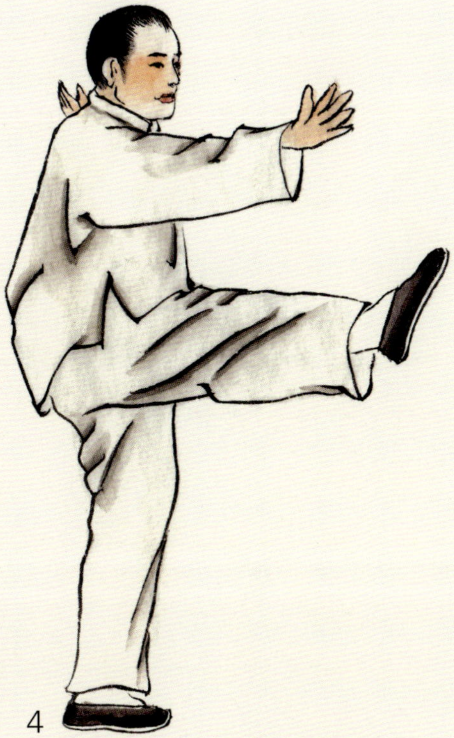

4

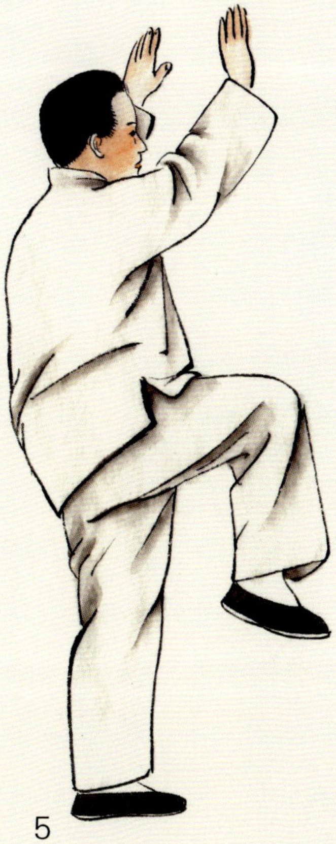

5

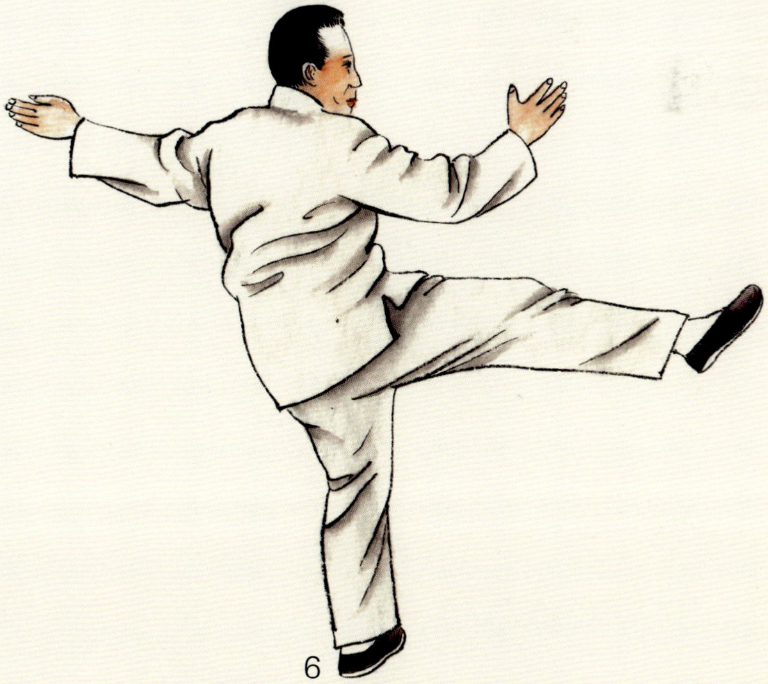

6

十六、转身蹬脚

16. Turn and kick

此式从正前方往左转向后方，转成一百八十度，然后把脚蹬出。

Turn left 180 degrees and kick.

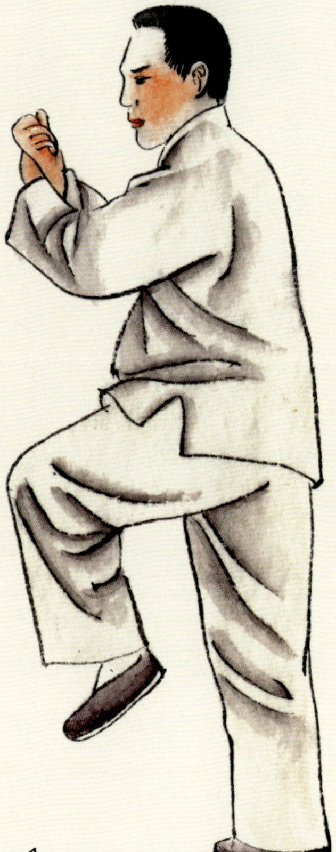

1

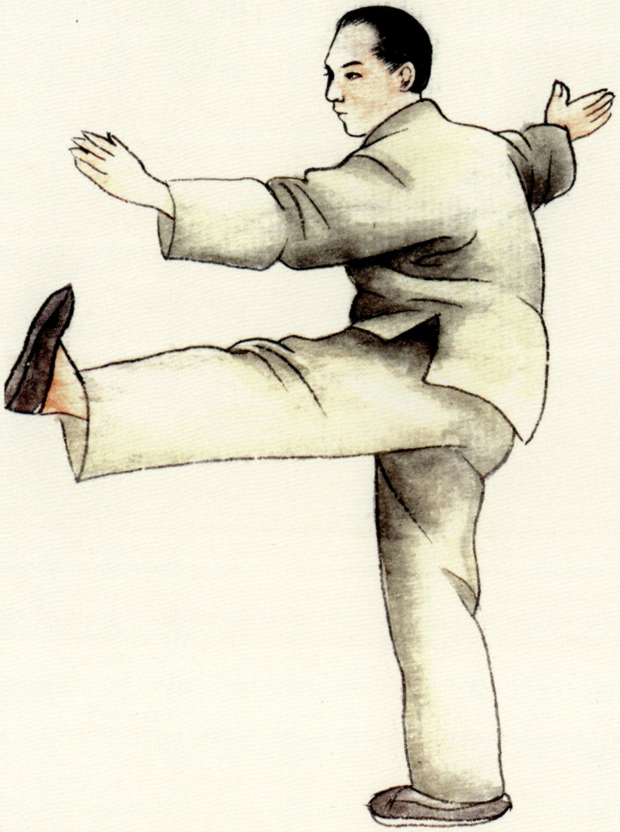

2

十七、进步栽锤

17. Advance and punch

此式以拗步前进，右拳犹如握一树苗，往左脚前方设想之深坑向下栽植。

Advance with “twist step” and bring the right fist downward as if planting a sapling in an imaginary pit in front of your left foot.

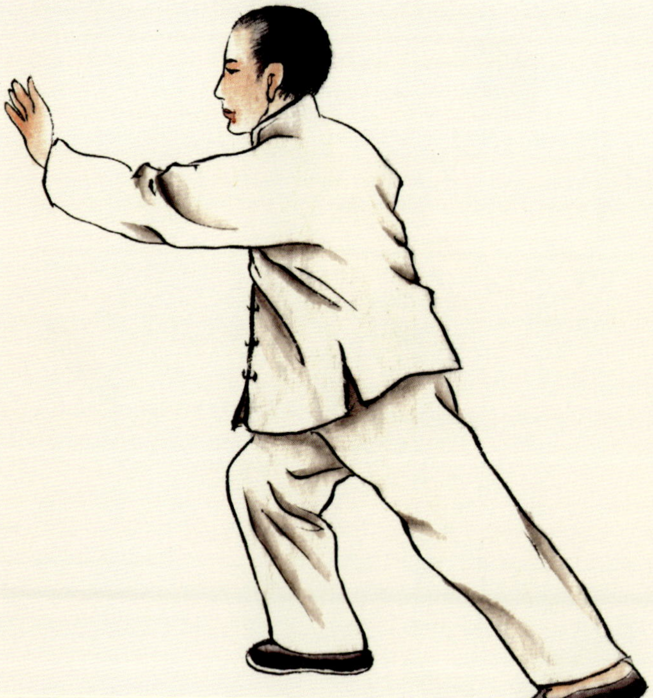

1

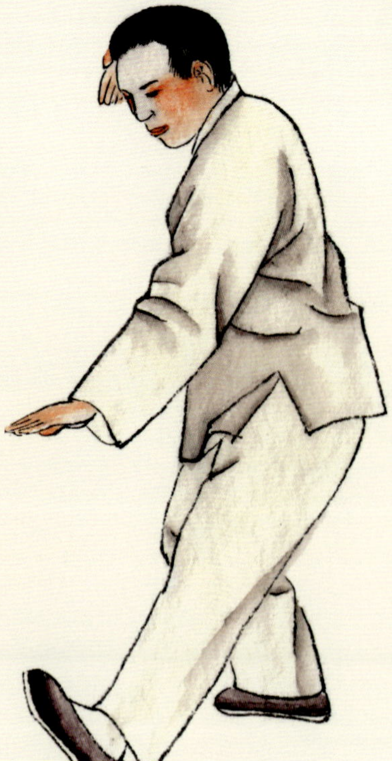

2

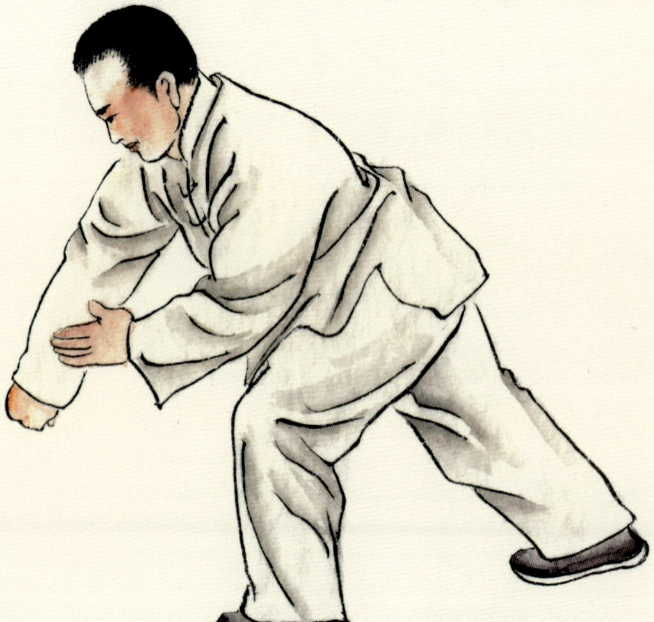

3

十八、翻身撇身锤

18. Turn and punch

此式指身体由前往后转一百八十度，用两臂之锤所产生的离心力，即向外撇出拳。

Turn 180 degrees and throw out your fists as if your two arms were two hammers.

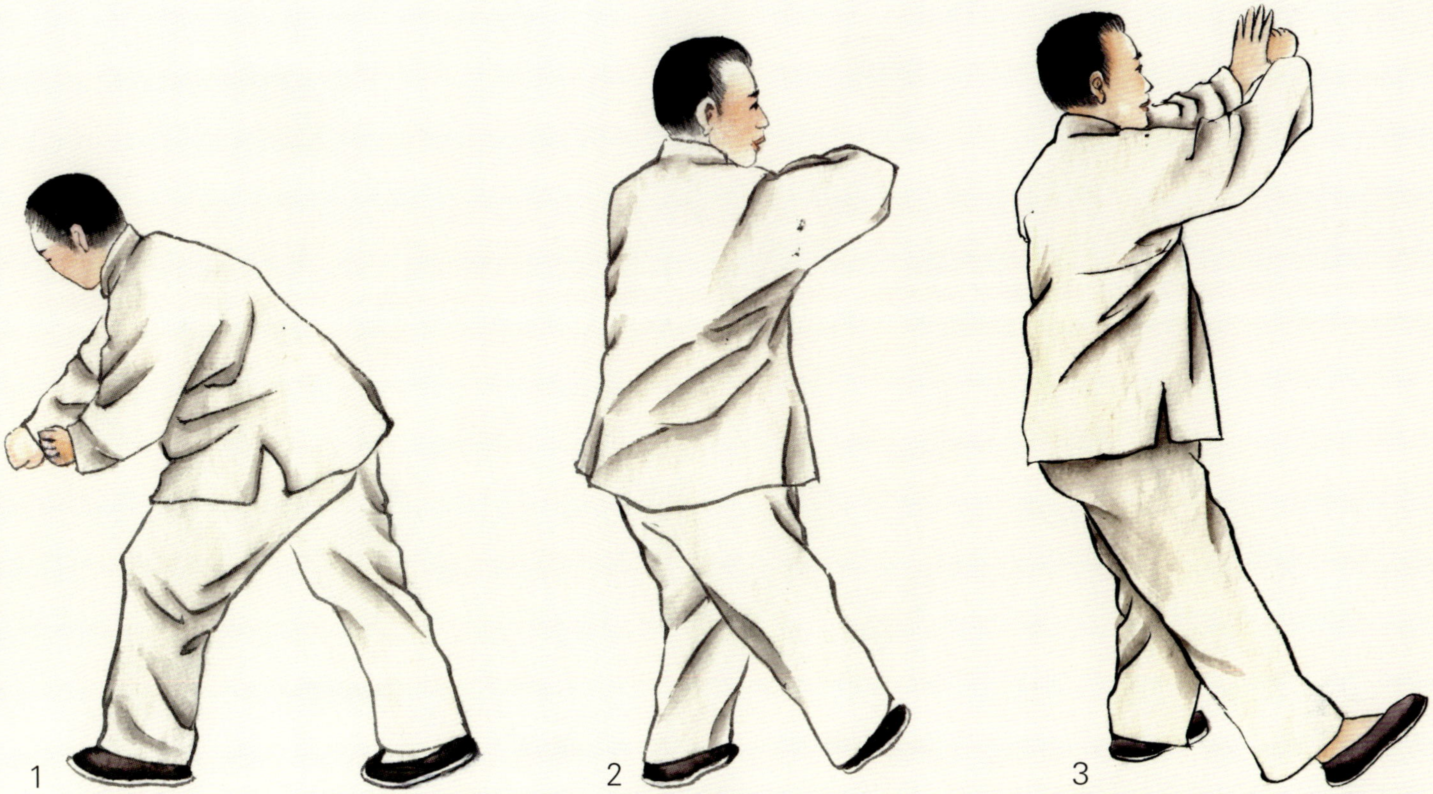

1 2 3

十九、二起脚

19. Raise feet one by one

此式指左右两脚逐步连续起落而言。

Your left and right feet rise and fall one by one.

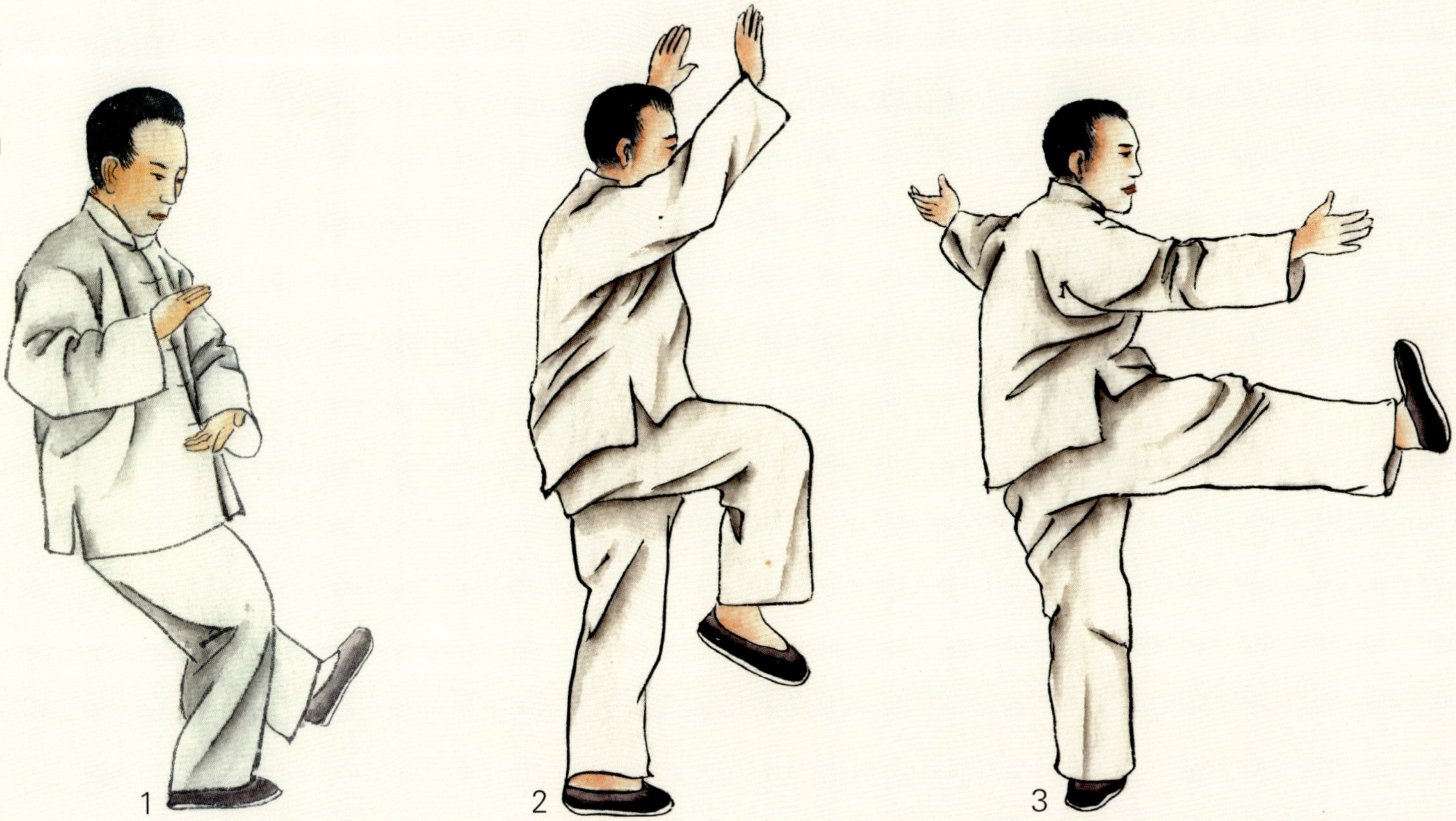

1 2 3

二十、左右打虎式

20. Beat the tiger this way and that

此式双拳并举，披身闪展，形如打虎。

Raise both fists and maneuver yourself this way and that as if fighting a tiger.

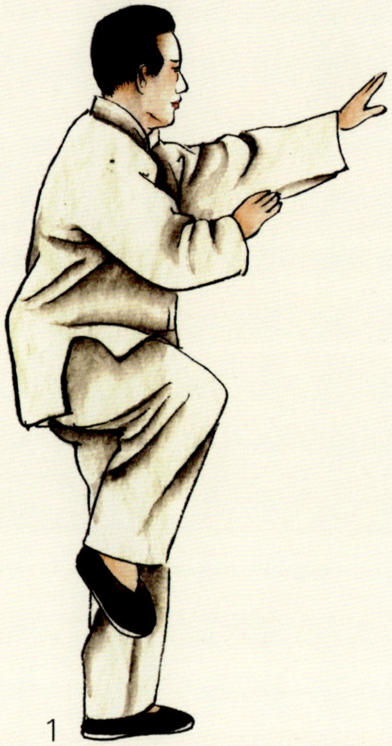
1

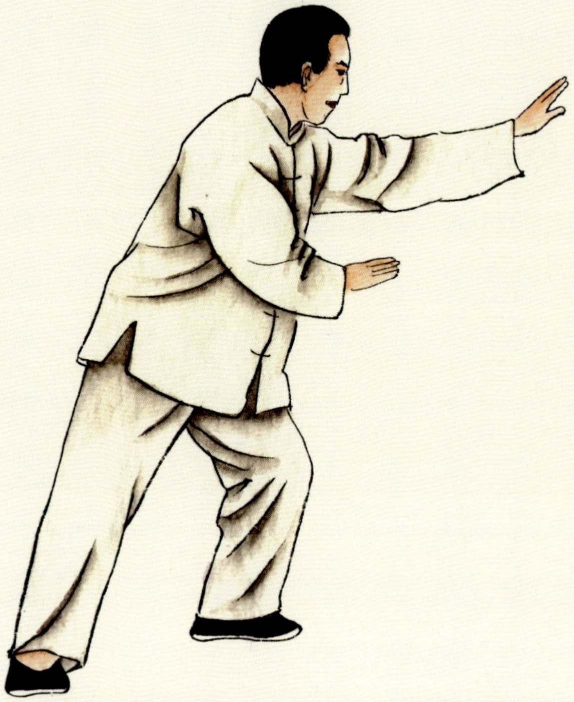
2

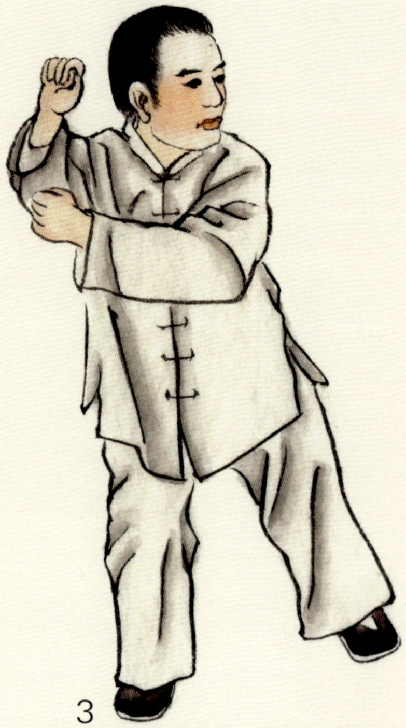
3

二十一、双风贯耳

21. Strike both ears

此式双拳对击直贯对方双耳。

In this movement, you bring your fists together to strike your opponents' ears.

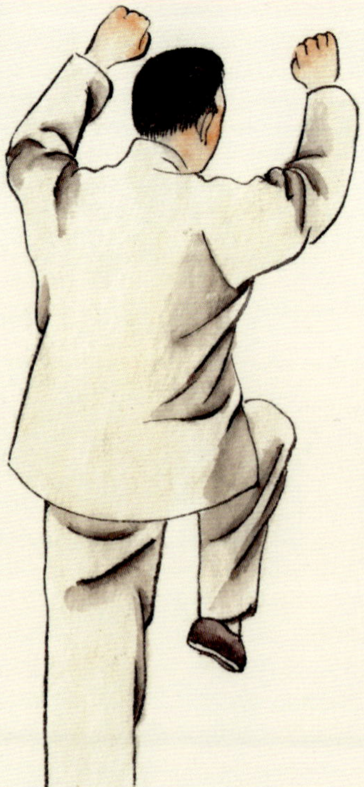
1

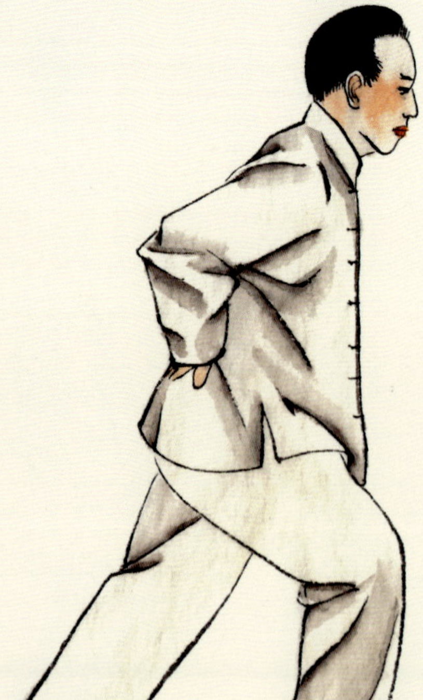
2

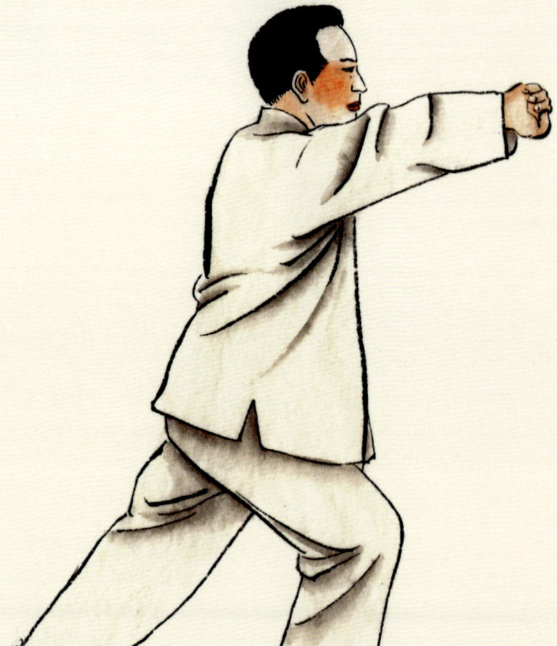
3

二十二、披身踢脚

22. Dodge and kick

此式指转身躲闪之后，以脚踢之之意。

Kick your opponent after turning to dodge.

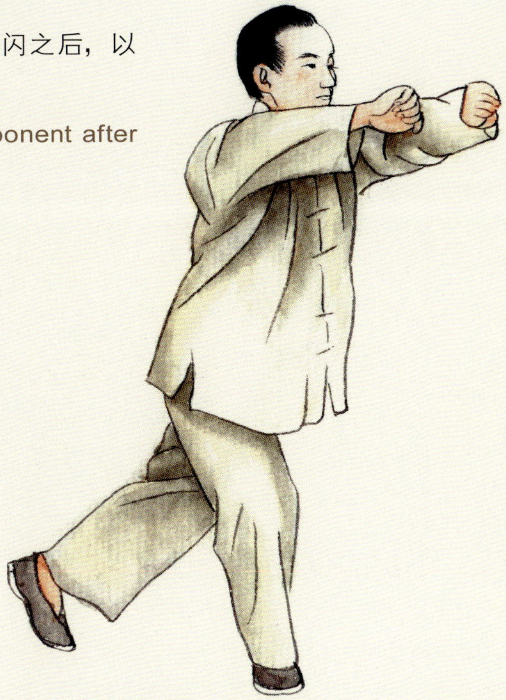

1

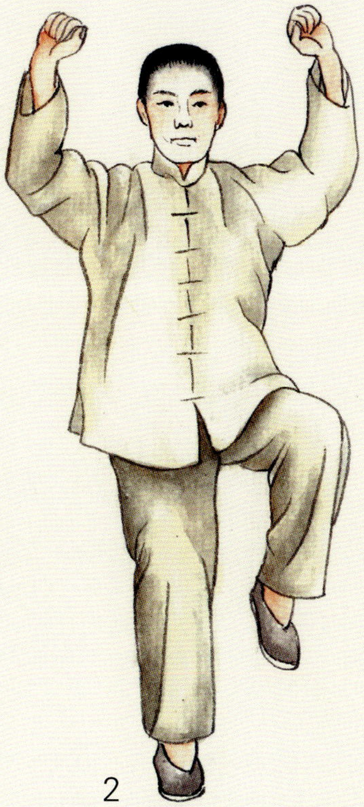

2

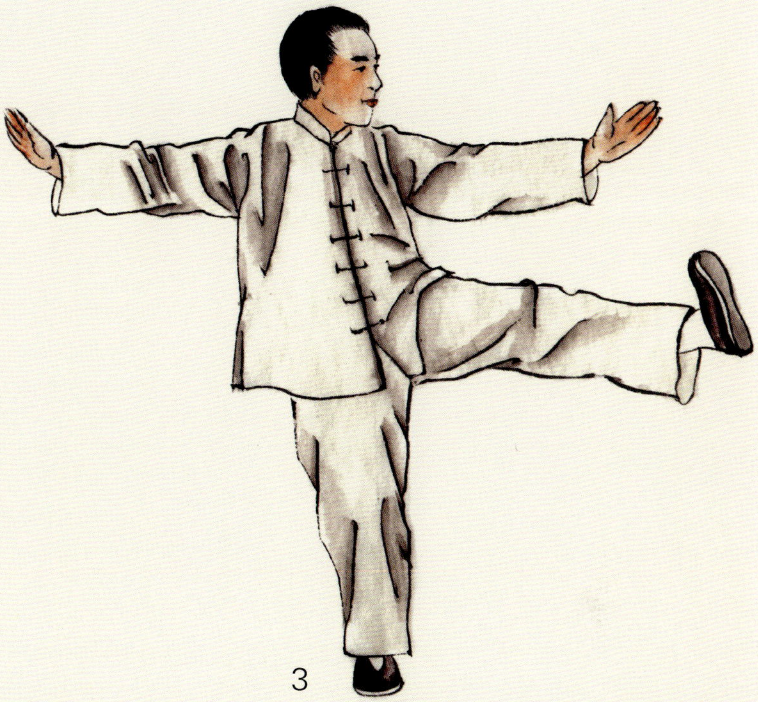

3

二十三、回身蹬脚

23. Turn and kick

此式指身体回旋一百八十度，而发腿蹬出之意。

Turn 180 degrees and kick.

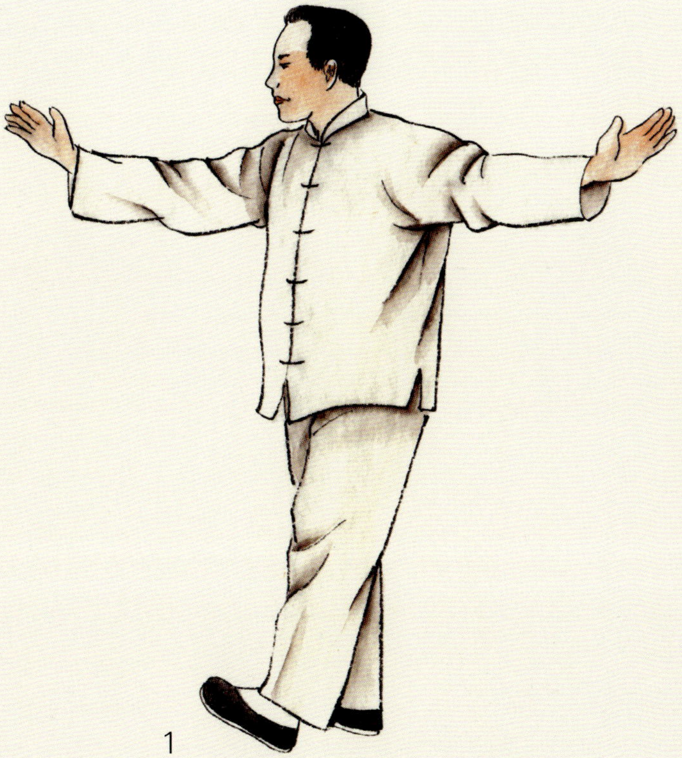

1

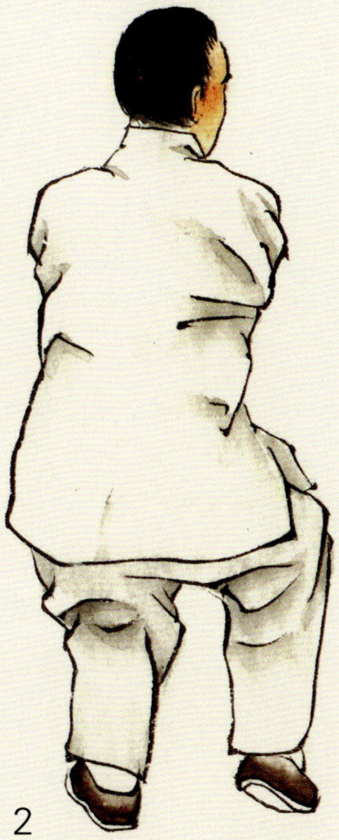

2

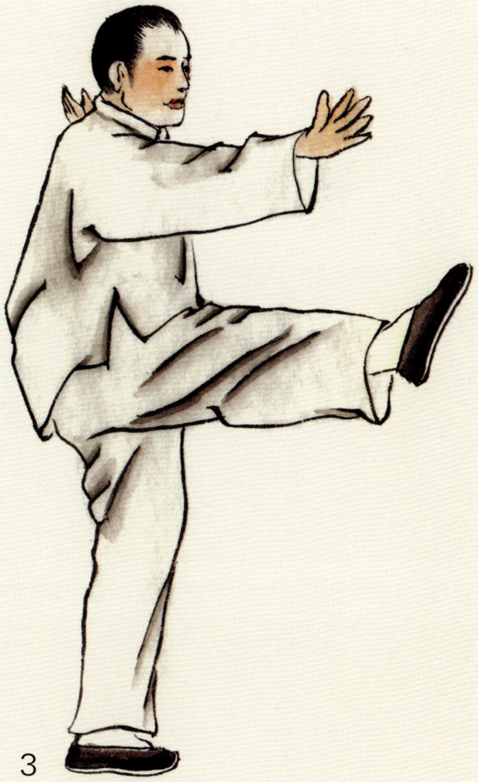

3

二十四、扑面掌

24. Lunge with palm forward

此式指顺步采掌，两掌交替滚旋，连扑带盖之意。

Advance and roll your hands by turns to pounce and strike.

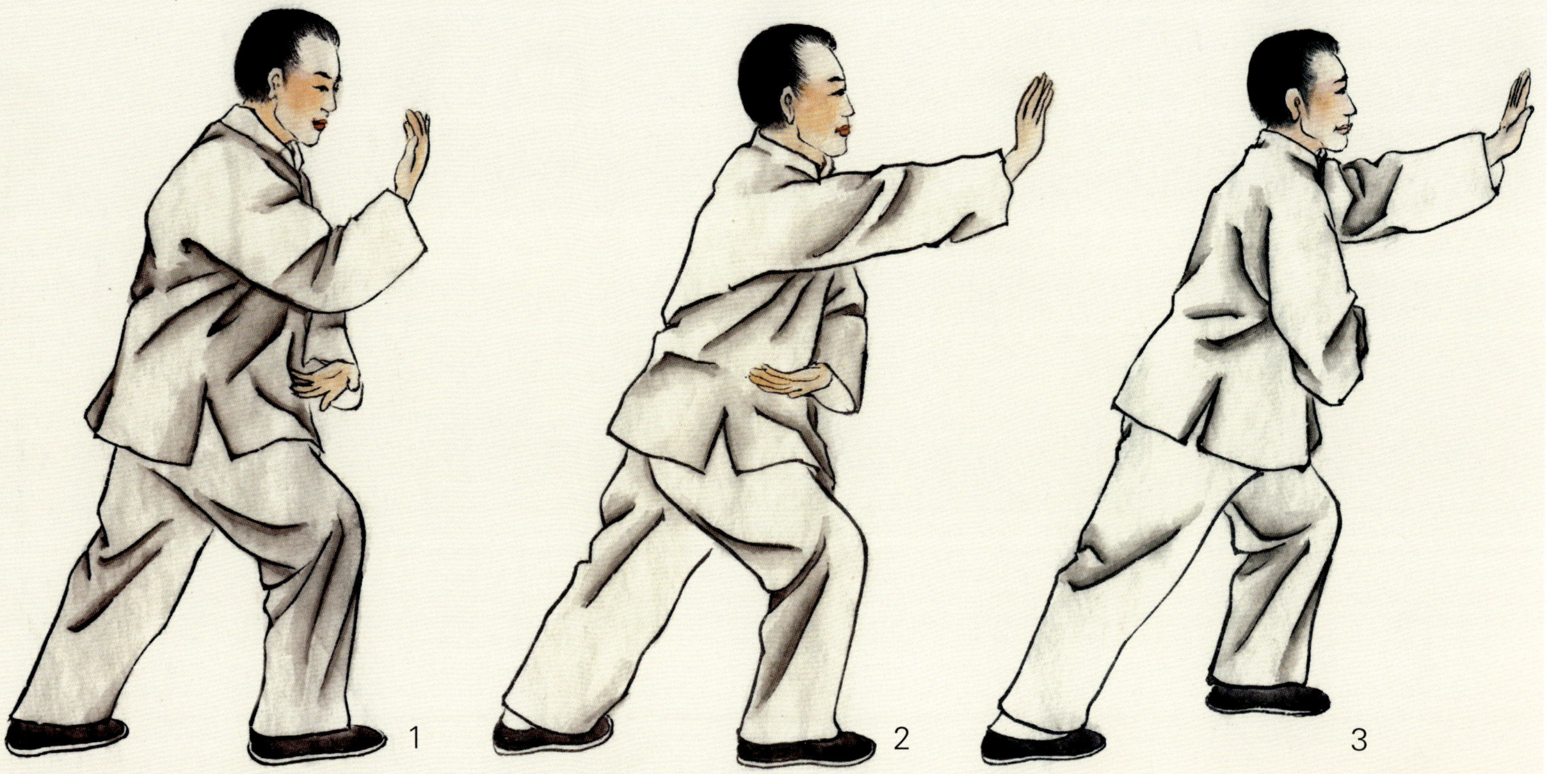

二十五、十字腿

25. Cross kick

此式指左臂与右腿所运转互相交叉如十字状，又拟风之摆莲。

Cross your left arm and right leg like 'a lotus swaying in the wind'.

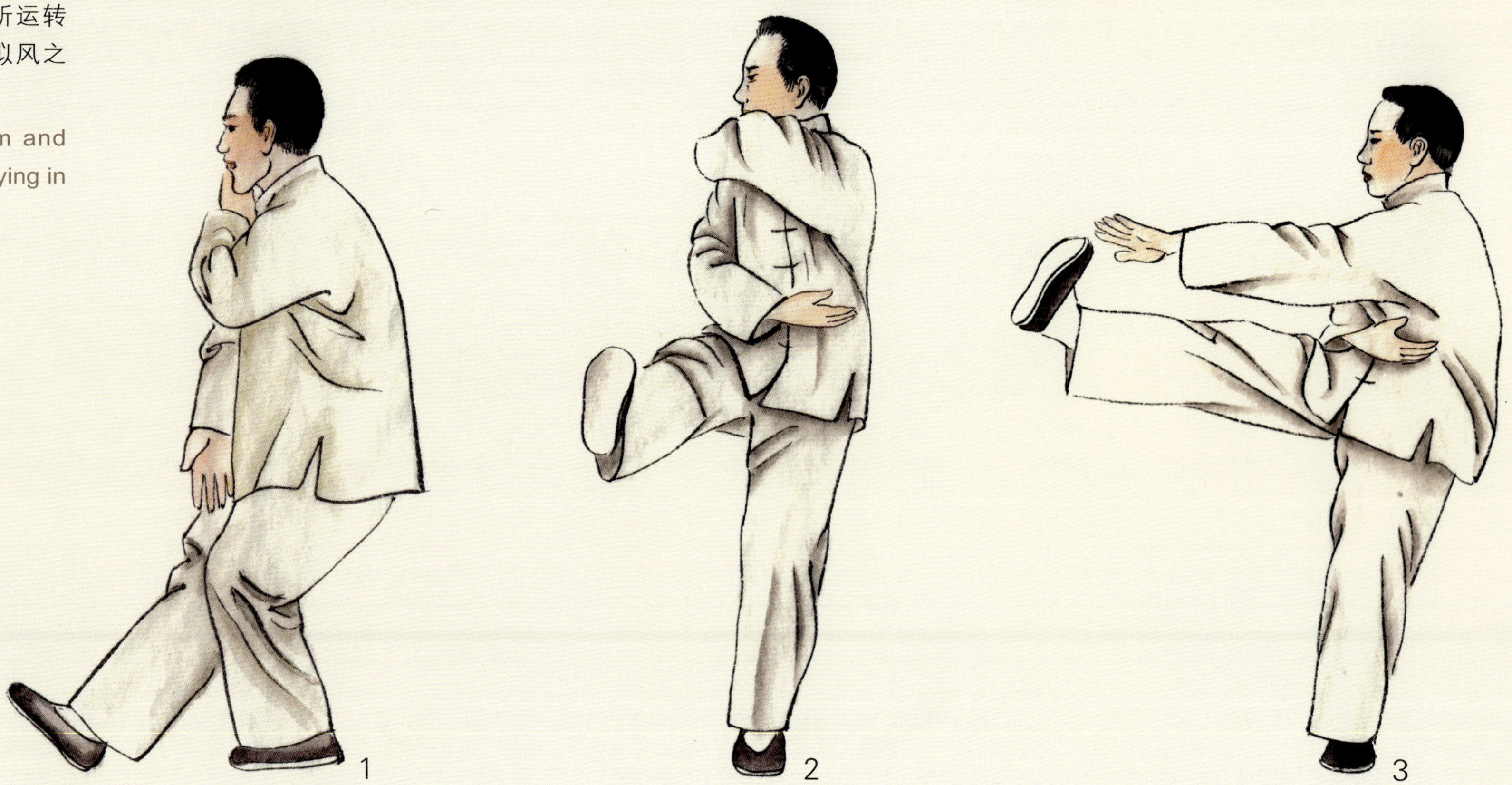

二十六、搂膝指裆锤

26. Brush the knee and punch at the crotch

此动作形势与搂膝拗步式相同，只是最后以掌改变为拳，向对方之下腹部进击。

This is similar to “brush knee and twist step”, except that at the end your hand turns into a fist aimed at your opponent's lower abdomen.

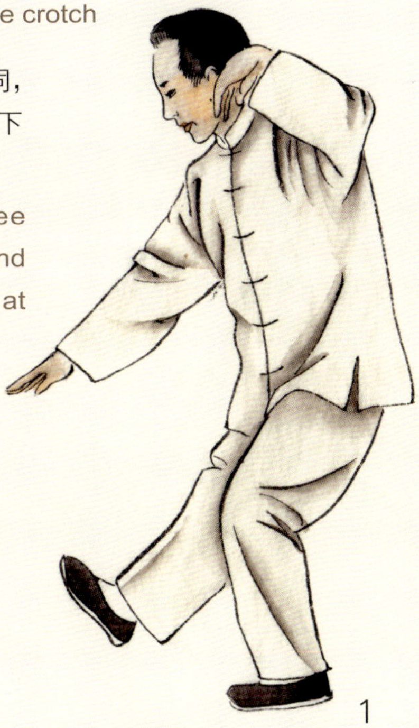
1

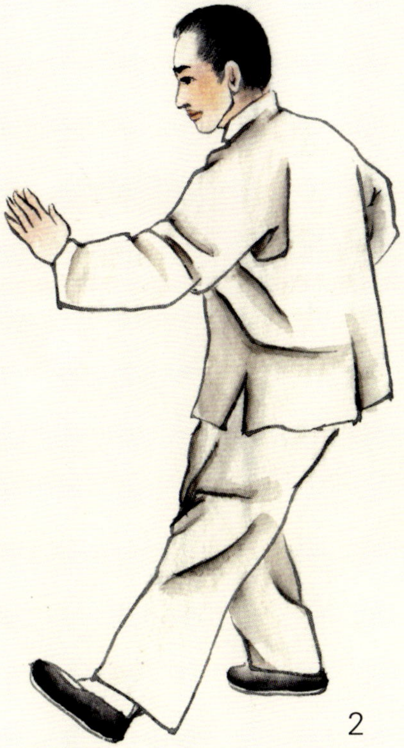
2

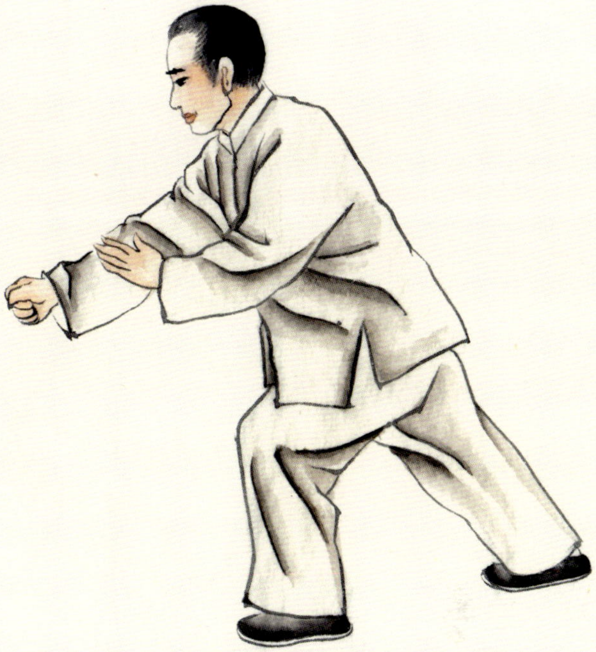
3

二十七、正单鞭

27. Front single whip

此式指以鞭根坐劲而力贯鞭梢之意。

Apply force as if on the handle of a whip in order to throw it out.

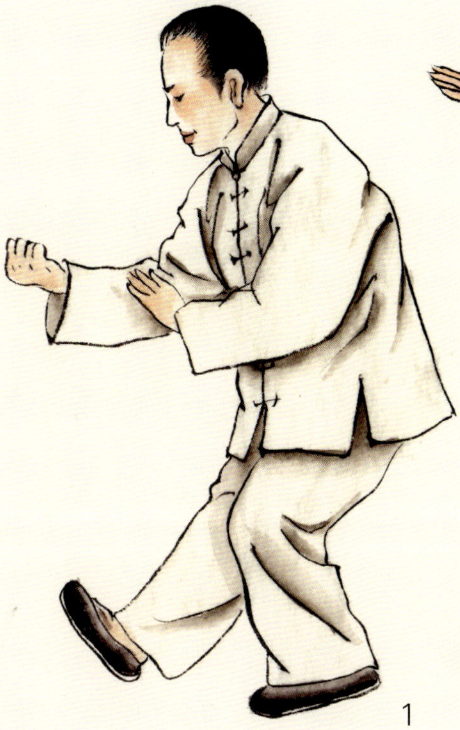
1

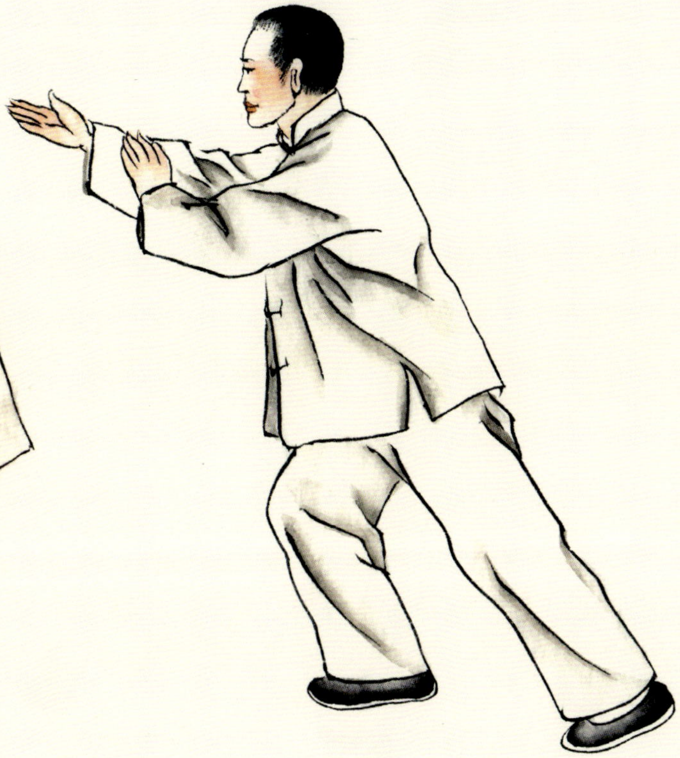
2

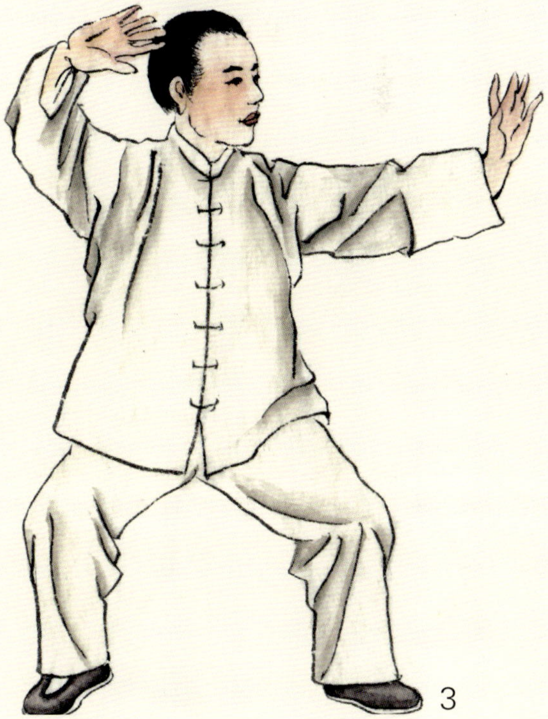
3

二十八、云手

28. Cloud hands

此式指两臂上下循环运转，其回旋缠绕之速度均匀和动作绵绵之姿态，就好像天空之行云一般。

Move your arms up and down in circles at an even speed and in a way suggestive of fleeting clouds in the sky.

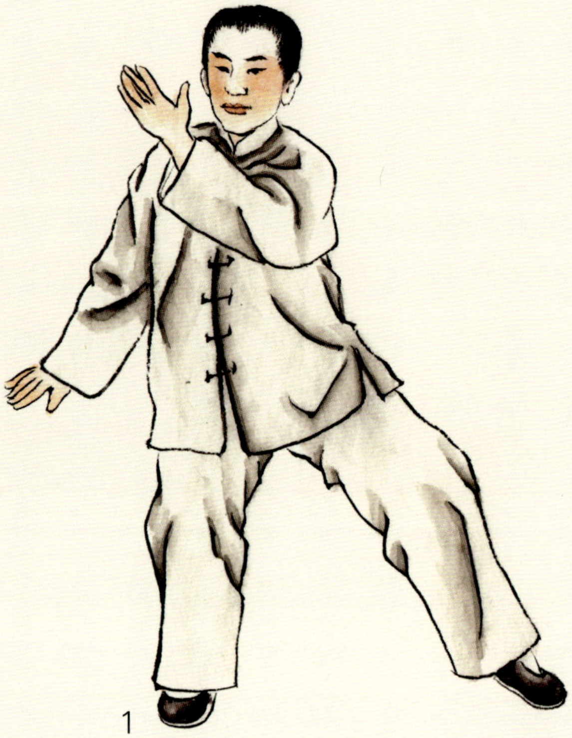

1

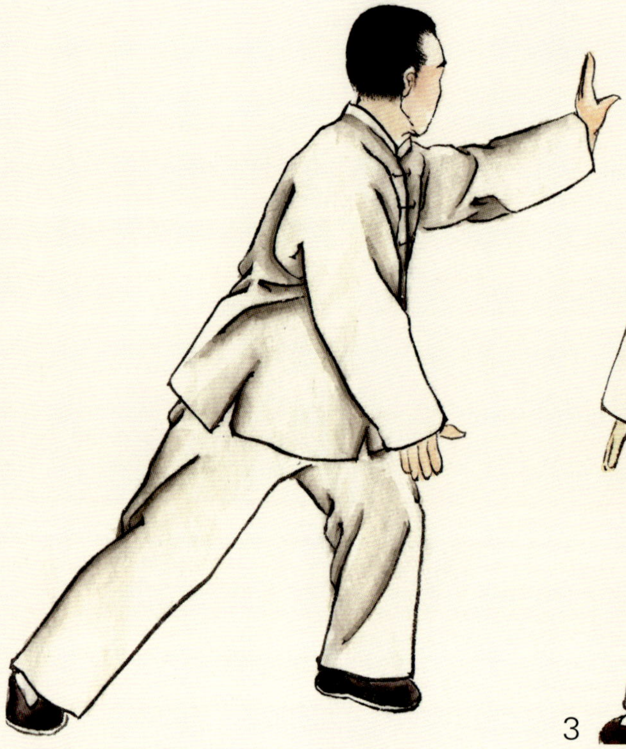

2

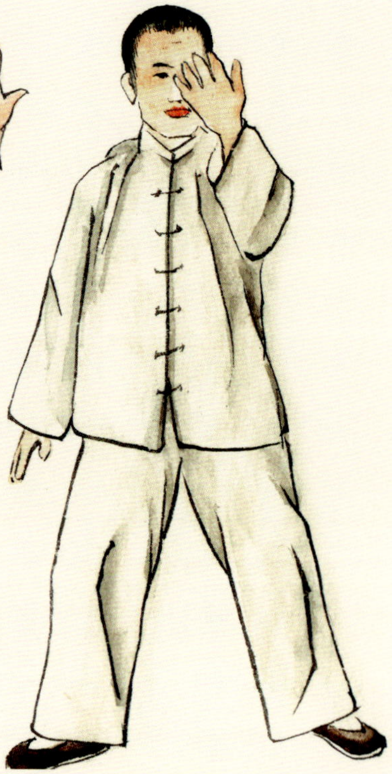

3

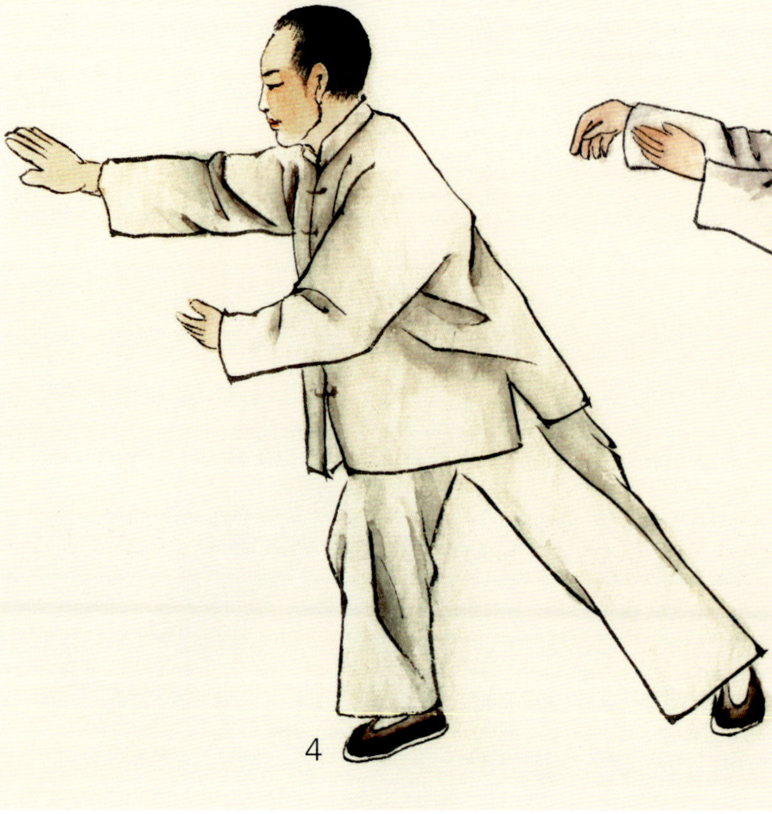

4

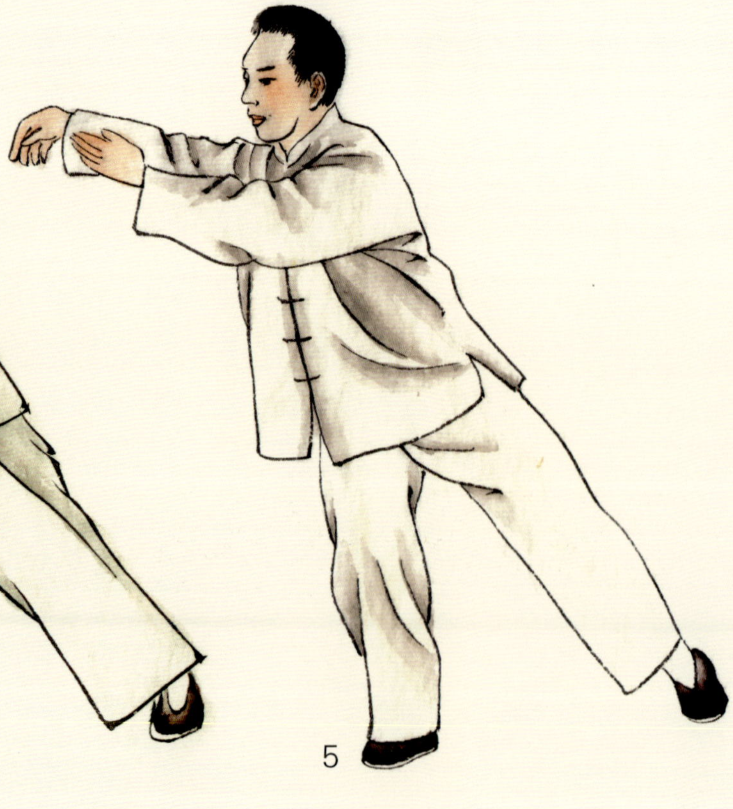

5

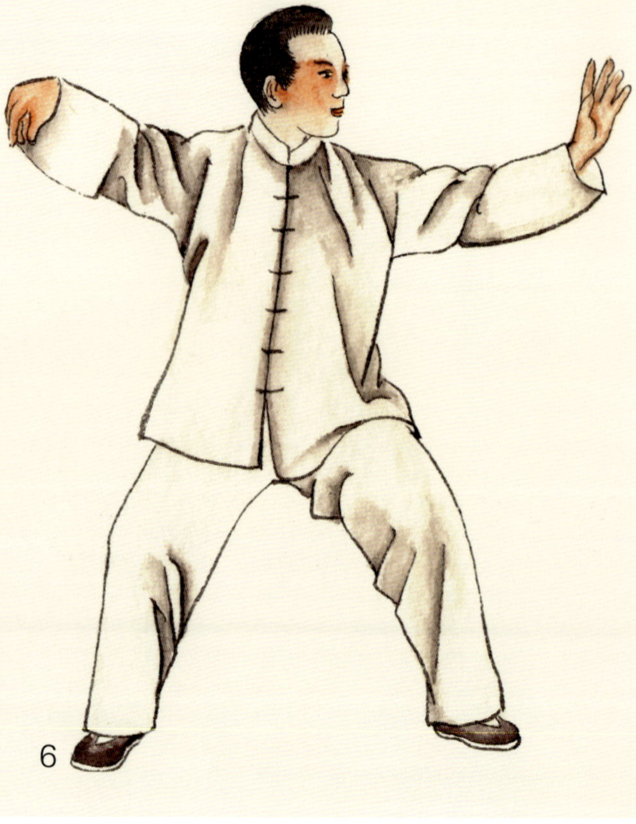

6

二十九、下式

29. Downward move

其式之形态好像鹰在空中盘旋，突然下落如捕兔之状。

This move resembles an eagle swirling in the sky and suddenly swooping down on a rabbit.

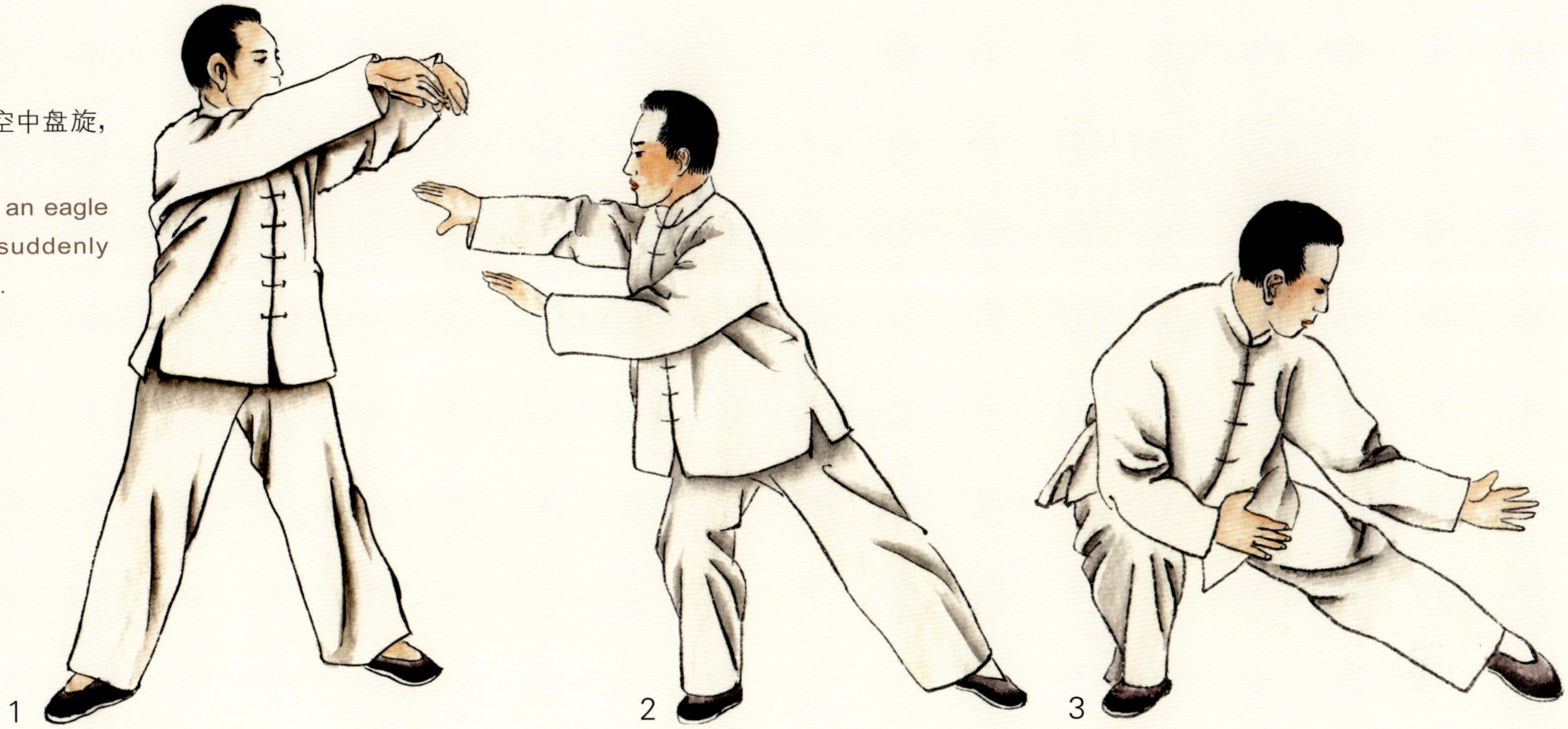

三十、上步七星

30. Step forward to form seven stars

此式突出了身上的七个部位，即头、肩、肘、手、胯、膝、足部。

This move highlights seven parts of the body: the head, the shoulders, the elbows, the hands, the hips, the knees, and the feet.

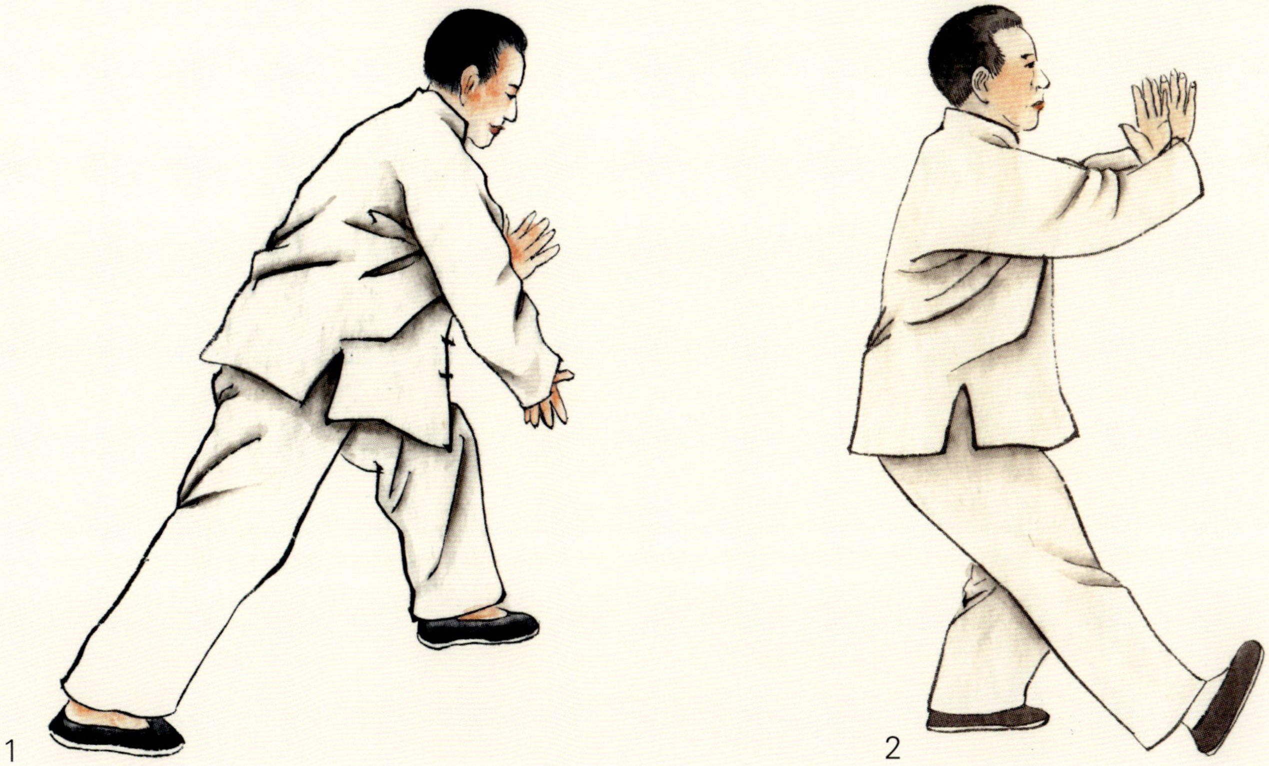

三十一、退步跨虎

31. Step back and straddle a tiger

此式坐身然后收左脚，脚尖虚沾地面成跨虚步，两臂分开，前掌后钩。

Lower your torso as if to sit down and move your left foot backward, with the tiptoe barely touching the floor. Spread your arms and bend the hand in front backward.

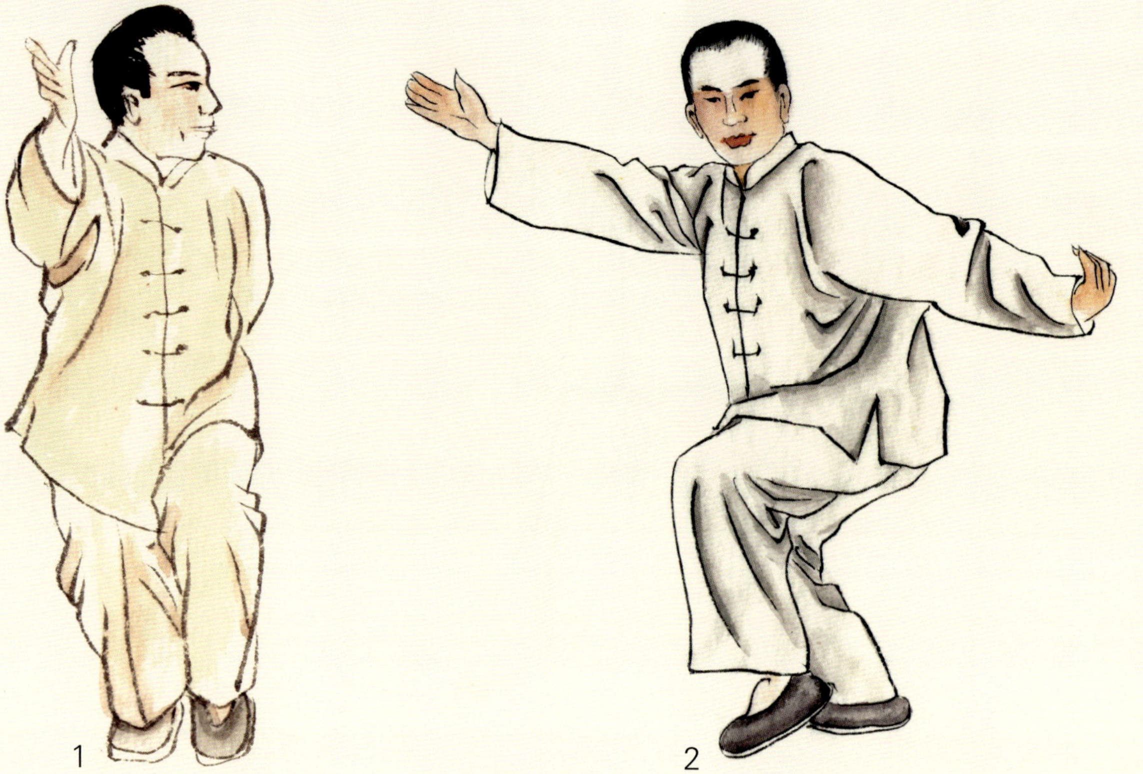

三十二、回身扑面掌

32. Turn around and lunge with the palm forward

此式指由前向后回转过身子以后，再发掌扑盖向前击之之意。

Turn around and push your hands forward to strike your opponent.

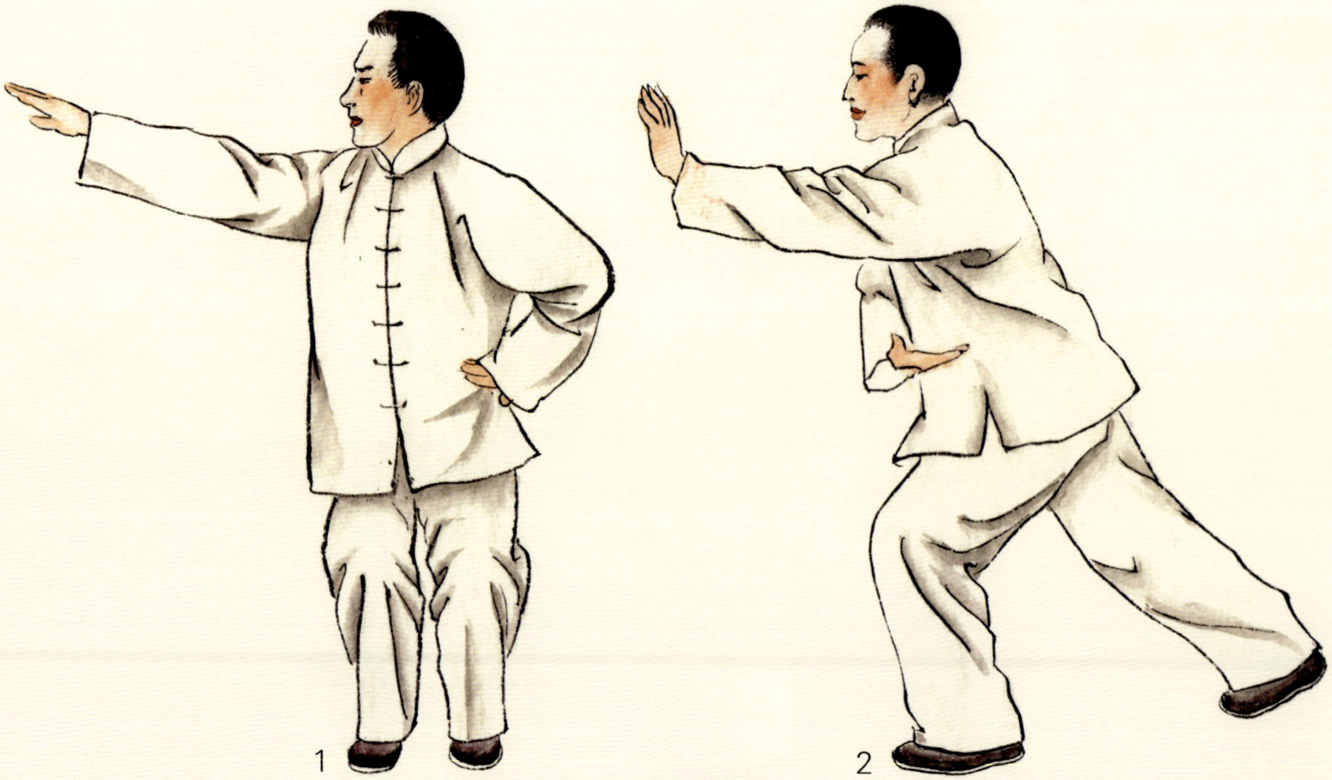

三十三、转角摆莲

33. Turn and sway lotus

此式指右脚之弧形运转与左右两掌逐递相触之动作，形若风之摆莲之摇的意思。

Move your right foot in a curve and touch it to your left hand and right hand one by one in a way suggestive of a lotus swaying in the wind.

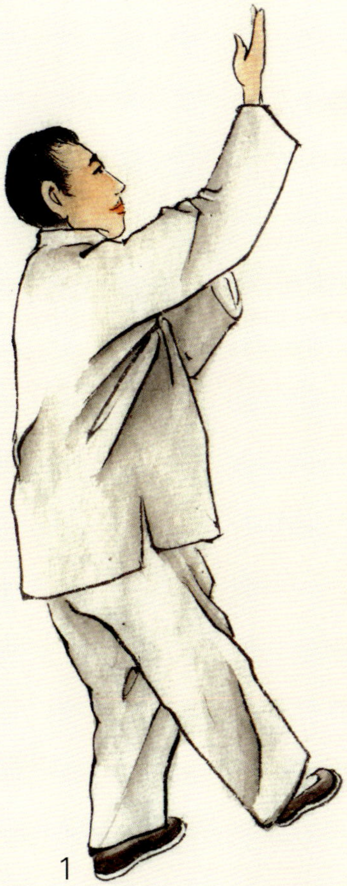

1

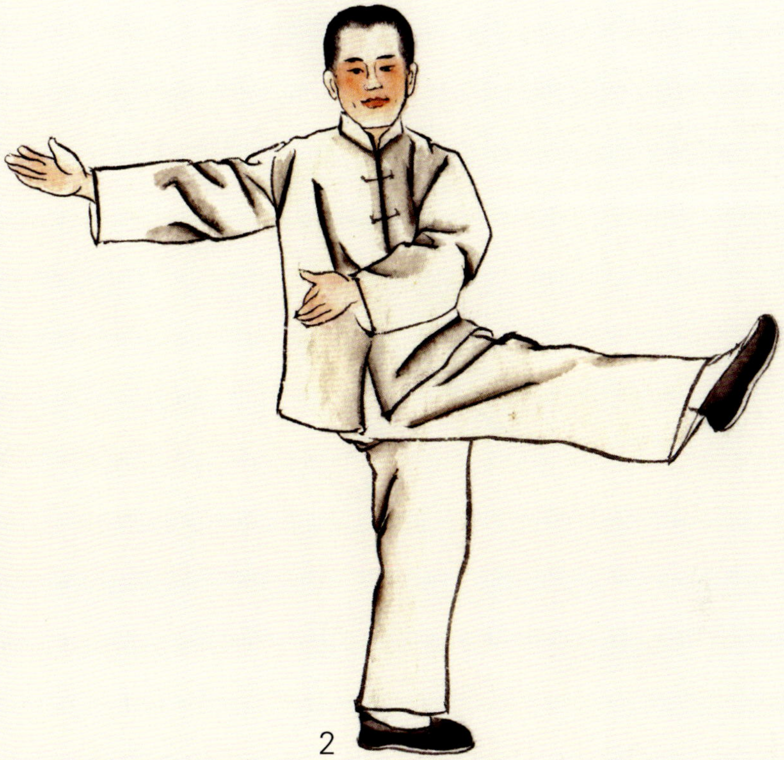

2

三十四、弯弓射虎

34. Draw the bow to shoot the tiger

此式好像握弓射箭，直射猛虎。

This move resembles drawing a bow and shooting an arrow at a tiger.

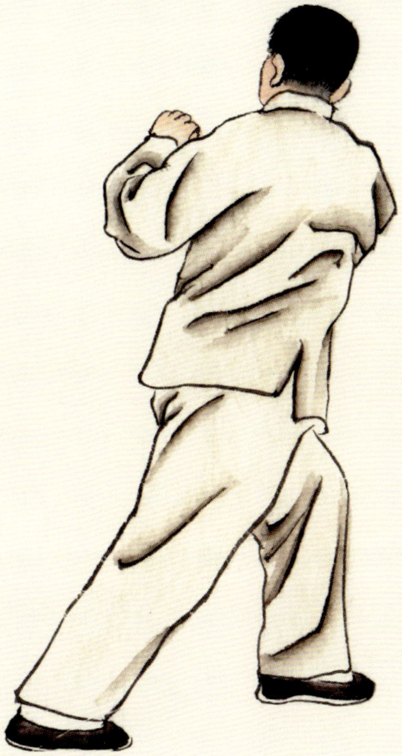

1

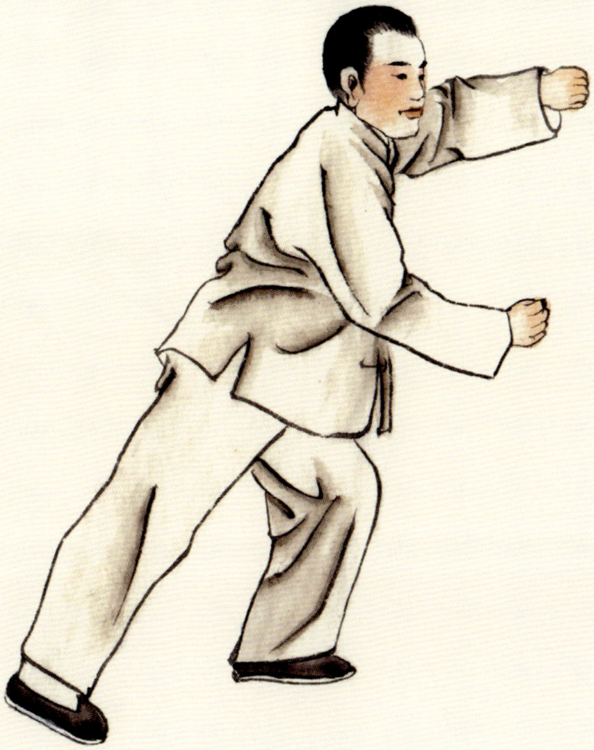

2

三十五、卸步搬拦锤

35. Turn body, deflect, parry, and punch

此式为撤步之同时将掌打出。

Strike with your hand while stepping back.

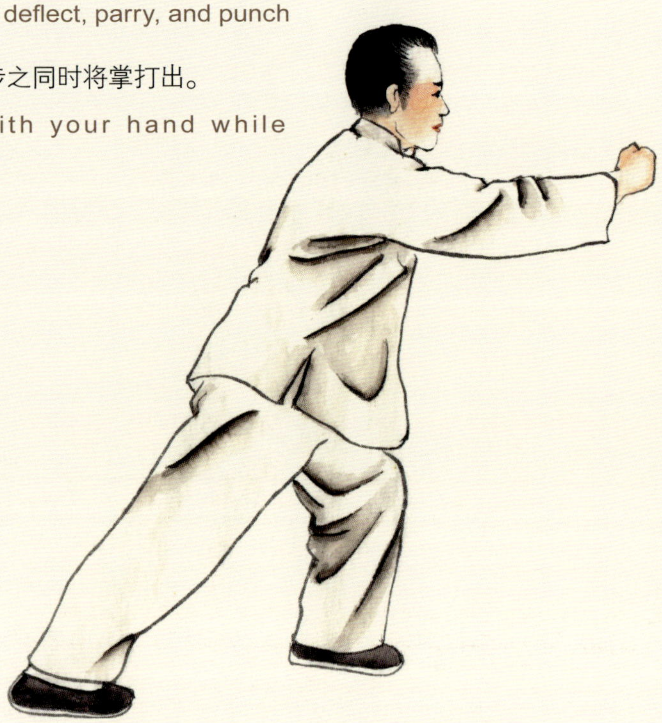

1

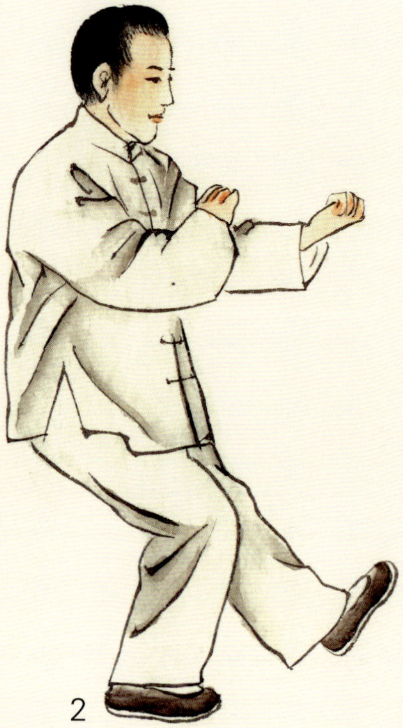

2

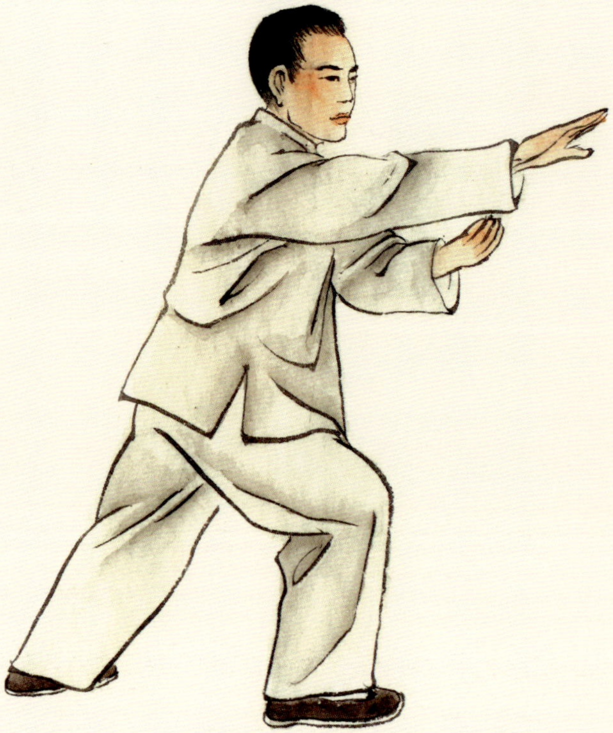

3

三十六 如封似闭

36. Appears sealed and closed

此式指两臂之交叉时形成斜十字状，好像封条一般。

Cross the arms like two paper strips used for sealing.

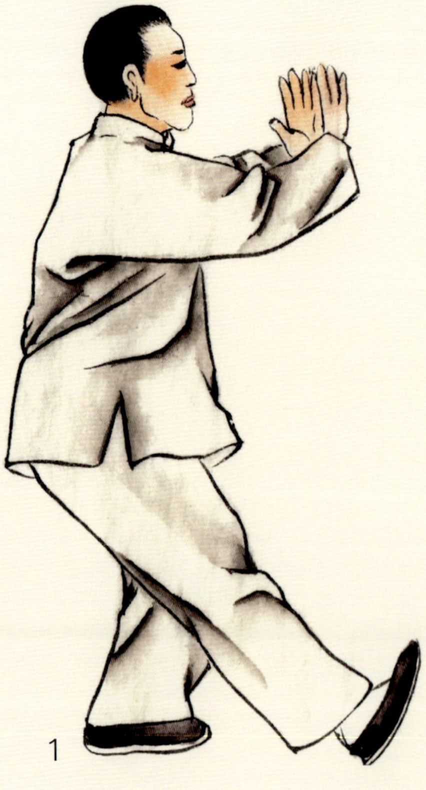

1

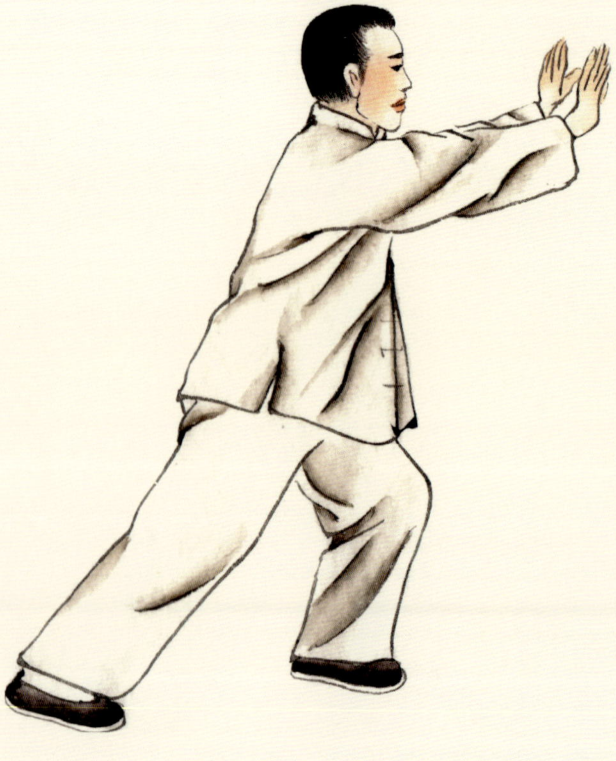

2

三十七、抱虎归山

37. Carry the tiger back to the mountain

此式动作是指两臂分开转身携抱，而后两掌合成十字于胸前，作为拳套终了之式，即恢复还原为起式状态。

Spread your arms, turn around, and bring your palms together in front of your chest as the closing posture, which is the same as the commencing posture.

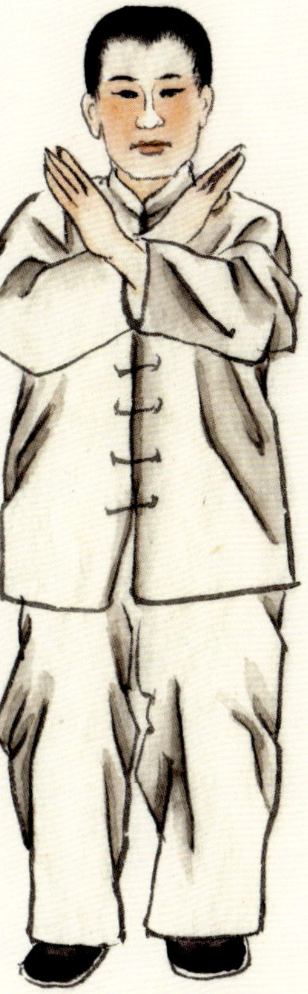

1

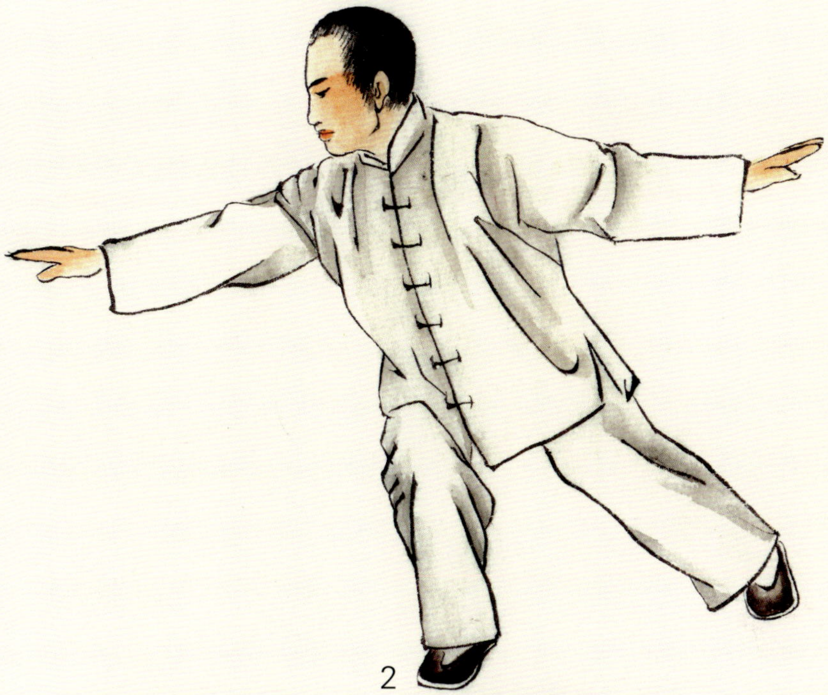

2

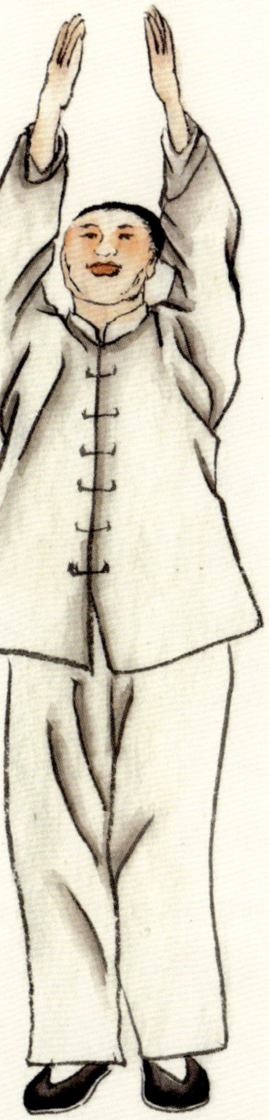

3

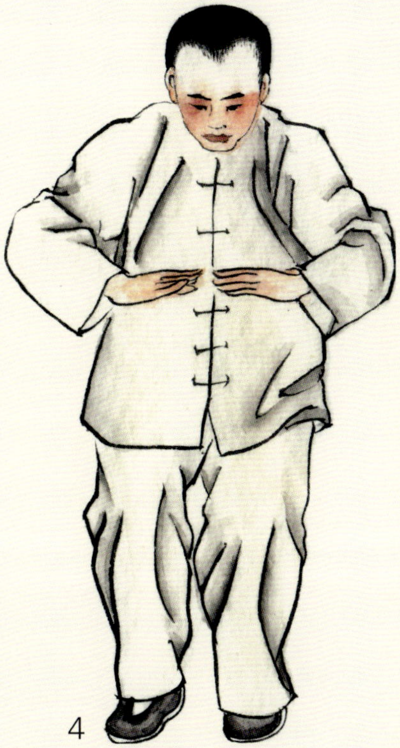

4

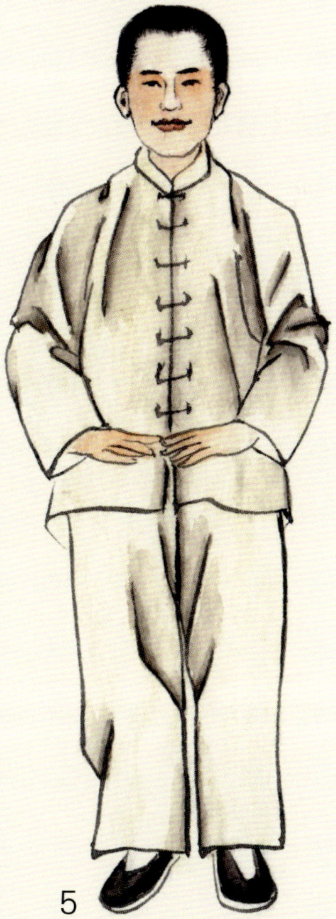

5

伍　正心养神

V. Mental Health

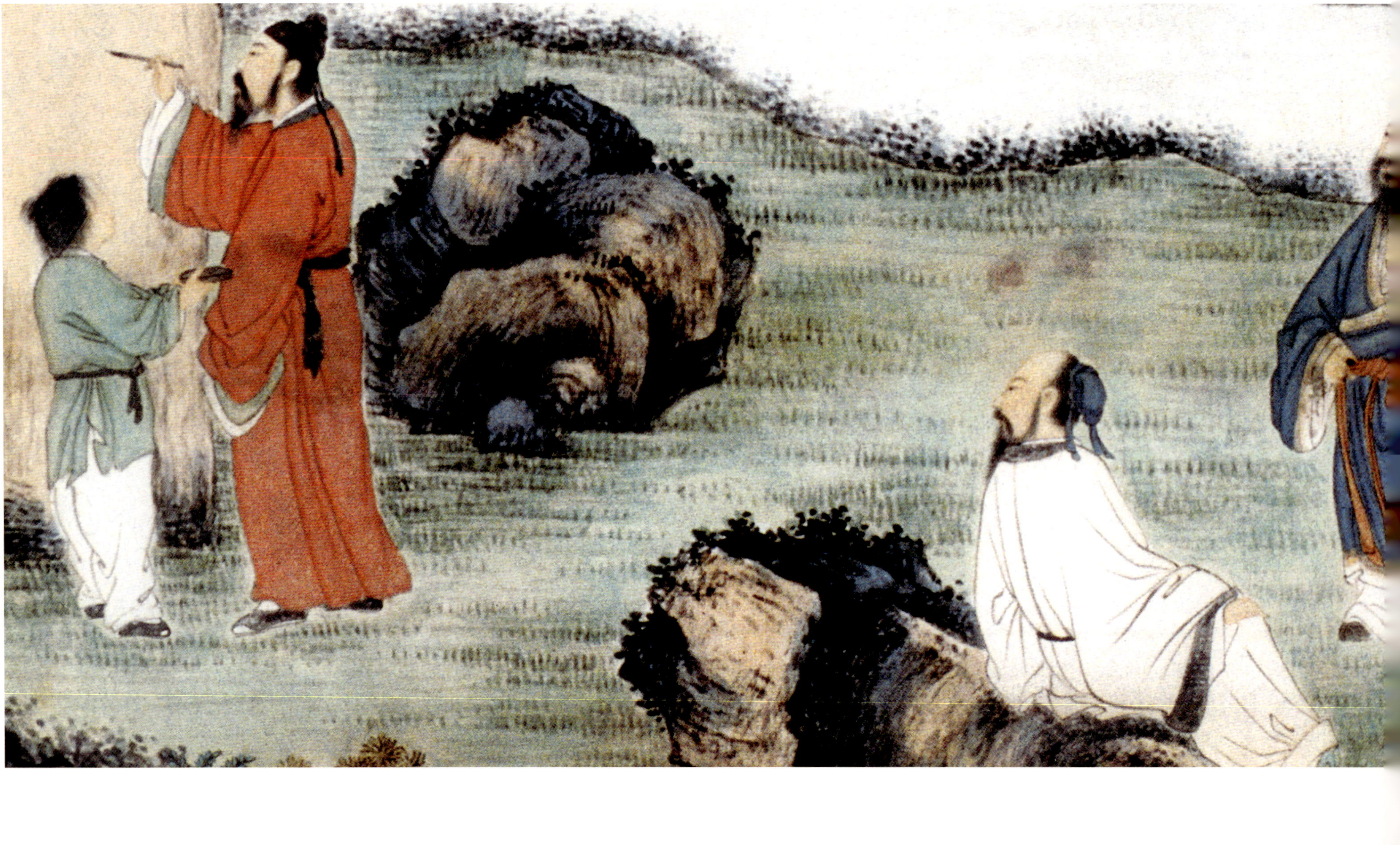

心理健康对身体健康至关重要。现代心理学中的认识、情感、意志即相当于中医中的“神”。养神有利于健康长寿，很多勤俭有为的人都身强体壮、享有高寿，养神需要人正心诚意，纯正心思。

Mental health is crucial to physical health. What is termed as ‘perception’, ‘emotions’ and ‘will’ are equivalent to ‘shen’, or the ‘spirit’, in Chinese medicine. The practice of nurturing the ‘spirit’ calls for sole-mindedness and sincerity and is conducive to health and longevity. That explains why those diligent and thrifty tend to enjoy physical and mental health and longevity.

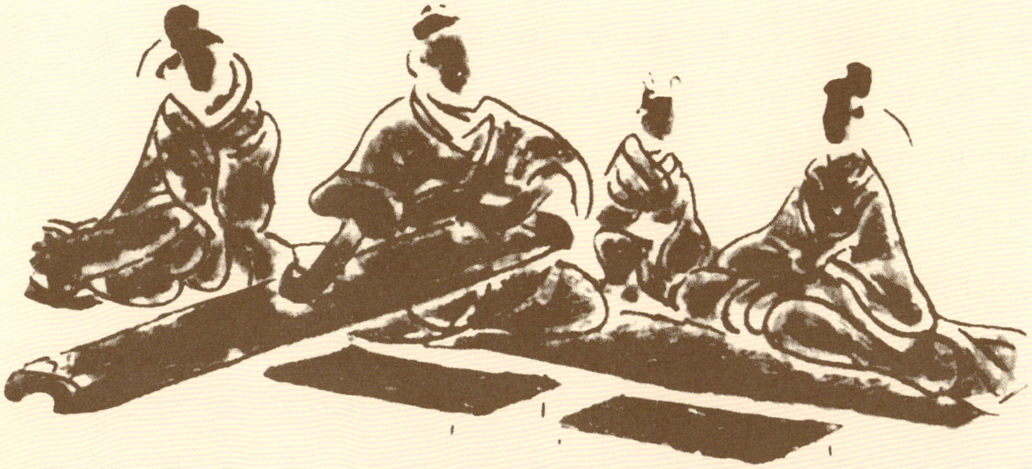

养神之道

The art of spiritual cultivation

养生之道，多种多样，简而言之，则可归之为养神与养形两大类。

Various as they are, regimens can be roughly divided into two categories: to nourish the spirit and to nourish the body.

“神”在人体居首要之位

Spirit, the premier component of human body

“神”是人生命活动现象的总称，它以精血为物质基础，包括精神意识、知觉、运动等。

Spirit is the aggregate of the phenomena of life activities and the epitome of all life activities.It includes the consciousness, perception and mental activities. The essence and blood are its material basis.

神
Spirit

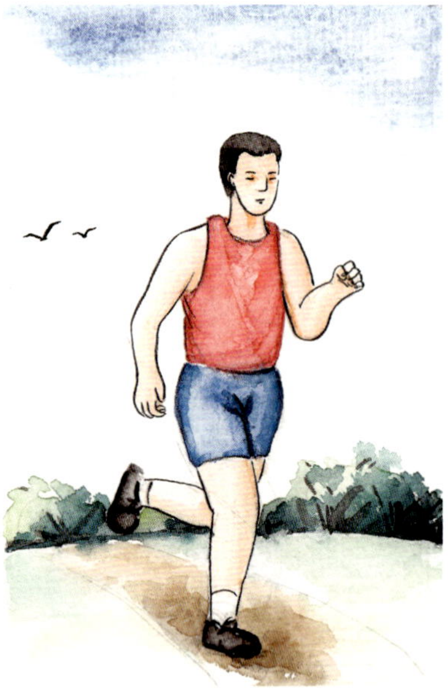

运动
Movement

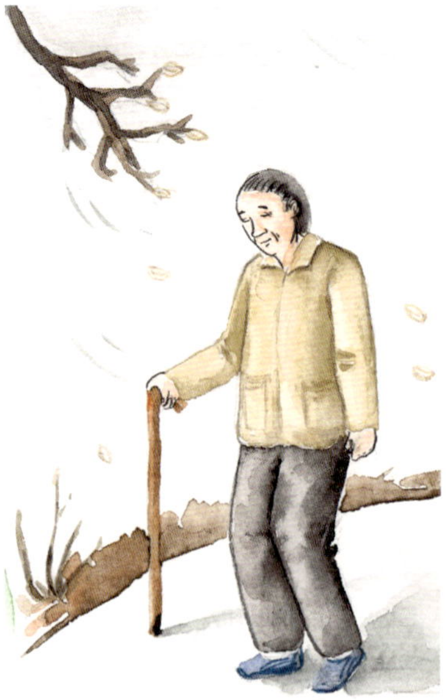

意识、知觉
Consciousness and perception

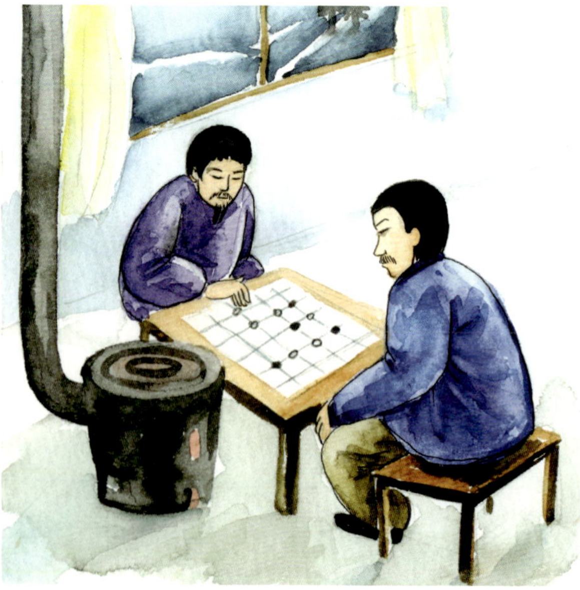

精神活动
Mental activity

中国传统养生学认为，在人体统一整体中，起统帅和协调作用的是心神，只有心神调节好了，生命活动才表现出各脏器组织的整体特性和整体功能，从而符合生命活动的规律。

According to the traditional Chinese theories on health preservation, the human body, which is a unified whole, is commanded and coordinated by the mind. Only when regulated by the mind can life show the overall traits, function, behavior and pattern of the organs and tissues.

形神一体

Union of body and spirit

整体观是中医“人与自然”观的核心，强调人与自然的共生关系。一体观也是中医的重要思想，强调“形与神俱”。

One of the basic characteristics of Chinese traditional medicine is its emphasis on the unity of man and nature. As to the human body itself, it emphasizes the integrated concept of “the unity of form and spirit.”

“神”控制和调节着“精”与“气”在人体内的正常运行，即所谓“神能驭气”。

Spirit (shen) controls and regulates the normal circulation of essence (jing) and qi in the human body. That is described by the phrase “the spirit has control over qi”.

“气”是人体内活力很强且不断运动的精微物质，是推动和调节人体生命活动的根本动力。“气”也是化生“神”的基本物质，气充则神旺。

Qi is a subtle substance in the human body, which is highly dynamic and keeps moving. It is the fundamental force to motivate and regulate the vital processes of the human body. It is also the fundamental substance for the generation of spirit, which cannot be lively without sufficient qi.

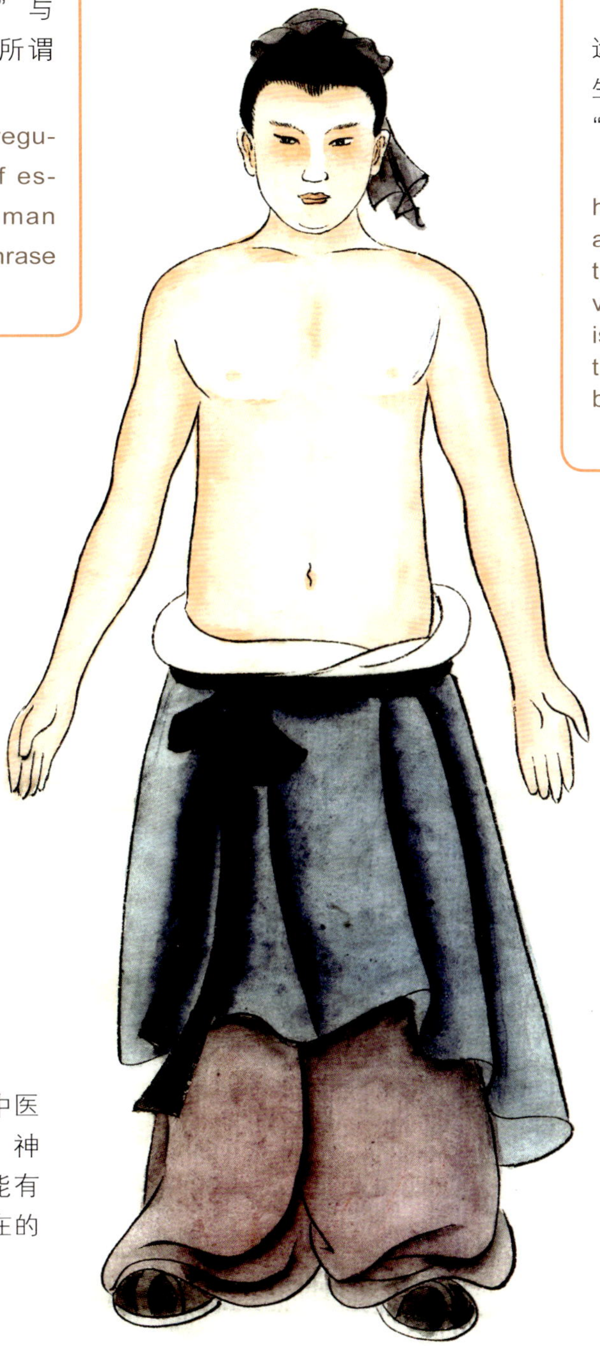

“精”是构成人之形体的最基本物质，也是化气生“神”的物质基础。“精”藏于脏腑之中而不妄泄，又受“神”和“气”的控制和调节。

Essence is the most fundamental substance for one's physical form and the material foundation for the generation of qi and spirit. On the other hand, it is thanks to the control and regulation by spirit and qi that essence is preserved in the internal organs without improper discharge.

精、气、神为人身“三宝”：精为基础，气为动力，神为主宰，三者一起构成“形”的有机整体。

Essence, qi and spirit are the 'three treasures' of the human body that make up the organic whole of the physical form, in which essence forms the foundation, qi provides impetus, and spirit has dominion over both.

对人而言，形体和精神并非彼此独立，毫无关联。中医认为，形与神相互依附，不可分离。形是神的藏舍之处，神是形的生命体现。神不能离开形体单独存在，有形才能有神，形健则神旺。神是形体的主宰，形神统一是生命存在的保证。

The union of the body and spirit means, in other words, the integration and union of the body and the spirit. The soul and the human body are interdependent and inseparable. The body is the abode of the spirit; the spirit reflects the life in the body. The spirit cannot exist independently without the body. When the body thrives, the spirit will flourish. On the other hand, once the spirit engenders, it dominates the body. The union of the body and spirit guarantees the existence of life.

养神的方法

Methods of spiritual cultivation

1 养神应不时御神

不能管理好自己心绪的人，很容易为贪图一时之乐，生活没有规律，久而久之必然会损害身心，出现早衰。

1. When cultivating your spirit, rein your spirit on a regular basis.

Those who do not control their spirit properly and indulge in momentary pleasures against the laws in life will have their physical and psychological health harmed. And their body will age prematurely.

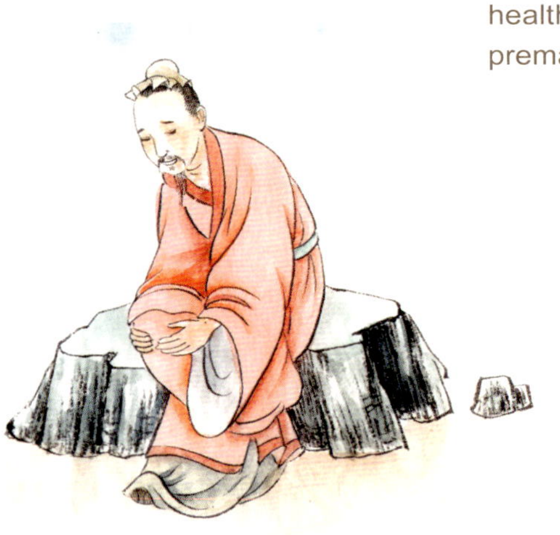

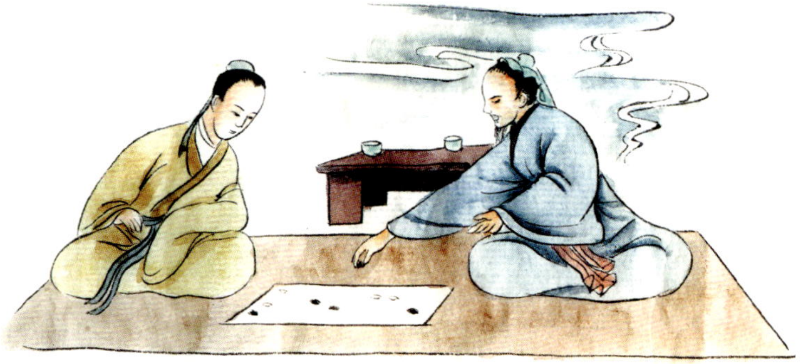

2 养神应高下不相慕

减少私心杂念，见素抱朴，少私寡欲。只有少私寡欲，精神才能守持于内。一个私心太重、嗜欲不止的人，必然无法拥有内心的宁静。

2. To cultivate your spirit, refrain from envying others.

Try to eliminate selfish ideas and personal considerations, revert and keep to simplicity, and clear your heart of desires. Only in this way can you keep your spirit from wavering inside. A man who is full of selfish ideas and consumed by desires cannot attain peace in the mind.

3 养神应抑目静耳

眼耳是神接受外界刺激的主要器官，其功能受着神的主宰和调节。目清耳静则神气内守而心不劳，若目驰耳躁，则神气烦劳而心神不宁。

3. To rein your spirit, see less and hear less.

The eyes and the ears are the main faculties for you to receive stimuli from outside. Their functions are dominated and regulated by the spirit. If you see less and hear less, your spirit will withdraw in recess and your heart will not be worried. If you see and hear too much, your spirit will be agitated and your heart worried. They cannot attain peace.

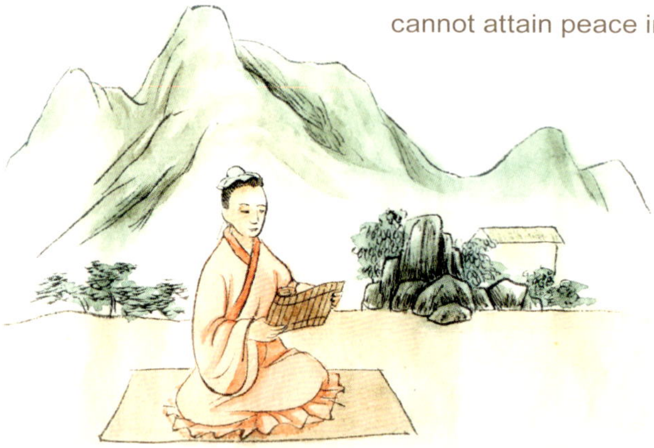

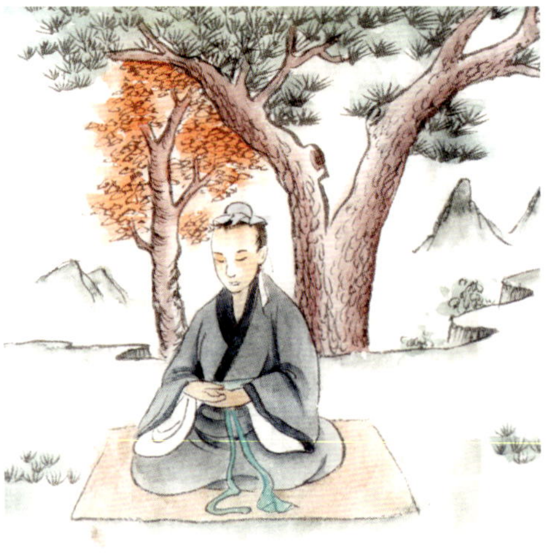

4 养神应凝神敛思

一如养生家孙思邈所说："多思则神殆，多念则志散，多欲则志昏，多事则形劳。"因此，人要有意识地凝神敛思，养护心神。

4. To cultivate your spirit, you should concentrate on meditation.

Concentrating your attention on meditation is a good way to keep your mind quiet and calm. Otherwise, as Sun Simiao, expert on health preservation in ancient China, puts it, "Think too much, and your essence will be exhausted; with too many worries, your spirit will be distracted; with too many desires, your mind will be confused; with too many affairs, your body will be tired."

清静养神

Repose in tranquility

清静，是指保持淡泊宁静的心理状态。欲使心神清静，关键是要做到“恬惔虚无”。即摒除杂念，畅遂情志，宁静淡泊，静养身心。“心乱则百病生，心静则万病悉去。”清静养神，以静制躁，有利于抗衰防老，所以心不可乱思，神不可过用，思太乱则伤，神过用则疲。清静养神的另一个重要方面是减少对名利和物质欲望。究竟名利和身体哪个重要？当然是身体。若患得患失，孜孜汲汲，唯名利是图，久而久之，必然会损伤心神，影响健康。

Tranquility is to keep a quiet state of mind. To achieve this, the key is to be indifferent to fame and wealth. That is, to eliminate distracting thoughts, to relax the mind, and to repose in quietness. “Fretting induces all kinds of illness, while tranquility keeps all diseases away.” Repose in tranquility and checking flippancy with quietness can slow down the aging process, so the mind should not be engaged in chaotic thinking, and the spirit should not be exploited excessively. Too much thinking is harmful, and excessive use of the spirit is exhausting. Another important aspect of quiet repose is to reduce the desire for fame and wealth and other material desires. Which is more important on earth, fame and wealth or one's health? Of course, the latter. If you worry about gain and loss, consider fame and wealth as your priority and ceaselessly pursue them, your mind and health will inevitably be damaged in the long run.

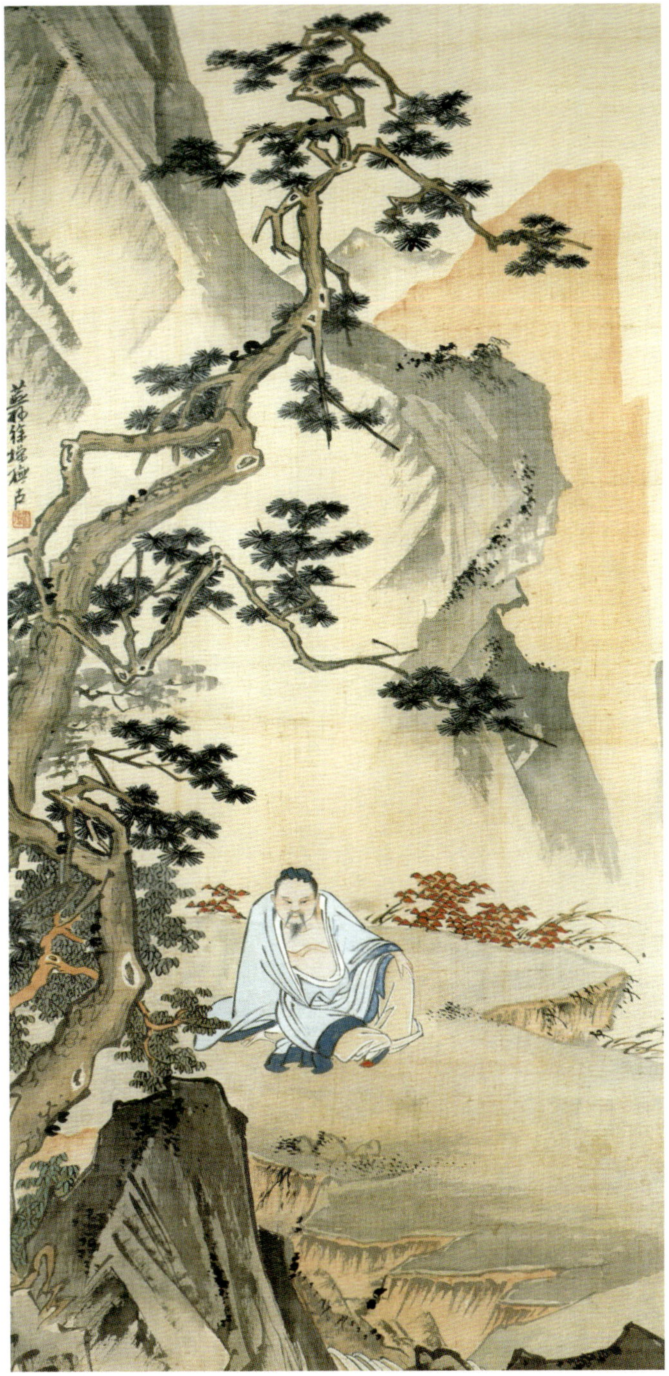

松下高士图

A Noble Hermit under the Pine

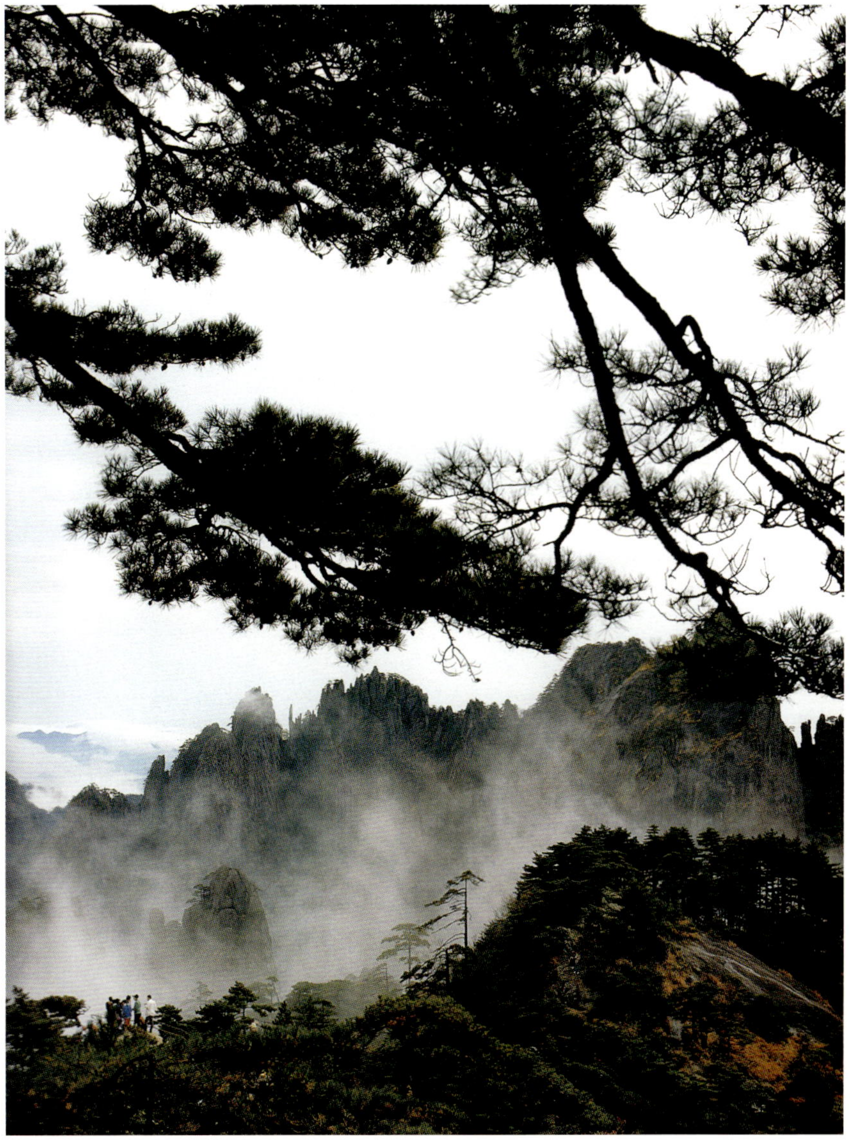

黄山松云

Pine trees amid clouds of Mountain Huangshan

怡情畅神

To relax the mood

怡情畅神，即经常保持愉快的情绪心境。人生的道路不可能一帆风顺，人难免会遇到一些不顺心之事，或失意悲伤，或愤怒激动。因此，人要锻炼意志，加强自我修养，及时排解烦恼，调节情绪，以便在面对挫折挑战时，心安不惧，神静不烦，始终保持乐观豁达的心态。这样不仅有益于身心健康，还有助于延年益寿。《素问·上古天真论》介绍的圣人养生之道，一是“无恚嗔之心”，二是“无思想之患”，三是“以恬愉为务”。

To relax the mood is to keep a happy state of mind. The road of one's life cannot always be smooth, and it is inevitable to meet some frustration, or sad, irritating things, which requires one to exercise one's will, to cultivate one's mind and develop a good character so that one can adjust one's mood, remain optimistic and unworried in the face of various troubles. This is not only good for physical and mental health, but is also the magic key to longevity. The regimens of the saints described in “How the Ancient People Keep Innate Essence” of the *Inner Canon* are as follows: first, “no resentment”, second, “free from too much thinking”, and third, “keep a happy and quiet state of mind”.

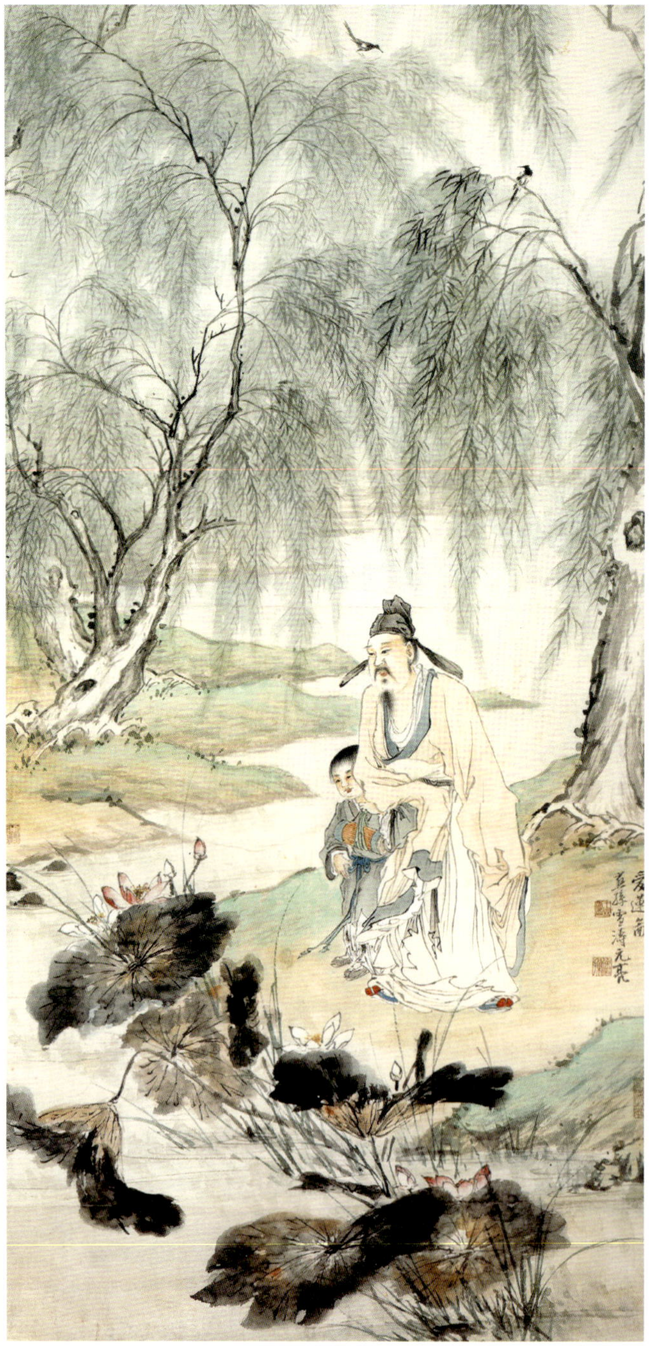

徐燕孙《爱莲图》
Xu Yansun *Admiring the Lotus Flowers*

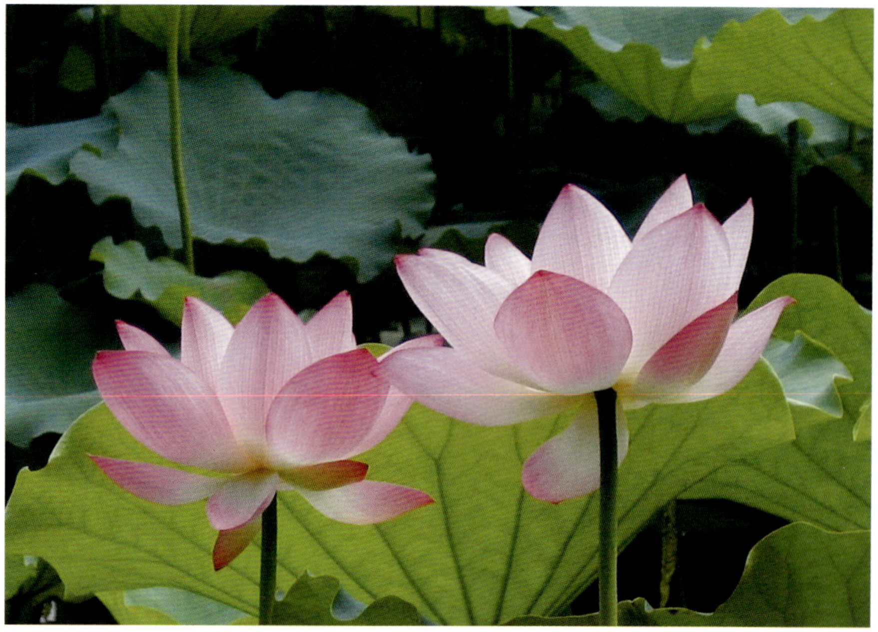

荷花
Lotus flowers

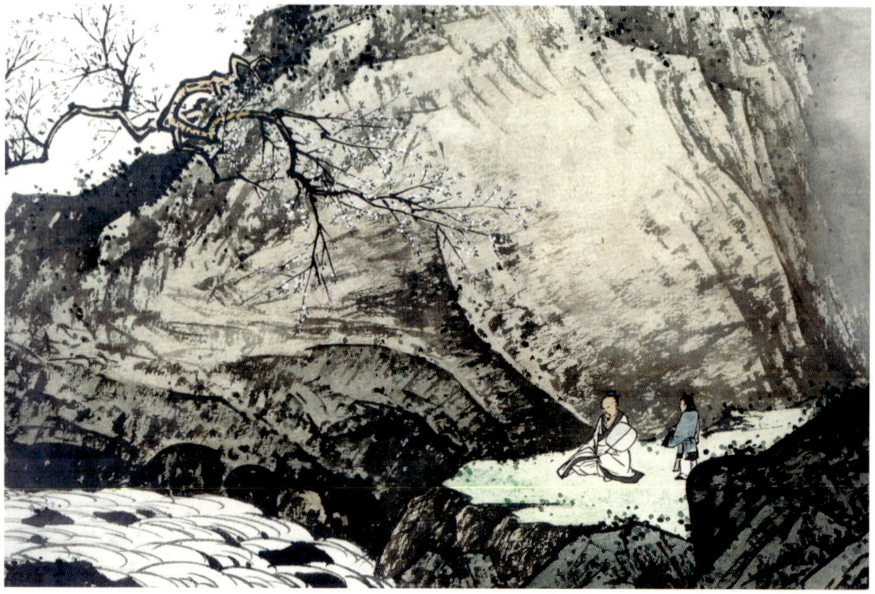

陈少梅《赏梅图》
Chen Shaomei *Admiring the Plum Blossoms*

怡情十乐

Ten joys to relax the mood:

要选择有益于身心的文体活动，健体怡情，如：

琴瑟乐；弈棋乐；书画乐；养花乐；散步乐；钓鱼乐；旅游乐；运动乐。

Choose sports or cultural activities that can improve your health and delight your mind, such as:

Playing a musical instrument, playing chess, painting, gardening, walking, fishing, traveling, and sports.

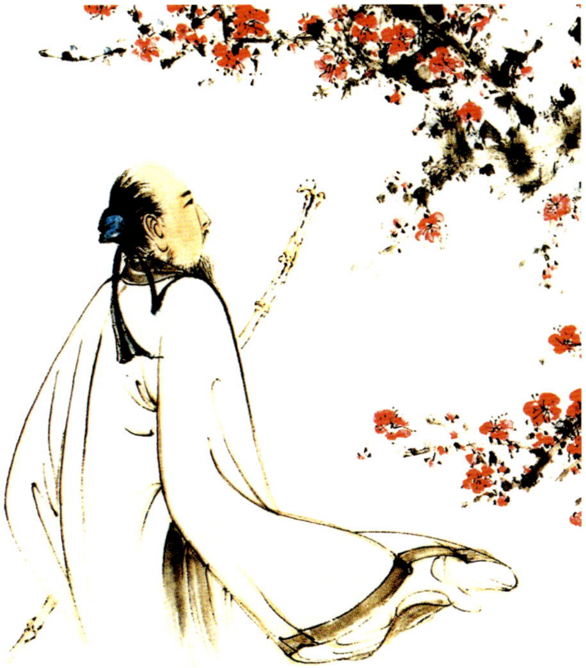

养花乐

The pleasure of gardening

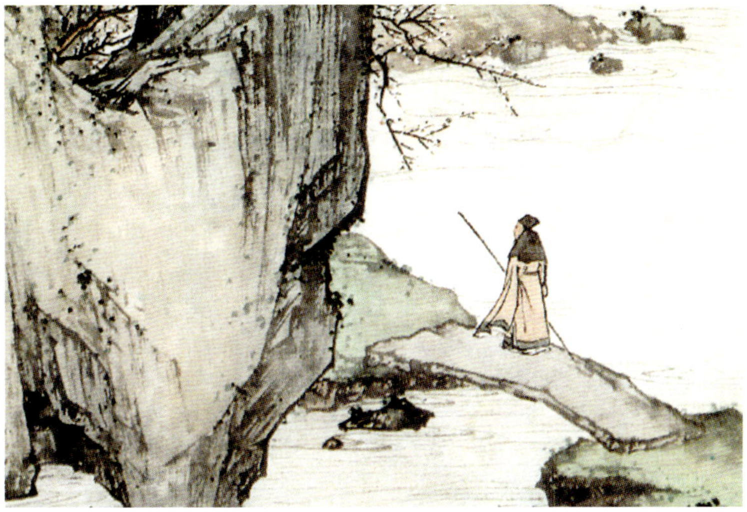

散步乐

The pleasure of walking

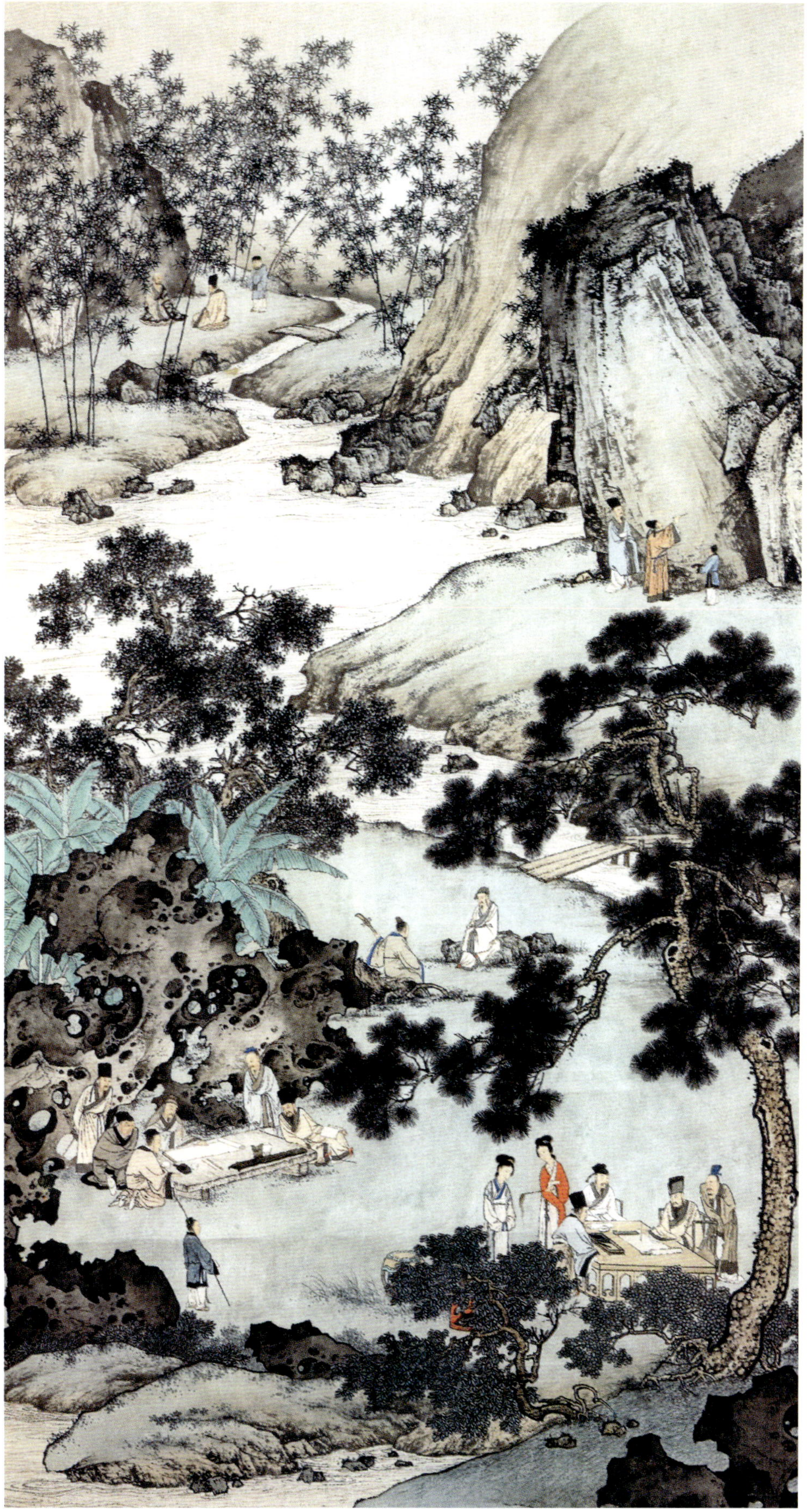

弈棋乐

The pleasure of playing chess

养心之道

Theories of spiritual cultivation

前人总结养心之道说："任意自适，不以外物伤和气，不敢做过当事，酌中恰好即止。"意思是处事恰如其分，绝不偏激，则情理得过，心安理得，自然有益于心身健康。

The way of mental cultivation has been summarized like this:"Adjust yourself, do not feel angry with outside things, do not overdo, and do everything in a proper way." Handling things appropriately and not going to extremes will induce peace of the mind, thus benefiting physical and mental health.

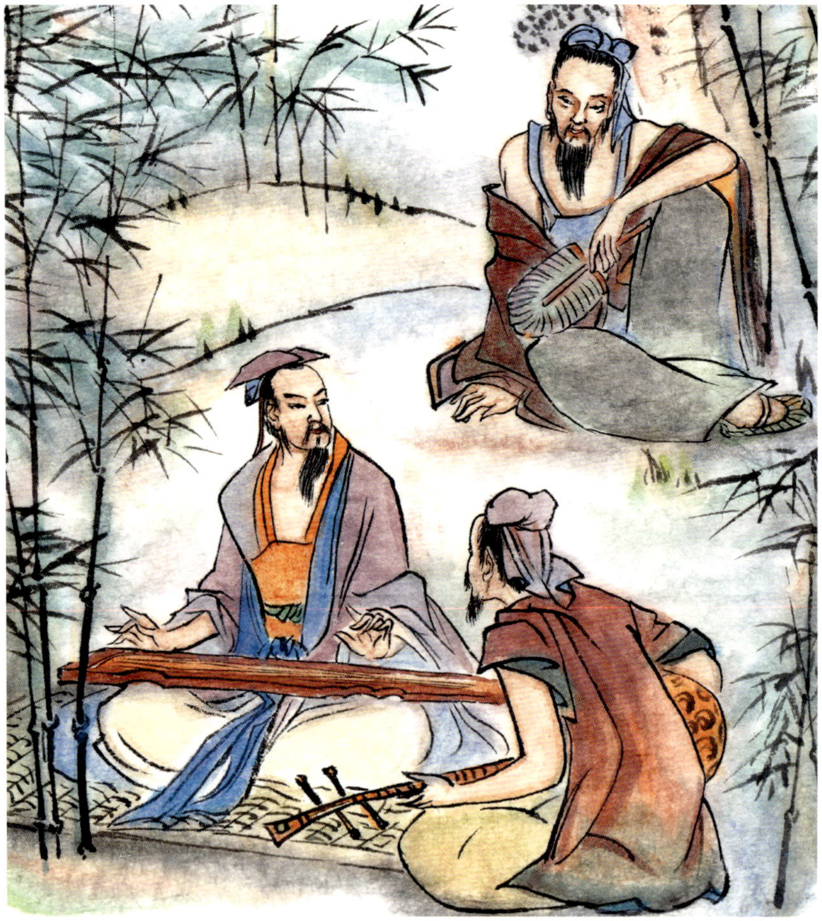

真实、达观

Be truthful and philosophical

魏正始年间(240年—249年)，嵇康、阮籍、山涛、向秀、刘伶、王戎及阮咸七人常聚在当时的山阳县(今河南辉县、修武一带)竹林之下，主张老庄之学，"越名教而任自然"肆意酣畅，世谓竹林七贤。

In the years of Zhengshi (240-249) during the Wei Dynasty, seven scholars, Ji Kang, Ruan Ji, Shan Tao, Xiang Xiu, Liu Ling, Wang Rong and Ruan Xuan, often gathered in a bamboo grove in Shanyang County (now around Huixian and Xiuwu in Henan). All advocates of the teachings of Lao Tzu and Chuang Tzu, they "pass over the Confucian ethical codes and revert to naturalness". This unrestrained and spontaneous bunch was referred to collectively as the "Seven Sages of the Bamboo Grove".

虚心慎行

Be modest and prudent

"人家最不要事事称意，常有些不足处才好，若人家事事足意，便有些不好事出来，亦消长之理然之"。常有不足之处，就会虚心慎行，祸患也就较难发生。

"One's desire should not always be gratified and it is better to have some discontent. If one's desire is always satisfied, something bad will soon occur as a common rule". If we are conscious of our deficiencies, we will be modest and prudent, and thus it is difficult for misfortune to befall.

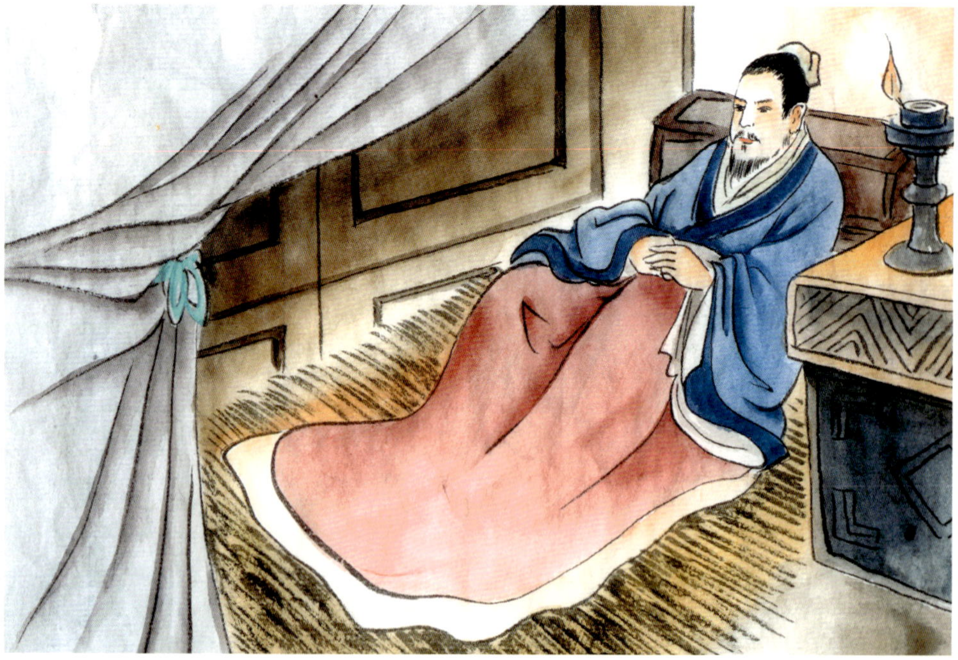

简单朴素

To lead a simple and plain life

生活越简朴，心胸越开阔，人知足，便不会有欲求不满的烦恼，对养生大有裨益。

The simpler your life is, the more broad-minded you are. Learn to be content, and then you will be free of worries incurred by desires. This is an effective way in health preservation.

厚德载物

Mental health cultivation

心脑开阔，宽宏大量，是讲究心理卫生的重要一环。而宽宏的气量，是可以通过学习、培养而形成的。怎么对待逆境，也是讲究心理卫生的重要课题。乐天者、识理者、意志坚强者，仍能善处逆境而乐之。

To be open-minded and generous is an important step towards mental health. Generosity can be cultivated through learning and training. How to treat adversity is also an important issue of mental health. In adversity, optimistic, rational and strong-willed people can still enjoy themselves.

古人的养心之论十分精彩

A variety of theories of spiritual cultivation proposed by the ancient Chinese are very impressive.

九字经：勿欺心，勿妄想，守廉耳。

Nine characters: primer no cheating, no wishful thinking, be honest and clean.

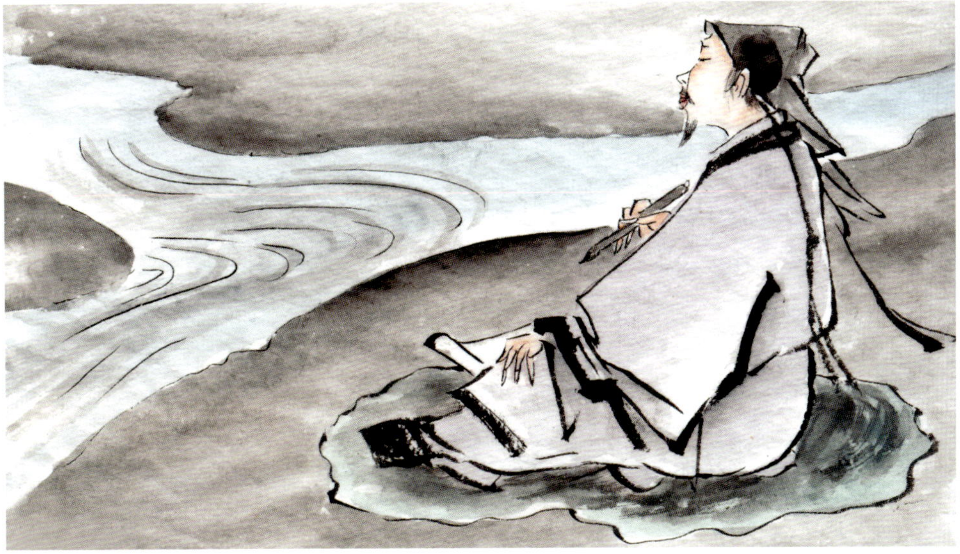

守廉图

Be honest and clean

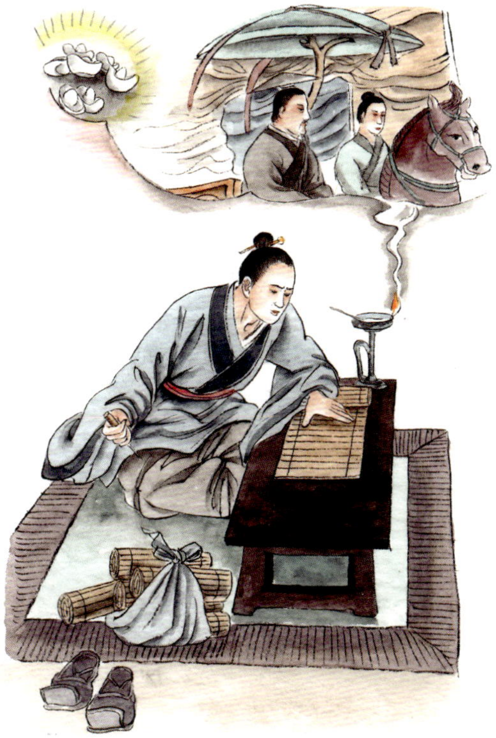

勿欺心

No cheating

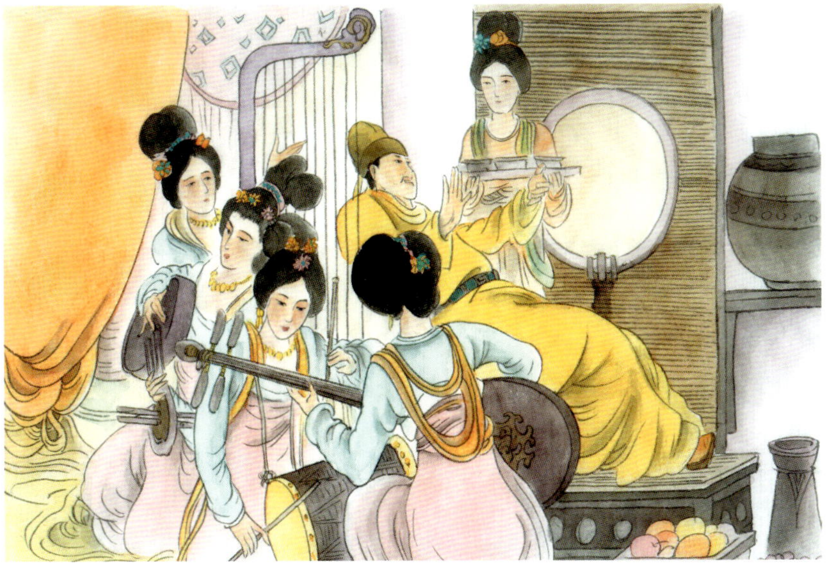

勿骄奢

Guarding against extravagance

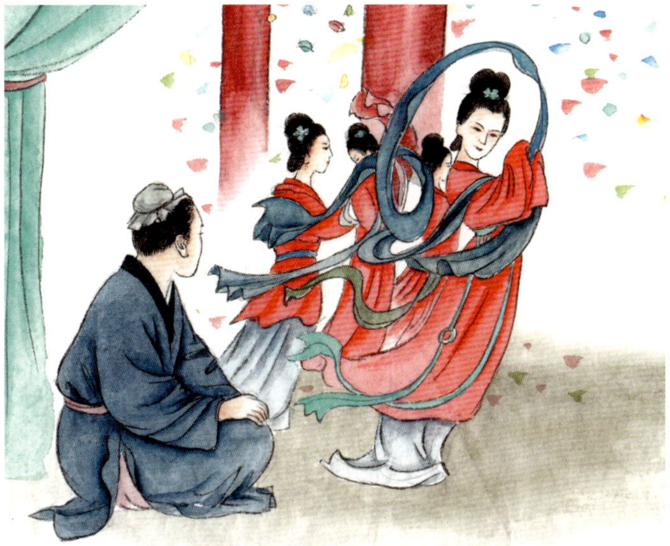

勿妄想

No wishful thinking

六字诀：曰忍，曰方便，曰依本分。

Six characters knack: tolerance, convenience, being fair and unprejudiced.

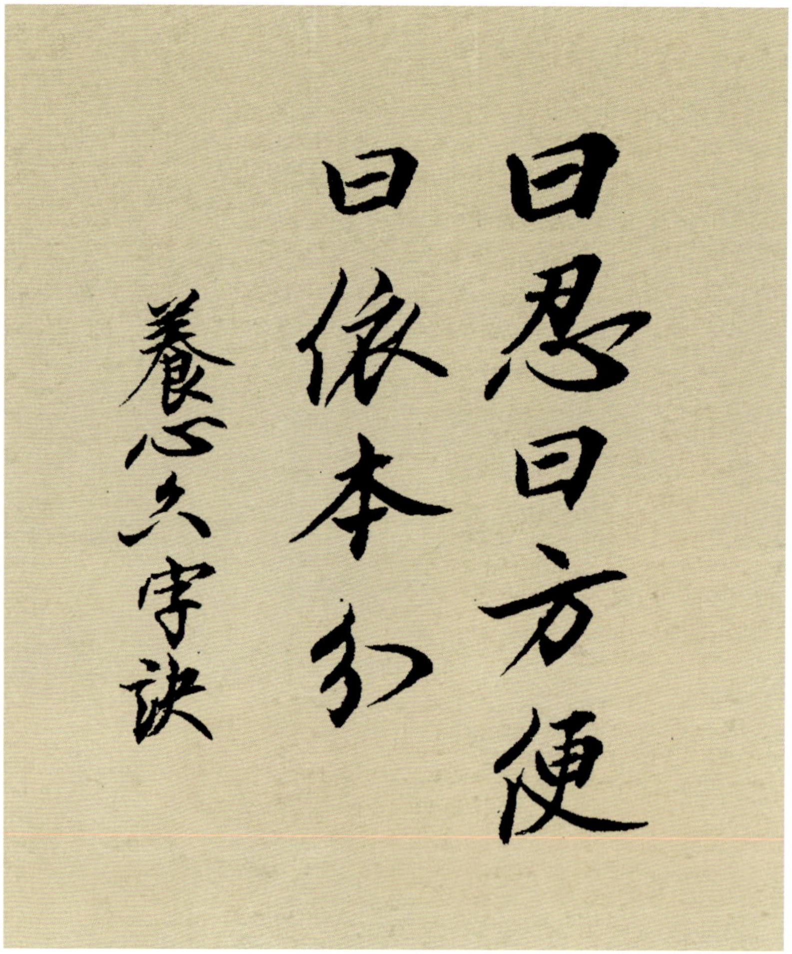

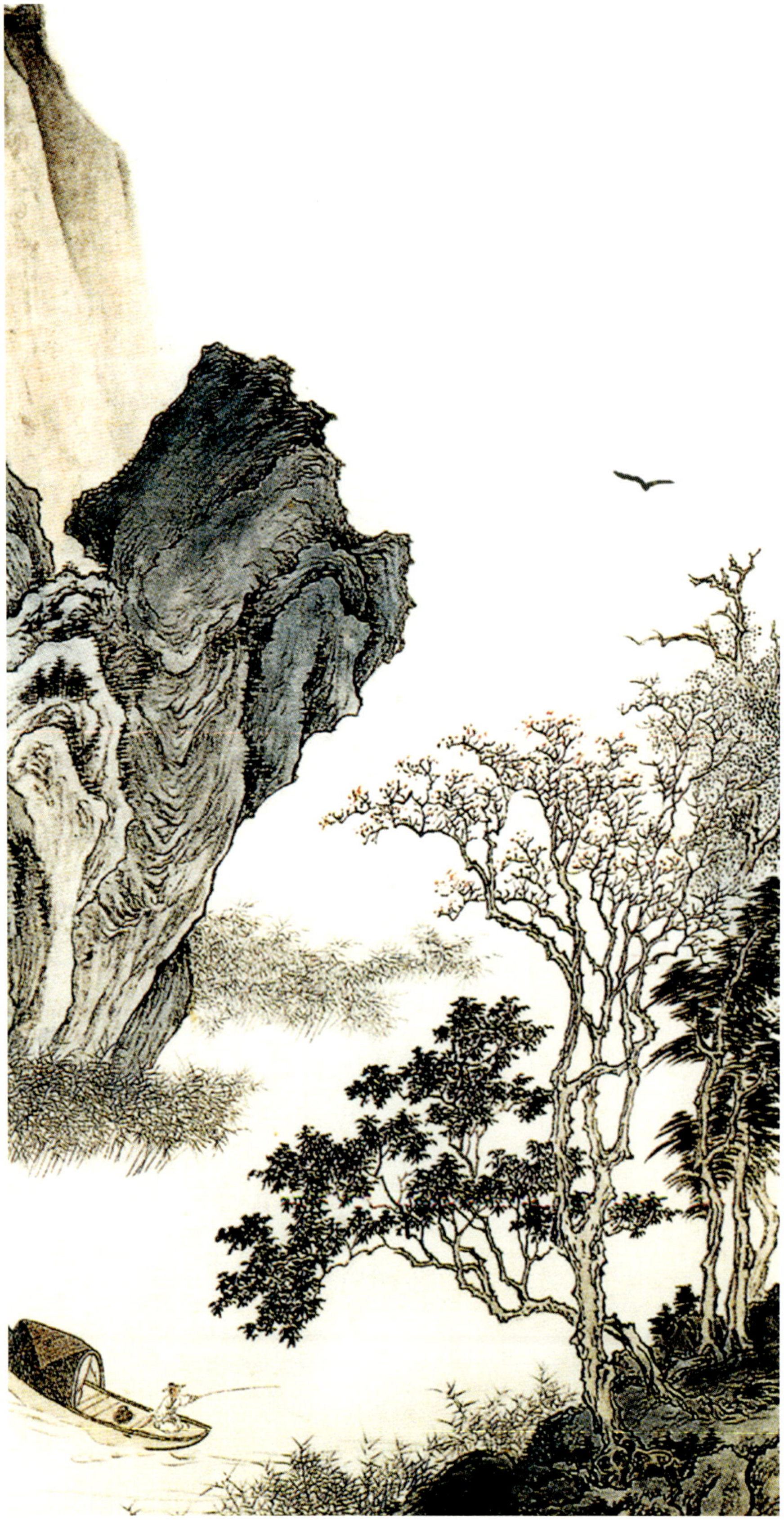

《渔父》
Fisherman

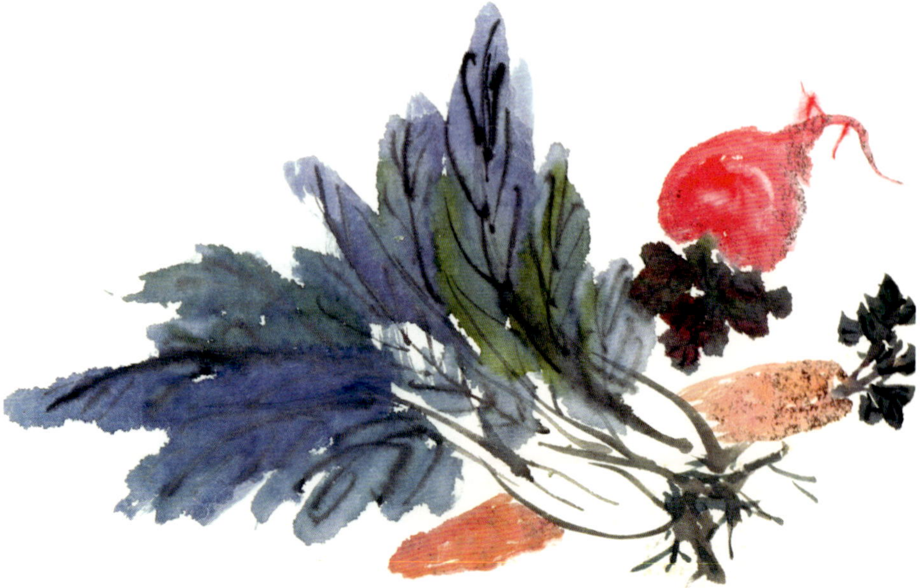

《菜根香图》
Enjoying the Taste of Vegetable Roots

四妙诚实汤：四妙者，熟思、审处、守口、防意也。治遇事轻易、言语粗率，岂惟免一朝之患，兼可免终身之忧。

Four wonderful ways to be honest: deliberation, prudence, weighing your words, and guarding against wishful thinking. If we avoid handling things in a hasty way or making careless comments, we can avoid not only trouble for the moment but also trouble for a whole life.

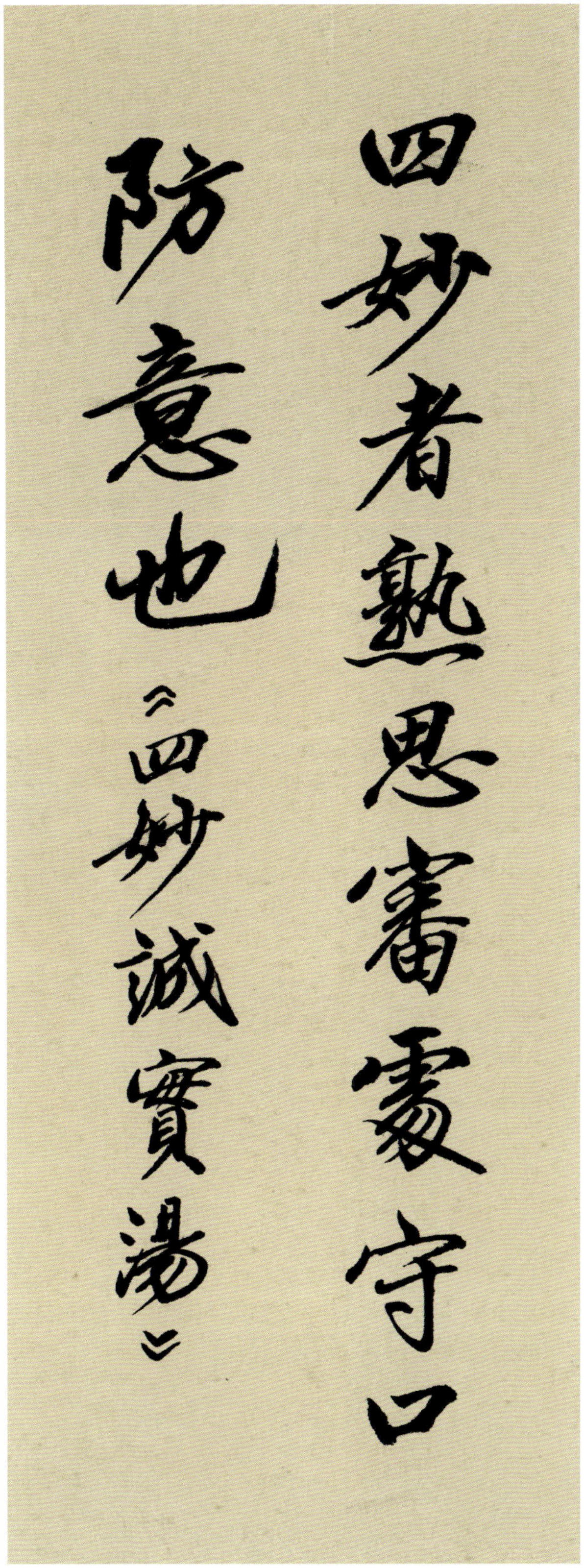

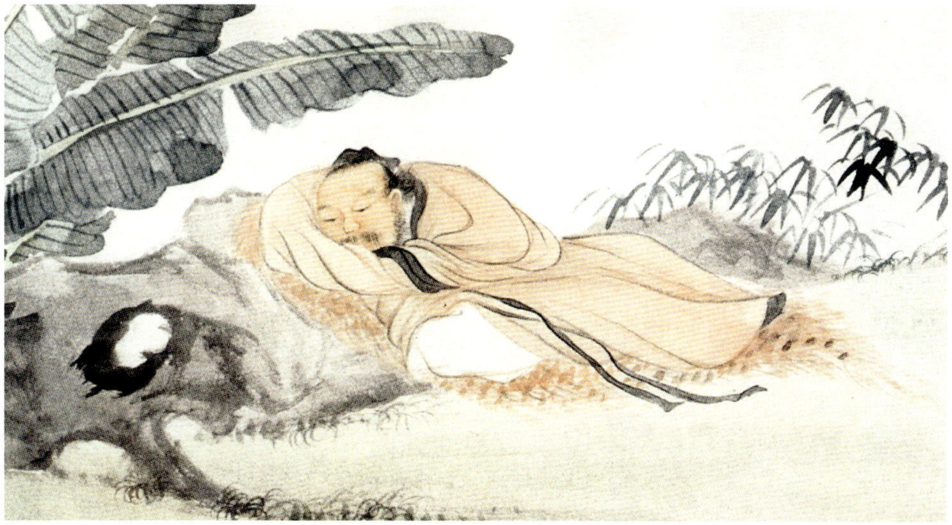

熟思图

Deliberation

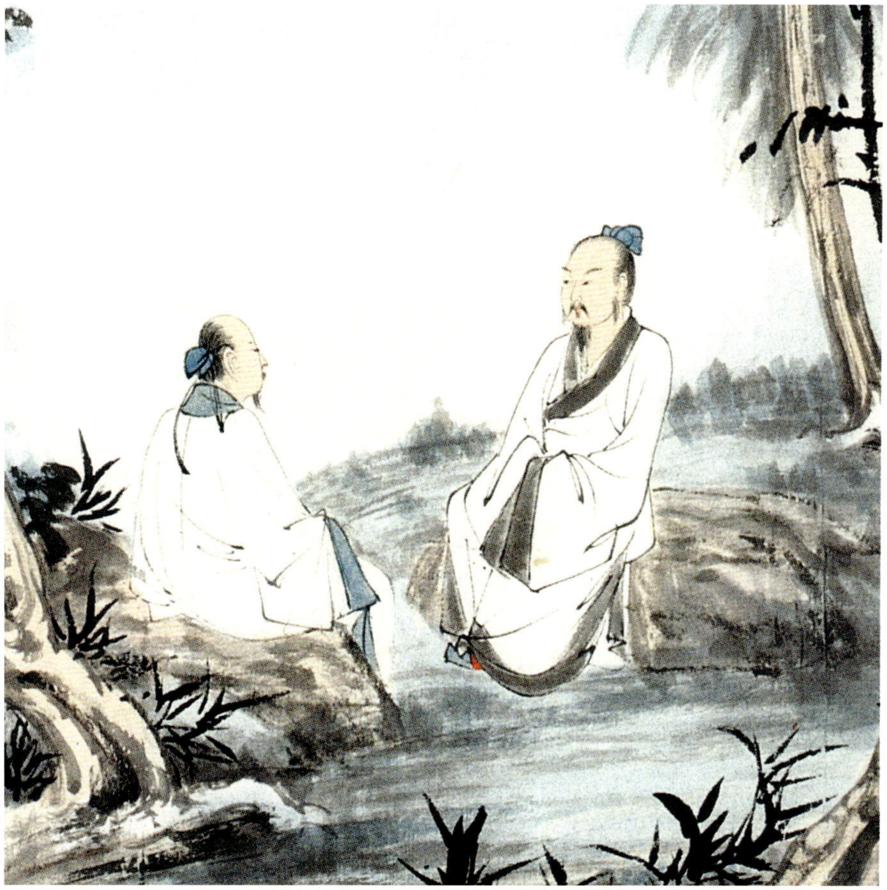

审处图

Prudence

和气汤：治一切客气、怒气、抑郁不平之气，先下一忍字，后下一忘字。

Recipe for mental tranquility: forbearance and forgetting are the two ingredients to disperse all kinds of anger, depression and feeling of injustice.

快活散：除烦恼，断妄想。

Skills to be cheerful: elimination of worries, giving up delusion.

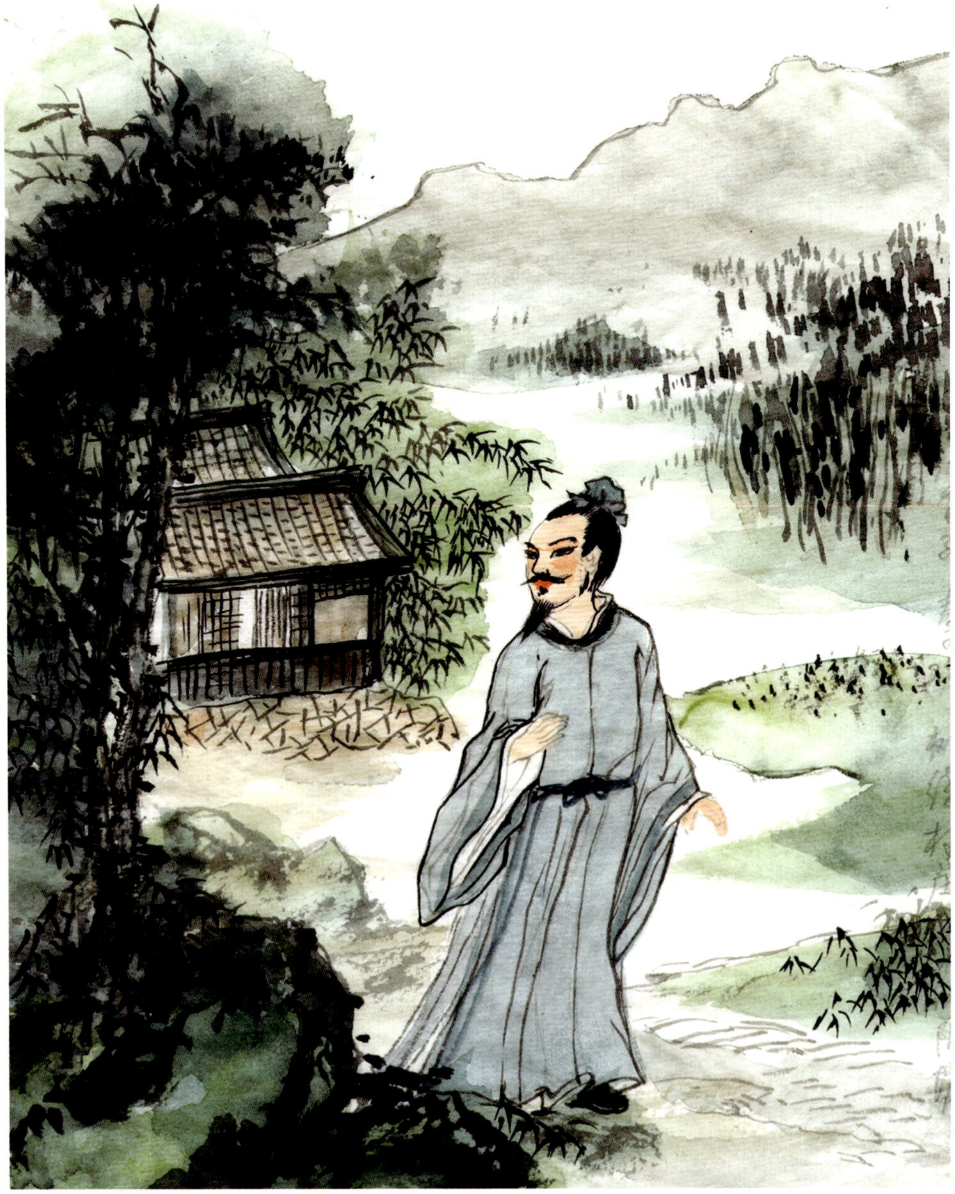

和气图

Mental tranquility

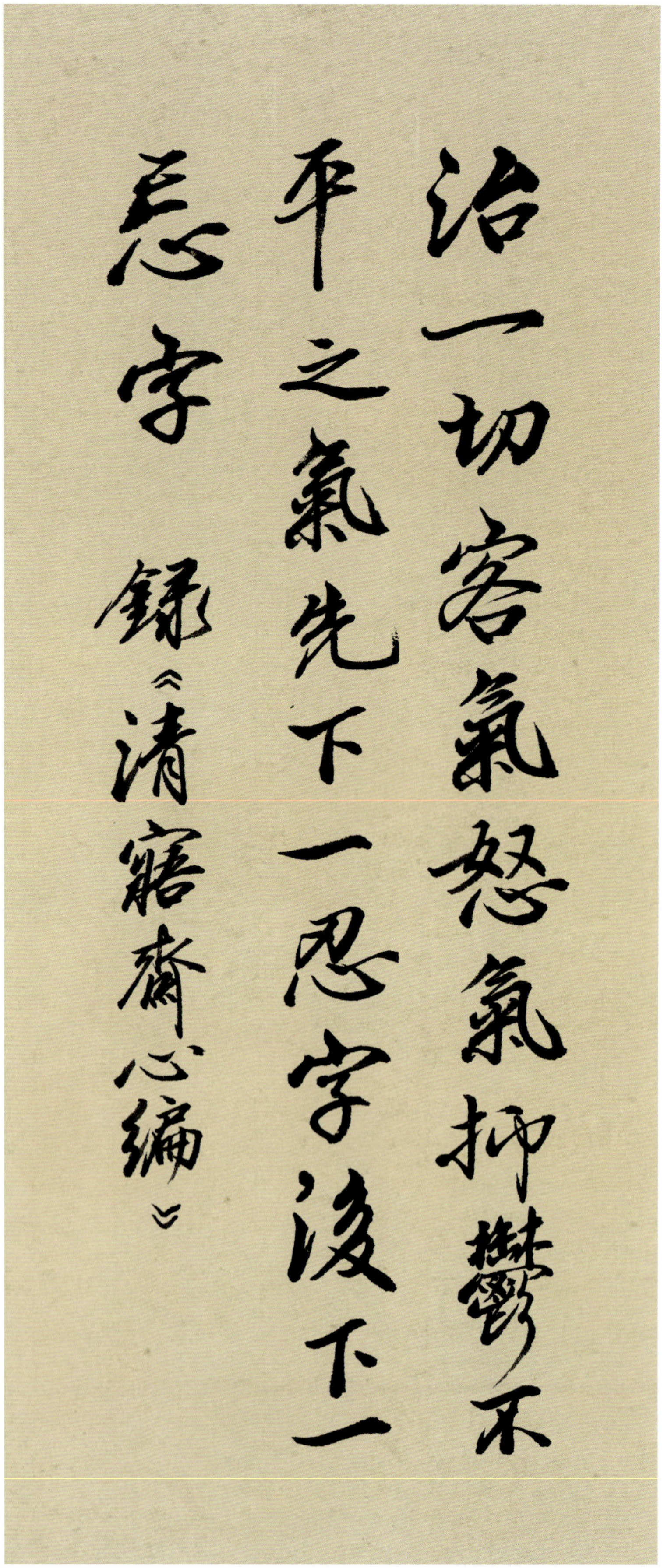

《黄帝内经》强调指出，养生要“志闲而少欲，心安而不惧，形劳而不倦”。

《黄帝内经》对心理卫生的要求有九条标准：

1. “心安而不惧”，“以恬愉为务”，“和喜怒而安居处”，“无为欣欣”。五志不过于心，发而中节，经常保持乐观心境。

Inner Canon of the Yellow Emperor points out that regimen depends on “an idle mind without desire, a peaceful heart without fear, and a laboring yet tireless body.”

Nine criteria for the mental health in the *Inner Canon of the Yellow Emperor*:

1. “A peaceful heart without fear”, “ keep a happy and quiet state of mind”, “to disperse anger with joy and to be contented”, “seeking no fame or profit”. All these criteria focus on the mind, which can be cultivated and controlled to keep optimistic.

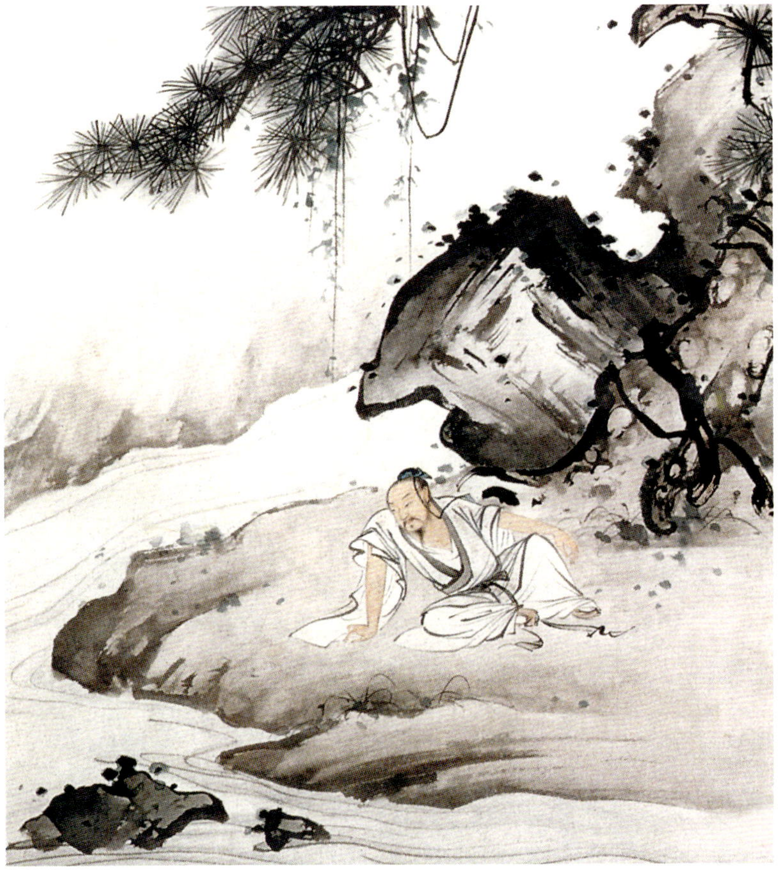

乐观图

Keep optimistic

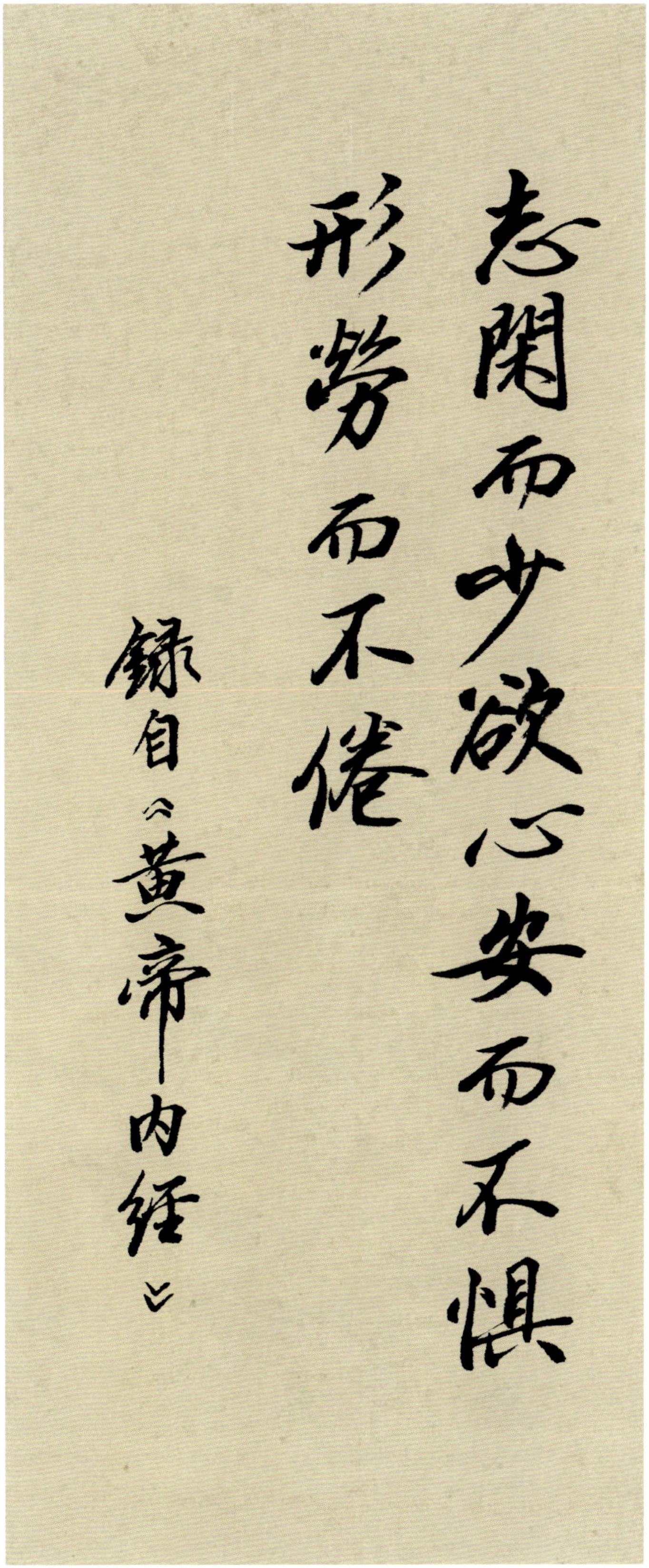

2. “志闲而少欲”，“不惧于物”，“无为惧惧”。欲有节而不恣于欲，志不贪，不妄求，心知足，不为物欲所累。

3. “无思想之患”，“不妄想”，“淫邪不能惑其心”，“不妄作”。即不妄想妄为。

2. “An idle mind without desire”, “no fear of things”, “no cares and worries”. One should restrain one’s desire instead of indulging in it, not be greedy, not seek uniqueness, feel contented, and free oneself from material desire.

3. “Free from too much thinking”, “no wishful thinking”, “sexual temptation cannot confuse the heart”, “no absurd acts”. One should guard against wishful thinking and irrational actions.

4. “志意和则精神专直，魂魄不散，悔怒不至”，“志意所为必当，则无悔怒，智以处物、治己，当循理而动也”。即意志坚强，循理而行。

5. “御神有时”，“勿伤于神”，“劳而不倦”，“起居有常”。即身心有劳有逸，有规律地生活。

4. “If the mind is harmonized, the spirit and soul will concentrate, free from anger or regret.” “Decisions should be properly made and then there will be no regrets or anger. One should handle things and treat oneself in a rational way, according to law.” In short, we should be strong-willed and act according to law.

5. “Live a regular life”, “do not do harm to the spirit”, “labor without getting tired”. That is, one should keep regular hours, combining work with leisure.

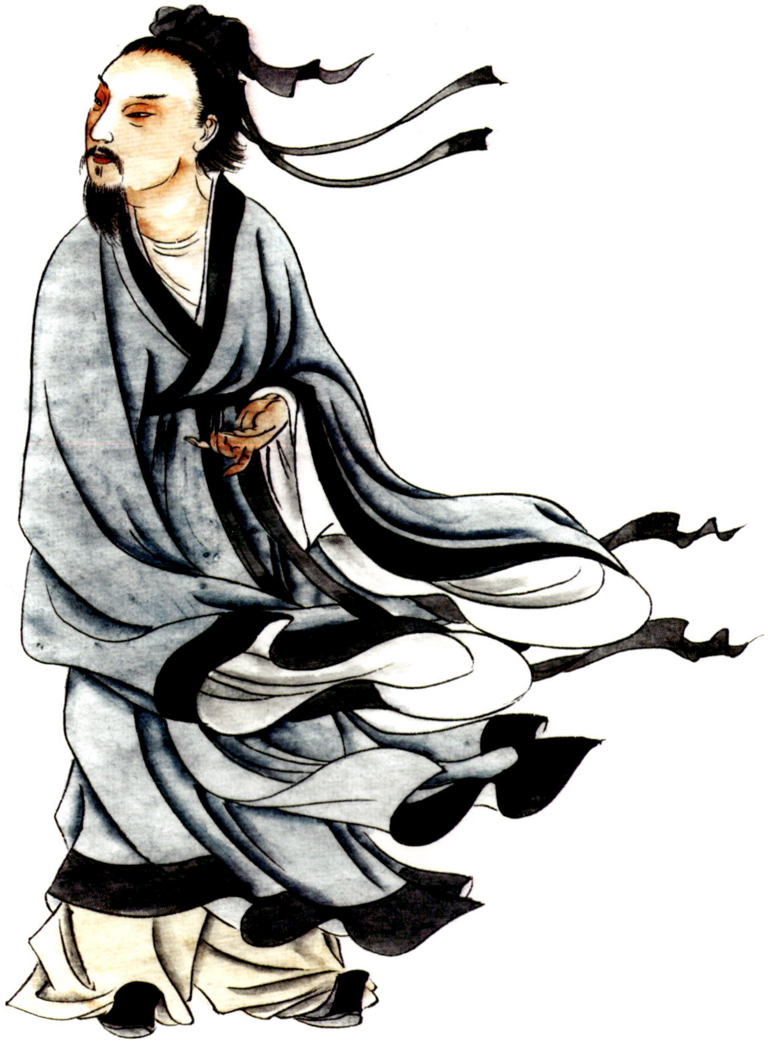

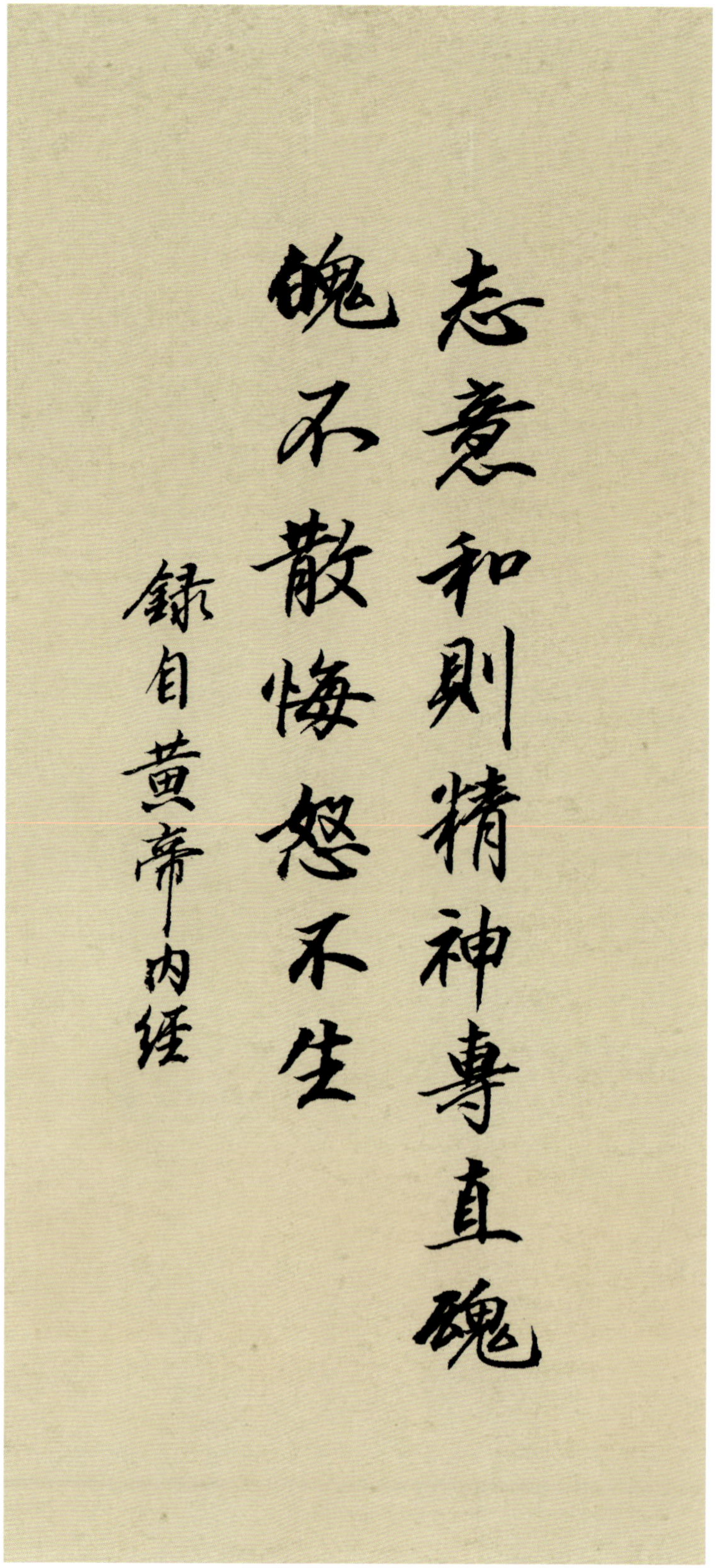

恬惔虚无图

Indifference to fame or fortune

6. “恬惔虚无”，“居处安静”，“静则神藏”。即心神宁静。

6. “Indifference to fame or fortune”,“ live a quiet life”,“ tranquility nourishes the spirit”. That is, one should keep a peaceful mind.

7. “乐其欲”，“善附人”，“好利人”，“尊则谦谦”。即热爱生活，人际关系良好。

8. “婉然从物，或与不争，与时变化”。即善于适应环境的变化。

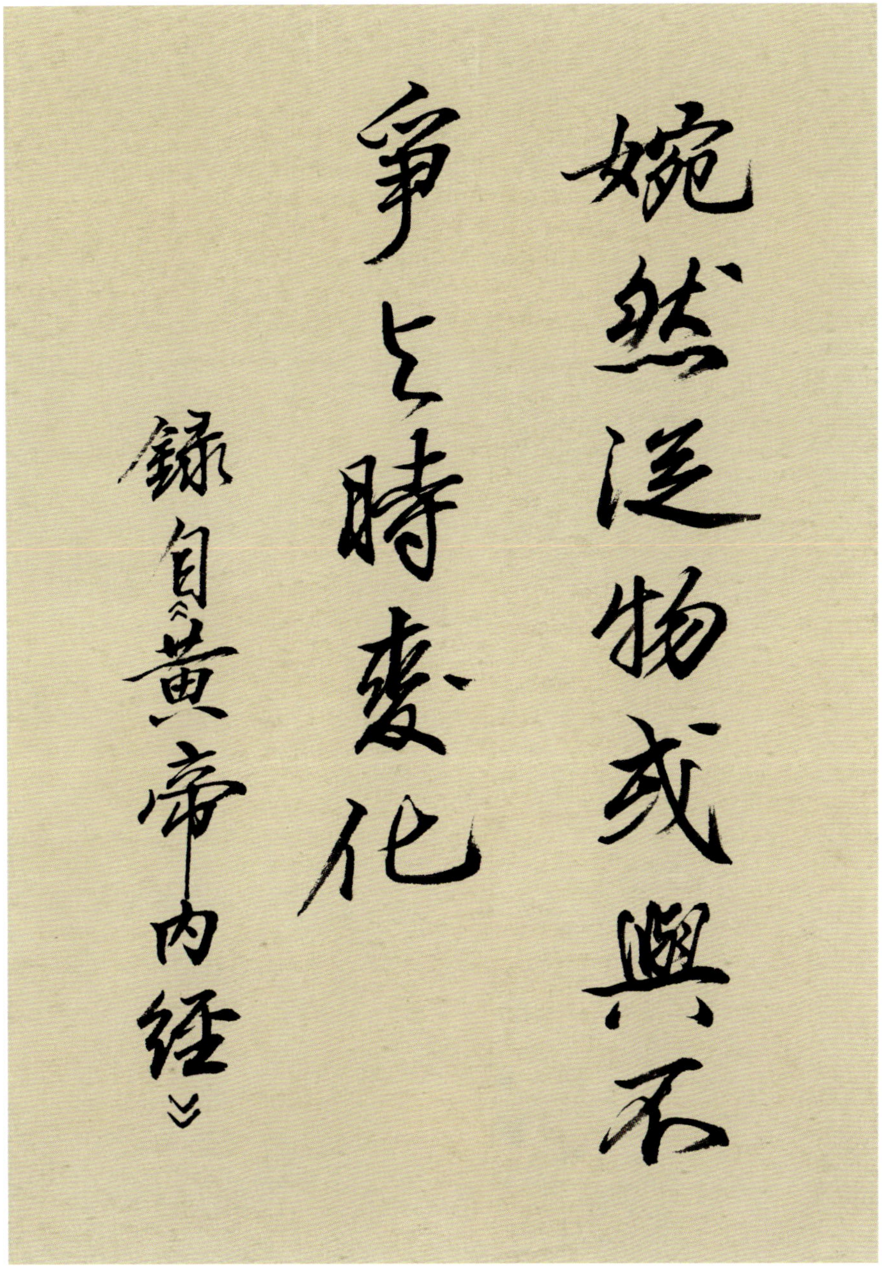

7. “Enjoy what you desire”, “be friendly to others”, “be generous to others”, “be modest and respectful”. That is, one should love life and establish good personal relations.

8. “Follow natural laws, do not compete with others, and change with the times.” That is, one should be good at adapting to changes in the environment.

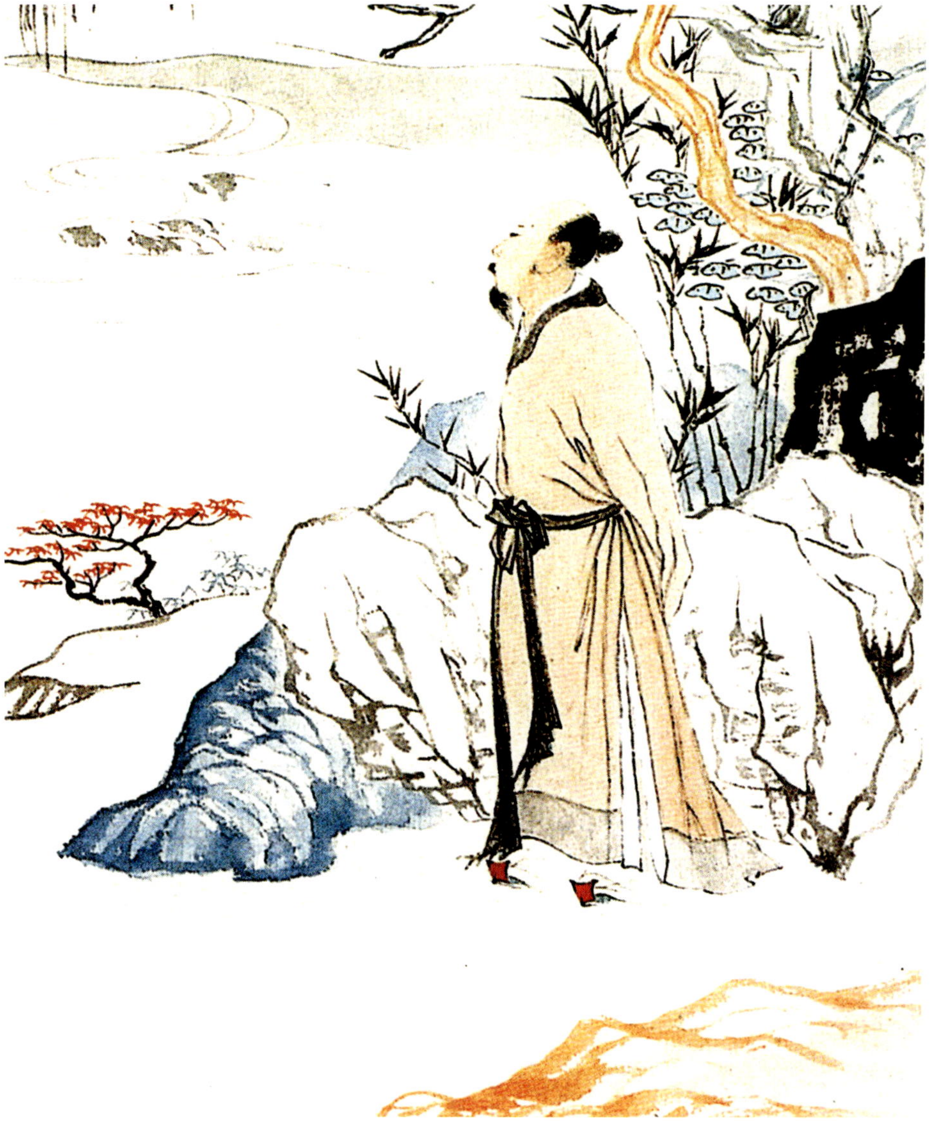

与时变化图

Change with the times

9. 善“节阴阳而调刚柔”。即善能涵养性格，陶冶气质，帮助人克服缺点（《黄帝内经心理学概要》）。

9. Good at “adjustment of yin and yang and integration of the rigid and the soft.” That is, one should have self-restraint, cultivate one’s character and overcome one’s own shortcomings (*The Psychology Summary of the “Inner Canon of the Yellow Emperor”*).

人的面部要经常擦洗，眼睛要经常揩抹，两耳要经常弹敲，牙齿要经常叩打，背部要经常保持温暖，胸脯要经常注意保护，腹部要经常按摩，脚底要经常揉搓，津液要经常吞咽，睡觉要经常曲身。

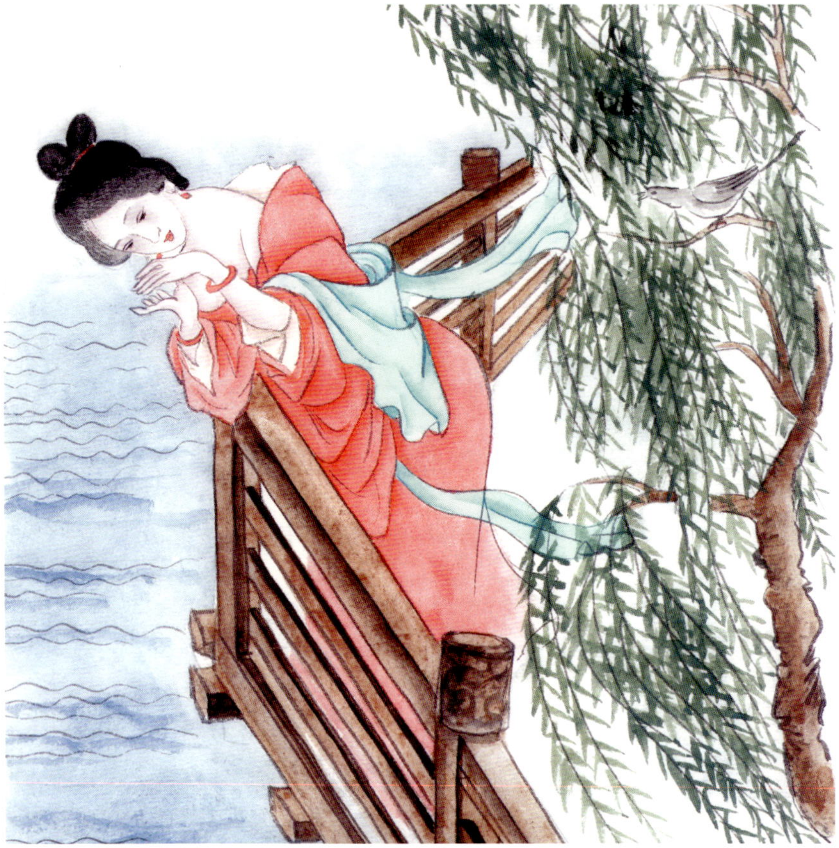

清代徐文弼说，真定梁先生每天晚上回到家，和人说话，一定要选择一些可喜可笑之事，与客人谈论，并时而抚须大笑，以释放劳累一天所积下的闷气，这是真心懂得了养生要诀。曾有一个乡人年过百岁，我向他请求长寿之道，他笑着说："我是个乡下人，不知道别的什么，一生中只知道高兴快乐，从来不知烦恼。"这难道是那些追逐名利的人所能做到的吗？

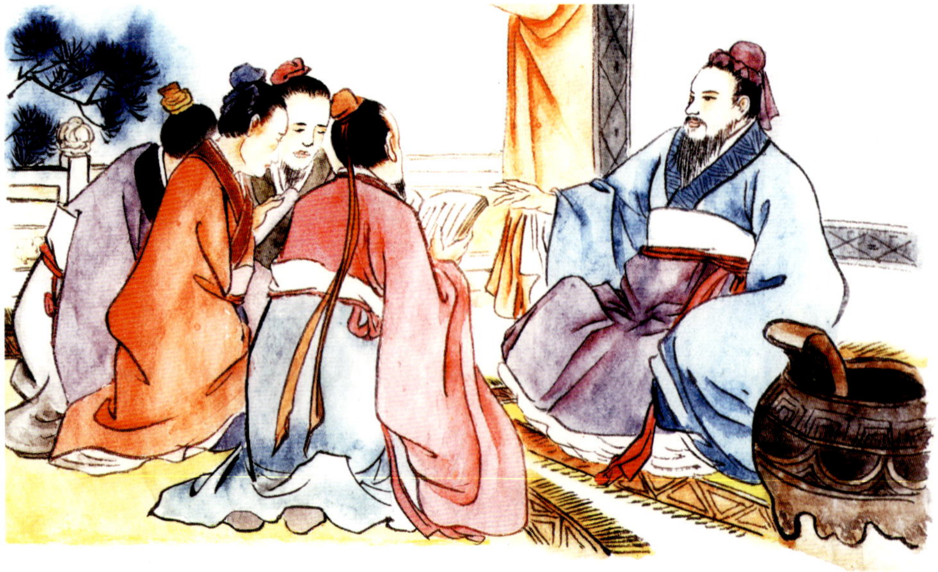

Do the following things frequently: wash your face, clean your eyes, drum your ears, click your teeth, keep your back warm, protect your chest, massage your stomach, rub your soles, swallow your saliva, and bend your body when sleeping.

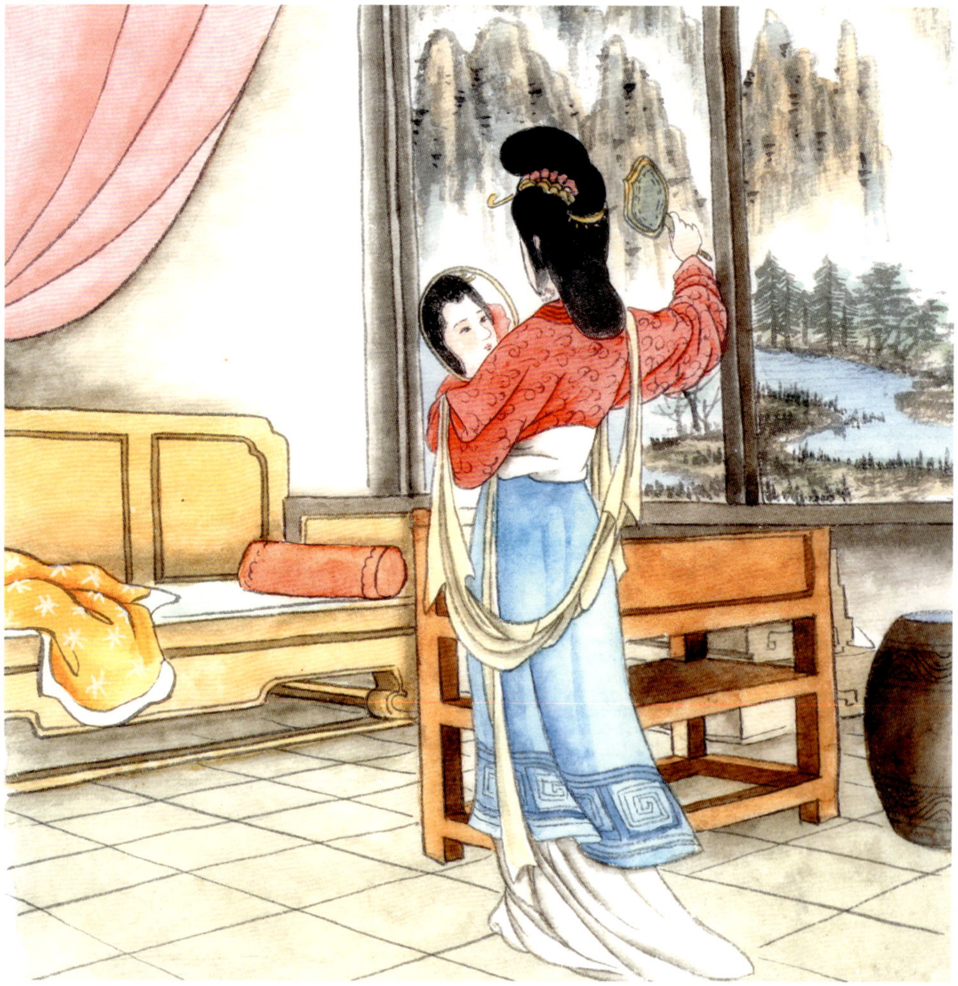

When he had visitors at home in the evening, Mr. Liang made a point of telling them something amusing or funny in his conversations, laughing while stroking his beard from time to time, in order to relieve the fatigue from working all day. He had grasped the essence of health preservation.

I know a countryman aged over a hundred. Once I asked him how to live a long life. "I'm just an ignorant countryman," said he with a smile, "The only thing I know is that throughout my life I've been happy and never worried." Can those who seek fame and fortune ever be capable of this? – Xu Wenbi (the Qing Dynasty): *The Truth about Longevity*

从前王右军说过：“我喜欢种植果树，因为其中有无限乐趣。我种的树，开一朵花，结一个果，看起来可爱，吃起来更甜。”右军可以说是自得其乐啊。陆放翁做梦到了仙人住处，得到两句诗：“长廊下瞰碧莲沼，小阁正对青萝峰。”便以为到了极为优美的景地。我住在禅房中，也有这种感觉，可以夸耀于放翁。

Wang Youjun (a master of calligraphy) said, “I’m fond of growing fruit trees because I can derive boundless pleasure from it. Each blossom on my trees looks lovely, and each fruit tastes sweet.” Here’s a man who indeed knew how to enjoy himself!

Once Lu Fangweng dreamed that he called on an immortal, who gave him two poetic lines: “The long corridor overlooks the green lotus pond/And the little pavilion directly faces Verdant Vine Peak.” He thought that an incomparable view. I had the same feeling when living in a Buddhist monastery, and I might boast of that to Fangweng.

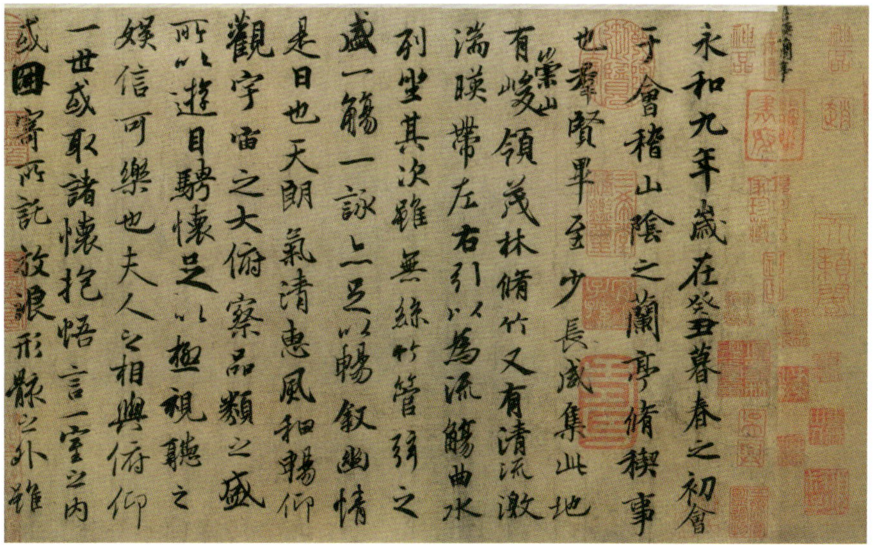

晋　王羲之《兰亭集序》

Jin Dynasty Wang Xizhi *Preface to the Orchid Pavilion*

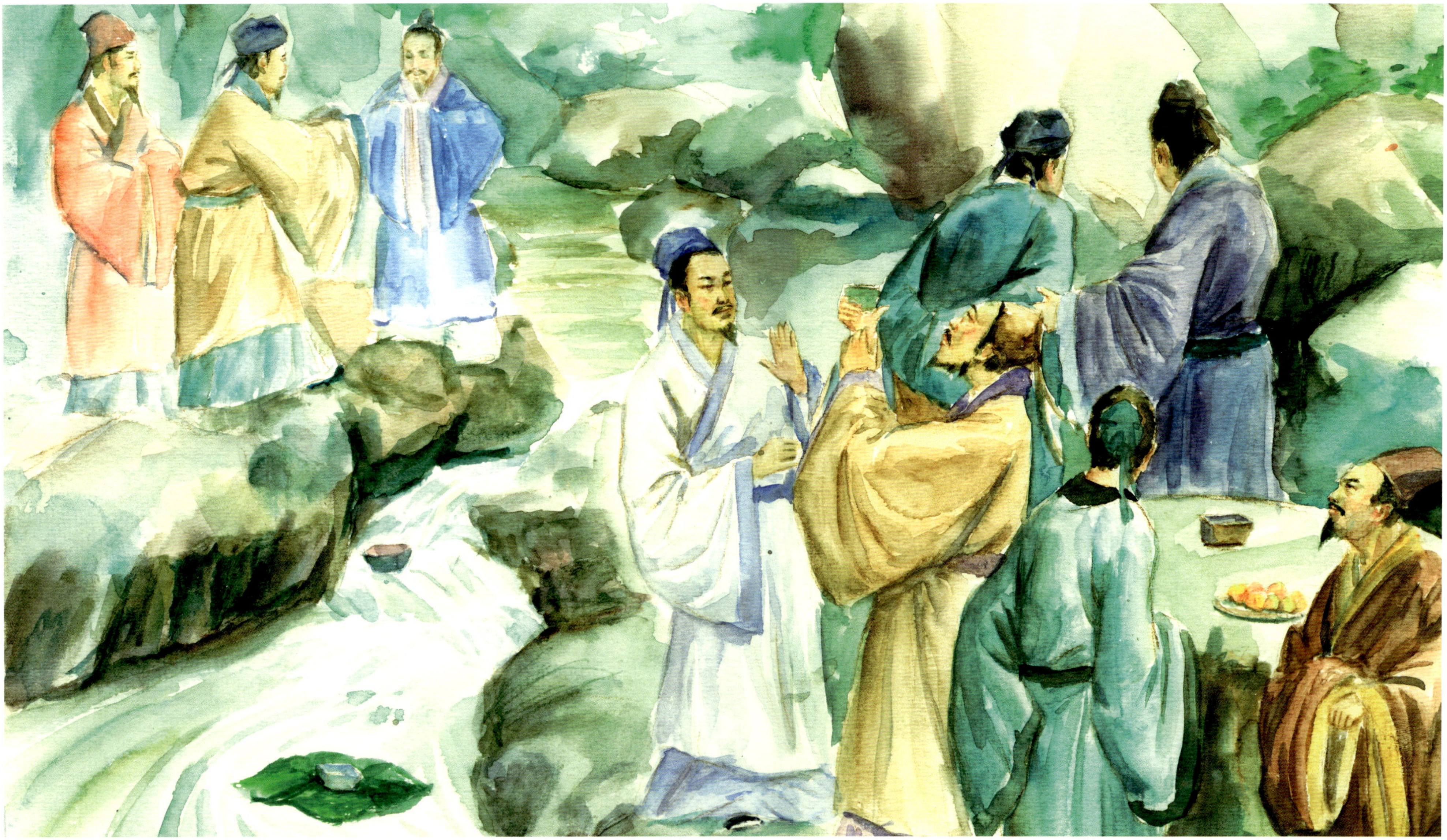

脑力劳动也益寿

Mental labor, no damage to life span

纵观古今中外名人，会发现发脑力劳动并不损寿。如大物理学家牛顿享年 85 岁、爱因斯坦 76 岁、生理学家巴甫洛夫 86 岁、电学家富兰克林和发明家爱迪生都是 84 岁，著名数学家、哲学家罗素竟活了 98 岁。中国历史上四大书法家颜、柳、欧、赵都是长寿者，颜真卿 76 岁、柳公权 87 岁、欧阳询 84 岁、赵孟頫 68 岁。又如，孙思邈 101 岁、朱丹溪 76 岁、叶天士 80 岁、钱乙 82 岁、齐白石 97 岁，等等。我国科学工作者曾对秦汉到 1949 年间的 3088 位科学家、艺术家、思想家、文学家的寿命进行了统计，结果发现他们的平均寿命是 65.18 岁，远高于解放前中国人口平均寿命（35 岁）。这些事实充分说明脑力劳动者并不是短寿者。

An overview of the histories of China and other countries has revealed that brain workers do not have a shorter life span.For example, Newton, the great physicist died at 85, Einstein, at 76, physiologist Ivan Pavlov, at 86, electrician Franklin and inventor Thomas Edison both at 84, and the famous mathematician and philosopher Bertrand Russell at 98. The four famous calligraphers Yan, Liu, Ou and Zhao in China's history all enjoyed long life: Yan Zhenqin lived 76 years, Liu Gongquan 87 years, and Ouyang Xun 84 years. Other famous figures also lived long, for example, Sun Simiao died at 101, Zhu Danxi at 76, Ye Tianshi at 80, Qian Yi at 82, and Qi Baishi at 97. Scientists have conducted a statistical analysis of life expectancy of 3088 scientists, artists, thinkers and writers from the Qin and Han dynasties to 1949, and the results reveal that the average life expectancy is 65.18 years old, much higher than the average life expectancy in China (35 years old) before the People's Republic of China was founded. These facts show clearly that the brainworkers are not short-lived.

长寿图

Longevity

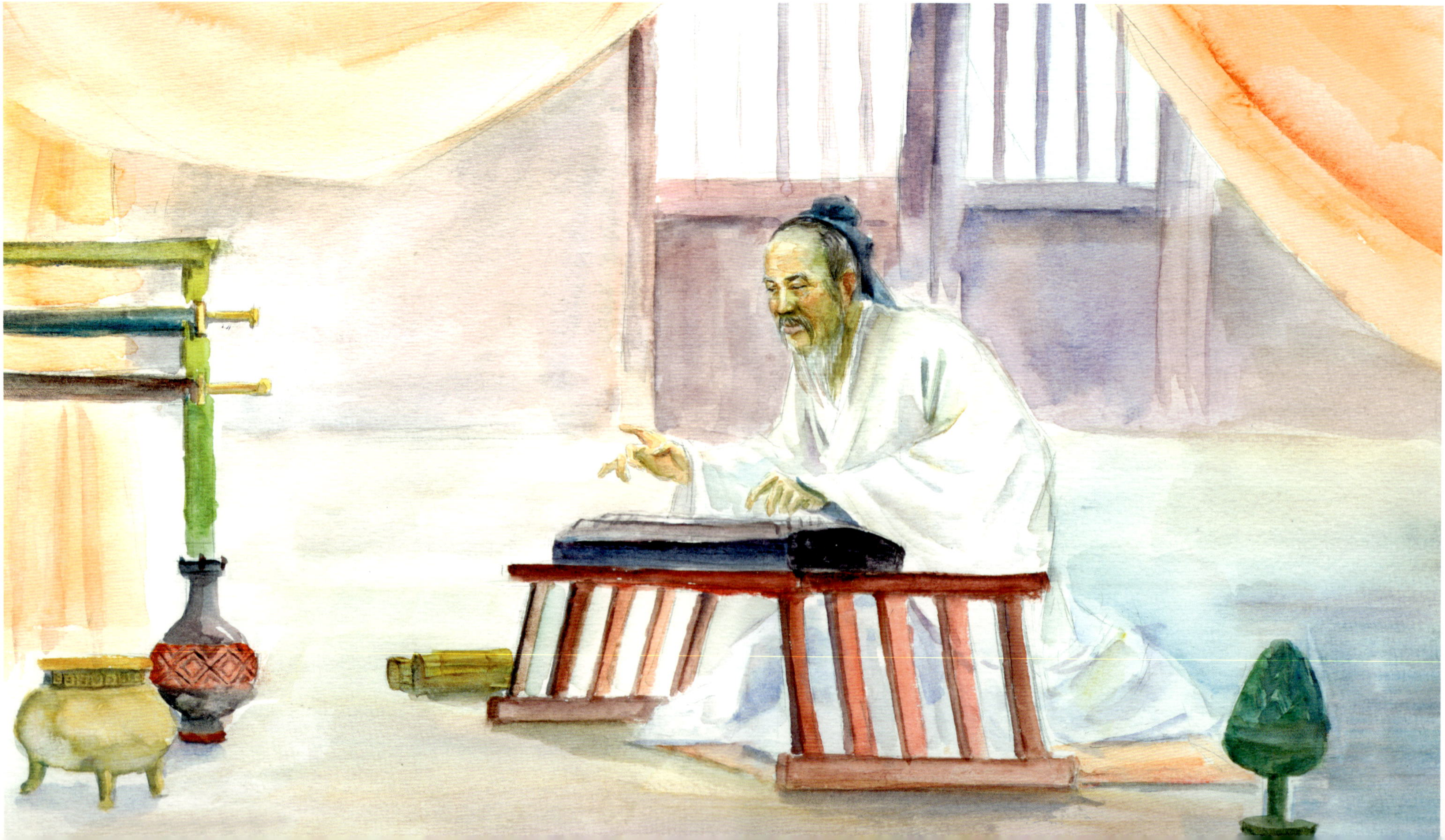

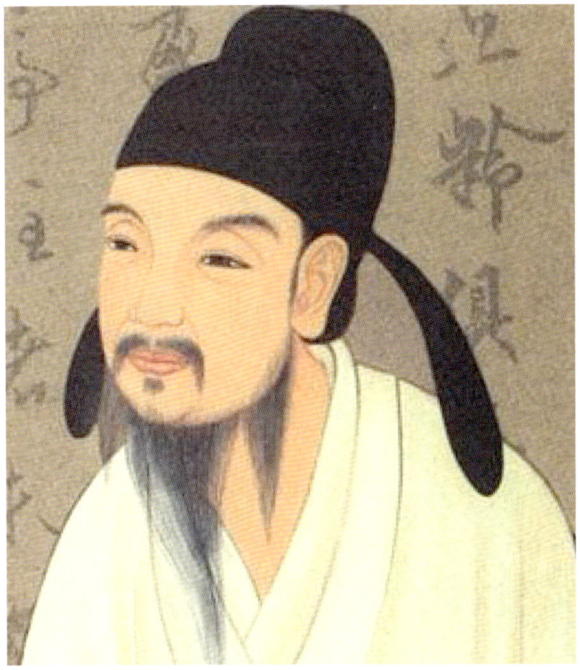

欧阳询享年 84 岁
Ouyang Xun lived 84 years

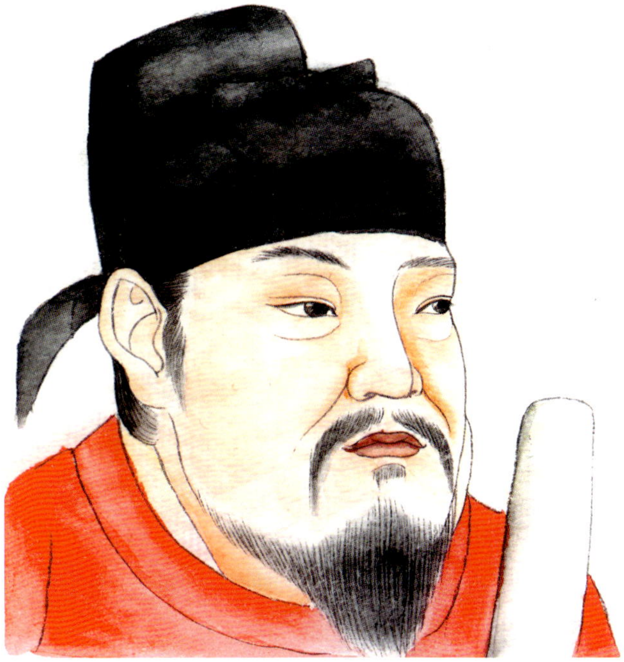

颜真卿享年 76 岁
Yan Zhenqin lived 76 years

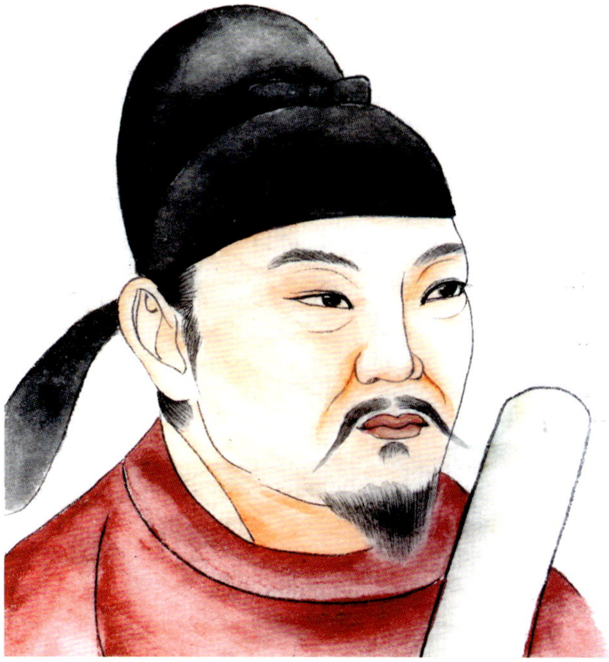

柳公权享年 87 岁
Liu Gongquan lived 87 years

脑力劳动者健康长寿的一个重要因素，就是积极的思维智慧活动能使心神安适。卫生者，就是保卫生命，维护生机之意也。脑力劳动能卫护心神，即讲究心理卫生，保持心理健康。

An important factor of health and longevity is the well-being of the spirit. To defend life is to protect life and maintain one's vitality. To defend the spirit is to pay attention to mental hygiene and keep mental health.

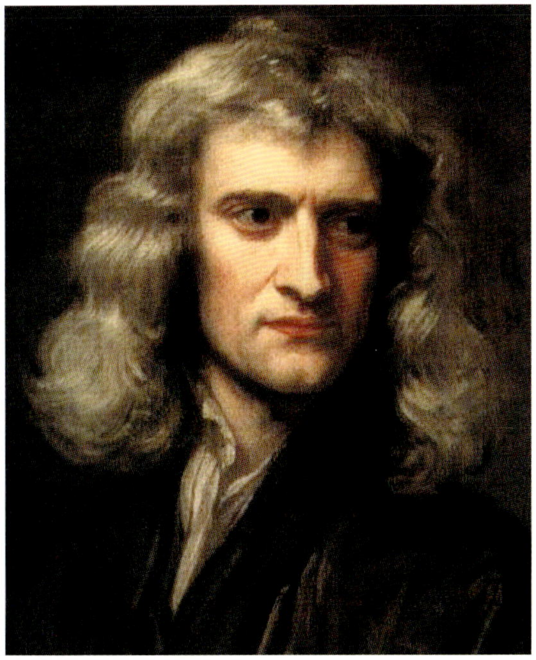

牛顿享年 85 岁
Newton lived 85 years

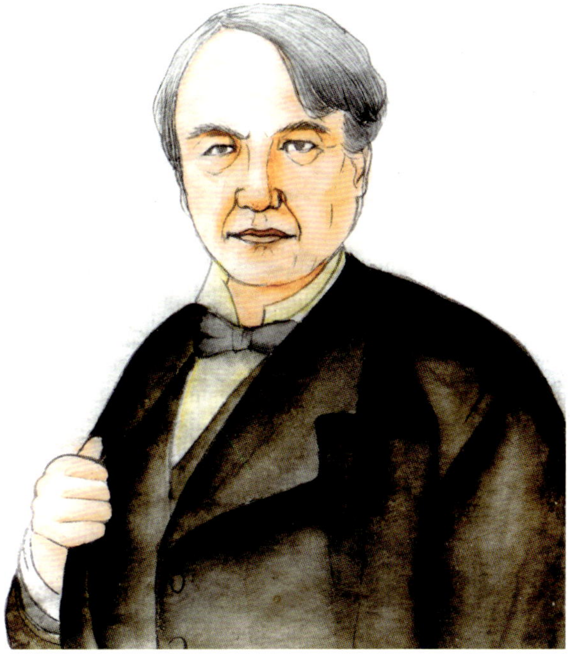

爱迪生享年 84 岁
Edison lived 84 years

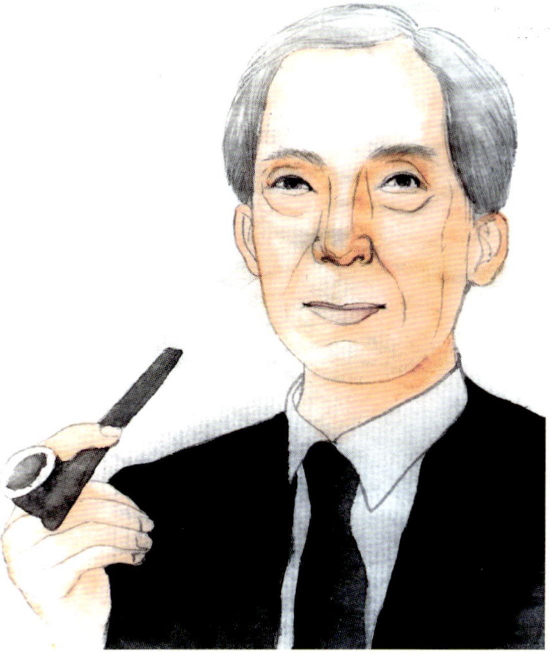

罗素享年 98 岁
Russell lived 98 years

陆　起居安适

VI.　Importance of Comfortable Living

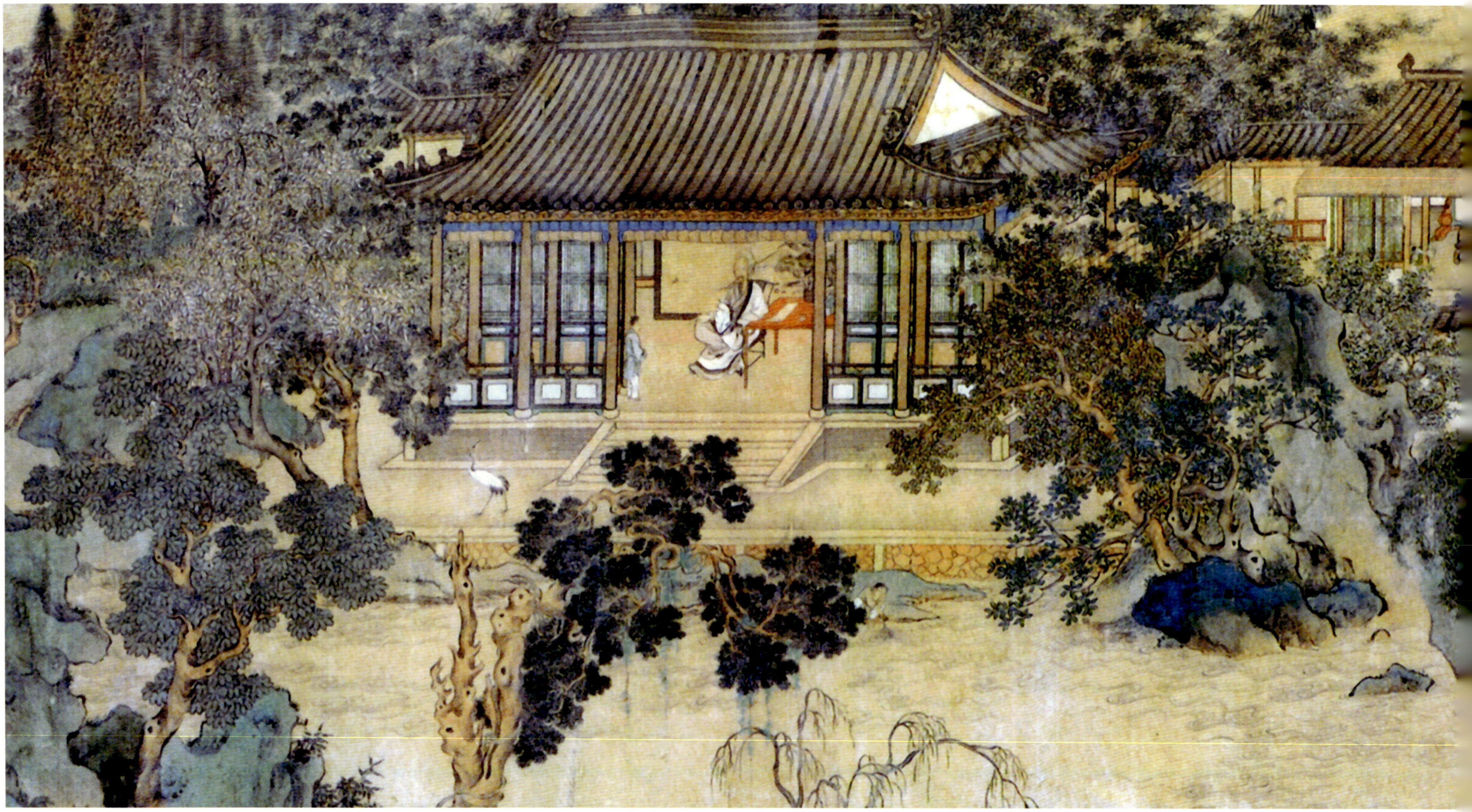

清新整洁的生活环境对人的养生大有裨益，起居之所要应让人心安气和，衣衾寝食应让人舒心适体。古人讲“天人相应”，人要在尊重自然中适应自然，利用自然规律。几千年来，中国人一直努力创造美好的居住环境。良好的生活习惯实际上反映着中国人的生存智慧。

The Chinese theories on health preservation stress the necessity of an environment conducive to health. A comfortable house may calm the mind; the ways we dress, sleep and eat can delight us. As a saying from ancient China puts it, ‘Man corresponds to Heaven’. We should adapt to Nature and make use of its laws while respecting Nature. Over thousands of years, we Chinese have been striving to create a livable environment in Mother Nature. Good habits in daily life are actually the epitome of Chinese people’s wisdom or perception of life.

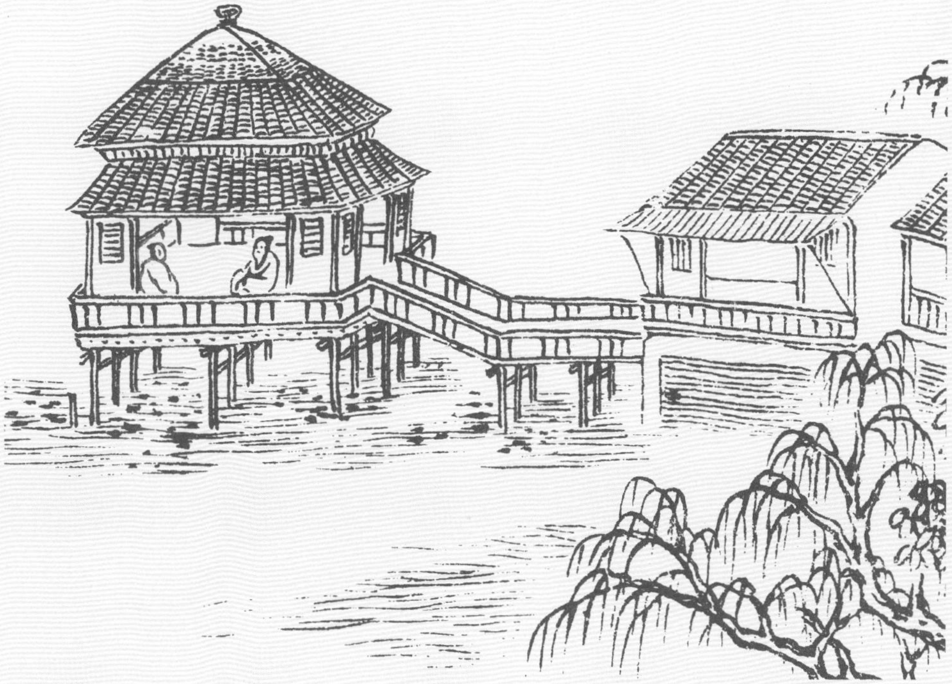

规律起居

Keeping regular hours

起居，主要指作息，也包括对各种日常生活细节的安排。中医学认为，起居有常，即生活有规律，是人能长寿的一个重要原因。

Everyday life mainly refers to work and rest, including arrangements of various living details. Chinese traditional medicine holds that keeping regular hours is an important reason for people to live longer.

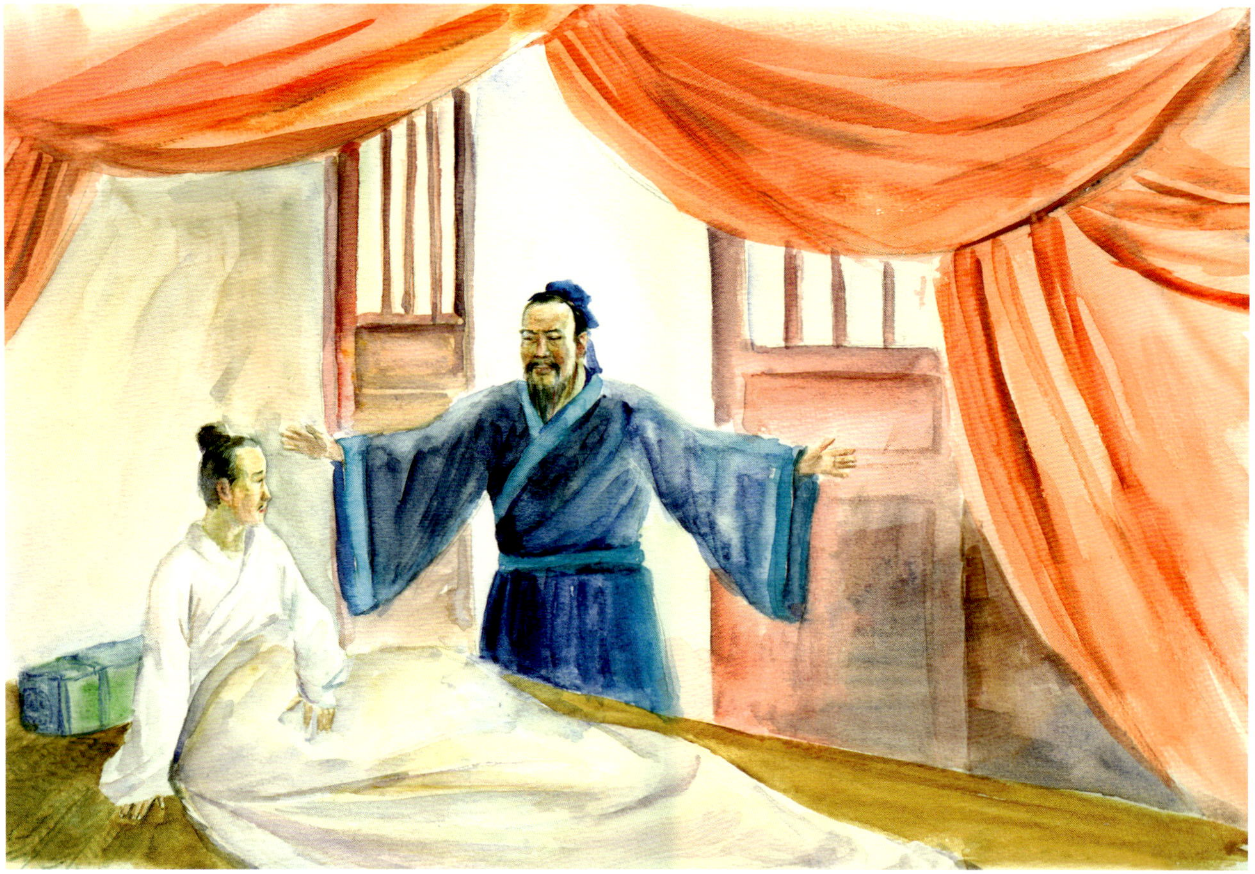

起居图

Daily life

起居调养：春季气候渐暖，该晚睡早起，披散长发，舒展形体，漫步庭院。同时，春天气候多变，应注意“春捂秋冻”。春天又是极适合锻炼身体的季节，应吐故纳新，练气以保精健体，怡情养性。

Everyday regimens: When the weather in spring is getting warmer, we'd better stay up late and get up early, let our hair fall about, stretch our body, and stroll in the garden. Meanwhile, since the climate in spring varies greatly, "we should not take off clothes too hastily in spring and should not wear too much clothes in autumn". Also, spring is the season most suitable for exercise, when we can renew our vitality and refresh our mind by practicing deep breathing.

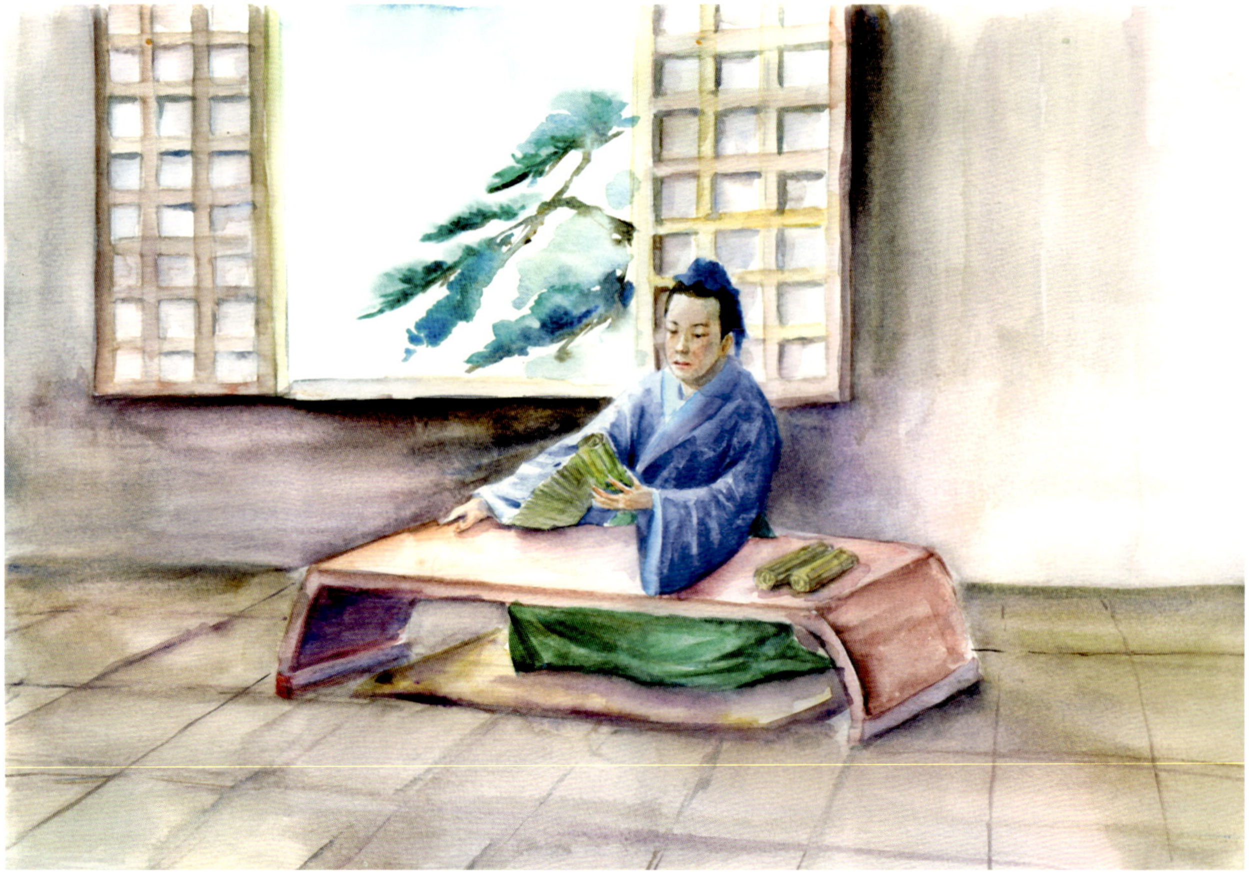

春季图

Spring

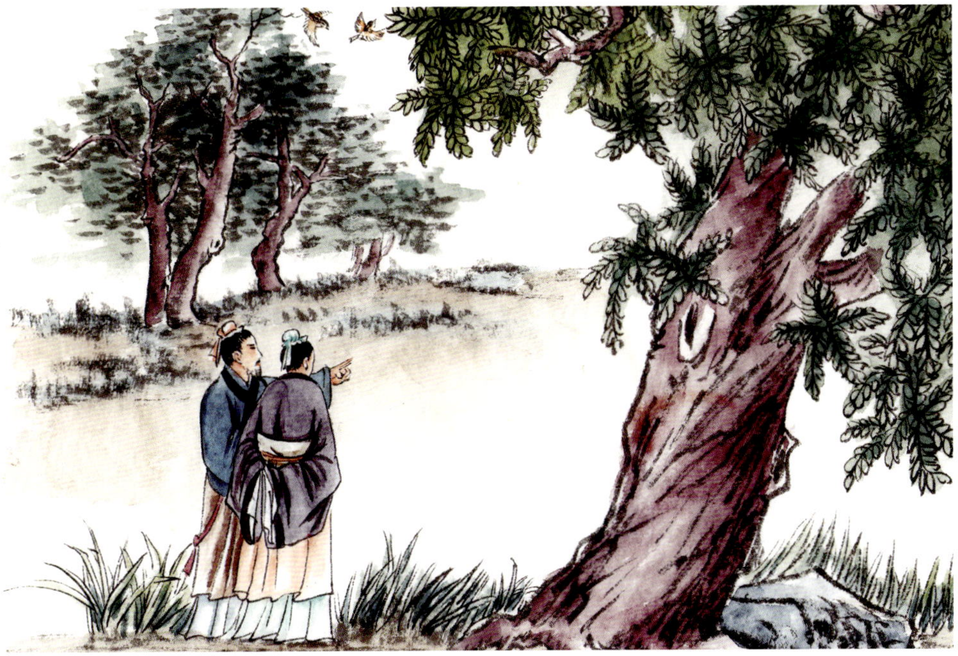

夏季图
Summer

夏季气候炎热，昼长夜短，可晚睡早起，适当午睡，以保存精力。夏季暑热偏盛，宜防“中暑”，但又忌当风而眠。夏天锻炼身体，可选择在清晨或傍晚。

In the hot summer when the day is long and the night short, we may take a nap after lunch to save energy. The summer heat is so prevailing that we should guard against "heatstroke", but we should avoid sleeping in the wind. In summer we'd better do physical exercise in early morning or evening.

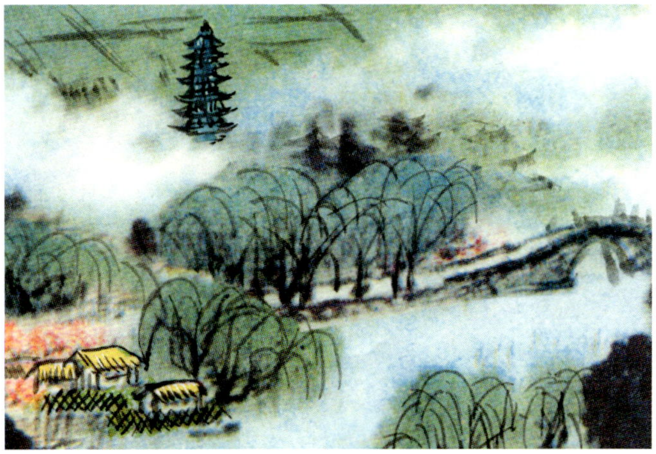

夏季图
Summer

秋季应“早卧早起，与鸡俱兴”，并注意补充体内的水分，避免大汗淋漓以伤津液。秋季气温亦多变，早晚温差较大，应注意随时增减衣着。

In autumn, we should "sleep early and get up early like a rooster", drink enough water and avoid too much sweating which may cause body fluid deficiency. The temperature in autumn is changeable with large difference between day and night, so we should change clothes accordingly.

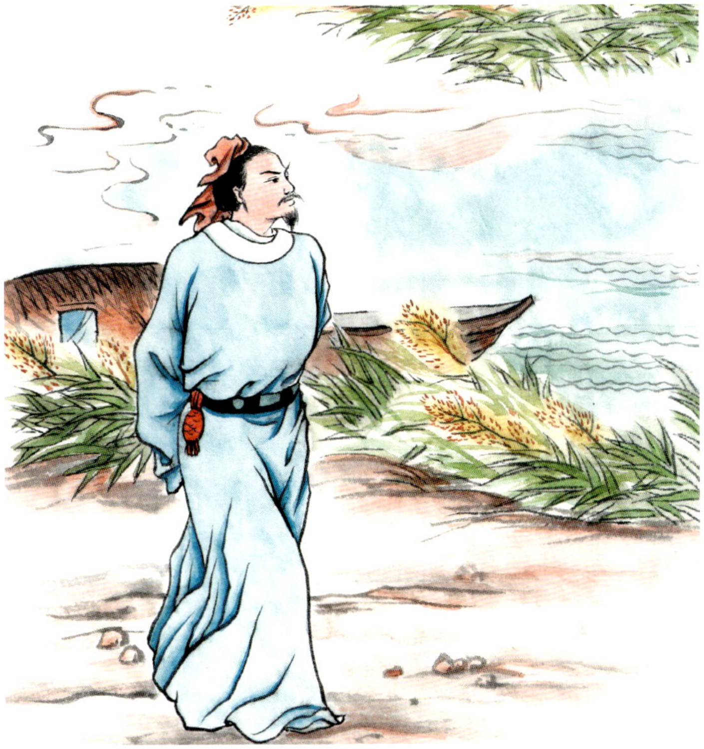

秋季图
Autumn

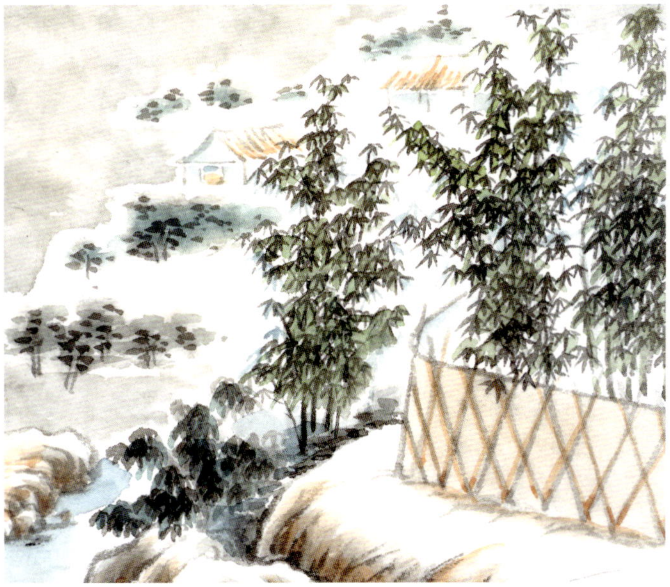

冬季图
Winter

冬季要注意避寒就暖、敛阳护阴，应“早卧晚起，必待日光”，防寒防风。此外冬季乃闭藏之时，因此更应固密心志，保精养神，故中医学尤其重视在冬季节制房事。

In winter the rule to follow is to avoid coldness and keep warm so as to protect the yang qi and yin qi. We should "sleep early and get up late until the sunlight comes out". "In winter one must protect oneself against coldness and wind". Moreover, as winter is the season for storage, we should restrain from over-exploitation of our energy and reduce sexual intercourse, which is especially emphasized in Chinese traditional medicine.

安于居处

Living in an agreeable environment

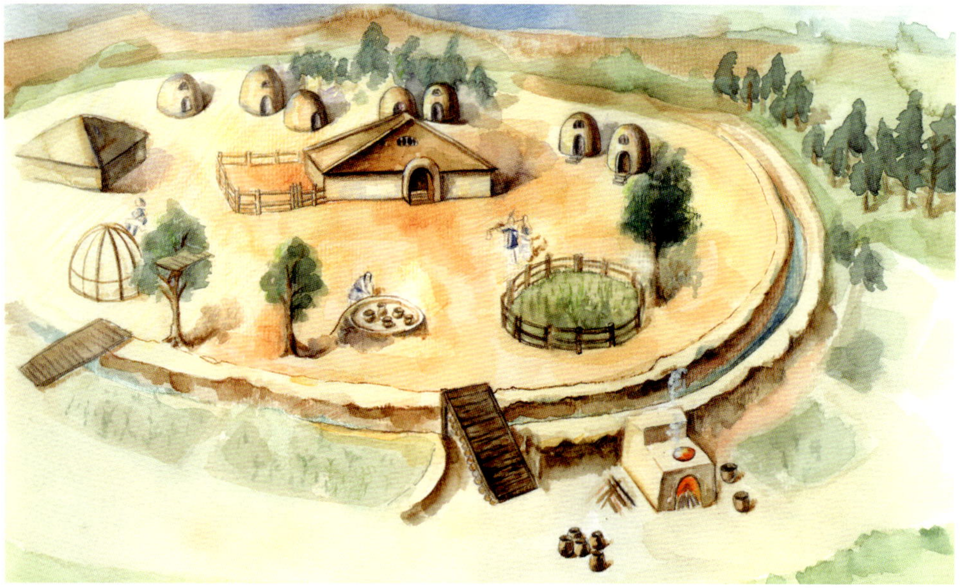

远古住宅

An ancient living place

住宅区土要坚润，水要甘美，忌污雾，污泥浊水，喧嚣嘈杂。住宅座北朝南是比较合理的，可充分利用太阳的光照，确保空气流通，冬暖夏凉。美化居住环境，实有利于健康长寿。

The place for residence should have firm earth and sweet water. The surrounding environment should be free from dirty smog, filth, mire, and noise. It is more desirable for the dwelling house to be seated in the north and to face up to the south, which can take full advantage of the sunlight, enjoy fine ventilation, and keep warmth in winter and coolness in summer. To beautify the living environment is conducive to health and longevity.

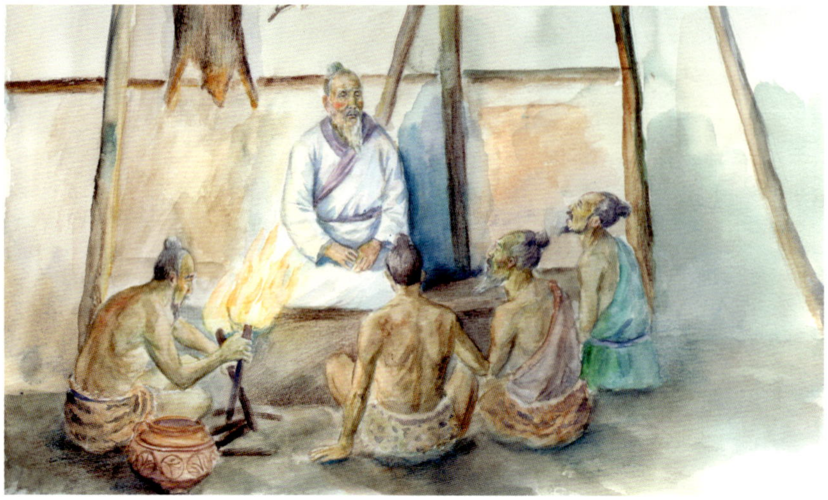

先民居处

Ancients in their lodging

居住在空气清新、气候寒冷地区的人多长寿，而那些住在空气污浊、气候炎热的地区的人则寿命相对短些。可见，中国人早在两千多年前就认识到了居处地理环境与寿命的关系。

People who live in regions with fresh air and cold climate usually live longer, while those who live in regions with polluted air and hot climate die earlier. In fact, as early as two thousand years ago, our ancestors realized the relationship between the dwelling place and the life span.

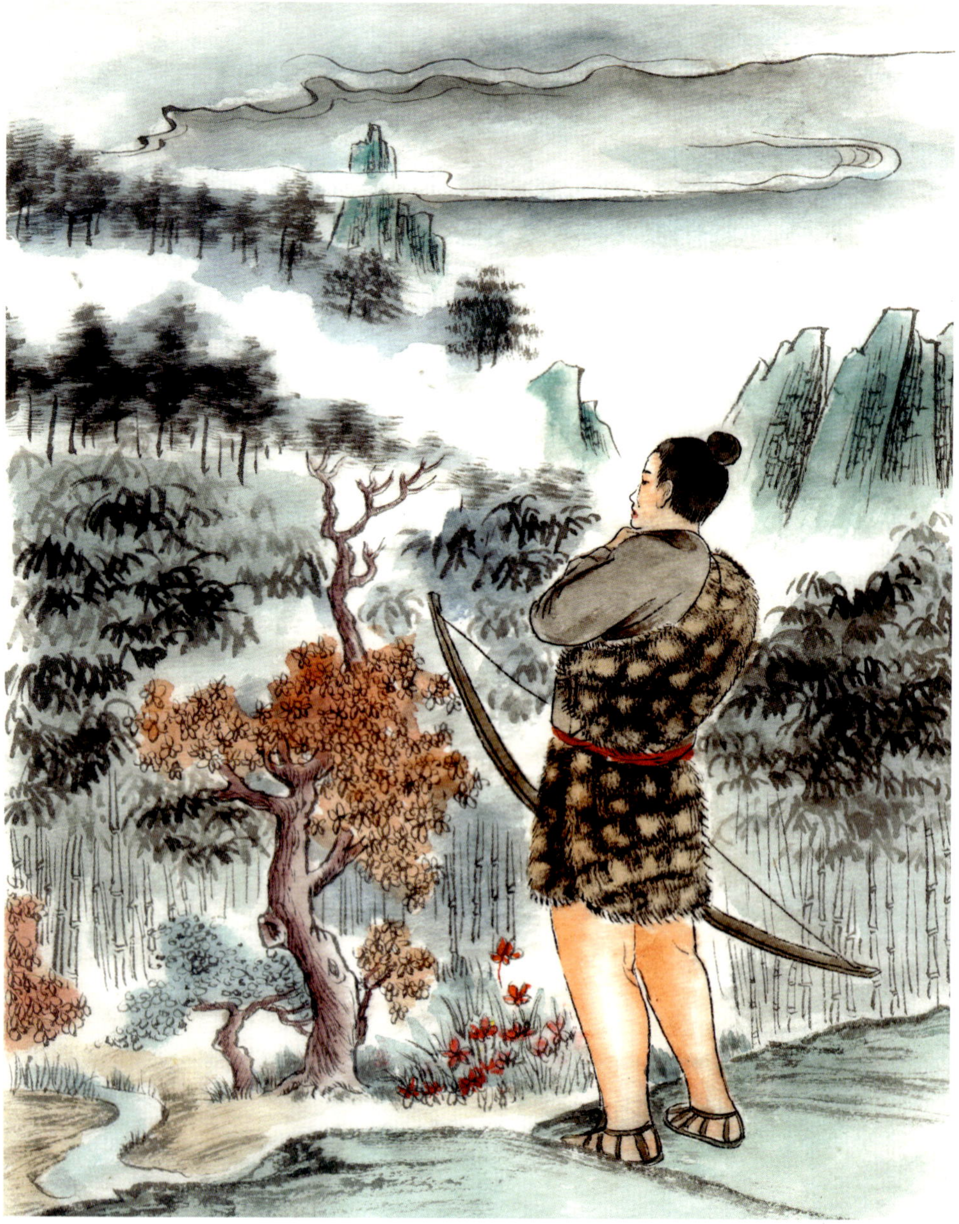

先民择居图

An ancient choosing a place to live

居室要保证光线充足，屋室的高度应该满足要采光的要求，并确保室内空气能自然流通（一般以每小时自然换气 2.5 至 3 次为宜）。除此之外，居室还应温暖舒适、干燥清洁，要注意卫生，防止污染。

The living room should have good sunshine. The height of room should meet the requirements for lighting and ventilation (It is most desirable to change air naturally 2.5 to 3 times per hour). We should pay attention to keeping the living room warm and comfortable, well lit, ventilated, and not too damp. It is necessary to keep the living room clean so as to avoid contamination.

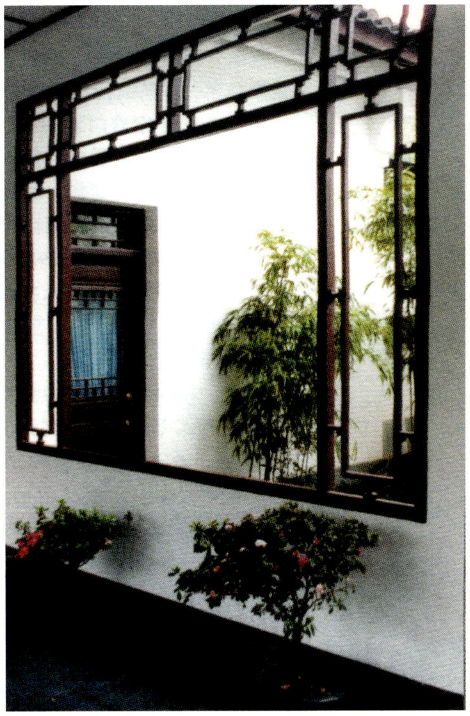

居室

A nice house

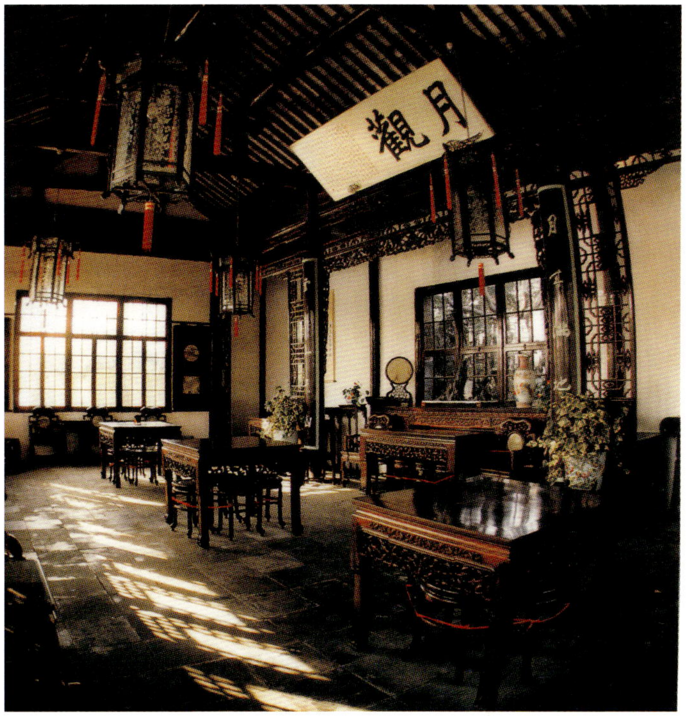

观月室

Moon-observing room

风寒湿三气杂至合而为痹也

The combined effect of Wind, Coldness and Dampness is aches or numbness in certain parts of the body.

风 Wind

寒 Coldness

湿 Dampness

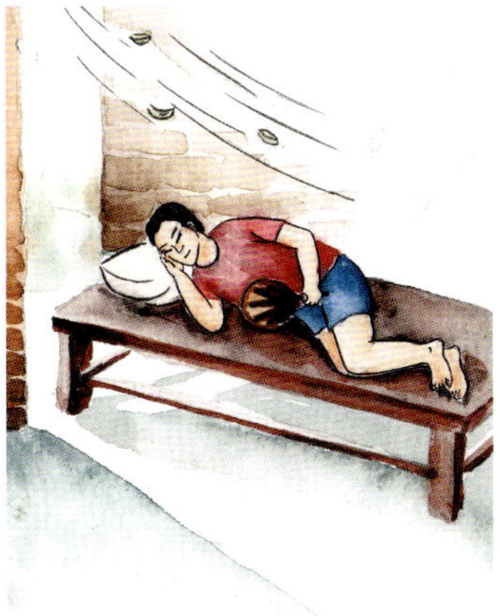

久卧当风

Lying long in a drafty place

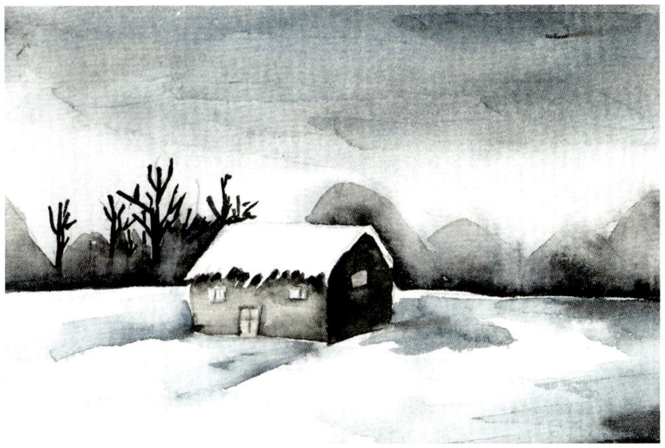

久居湿地

Living long in a humid place

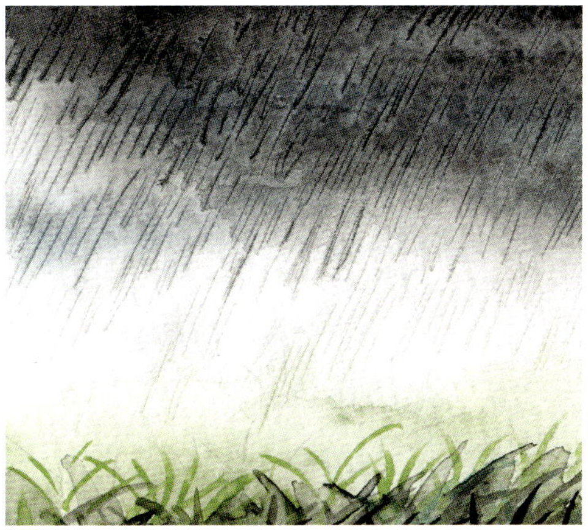

水中作业

Working in the water

应将家中阳光最充足、空气最流通的房间辟为卧室。每天起床后不要急于叠被，让水分、气体充分散发和逸出，被子等物最好经常晒一晒。

We should make the sunniest room with best air circulation our bedroom. It is advisable not to hastily make bed every day after getting up and let the moisture and smell fully emit. Quilts and other bedclothes should often be sunned.

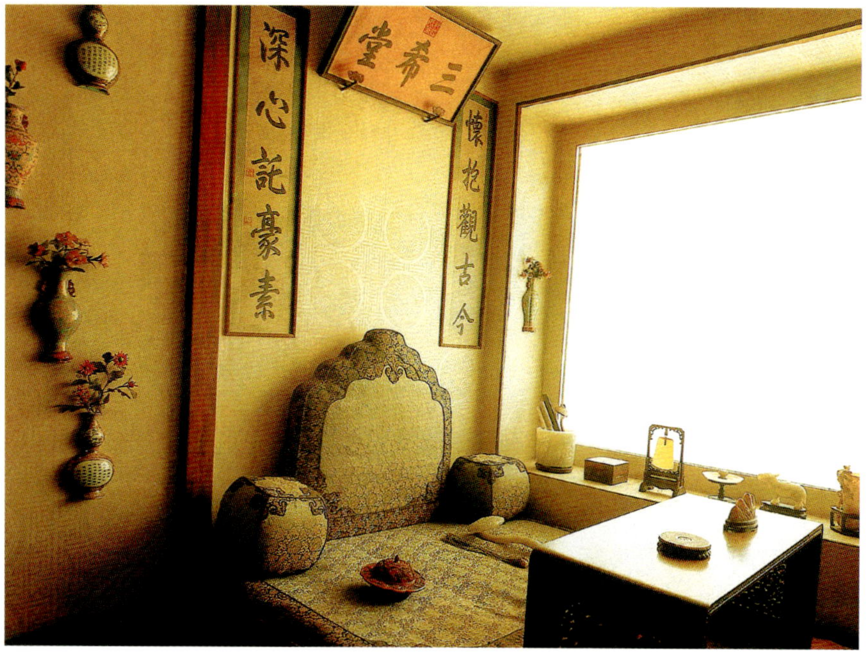

北京故宫三希堂

The Hall of Three Rare Treasures in the Palace Museum, Beijing

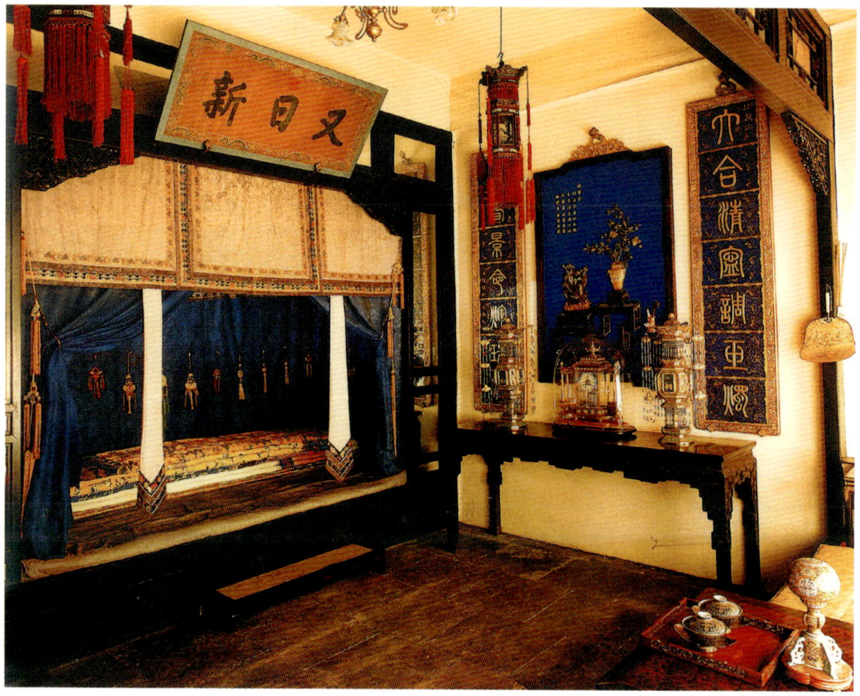

故宫皇帝寝宫

The imperial bedroom in the Palace Museum

优美舒适的居室对人的心理、生理都大有好处，居室的色彩就能直接影响人的精神和情绪。如黄色可增加房间的宽阔感，给人以典雅高贵的感觉；嫩绿、浅蓝等色彩使人产生安闲、幽雅感；卧房布置成浅粉色调则会帮助人在慰藉和温馨的气氛中安然入睡。

A pleasant room will have good effects on one's psychology and physiology. For example, colors can directly affect people's spirit and emotion: yellow can make the room seem bigger, giving people an elegant and noble feeling; light green and light blue make people feel relaxed and produce a leisurely atmosphere; a light pink bedroom induces a sound sleep in a comforting and warm ambience.

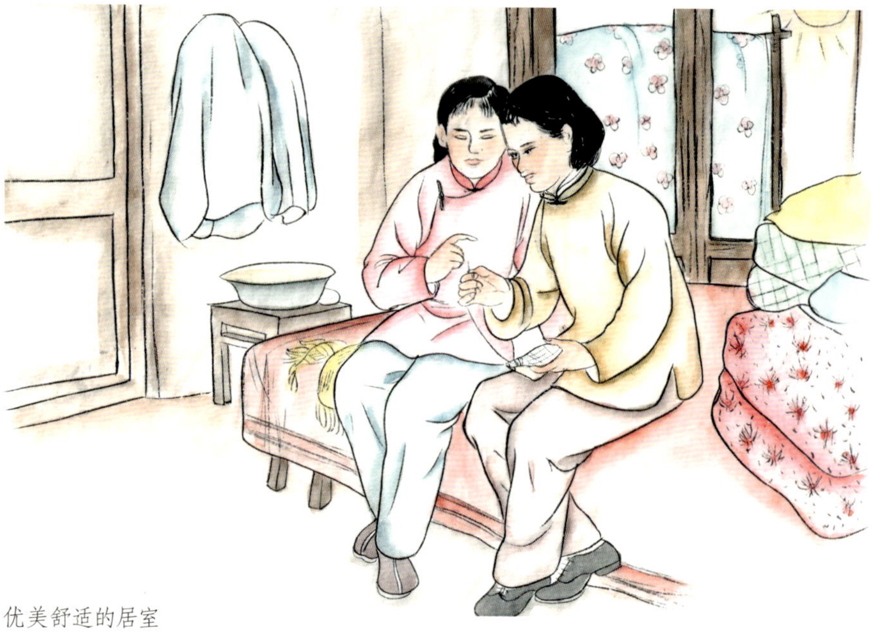

优美舒适的居室

A pleasant room

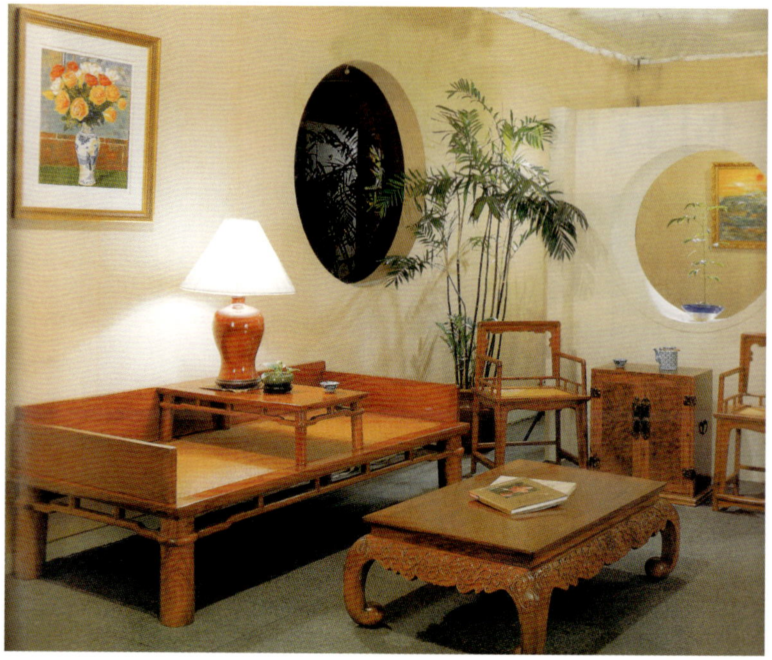

优美舒适的居室

A pleasant room

睡眠与梦境

Sleep and dream

睡眠，是起居的一个重要方面。越来越多的资料表明，睡眠与长寿有着密切关系，故欲求长寿，不可不重视睡眠。

古人有诗曰“华山处士如容见，不觅仙方觅睡方”，民谚云“会吃不如会睡”，“吃人参不如睡五更”。

Sleep is an important aspect of everyday life. More and more data indicate that sleep has a close relationship with longevity, so we cannot neglect the quality sleep if we want to live a long life.

An ancient poem said, “If the reclusive of Huashan can grant me a meeting, I’ll ask for his recipe for sleep instead of recipe for becoming an immortal.” As folk sayings go, “Eat well is not as good as sleep well”, and “A sound sleep till the fifth watch of the night is better than eating ginseng.”

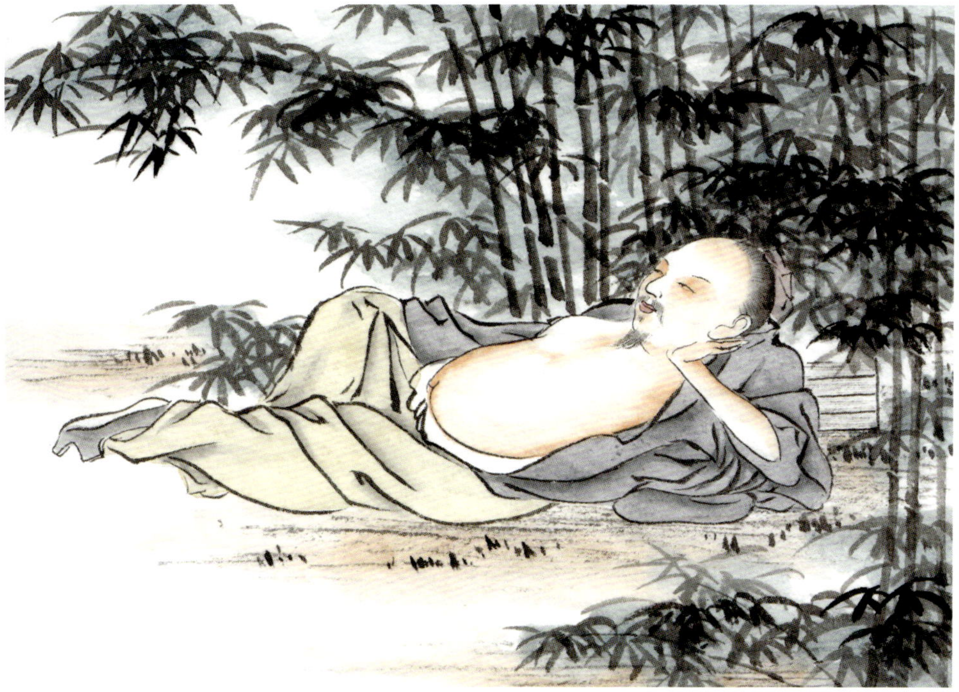

觅睡图

Try to have a sound sleep

做梦是睡眠中常有的现象。在睡眠时，大脑皮质神经细胞绝大部分已处于抑制状态，而获得休息的机会。但抑制有深、浅之别，其区域也有大、有小。当大脑皮质处于局部的、不完全的、或含有兴奋点（区）的抑制状态时，周围环境与身体内部的刺激传向大脑，便可以产生不正确的反应。而强弱、范围、久暂不等的脑细胞群的活动，就可以产生形形色色，变幻莫测的梦境。由此可见梦是人在睡眠状态下的一种特殊的意识活动，由于它发生的不自觉，内容虚幻离奇，所以一直是现代科学重点研究的对象，而梦在医学上也有其重要的地位。

Dreams are a common phenomenon in sleep. In sleep, the neurons at the cerebral cortex are in an inhibitory state. Thus sleep is an opportunity for rest. However, the degree of inhibition may vary in depth and area. When the inhibitory state is partial, incomplete or with active points, when stimuli from the surroundings or inside the body are transmitted to the brain, it may give incorrect responses. The activities of neuron groups varying in degree, scope and time length may give rise to dreams of various sorts. Therefore, it can be seen that dreams are a special conscious activity in sleep. Because of their involuntariness, transience and oddity, they have been a focus of scientific research in modern times and played an important role in medicine.

中国古代哲学家庄子曾经梦见自己变成了一只无拘无束的蝴蝶。（见右图）

Chuang Tzu, ancient Chinese philosopher, once dreamed that he turned into a free butterfly.

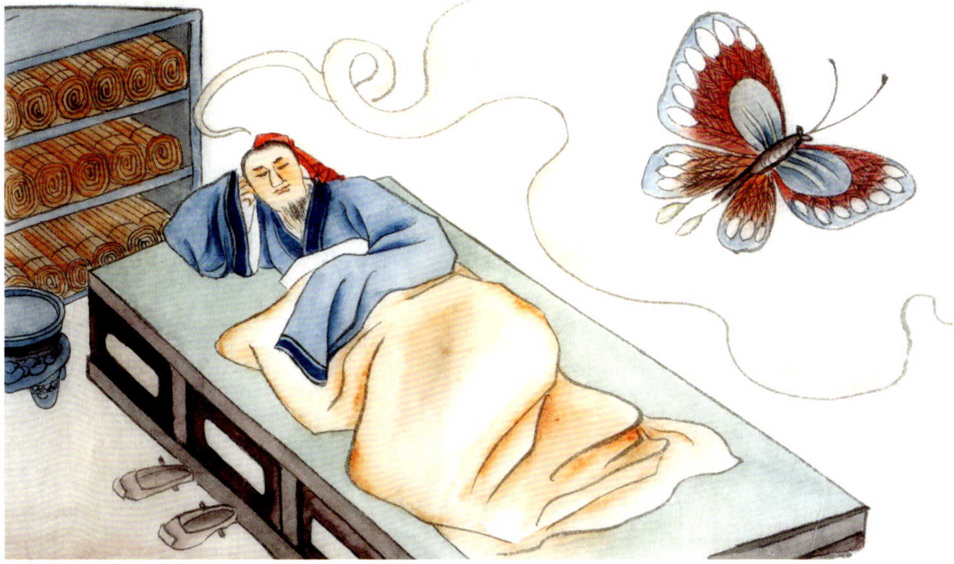

人的感知、记忆、思虑、情感、性格都会影响梦的产生及梦的内容。其中最重要的因素是思虑、情感、性格。

Occurrence of dream and its content are influenced by a wide number of factors including people's perceptions, memories, worries, emotions, as well as their personalities; among them the last three are the most important factors.

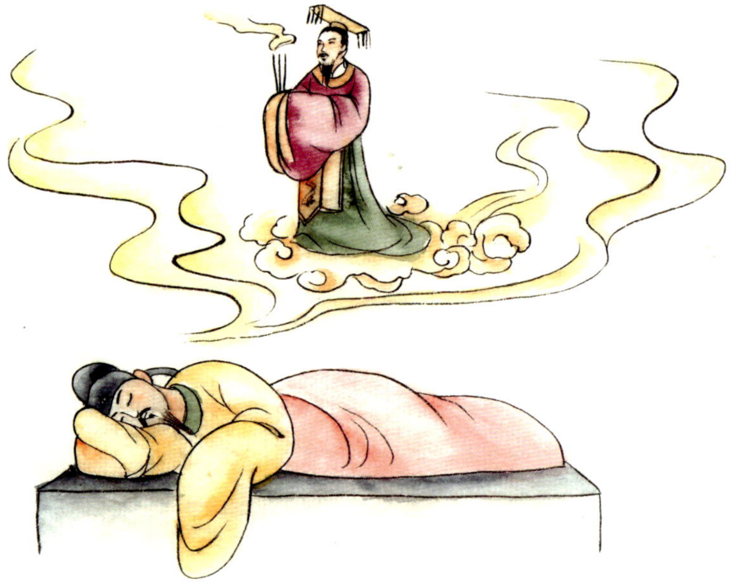

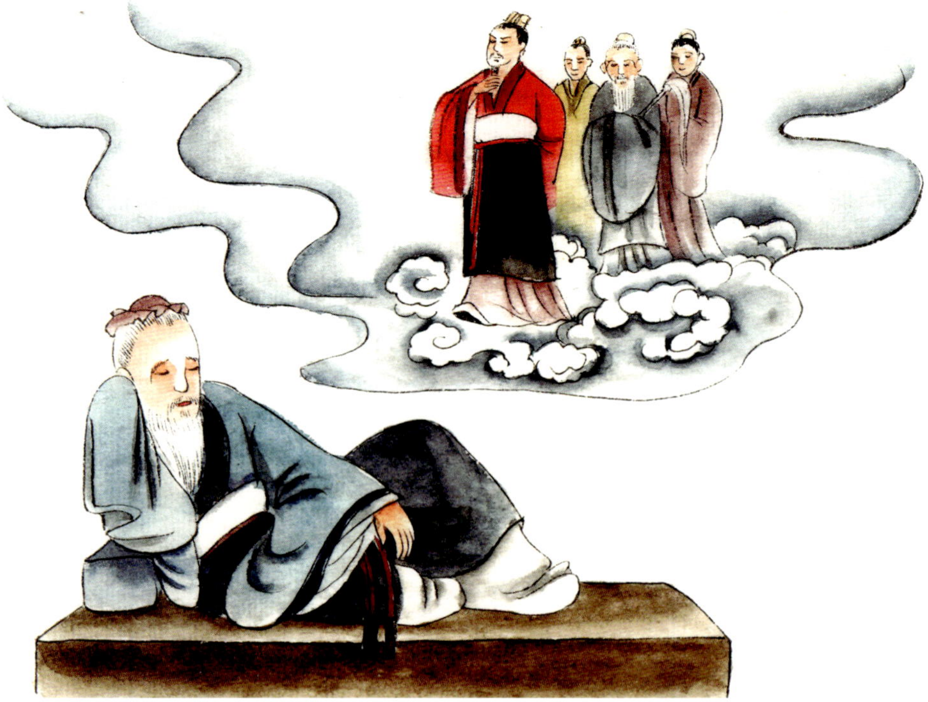

“昼无情念，夜无梦寐。”由此可见，情感是致梦的一个重要因素。

“好仁者多梦松柏桃李，好义者多梦刀兵金铁，好礼者多梦簠簋笾豆，好智者多梦江湖川泽，好信者多梦山岳原野。”古人认为人的性格对梦的内容有很大影响。

“There would be no dreams at night without emotions and thoughts during the day.” That is to say, emotions are another important cause of dreams.

Those interested in benevolence tend to dream of pines, cypresses, peaches and plums; those interested in righteousness tend to dream of weapons and battle; those interested in rites tend to dream of ritual vessels; those interested in wisdom tend to dream of rivers, lakes and marshes; those interested in faith tend to dream of plain and mountains. Ancient people also believed that one's character had a great influence on what he would dream of.

“孔子生于乱世，日思周公之德，夜即梦之。”日有所思，夜有所梦，古人认为“昼想”与“夜梦”密切相关。人们的夜间之梦其实就是白日之“思”的延伸。另外，梦既可由思虑引起，也可由感知、记忆引起。人的整个认知过程都可以成为梦境的来源。

“Confucius was born in chaotic years. In the day he thought of the virtues of Duke of Zhou, and at night he dreamt about them too.” As a Chinese saying goes that one dreams at night what he thinks in the day, ancient Chinese people believed that there was a close tie between the two, and what one dreamt at night was actually the continuation of what he thought in the day. Moreover, just as people's thoughts can lead to dreams, so can their perceptions and memories. As a matter of fact, every process in human being's perception serves as the source of dreams.

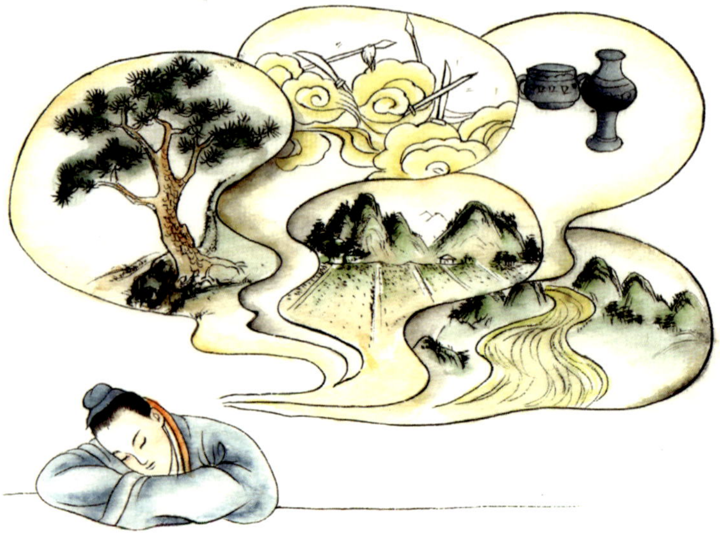

中医梦诊

Diagnosis through dreams in traditonal Chinese medicine

所谓梦诊就是依据患者对梦的自述，四诊合参，进行诊断、治疗。

Diagnosis through dreams refers to the method of diagnosing the patient through his description of his dreams. The doctor will then incorporate the other three traditional diagnostic methods and make the final diagnosis and treatment plan.

步骤1 step 1 → 辨生理梦与病理梦 Distinguish physiological dreams from pathological dreams

步骤2 step 2 → 辨梦因 Analyze the reason of dreams

步骤3 step 3 → 辨梦量 Analyze the number of dreams

步骤4 step 4 → 辨梦境 Analyze the content of dreams

梦预示着五脏的虚实

Dreams indicates the conditions of your five viscera

1 梦见山丘烟火弥漫 Dreaming of a hill with pervasive smoke and fire →

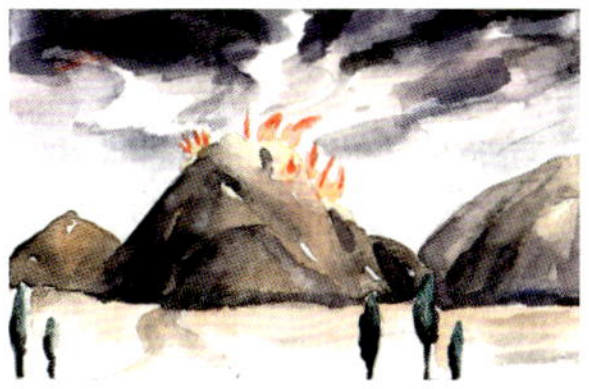

→ 邪气犯心 Evil factors are affecting the heart

2 梦见丘陵和巨大的湖泽 Dreaming of hills and a vast lake →

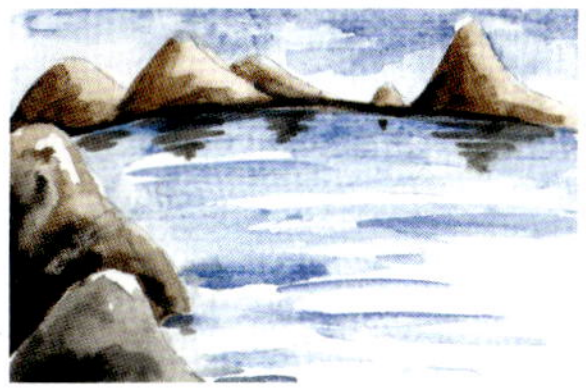

→ 邪气犯脾 Evil factors are affecting the spleen

3 梦见飞扬、腾越或金属 Dreaming of something rising or flying upward, or metal →

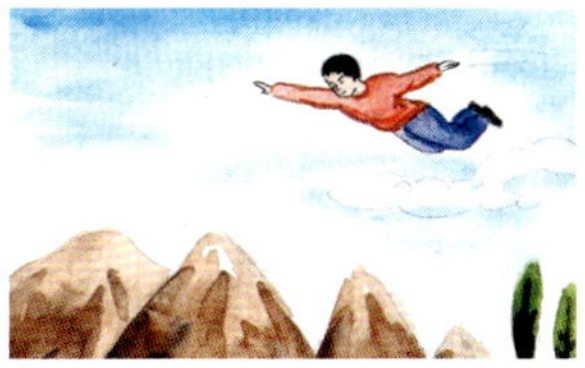

→ 邪气犯肺 Evil factors are affecting the lungs

4 梦见浸没在水潭中 Dreaming of being immersed in a pool →

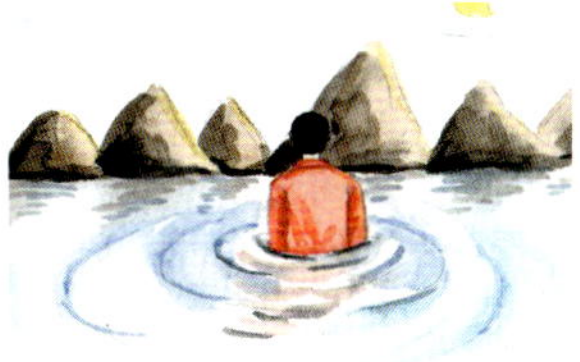

→ 邪气犯肾 Evil factors are affecting the kidneys

5 梦见大火灼身 Dreaming of being burned by a blazing fire →

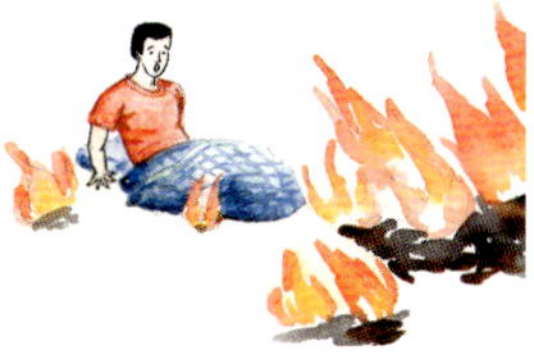

→ 邪气犯肝 Evil factors are affecting the stomach

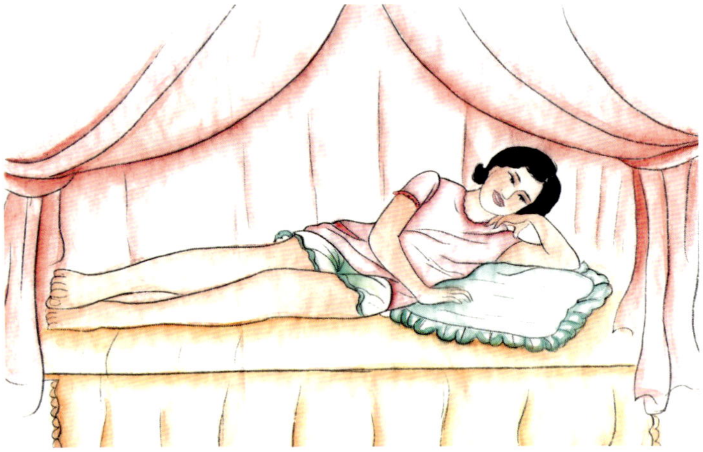

睡前要放松
Relax before sleep

就寝前必须保持心境平和、精神松弛。卧室要安静、干净卫生、空气清新。理想的睡姿是侧身屈膝，以使精气不散。

Before going to bed one must have a peaceful mind and a relaxed mood. Clean bedroom with fresh air. It is generally believed that the ideal sleeping position is to lie on one's side with the body bent, which will keep one's vitality.

中医养生学提倡睡“子午觉”。“子”是指 23 点至 1 点，这段时间基本上所有人都在休息。而“午”是指 11 点至 13 点，中医认为此时睡觉，可以顺应阳气的升发，有利于身体健康。

The regimen theory of Chinese traditional medicine proposes to sleep from 11 p. m. to 1 a.m, a period of the day when almost everyone rests, and from 11 a.m. to 1 p.m, just at noon. Chinese traditional medicine holds that sleep at these two periods is in line with the ascending of yang qi, which is conducive to good health.

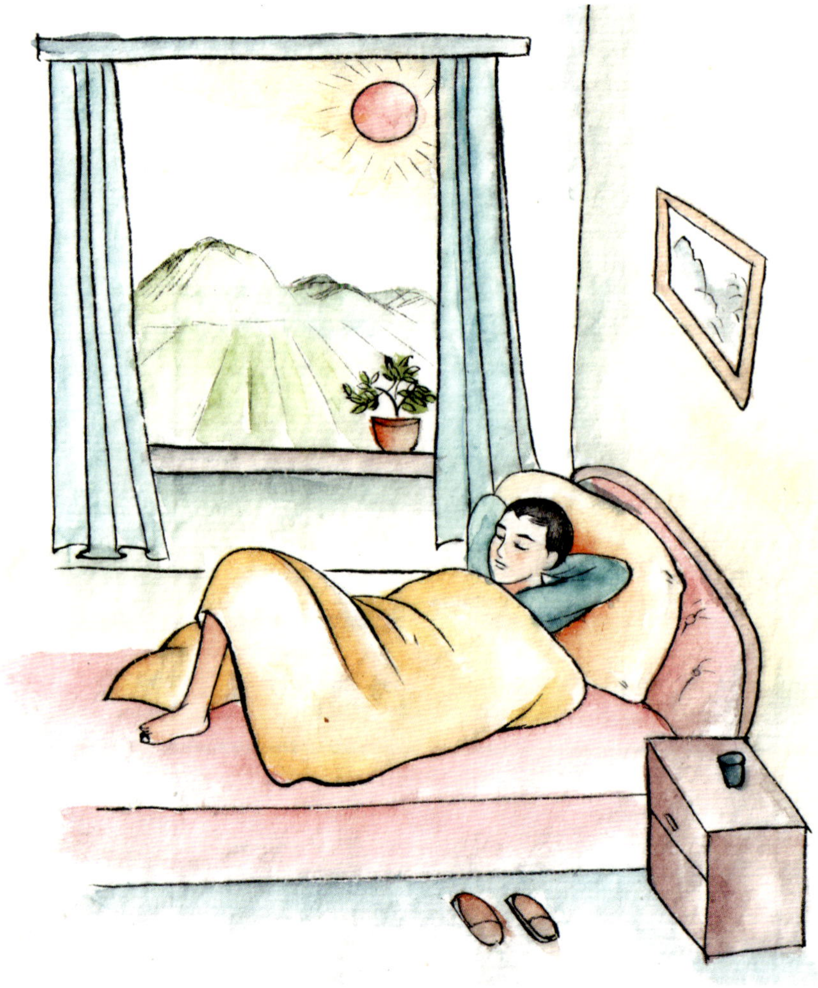

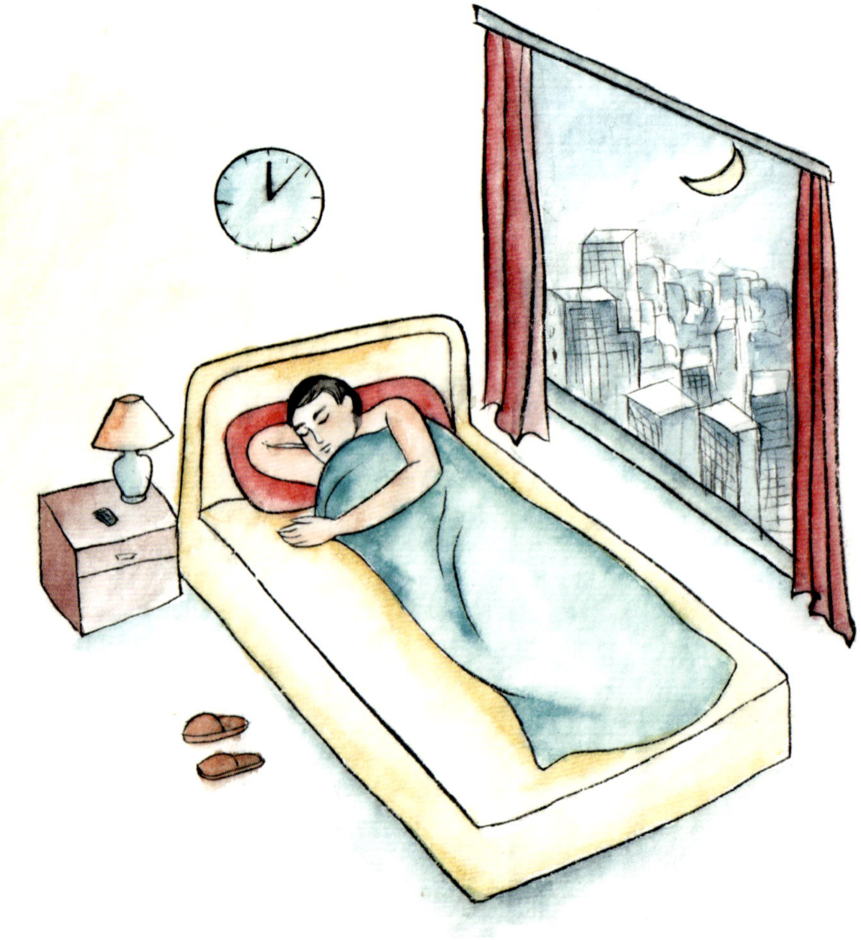

睡眠养生三法

Three ways to preserve health through sleep

1. 清静安眠法

1. Calming the mind

“先睡心，后睡眼”，心静神安方能入睡。在睡前半小时最好不要思考问题，可以做一些如散步、听轻音乐等有助于大脑放松的活动，以使自己尽快入睡。

“Calm your mind before closing your eyes”, for you cannot sleep without a tranquil mind. You'd better stop pondering over anything half an hour before sleeping. Instead, you may do something to relieve tension, such as taking a walk or listening to light music, which can help you to fall asleep more quickly.

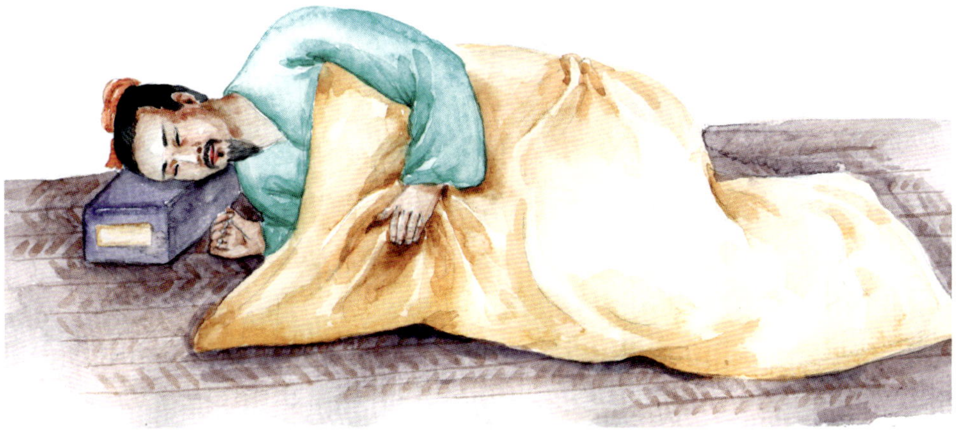

清静安眠

Calming the mind

2. 按摩安眠法

2. Massaging

仰卧揉腹：每晚入睡前，仰卧在床上，意守丹田（肚脐下 4 横指），先用右手按顺时针方向绕脐稍加用力揉腹，一边揉一边默念计数，计数 120 次。再换用左手逆时针方向同样绕脐揉 120 次。仰卧于床上做细而均匀的深呼吸 30 次，全身放松，意守丹田也可入睡。

Rubbing your stomach while lying on your back: every night, before sleeping, lie on your back in bed and concentrate your mind on your dantian (four fingers below the navel). Rub your stomach with your right hand, clockwise around the navel and with a little force, while silently counting to 120. Switch to your left hand, and rub your stomach counter-clockwise, again for 120 times. The third method: lying on your back in bed, draw a gentle and even deep breath for 30 times; relax your whole body and concentrate your mind on your dantian.

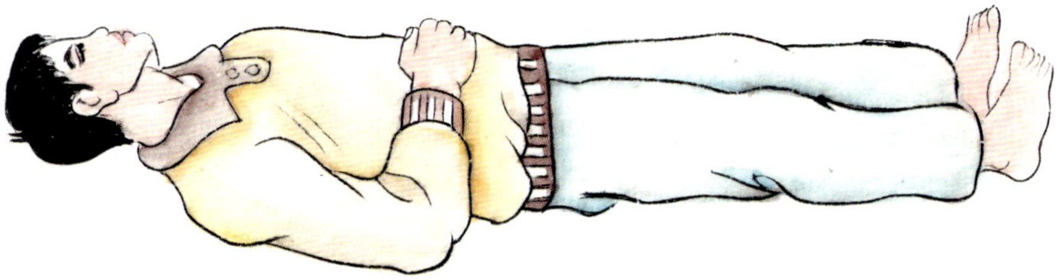

按摩安眠法

Massaging

失眠者如果能长期坚持，对上半夜进入深睡有良好作用。如下半夜醒后再不能入睡，可按上述方法各揉腹 60 次，对再次入睡也有一定作用。

If you suffer from insomnia, persistence in this method can give you a sound sleep before midnight. If you wake up after midnight and remain sleepless after that, you may try to fall asleep again by rubbing your stomach for 60 times with the first method and for another 60 times with the second one.

睡前饮茶或咖啡，茶叶和咖啡中含有咖啡碱等物质，这些物质会刺激中枢神经，使人兴奋，若睡前喝茶，特别是浓茶，中枢神经会更加兴奋，使人不易入睡。

If people drink tea or coffee before going to sleep, the caffeine contained in tea and coffee will irritate the central nervous system and lead to excitement. Tea, especially strong tea, if taken before sleep, will cause the central nervous system to become excited and therefore make people hard to fall asleep.

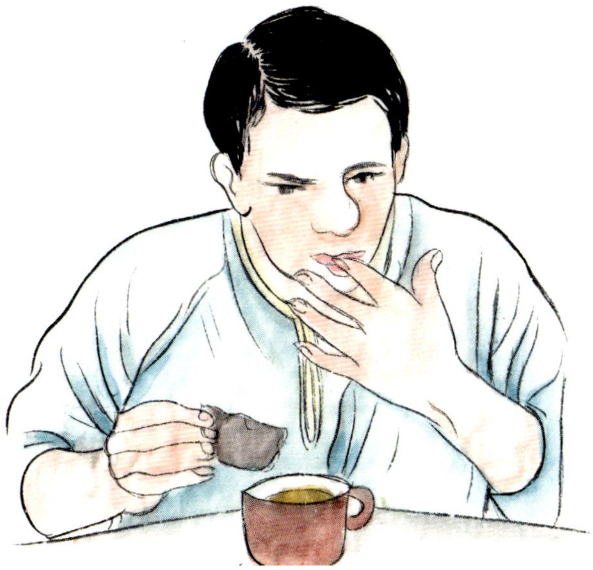

3. 饮食安眠法

3. Food therapy

失眠者可适当选用一些有利于睡眠的药膳，或睡前饮用 1 袋牛奶，以改善睡眠。但切忌睡前饮食过饱。睡前亦不可饮用茶、酒、咖啡等刺激性饮料。

An insomniac may eat certain therapeutic foods that can aid sleeping, or drink a carton of milk before going to bed to sleep better. Never eat too much or take any stimulating beverage, such as tea, liquor and coffee before you go to bed.

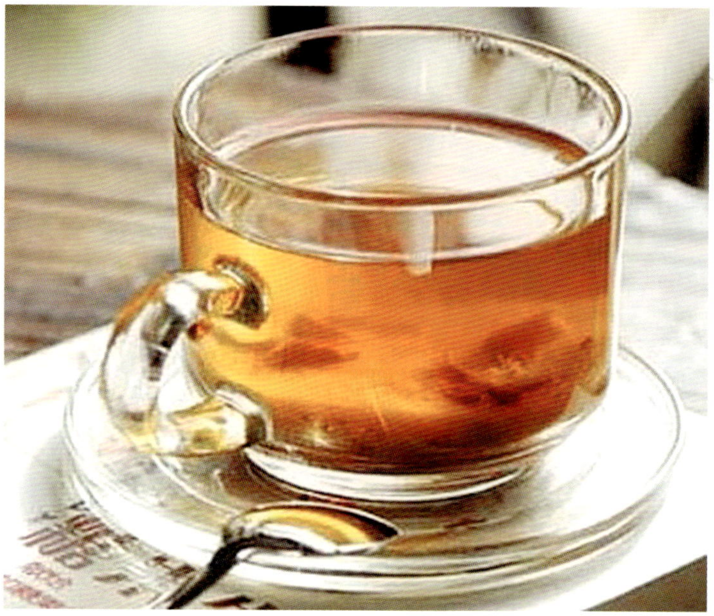

药膳可用：

1. 龙眼冰糖茶：龙眼肉 25 克，冰糖 10 克。把龙眼肉洗净，同冰糖放入茶杯中，冲入沸水，加盖闷一会儿，即可饮用。

Here are two kinds of therapeutic food to choose from:

1. Longan and crystal sugar soup: Use 25g of longan flesh and 10g of crystal sugar. Wash the longan flesh and put it together with the crystal sugar in a tea cup. Fill the cup with boiling water and put the lid on. You may drink the soup after a while.

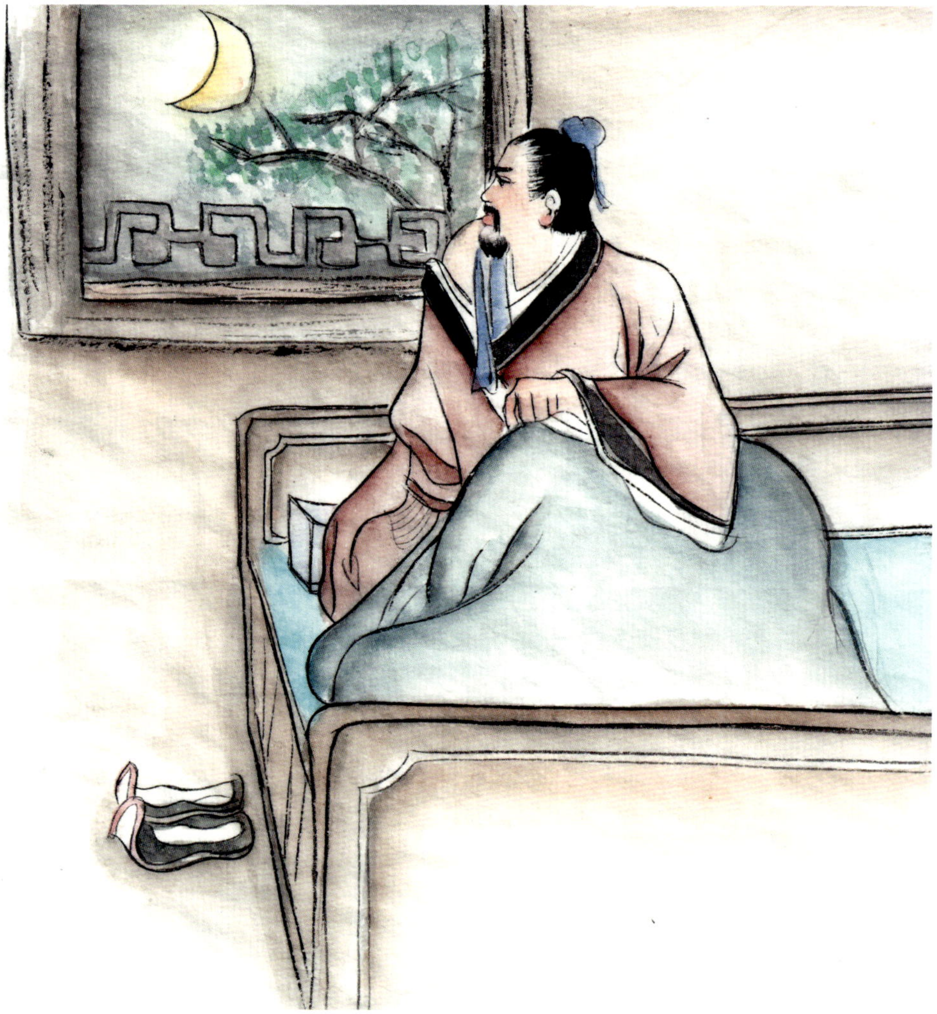

辗转失眠

Suffering from insomnia

2. 远志枣仁粥：远志 10 克，炒酸枣仁 15 克，粳米 75 克。粳米淘洗干净，放入适量清水锅中，加入洗净的远志、酸枣仁，用大火烧开后转小火煮成粥，可作为夜餐食用。

2. Polygana and wild jujube congee: Use 10g of polygana, 15g of stir-fried wild jujube, and 75g of jingmi (polished round-grained rice). Wash the rice and put it into a pot filled with an appropriate amount of clean water, and add washed polygana and wild jujubes. Boil the mixture first in high heat and then stew it into congee with low heat. The congee can be taken as a night snack.

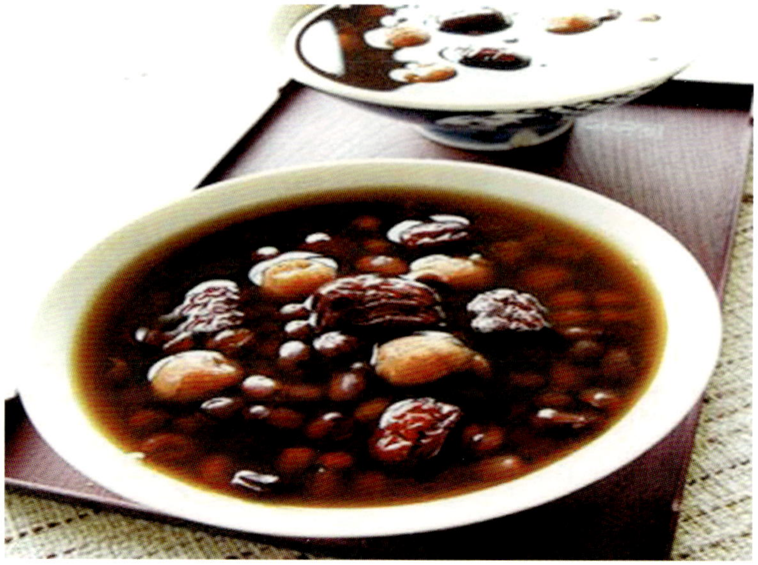

远志枣仁粥

Polygana and wild jujube congee

睡眠养生要注意睡眠姿势的选择。古人对睡眠的要求是卧如弓，右侧卧势。这样的睡眠姿势，不压迫心脏部位，有利于心肺功能活动和肠胃的机械消化。对于睡眠的方向，春夏头宜向东，秋冬头宜向西。睡眠的时间成人每天不低于 6 小时，除应强调夜间睡眠外，还应坚持午睡。足够的睡眠时间和良好的睡眠质量是睡眠养生的关键。

To preserve health through sleep, one should also choose the proper posture. The traditional requirement is to sleep on your right flank and bend your body like a bow. This posture, which exerts no pressure on the heart, is good for digestion as well as the function of the heart and lungs. As for where to put your head, it should be in the east in spring and summer, and in the west in autumn and winter. An adult should sleep for no less than six hours a day, not only during the night but also at noontime. Enough time and good quality are essential for health preservation through sleep.

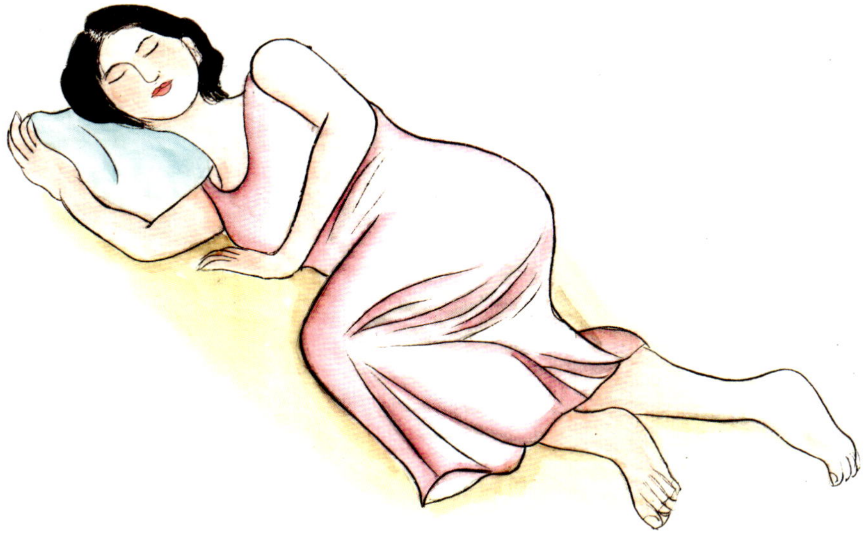

睡如弓姿

To pose like a bow while sleeping

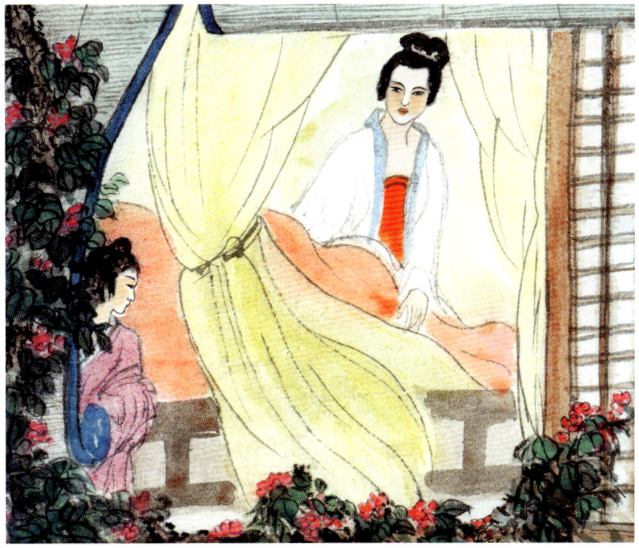

充足睡眠

Sufficient sleep

睡眠养生有以下禁忌。

睡眠切忌蒙头，俗语说："睡觉不蒙首，活到九十九。"蒙头大睡易使人呼吸困难，吸入不洁之浊气，有损健康。

When sleeping, do not cover your head with the quilt. As the saying goes, "Keep your head out of the quilt, and you'll live to the age of ninety-nine." Covering your head while sleeping can make you breathe with difficulty and inhale unclean air, which are detrimental to health.

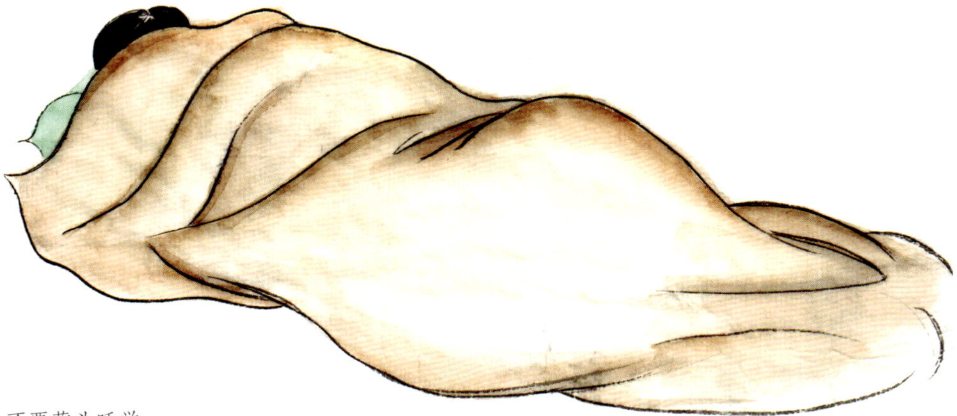

不要蒙头睡觉

Don't sleep with the head enveloped.

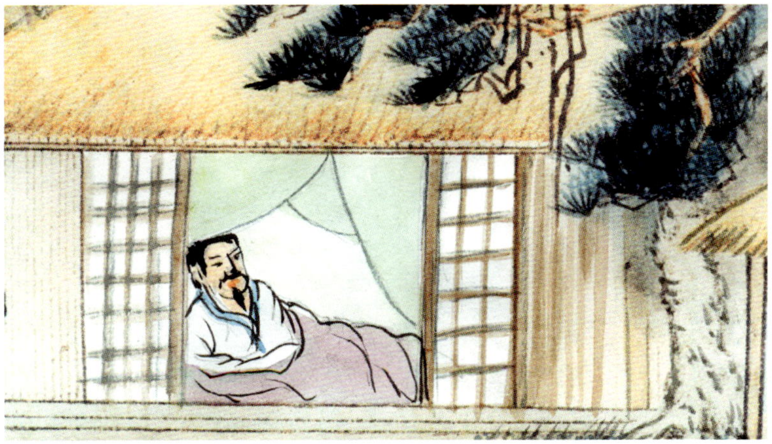

胃不和，则卧不安

Dysfunction of stomach will lead to uneasy sleep

睡前吃得过饱，胃肠要加紧消化，装满食物的胃刺激大脑。大脑有兴奋点，人便不会安然入睡，正如中医所说"胃不和，则卧不安"。

Overeating before sleep will increase the burden of the intestines and stomach whose job is digesting the food, and thereby irritate the brain. Once the brain becomes excited, it will be difficult for people to fall into a sound sleep. This is what the traditional Chinese medicine describes as "dysfunction of stomach will lead to uneasy sleep".

科学起居要注意肠中常清

Purge your bowels of waste

唐代医药家孙思邈在《千金要方》中记述道："便难之人，其面多晦。"历代医学家也有"想长寿，肠须清"之说，此话有一定的科学道理。有些人因肠中食物积滞而容易生毒疮，很多肠胃病甚至癌症都由此而发，适度的饥饿会对人的自主神经、内分泌和免疫系统造成冲击，进而通过重新调整人机体生理内环境功能，来提高人体承受生理负担的能力，使各种心身疾病得到缓解。可以说保健祛疾，排毒第一。

In *Prescriptions Worth a Thousand Gold for Emergencies*, Tang medical scientist Sun Simiao wrote, "Those who suffer from constipation tend to have a dark complexion." Other medical scientists of past ages also remarked that one who wants to live a long life must purge his bowels of waste. These words have a ring of truth. If food stays too long in one's bowels, it is likely to cause noxious sores, many kinds of intestinal and stomach troubles, and even cancer. A proper degree of hunger, which stimulates the autonomic nervous system, the endocrine system and the immune system, can enhance the human body's ability to bear physiological pressure and improve various mental and physical conditions by readjusting the internal environment. Thus we can say that purging your bowels is of primary importance for health protection and disease resistance.

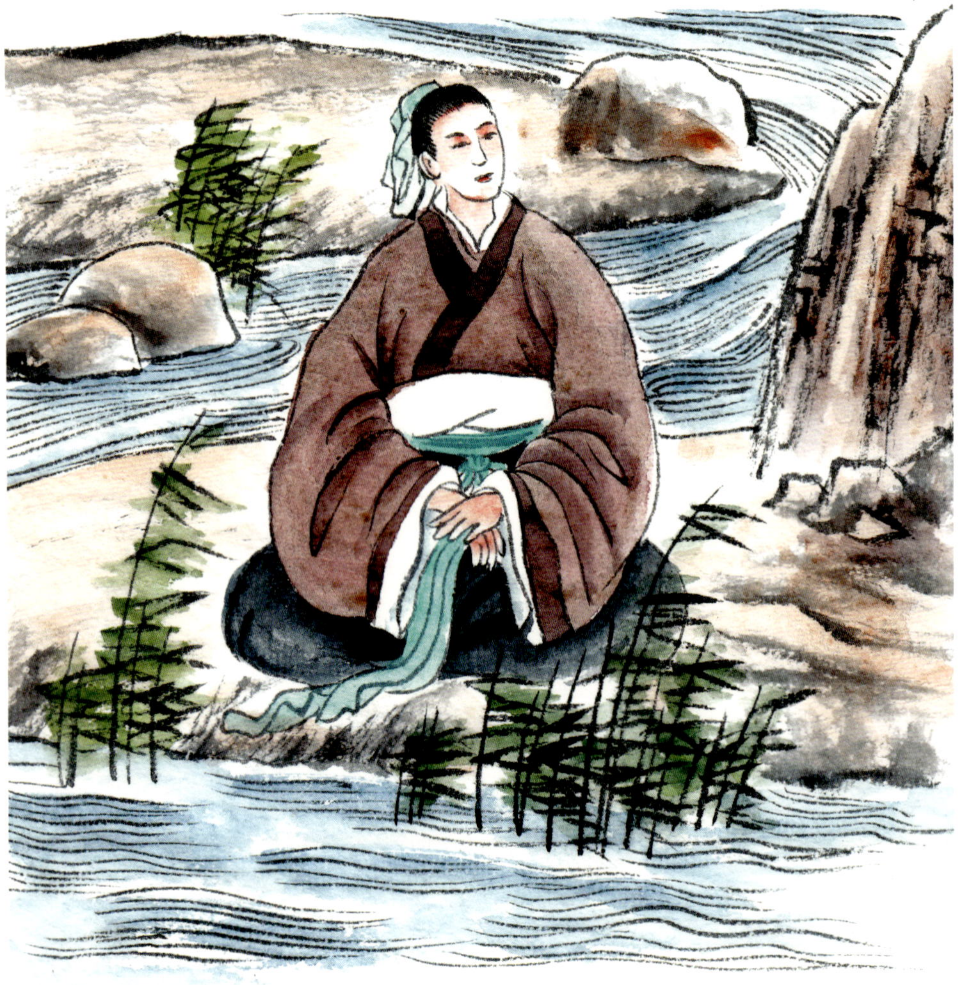

想长寿，肠须清

To live a long life one must purge his bowels of waste

人可以通过这些方法增强肠胃活动能力：

1. 饮水跑步排便法
2. 按摩排泄通便法
3. 饮食调养通便法
4. 服用药物通便法

One can improve bowel movements by

1. drinking water and running
2. massaging
3. dietary regulation
4. taking medicine

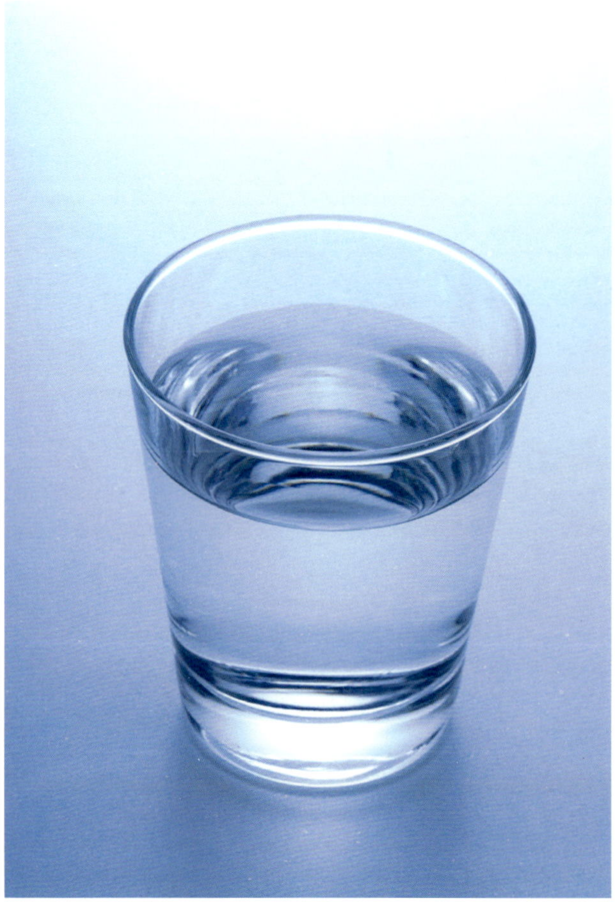

最好的饮用水可以润肠

Live water does good to life, and high-quality drinking water nurtures the intestines.

肠胃运化食物图解

Illustrations of food digestion

受盛与化物

Receiving and digesting the food

受盛
Receive

1 小肠是接受经胃初步消化饮食物的盛器。

1. The small intestine is a container for the partially digested food from the stomach.

2 经胃初步消化的饮食物在小肠内必须有相当时间的停留，以利于进一步消化和吸收。

2. The partially digested food from the stomach will stay in the small intestine for a certain period of time for further digestion and absorption.

泌别清浊

Absorb the nutritional and pass the waste

泌别清浊
Absorb the nutritional and pass the waste

营养 nutrition	残渣 waste	经过小肠消化后的饮食物，分别为水谷精微和食物残渣两个部分。 Food digested by the small intestine can be divided into two parts: nutritional food essence and waste.
吸收营养 absorb nutrition	输送残渣 transmission of waste	将水谷精微吸收，把食物残渣向大肠输送。 The nutritional food essence is absorbed, while the waste is transported into the large intestine.
吸收营养 absorb nutrition	吸收水液 absorb the water	小肠在吸收水谷精微的同时，也吸收了大量的水液。 When the small intestine absorbs the nutritional food essence, it also takes in a large quantity of water.

受盛
Receive

胃初步消化的饮食物
The partially digested food from the stomach
→ 停留于 stay at →
小肠
The small intestine
→ 传化为 change into →
水谷精微
Nutritional food essence

A

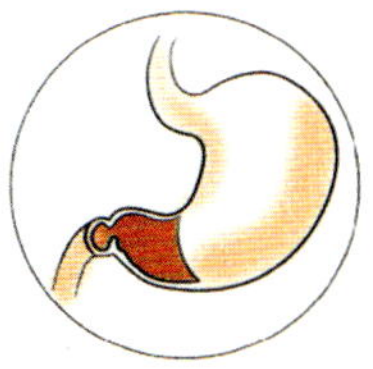

幽门：小肠与胃相连接处称为幽门。

Pylorus: the part which connects the stomach and the small intestine.

B

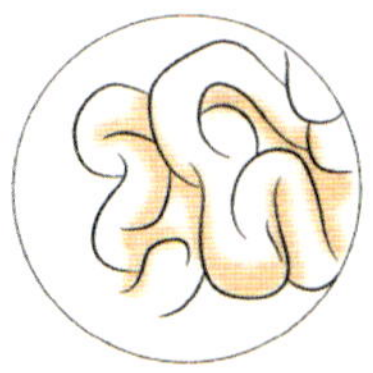

阑门：与大肠相连接处称为阑门。

Ileocecal valve: the part which connects the small intestine and large intestine.

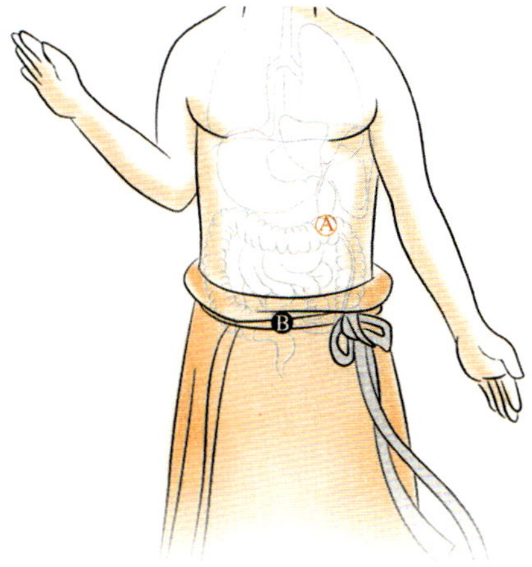

《灵枢·肠胃》说："小肠后附脊，左环回周叠积，其注于回肠者，外附于脐上，回运环十六曲，大二寸半，径八分分之少半，长三丈二尺。"

According to the description in the volume of *Stomach and Intestines* from *Classic of the Miraculous Pivot*, the small intestine is attached to the spine, and then goes left zigzagging into sixteen turns until the ileum reaches the naval. Its length is about three zhang and two chi (approximately 10.6 meters), and about 2.4cm in diameter.

大肠居于腹中，上口在阑门处与小肠相接，下口紧接肛门(魄门)。其上中部绕行于腹部之左右，先升后降，下部管腔扩大，沿脊之下部下行至魄门(即肛门)。

The large intestine is located in the abdomen, its upper opening connected with the small intestine through the ileocecal valve while its end connected with the anus. Its upper and middle part circles around the abdomen, first rising up and then going down, while its lower part broadens and goes along the spine to the anus.

传送食物的糟粕，使其排出体外

The large intestine: to transport the food waste and defecate

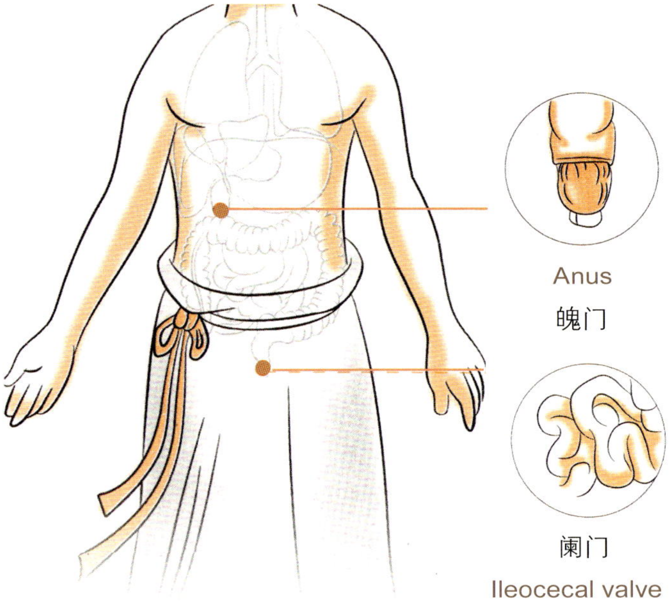

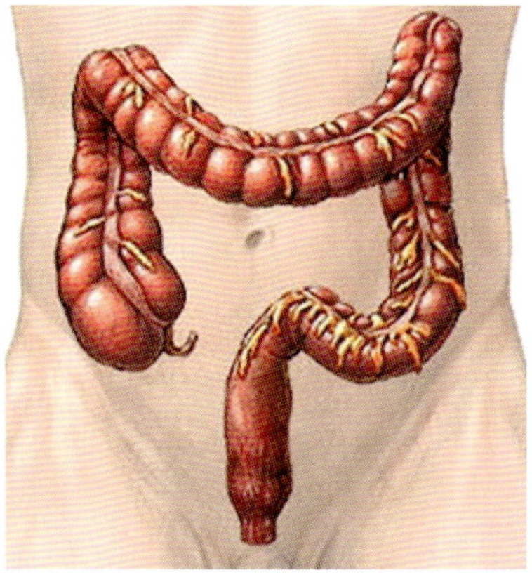

大肠
The large intestine

回肠
Circled intestine

大肠的上中部绕行于腹部之左右，先升后降，所以古人称为“回肠”。《黄帝内经》说：“回肠大四寸，径一寸寸之少半，长二丈一尺，受谷一斗，水七升半。”

The upper and middle part of the large intestine circles around the abdomen, first rising up and then going down, forming a shape of a Chinese character (meaning circle). Thus it is named by ancient Chinese as “circled intestine”. According to the *Inner Canon of the Yellow Emperor*, the circled intestine is four cun (about twelve centimeters) large, and extends about two zhang and one chi (about seven meters) with a diameter of about three centimeters. The volume of the circled intestine can be measured by one dou of grain (approximately 6.25 kg) or seven and a half sheng of water (about 4.7 kg).

广肠
Broad intestine

大肠下部管腔扩大，沿脊下部下行至魄门(肛门)，故古人称为“广肠”。《黄帝内经》说：“广肠大八寸，径二寸寸之大半，长二尺八寸，受谷九升三合八分合之一。”

The lower part of the large intestine broadens and goes along the spine to the anus. Thus the ancient Chinese people named it as “broad intestine”. According to the *Inner Canon of the Yellow Emperor*, the “broad intestine” is eight cun (about twenty-four centimeters) large, and extends about two chi and eight cun (about ninety centimeters) with a diameter of about seven centimeters. The volume of the “broad intestine” can be measured by nine sheng, three he and eight fenhe of grain (about 5.8 kg).

名词解释 Explanation of Terms

魄门

大肠与小肠之会称为阑门，此处能阻止小肠内的精微物质流入。

Anus

The ileocecal valve is where the small intestine and large intestine meet. It functions to prevent the nutrients in the small intestine from flowing into the large intestine.

阑门

即肛管与肛门及其周围的括约肌组织，有控制粪便排出的作用。

Ileocecal valve

The anal canal, anus and musculus sphincter around it function to control the defecation.

名词解释 Explanation of Terms

回肠

回肠是大肠的上段部分，上接小肠，下接广肠，它包括解剖学中的盲肠、升结肠、横结肠和降结肠。

Circled intestine

The circled intestine refers to the upper part of large intestine. It connects the small intestine and the broad intestine. It includes the cecum, the ascending colon, transverse colon, and descending colon in modern anatomy.

广肠

广肠是大肠的下段部分，上接回肠，下端终于魄门，它包括现代解剖学中的乙状结肠和直肠。

Broad intestine

The broad intestine refers to the lower part of the large intestine. It connects the circled intestine and ends at the anus. It includes the sigmoid colon and rectum in modern anatomy.

科学起居要防“五劳七伤”

To avoid the “five fatigues” and “seven harms”

《素问·宣明五气篇》提出的“五劳所伤”，即久视伤血，久卧伤气，久坐伤肉，久立伤骨，久行伤筋。视、卧、坐、行、立是人体的五种体态和功能活动，这五种体态功能，既不能长时间地不活动，又不能活动过度，否则都会影响人体健康。

“七伤”见《诸病源候论·虚劳候》，七种劳伤为：大饱伤脾；大怒气逆伤肝；强力举重，久坐湿地伤肾；形寒，寒饮伤肺；忧愁思虑伤心；风雨寒暑伤形；大恐惧，不节伤志。

1. 久视

属神劳太过的一种形式。看报、看电视不宜过久，一般 1 小时左右，就休息片刻，或走动或眺望远方，以减少眼睛的疲劳损伤。

1. Seeing for too long

This is a kind of mental fatigue. Do not read or watch TV for too long. Take a break, walk about, or look into the distance every hour to relieve the strain of your eyes.

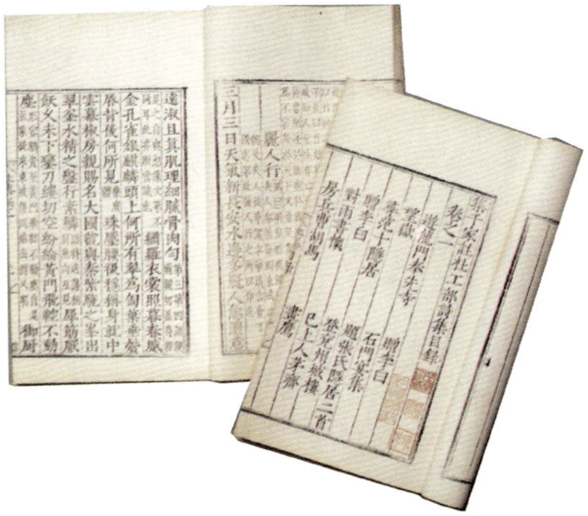

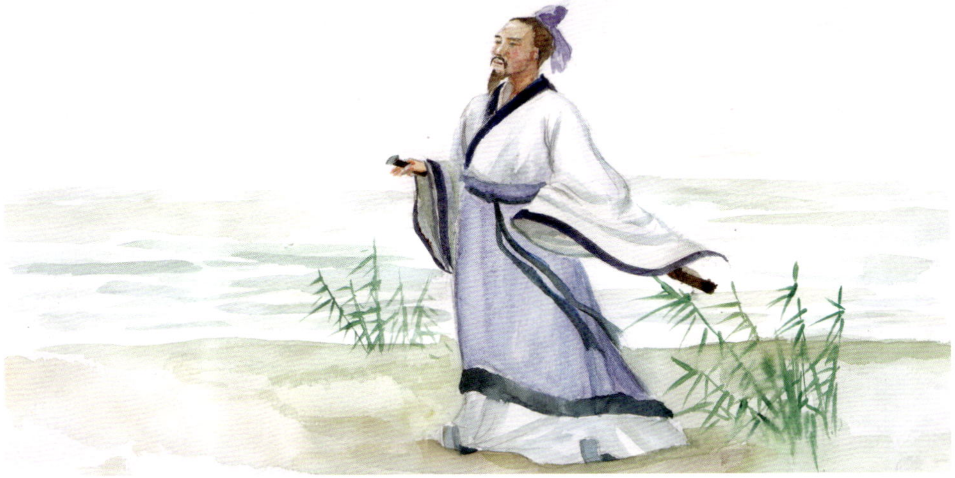

The chapter “The Exposition of the Five Qis” of the *Inner Canon* puts forward the concept of “harm from five kinds of fatigue”–seeing for too long harms blood, lying in bed for too long harms vital energy, sitting for too long harms flesh, sitting for too long harms bones, and walking or running for too long harms tendons. Seeing, lying, sitting, walking and standing are five functions of the human body. Long inactivity or too much activity in any of these five functions will affect one’s health.

“Seven harms” is discussed in “The Symptoms of Exhaustion” in *Treatise on Causes and Symptoms of Various Diseases*, which means: eating too much harms the spleen; fury and depression harm the liver; lifting heavy weights or sitting on wet ground for long harms the kidneys; cold and cold drinks harm the lungs; sorrows and worries harm the heart; extreme weather harms the body; fright and indulgence harm the spirit.

2. 久坐

属形劳太过的一种形式。人应适当多走路，勤活动，这样才能改善血液循环，加强肌肉锻炼，使自己胖瘦适宜，达到自我防病、保健及延年益寿的目的。

2. Sitting for too long

This is a kind of physical fatigue. Walk and exercise more to improve blood circulation. Intensify the exercise of your muscles to keep your figure. These will help to resist diseases, protect your health, and prolong your life.

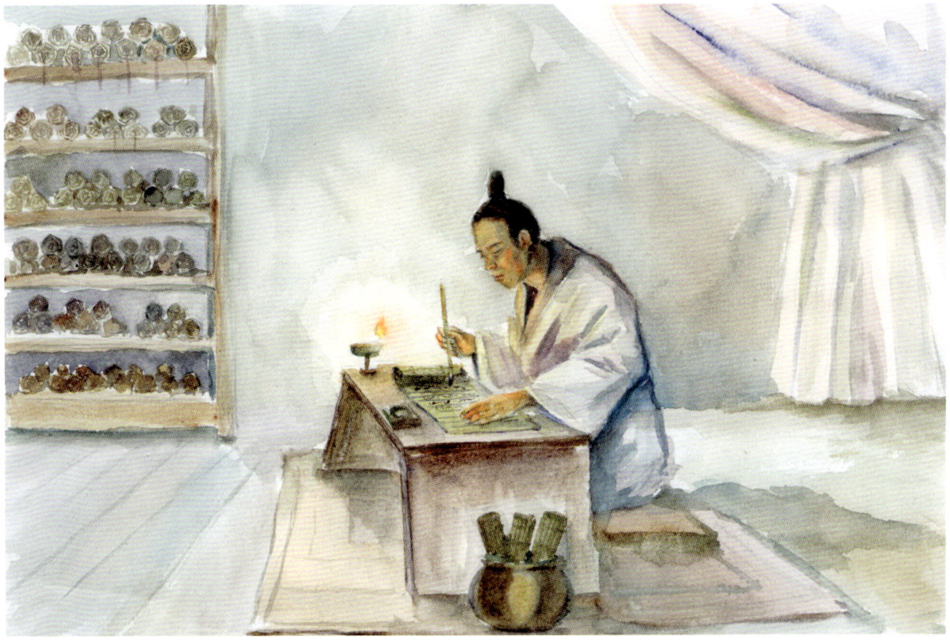

3. 久立

属形劳太过的一种形式。如果长时间站着不动，骨骼的弹性与韧性就会减弱，脆性变大，一旦受到外力的冲击就使部分组织和细胞的营养失调，出现气滞血凝，导致某些骨骼关节发生畸形或活动障碍，因此站立时间不可过久。

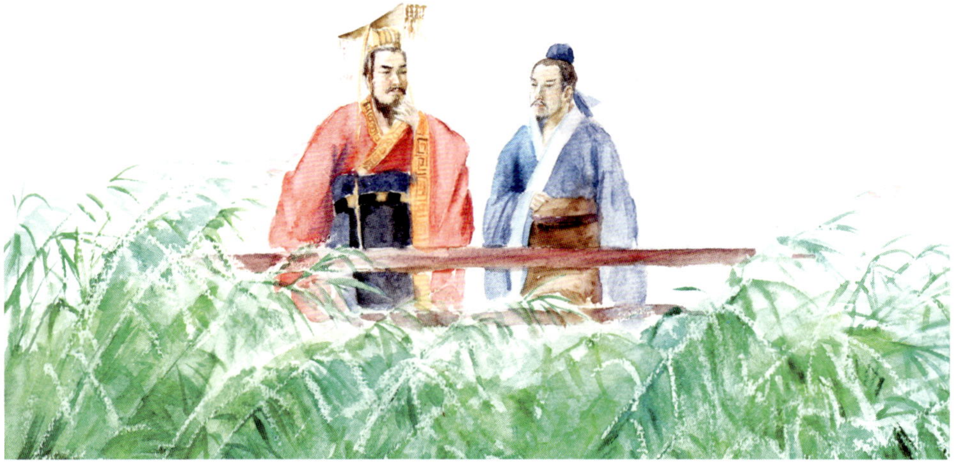

3. Standing for too long

This is a kind of physical fatigue. Standing for too long can make your bones less elastic and tough and more fragile, so that any impact from an external force will cause malnutrition in some tissues and cells as well as the stagnation of blood and vital energy, deforming some joints or making them difficult to move. Therefore it is inadvisable to stand for too long.

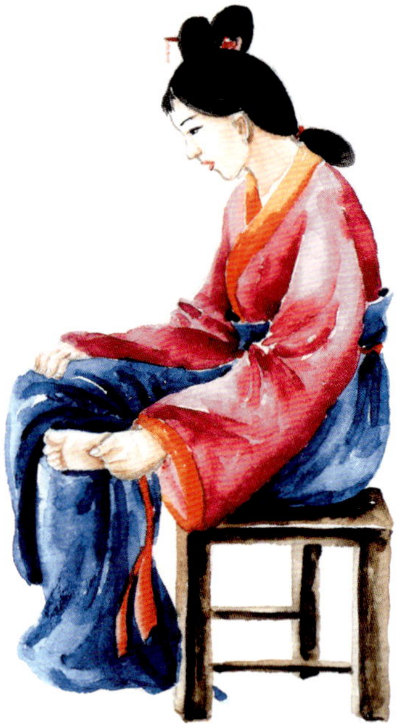

久立后，要按摩脚
Massage the feet after standing long

4. 久行

属形劳太过的一种形式。长时间远距离地奔走或跑步，就容易使肢体、特别是下肢关节周围的韧带等筋腱组织扭伤或劳损，招致疾病。因此，行走散步要适度，注意使全身放松，调匀呼吸，脚步均匀，“行不宜急”方能“气血畅通，百脉流通，内外协调”，健康持久。

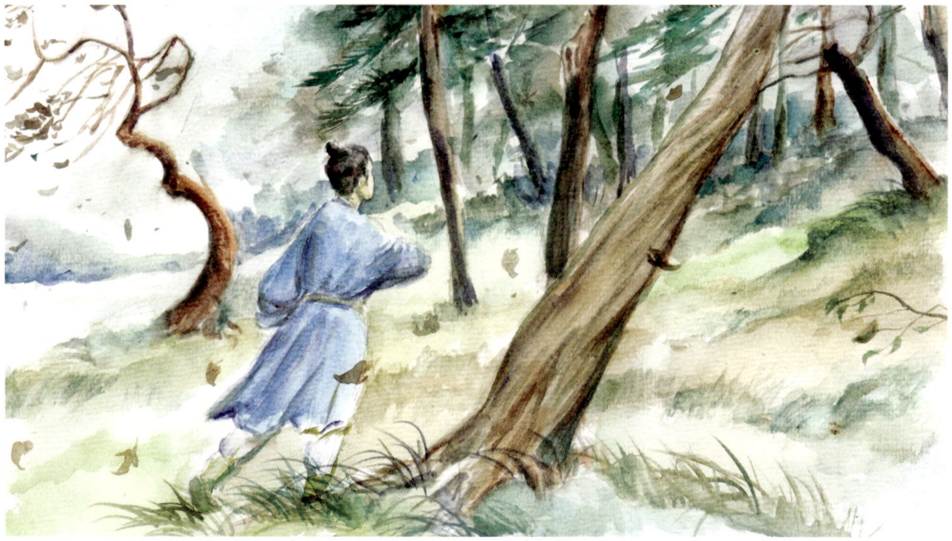

4. Walking or running for too long

This is a kind of physical fatigue. To walk or run for a long time and distance is likely to sprain or strain ligaments and other tendons, especially those around the joints of your legs. So one should not walk too much. When walking, relax your whole body and take even breaths and steps. Only by walking without haste can your blood and vital energy flow without obstruction through all the channels, bringing about a harmony between the internal and the external of your body, which can ensure lasting health.

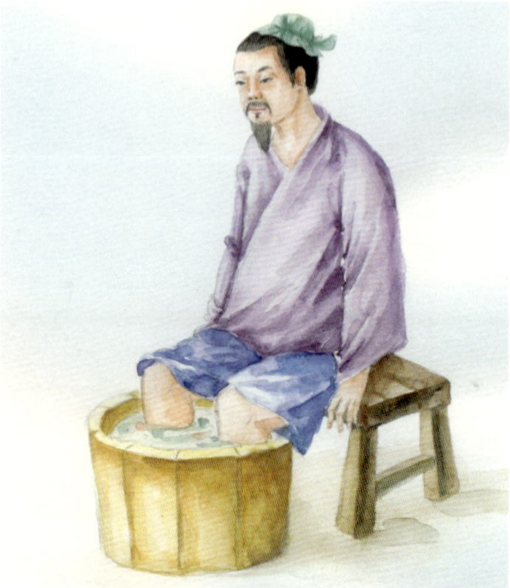

久行后，要泡足和腿
Soak the feet and legs after a long walk

5. 久卧

属安逸太过的一种形式。传统医学注重人体的“精、气、神”。气是维持生命的能源，养气有助于延寿，提高生命质量。人们经常躺着休息，若不进行肢体的活动，不仅肢体筋骨器官司窍之气会渐趋衰弱，内脏各腑脏之气也会受到损害，致使人身体懒散，精神萎靡不振。长此以往，必大大危害人的健康。

5. Lying in bed for too long

This is an instance of excessive ease and comfort. Traditional medicine emphasizes a person's essence (jing), qi, and spirit (shen). Qi is the energy that sustains life. To nurture qi, therefore, can help to prolong your life and improve its quality. If you lie in bed to rest or sleep too much, without doing any exercise, it will not only weaken the qi of your bones, muscles and orifices, but also affect the qi of your internal organs. This will lead to indolence and lethargy and, over time, a serious deterioration of health.

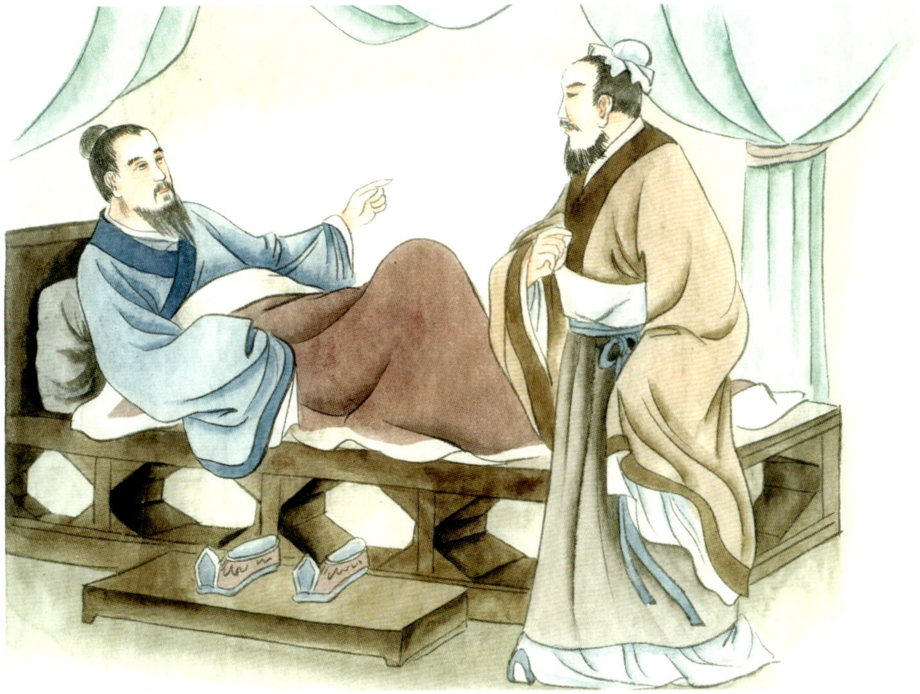

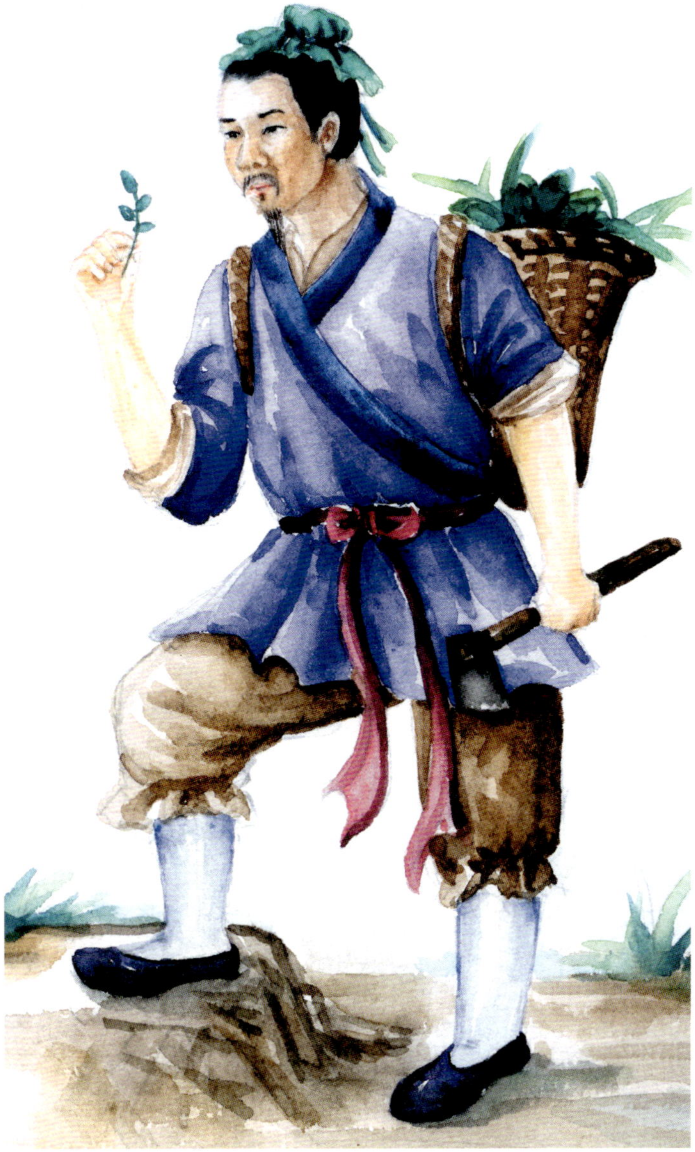

采药养气图

Gathering medicinal herbs to nurture the internal qi

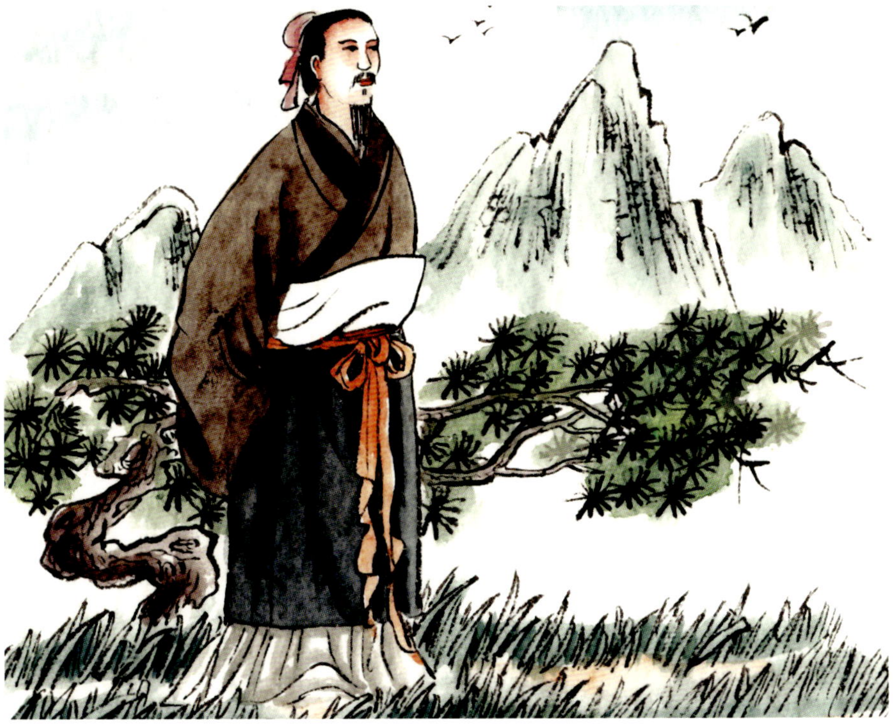

久卧要行走

Walk after lying long

柒 食 养

VII. Dietary Regimen

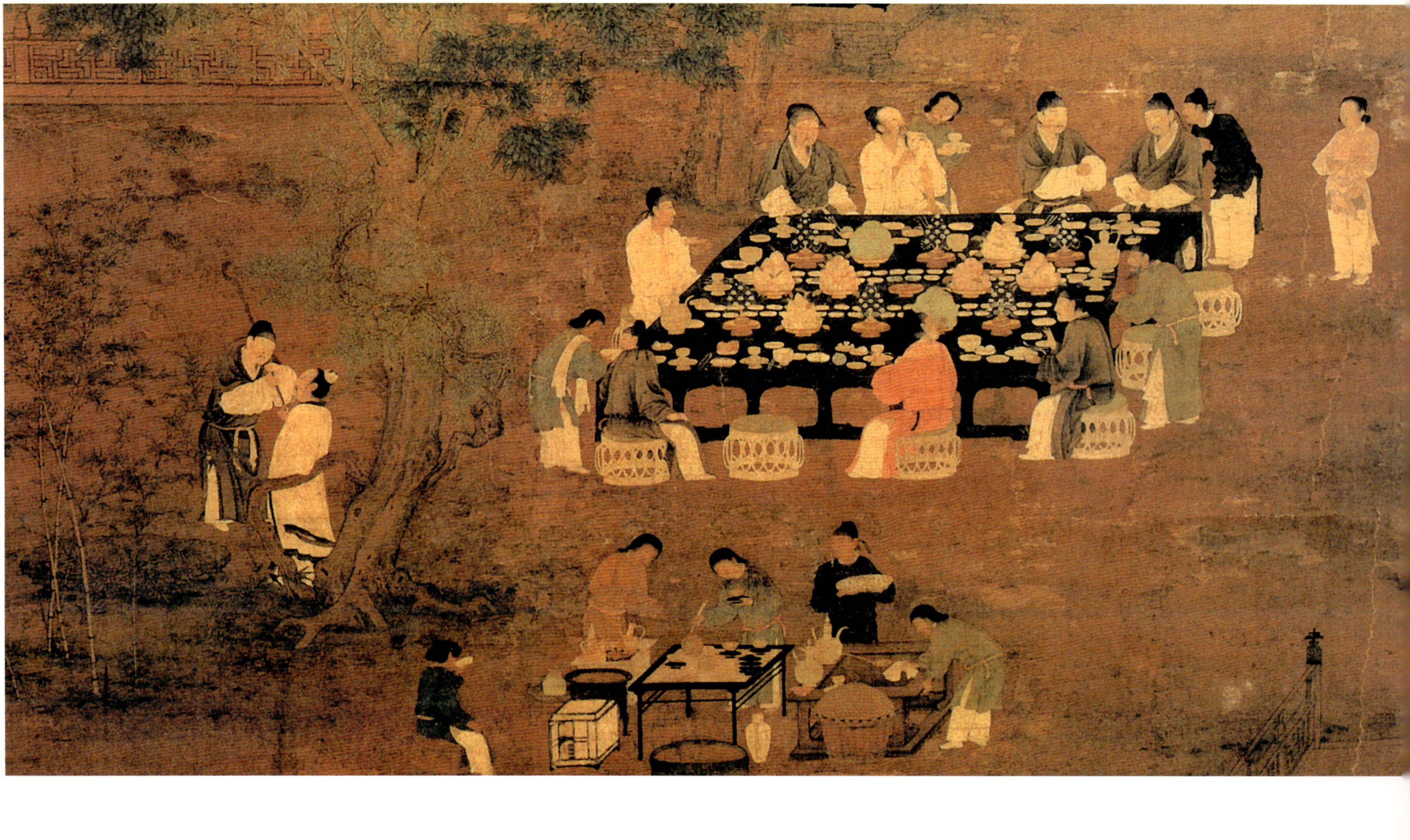

古人说："主身者神，养气者精，益精者气，资气者食。食者生民之天，活人之本也。"明确指出了食物是人体三宝——精、气、神的基础。本篇还包括了饮，即饮水、饮茶。

As ancient Chinese put it, "Spirit dominates the body, essence nurtures qi, qi promotes/supports essence, and food builds up qi. Food is heaven for the people and is fundamental to life." This observation makes it clear that food is the basis for the Three Treasures of the Body, i.e. essence, qi ('inner energy') and spirit. This chapter also covers drinking, i.e. drinking water and tea.

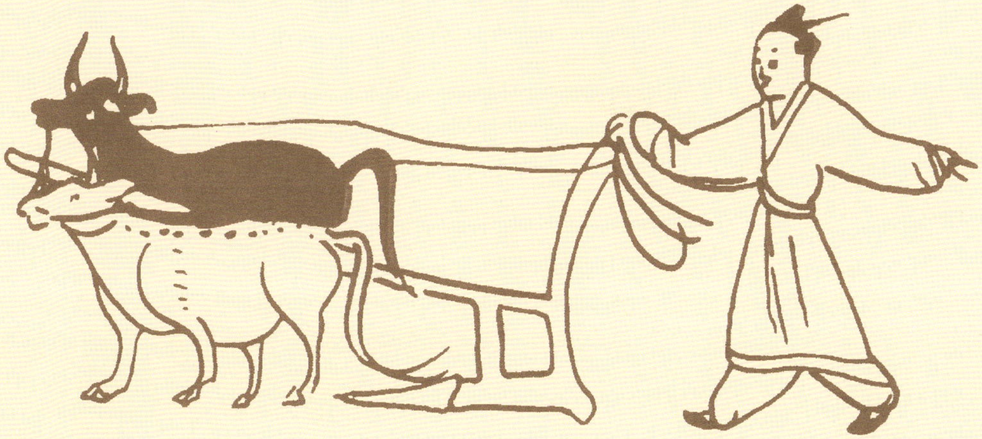

食养是中国医学宝库中重要组成部分，为中华民族的防治疾病、养生保健都做出了贡献。

饮食是人体营养的主要来源，是维持人体生命活动的必要条件。饮食调理得当，不仅可以保证人体功能正常，提高机体的抗病能力，还可以治疗某些疾病。相反饮食不足或饮食不当，则可诱发某些疾病。

Diet is an important part of Chinese traditional medicine, which contributes to disease prevention and health care of the Chinese nation.

Food and drink are the main source of nutrition for the human body and a necessary condition for the continuation of life. To eat and drink properly can not only enable the human body to function normally and be more resistant to illness, but also cure some diseases. On the other hand, insufficient or improper food and drink can cause certain diseases.

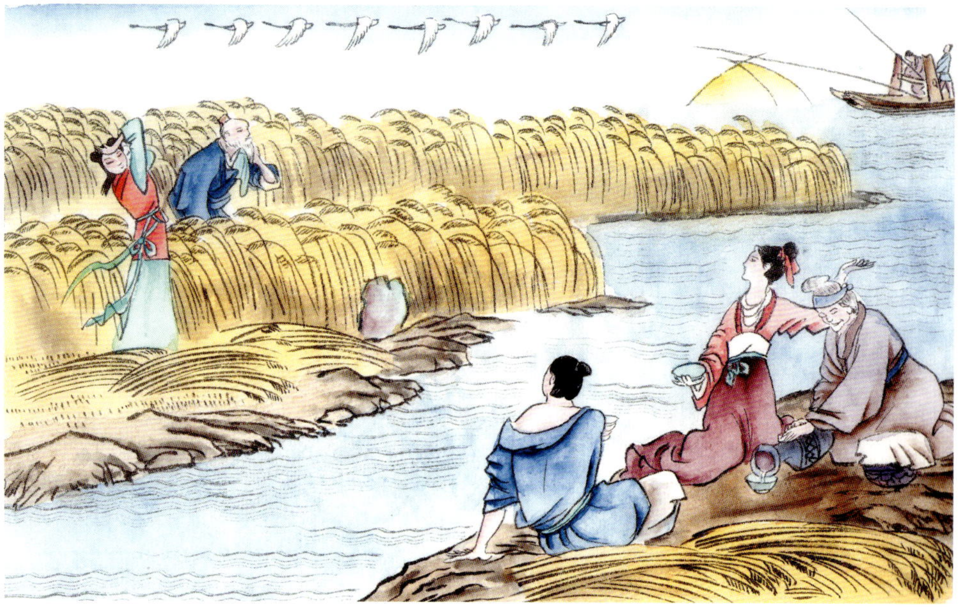

先民稼穑图

Ancient people planting and harvesting

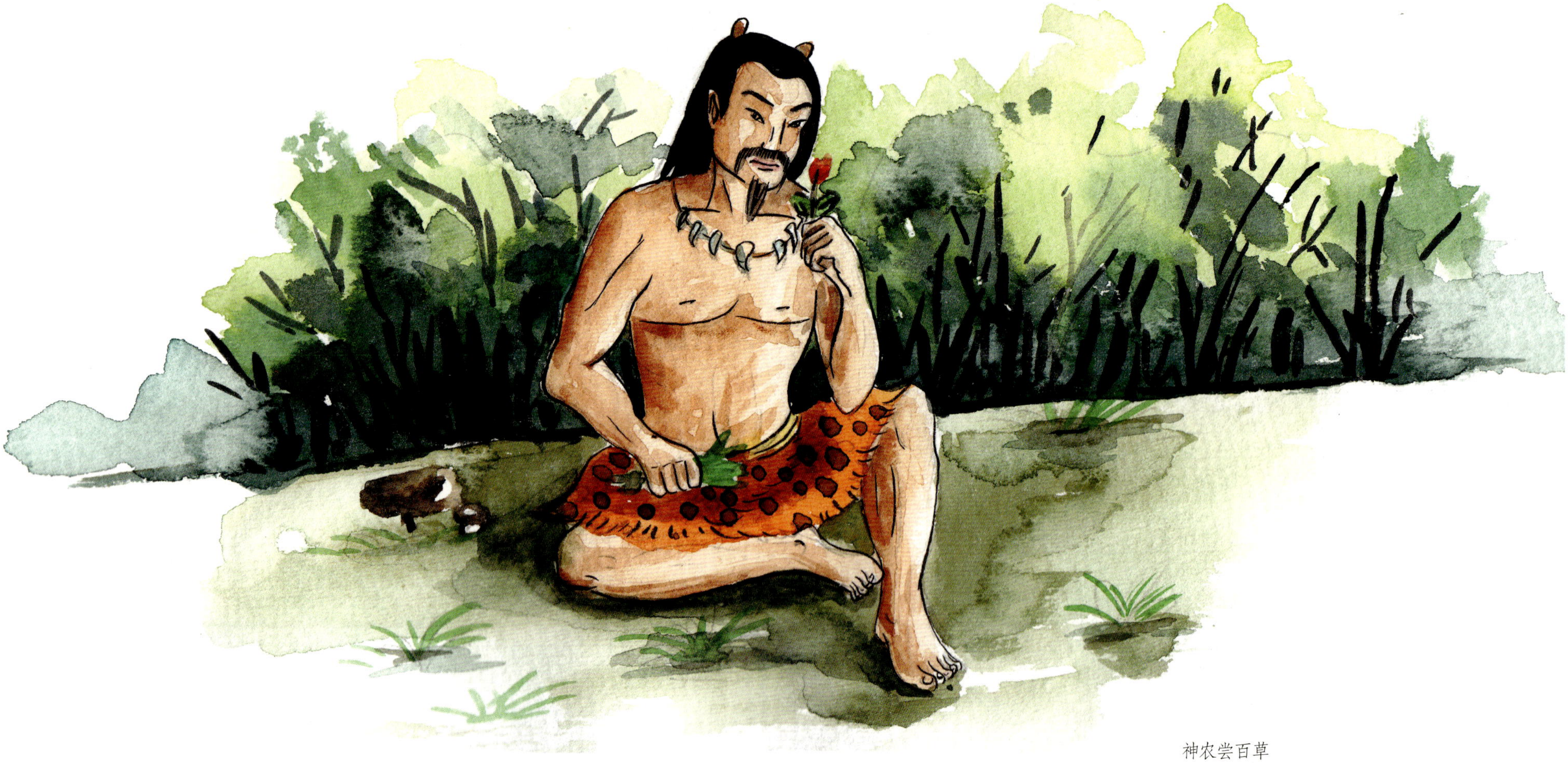

神农尝百草

Sheng Nong — the Divine Cultivator — tasting the medicinal herbs

调和五味

Balancing the “five tastes”

中医强调食五谷以养人。古人早就认识到各种食物中所含的营养素不同，只有做到使各种食物合理搭配，才能使人体得到各种不同的营养素，满足各种生理功能的基本要求。粮谷、肉类、蔬菜、果品等是饮食主要的组成内容，人们必须根据需要兼而取之，才能称之为合理的营养，有益于人体健康。这就是古人强调的“杂食五谷，粗细搭配”原则。

Traditional Chinese Medicine stresses the body-nourishing effect of the five crops. Ancient Chinese realized that different foods contain different nutrients and satisfy various physiological needs. Grains, meat, vegetables and fruits are the main components of a diet. People should keep a varied diet suiting their respective needs. Only in this way can they get the nutrition they need, and improve their health. This actually accords with ancient Chinese’s dietary principle of “keeping a varied diet and combining coarse and refined grains”.

五谷为养

The “five grains”, a source of nutrition

谷类是人体的主食，是人体必需的碳水化合物与热量的主要来源。五谷一般是指黍、稷、麦、稻、豆。

Grains are the staple food for humans, and the main source of carbohydrate and caloric power indispensable to the human body. The five crops generally refer to millet, soybean, wheat, barley and rice.

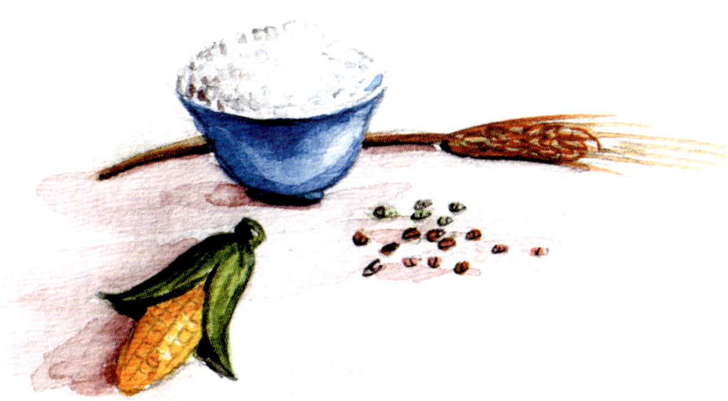

五菜为充

The “five vegetables”, indispensable nutrients

蔬菜富含多种微量元素和纤维素，是饮食中不可缺少的辅助食品。一般是指葵、韭、藿、薤、葱五种。

Vegetables are rich in many trace elements and nutrients. They are indispensible supplementary foodstuff. The “five vegetables” generally refer to cluster mallow, leek, betony, shallots and green onions.

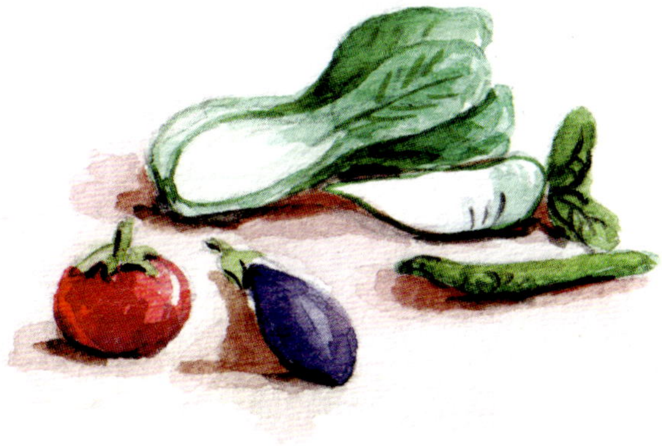

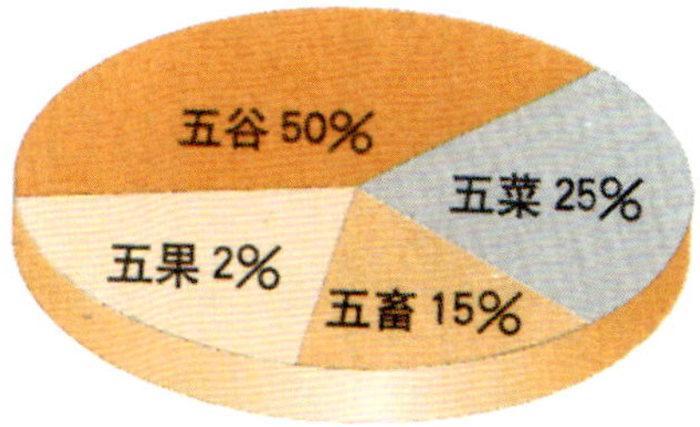

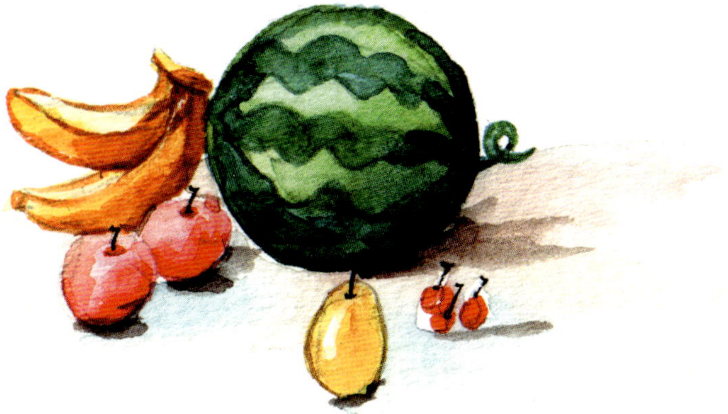

五果为助

The “five fruits”, essential food supplements

水果富含维生素、糖和有机酸等，是助消化、平衡饮食的辅助食物。五果一般指枣、李、杏、栗、桃。

Rich in vitamins, sugar and organic alcohols, Fruits are subsidiary foods aiding digestion and balancing the diet. The five fruits generally refer to date, plum, apricot, chestnut and peach.

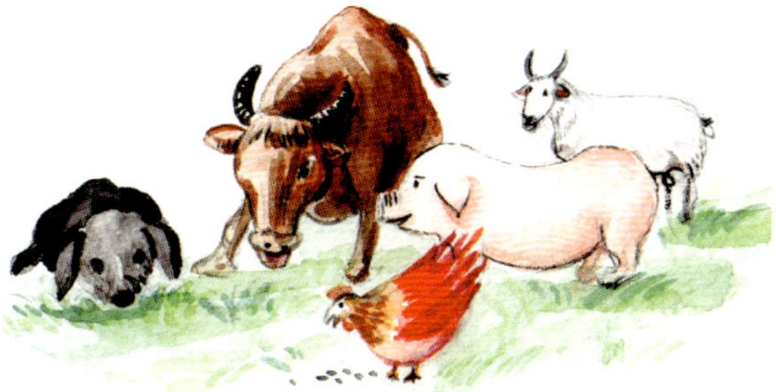

五畜为益

Meat of the “five domestic animals”, health boosters

肉食多含高蛋白、高脂肪、高热量和人体必需的氨基酸，是人体修补组织与增强抗病能力的重要营养物质。

Meat is rich in protein, fat, calorie, and amino acid necessary to the human body. It supplies important nutrients for improving the human body’s rehabilitative capacity and disease resistance.

四季饮食

Diets of the four seasons

“食”，主要指进食，而“饮”，则包括饮水、饮酒、饮茶等。“有节”则是强调食和饮水必须有节制，有规律。

“Eating” mainly refers to eating food, while “drinking” refers to drinking water, alcohol, tea and so on. “Restraint” stresses moderate and regular eating and drinking.

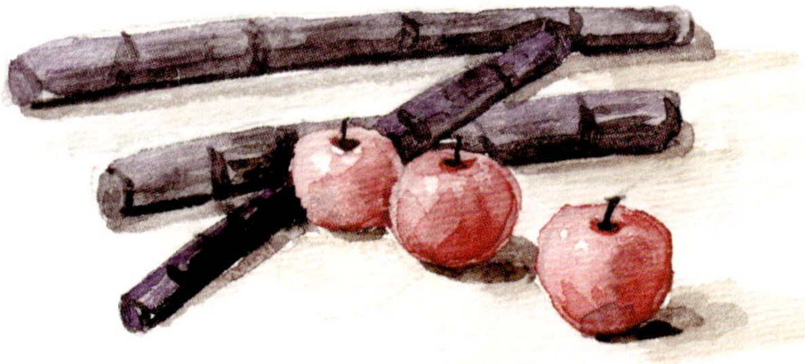

春季饮食

Foods for spring

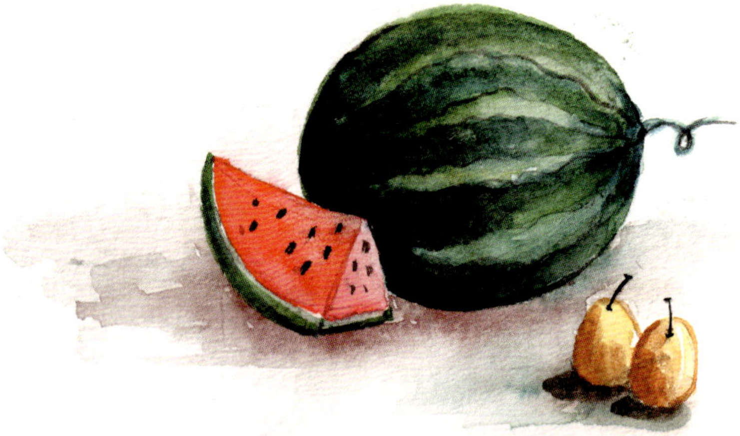

夏季饮食

Foods for summer

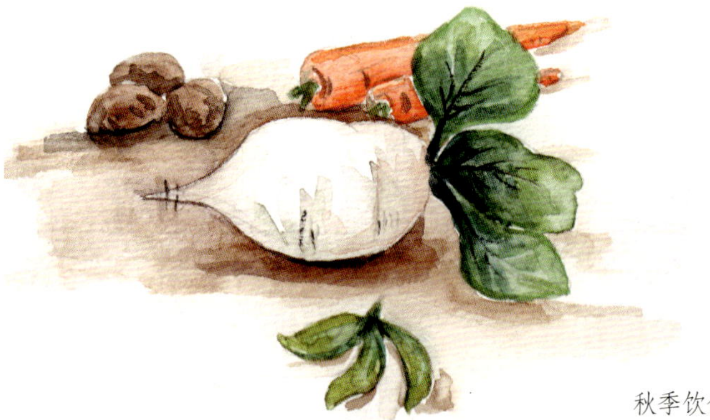

秋季饮食

Foods for autumn

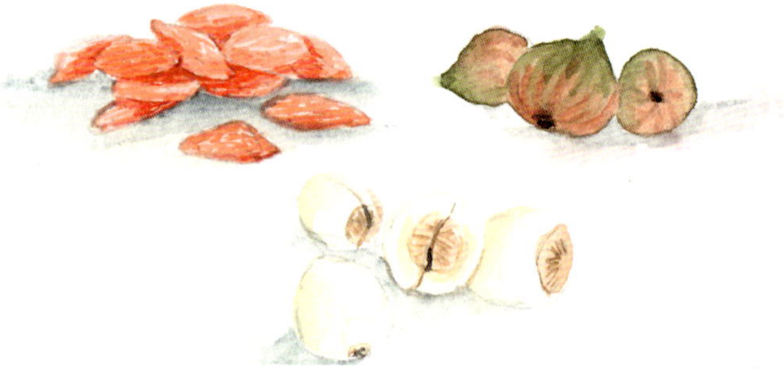

冬季饮食

Foods for winter

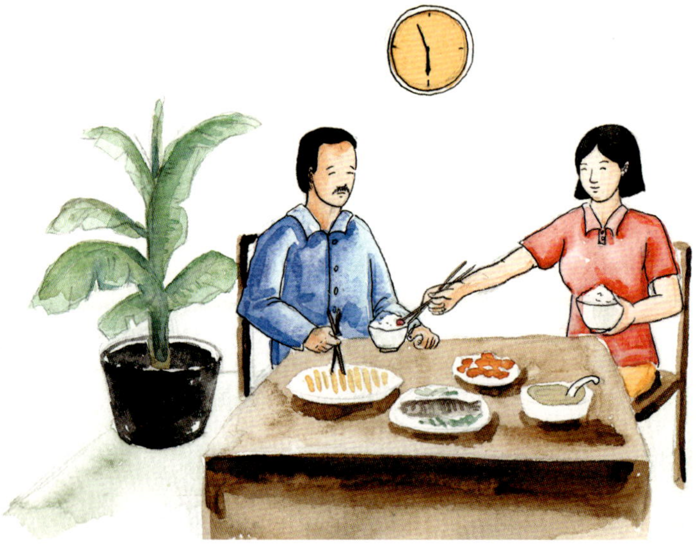

饮食有节

To have a moderate diet

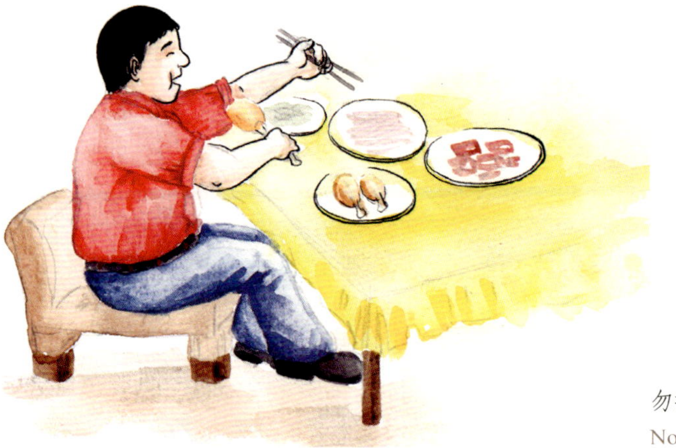

勿挑食

Not to be a picky eater

饮食是营养人体、维持生命的物质基础，历来就有“药补不如食补”的说法。

食养的原料，主要是指进行食养所需要的食物与中药。食物则种类繁多，有动物类、植物类、禽蛋类等。

Food is the material basis for nourishing and sustaining life. Just as the saying goes, “Diet cures more than doctors.”

Dietary raw materials mainly refer to food and medicine for the dietary needs. There are a wide variety of foods, such as animals, plants, and eggs.

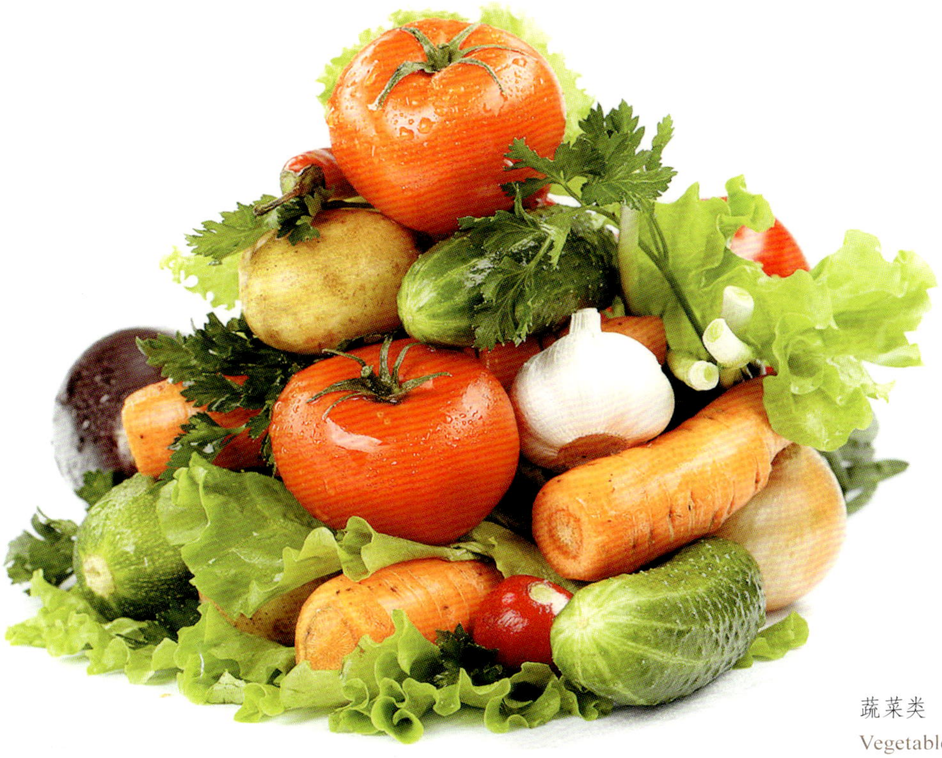

蔬菜类
Vegetables

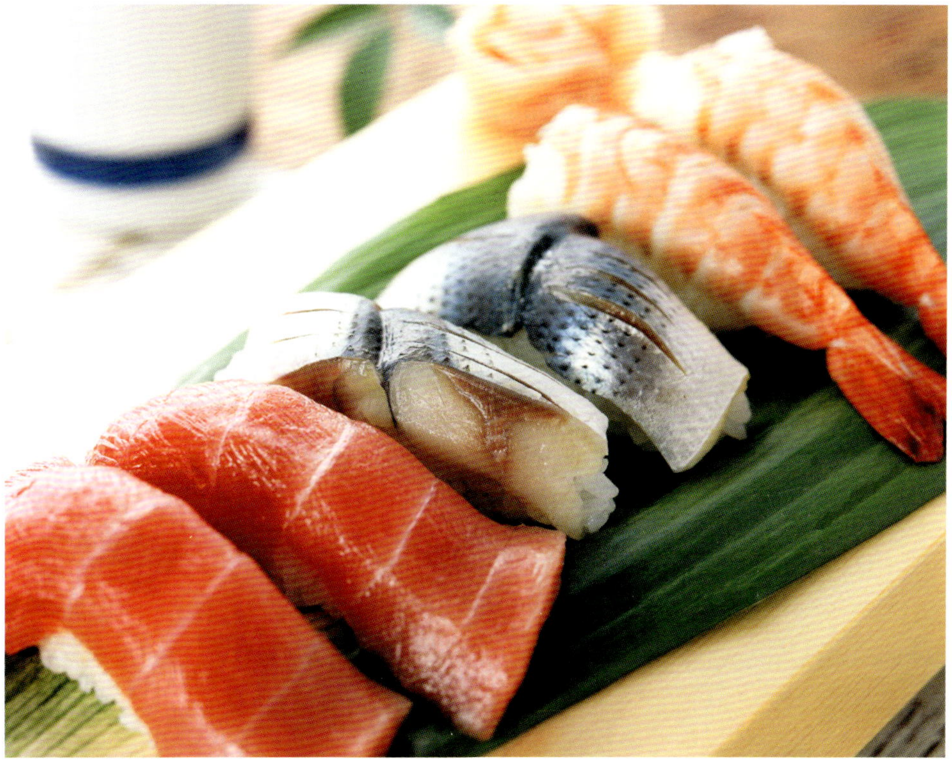

肉食类
Meats

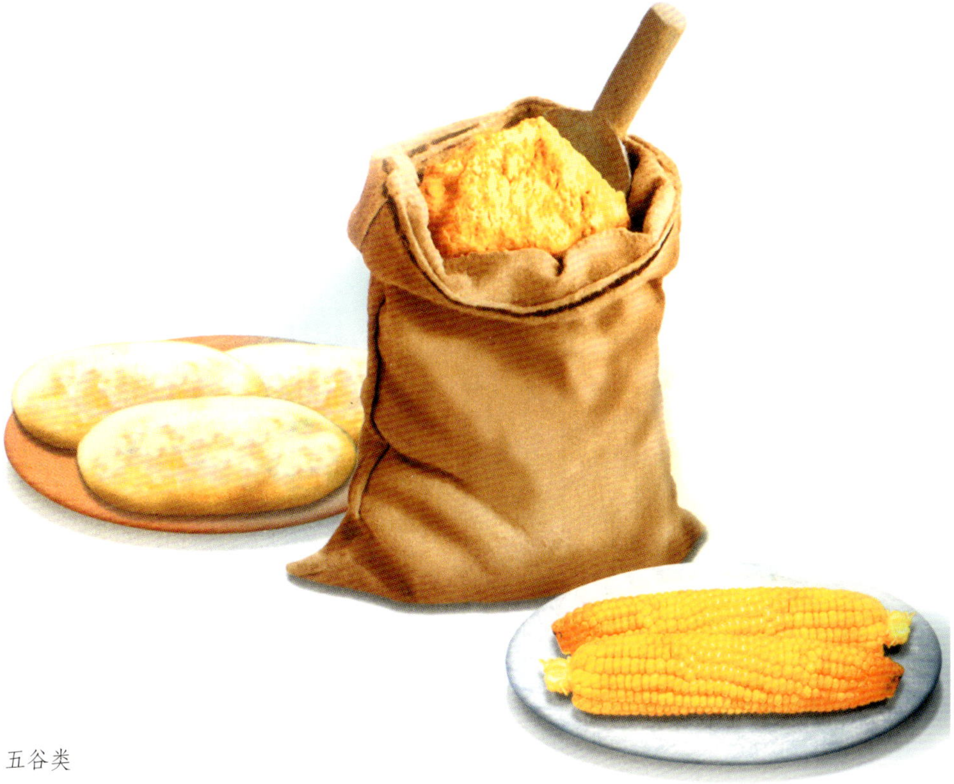

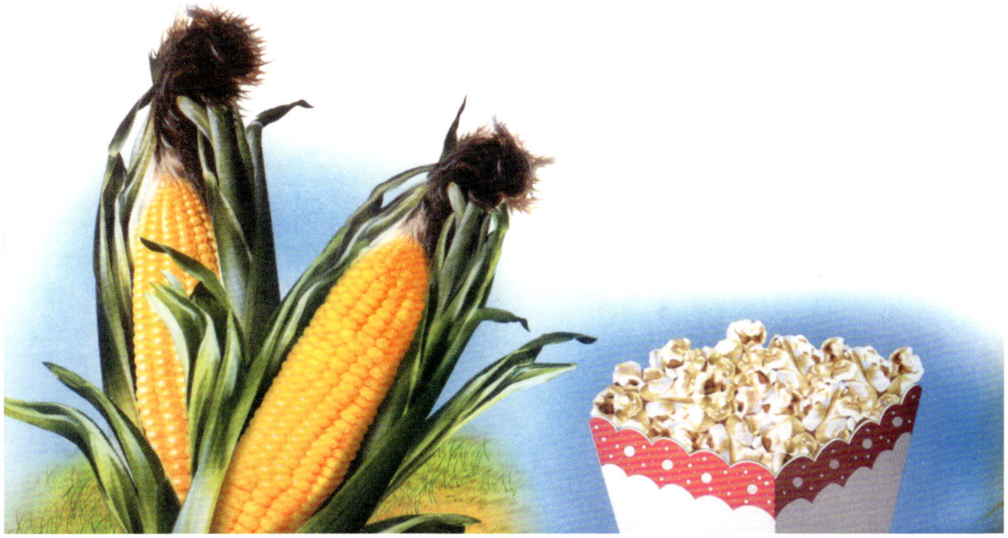

五谷类
Cereals

养气、血、阴、阳的食养品

Foods for the nourishment of qi, blood, yin, and yang

养气、血、阴、阳的常用食物有：鸡、鸭、鱼、兔肉、羊肉、海参、牛肉、猪肝、萝卜、灵芝、燕窝、甲鱼、小麦、绿豆、鸽蛋、西瓜、鸡蛋、雪梨、羊肝、狗肉、猪肚、猪肘、鹿肉、麋角等。

Foods commonly used for the nourishment of qi, blood, yin, and yang are: chicken, duck, fish, rabbit, lamb, sea cucumber, beef, pork liver, radish, ganoerma, cubilose, turtle, wheat, mung bean, pigeon eggs, watermelon, eggs, pear, jemmy, pig tripe, pork leg, venison, elk horn, etc.

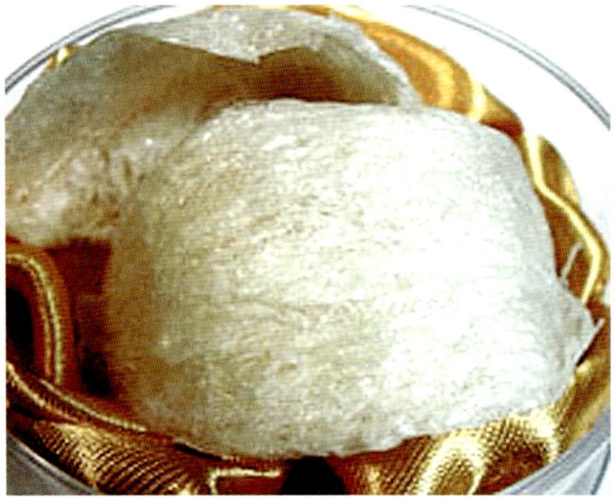

中医认为燕窝养阴润燥、益气补中，治虚损、咳痰喘、咯血、久痢，适宜于体质虚弱，营养不良人群，可促进免疫功能，有延缓人体衰老、延年益寿的功效。

Traditional Chinese Medicine believes that the bird's nest can cultivate yin energy and relieve dryness, increase inner energy and tonify the internal organs, treat physical weakness, cure coughing, expectoration & panting, hemoptysis and protracted dysentery. Suitable for the weak and ill-nourished, it can slow down the aging process, and prolong life.

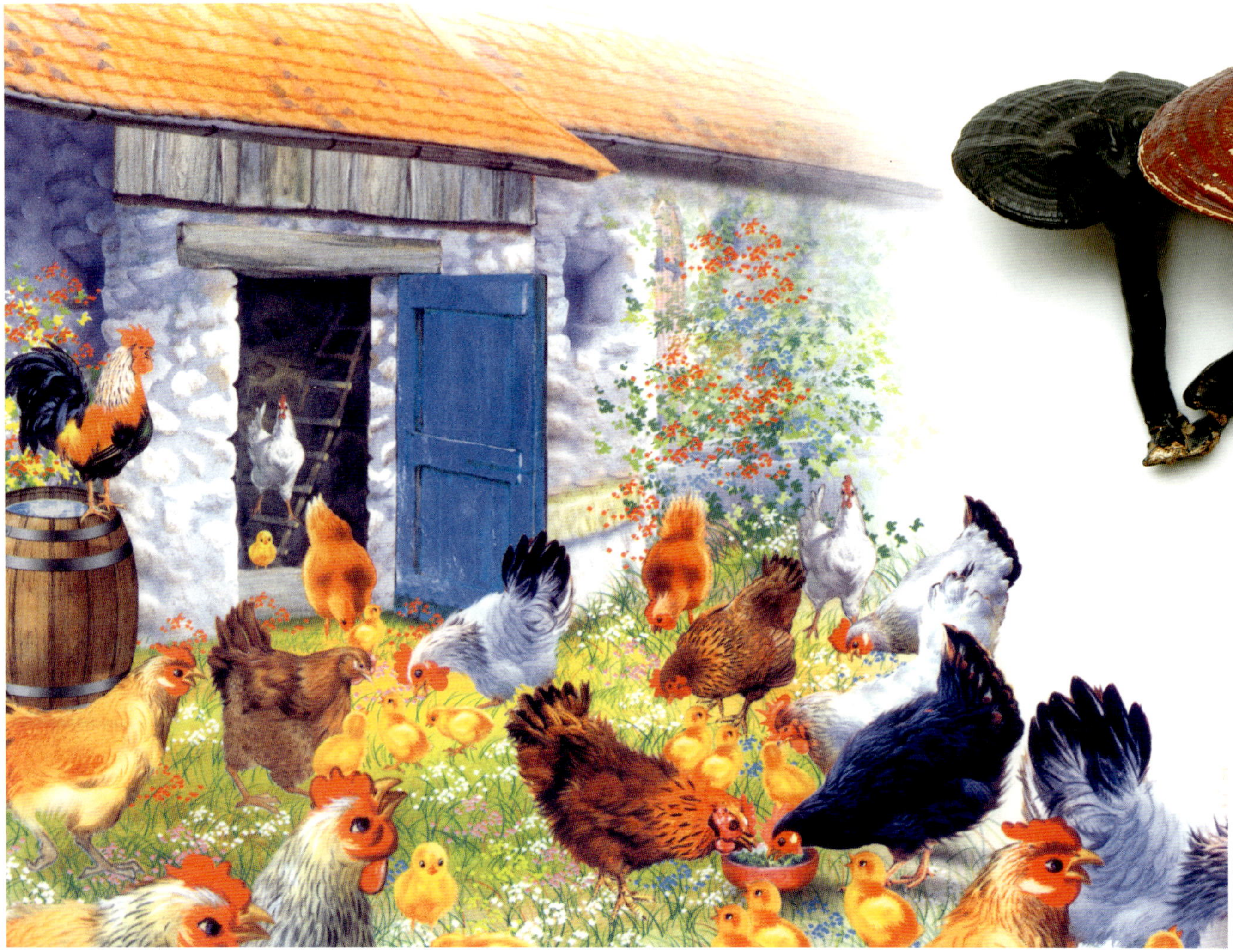

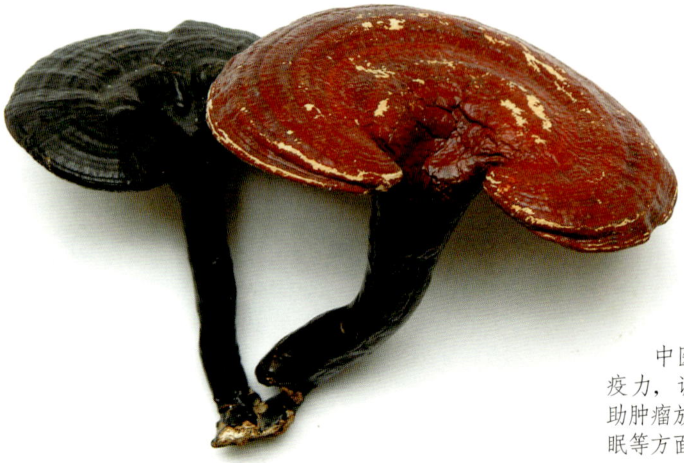

中医认为灵芝在增强人体免疫力，调节血糖，控制血压，辅助肿瘤放化疗，保肝护肝，促进睡眠等方面均具有显著疗效。

Traditional Chinese Medicine believes that ganoderma can significantly strengthen the immunity of the human body, regulate its blood sugar levels, control the blood pressure, aid the radiation treatment of tumors, guard and tonify the liver, and improve sleep.

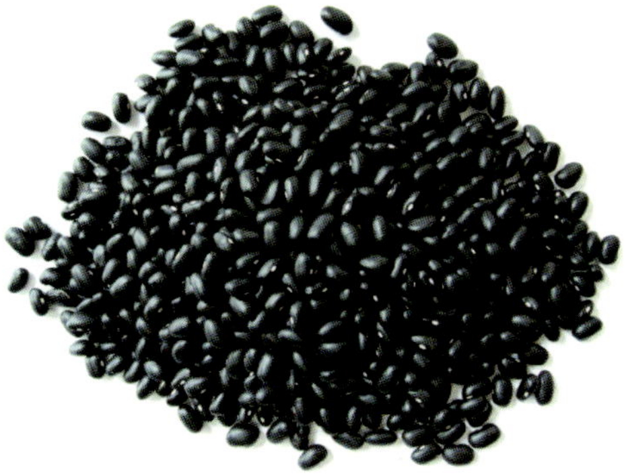

黑豆是植物中营养最丰富的保健佳品。中医认为黑豆能够补肾养气。黑豆营养丰富，黑豆中的蛋白质、不饱和脂肪酸和粗纤维的含量很高，它还含有丰富的对人体有益的微量元素。常食黑豆，能软化血管，滋润皮肤，延缓衰老。

Black beans are most nutritious health-preserving food of all plants. Traditional Chinese Medicine believes that they can tonify the kidney and build up inner energy. They are rich in protein, unsaturated fatty acid and cellulose; they also contain abundant trace elements beneficial to the human body. Eating black beans regularly can soften blood vessels, nourish the skin and slow down the aging process.

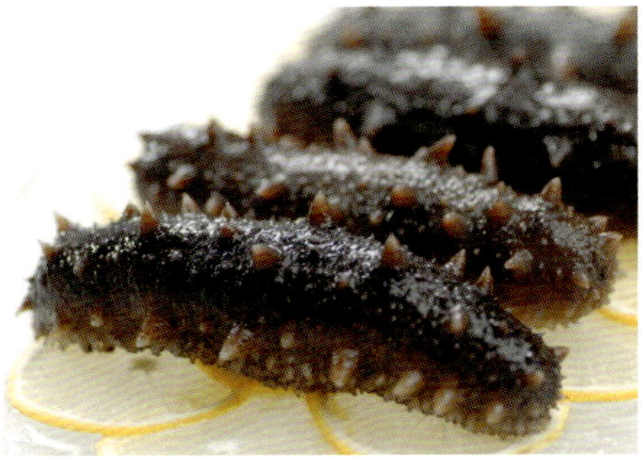

中医认为海参能够补肾养血。现代研究表明，海参具有提高记忆力、延缓性腺衰老、防止动脉硬化、糖尿病以及抗肿瘤等作用。

Traditional Chinese Medicine believes that sea cucumber can strengthen the kidney and improve blood-generating capacity. Modern studies have proven that sea cucumber can improve memory, slow down the aging of sex glands, prevent the hardening of arteries and help resist diabetes and tumors.

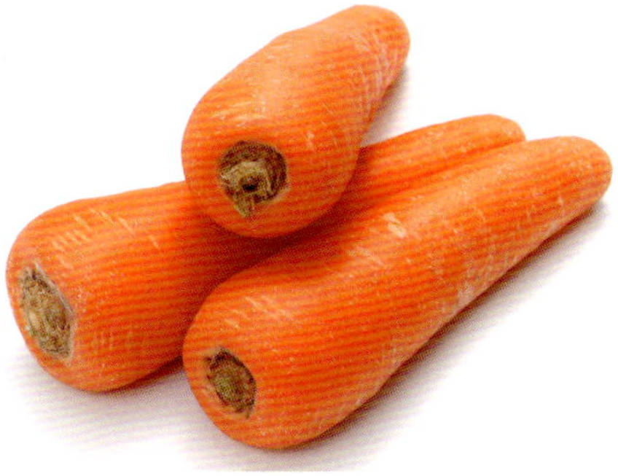

中医认为胡萝卜有健脾和胃、补肝明目、清热解毒、壮阳补肾的功效。现代研究表明，胡萝卜中维生素含量非常丰富，另含果胶、淀粉、无机盐和多种氨基酸，有助于预防心脏疾病和肿瘤。

Traditional Chinese Medicine believes that carrots can invigorate the spleen and stomach, strengthen the liver, improve eyesight, clear internal heat and toxic substance, improve sexual capacity and benefit the kidney. Modern studies have proven that carrots contain rich vitamins, as well as pectin, starch, inorganic salt and amino acids. They help prevent heart diseases and tumors.

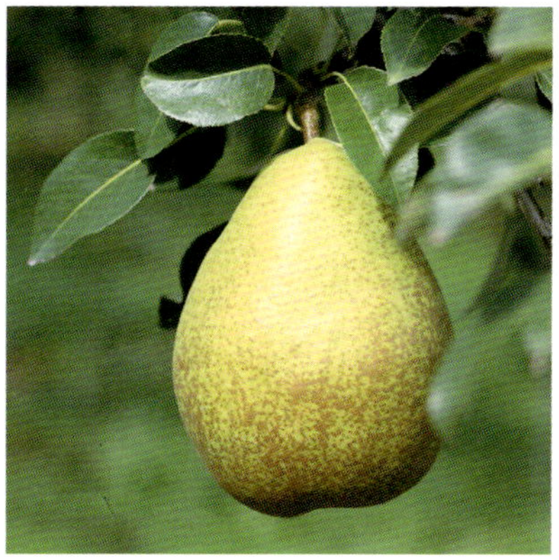

中医认为雪梨能养阴清肺，除烦止咳。雪梨的营养价值丰富，梨中含较多的糖类物质和多种维生素，可以帮助保护心脏，减轻疲劳，降低血压。而所含的配糖体及鞣酸等成分，则对咽喉有养护作用。

Traditional Chinese Medicine believes that pears can cultivate yin energy, clear lung-heat, relieve anxiety and suppress coughing. Very nutritious with abundant sugar and vitamins, they help protect the heart, relieve fatigue, and reduce blood pressure. The glycoside and tannic acid they contain are beneficial to the throat.

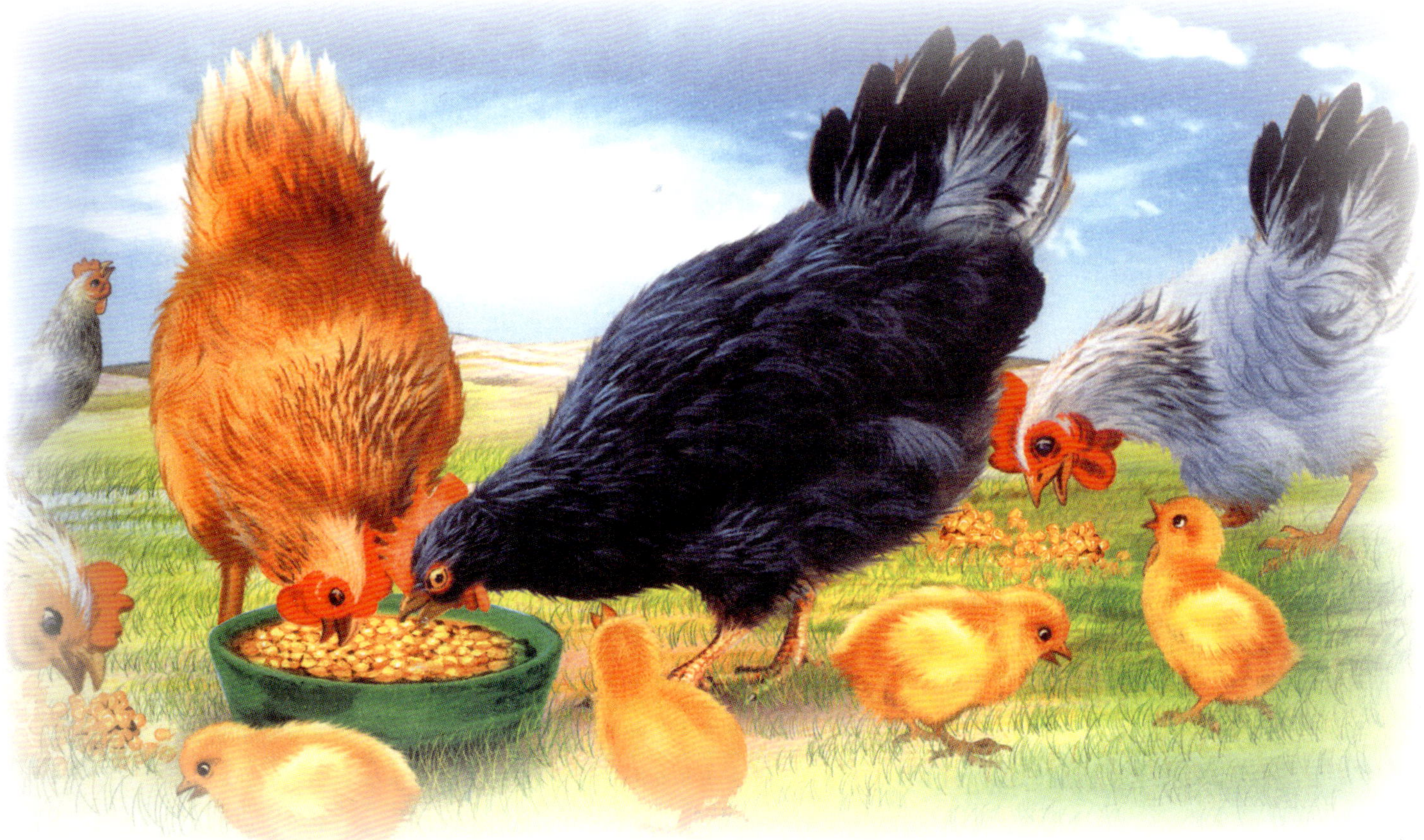

养心、肝、脾、肺、肾的食养品食物

Foods for the nourishment of heart, liver, spleen, lungs and kidneys

养心、肝、脾、肺、肾而常用的食物有：动物的肉、心、肝、肚、肾、鞭、脑髓、肺等。

Foods commonly used for the nourishment of heart, liver, spleen, lungs and kidney are: animal flesh, heart, liver, stomach, kidney, penis, encephala, lungs, turtles, etc.

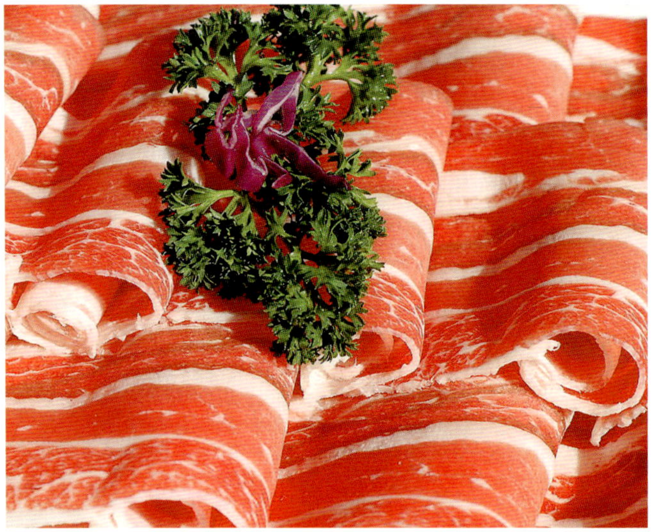

中医认为羊肉能补虚劳，祛寒冷，温补气血。

Traditional Chinese Medicine believes that mutton can reinforce insufficiency, dispel coldness, and warm up and supplement the qi and blood.

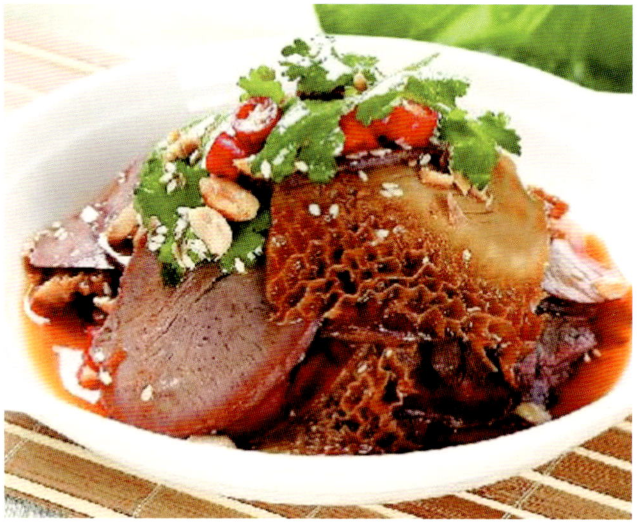

中医认为牛肚补虚，益脾胃，治病后虚羸，气血不足。

Traditional Chinese Medicine believes that beef tripe can reinforce insufficiency, benefit the spleen and stomach, improve rehabilitative weakness, and treat insufficiency in qi and blood.

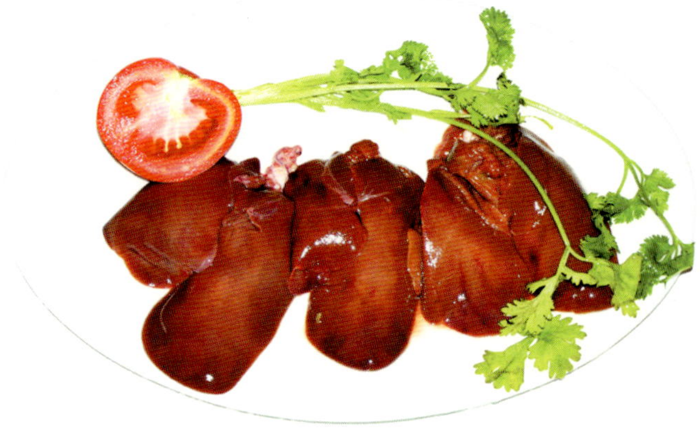

中医认为羊、鸡、鸭肝可补肝、明目、养血。

Traditional Chinese Medicine believes that duck liver can benefit the liver, improve eyesight and nourish the blood.

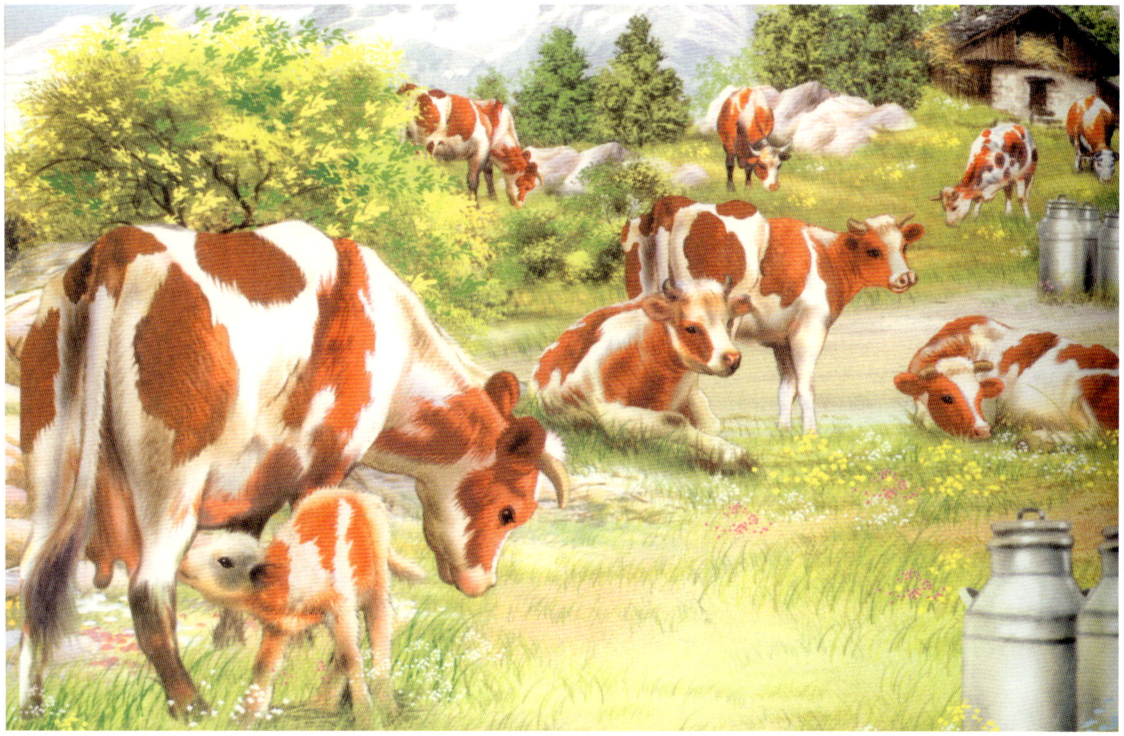

养筋、骨、肤、发、齿的食养品常用食物

Foods for the nourishment of tendons, bones, skin, hair and teeth

养筋、骨、肤、发、齿的常用的食物有：动物的骨、肾、肉、尾及牛肉、燕窝、蛋、冰糖、蜜糖、花生等。

Common foods that nourish tendons, bones, skin, hair and teeth: the bones, spleens, meat, tails of animals, beef, bird's nets, eggs, crystal sugar, honey, peanuts, etc.

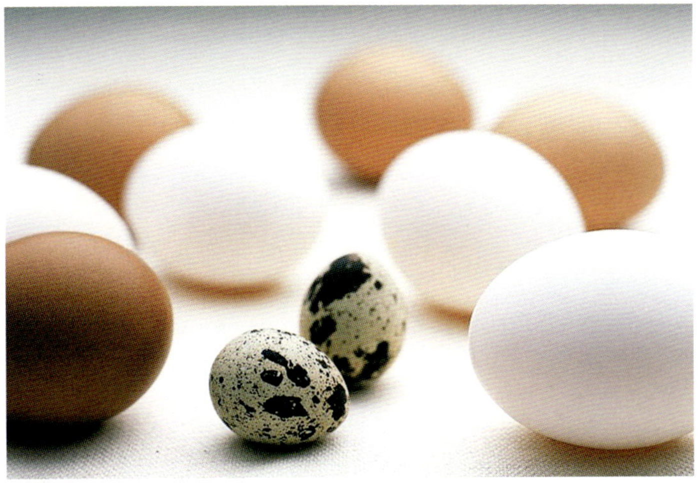

蛋清和蛋黄分别约占总可食部的2/3和1/3。蛋清中营养素主要是蛋白质，不但含有人体所需要的必需氨基酸，且氨基酸组成与人体组成模式接近，全蛋蛋白质几乎能被人体完全吸收利用，是食物中最理想的优质蛋白质。

The white and yolk account 2/3 and 1/3 of the edible part of an egg. The chief nutrient in the egg white is protein. Not only does the white contains the amino acids indispensable to the human body, but also the composition of the acids are similar to those in the human body. Thus, all the protein in the egg can be almost completely absorbed by human body. It is an ideal source of protein among all foods.

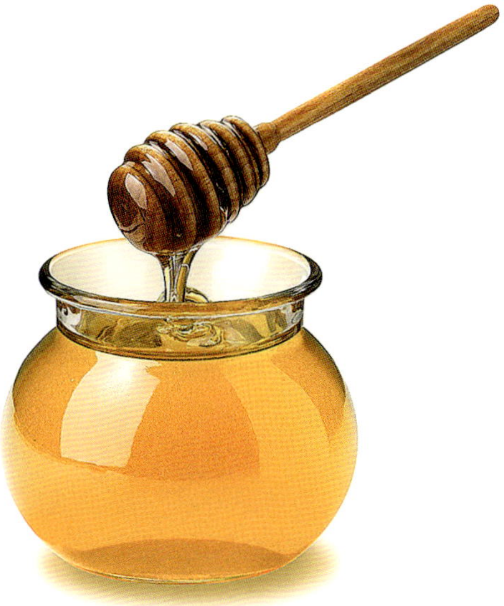

蜂蜜是一种营养丰富的天然滋养食品，含有多种无机盐和维生素、铁、钙、铜、锰、钾、磷等有机酸以及有益人体健康的微量元素，具有滋养、润燥、解毒之功效。

Honey is a nutritious natural food that contains inorganic salts, vitamins, organic acids (iron, calcium, copper, manganese, kalium and phosphor) and trace elements beneficial the human body. It can nourish the body, relieve dryness and remove toxic substance.

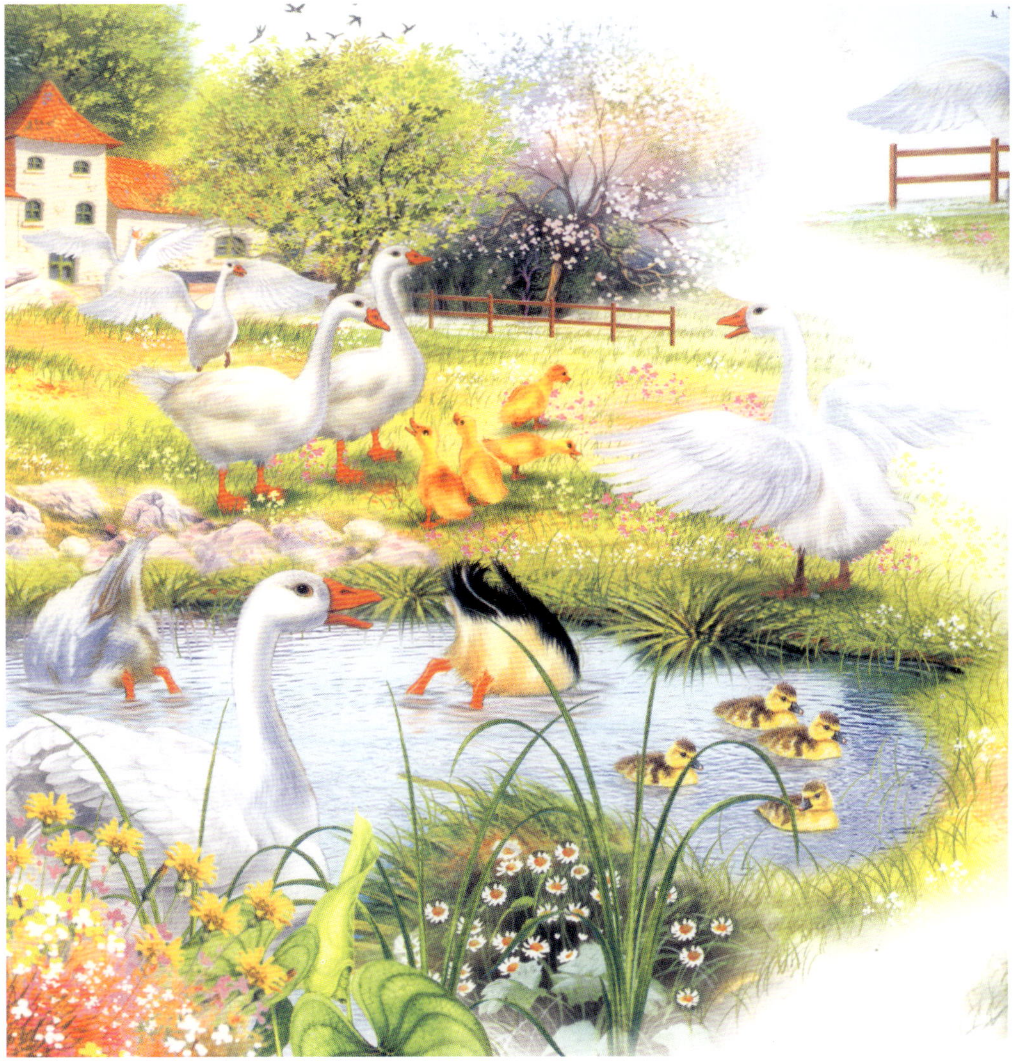

饮食有节

Moderate diet

人所饮所食必须通过脾胃的受纳、运化，始能化生为气血，营养身体，维持生命。饮食太过，反而增加脾胃负担。

中国儒家养生讲："食不厌精，脍不厌细。"意思是指粮食舂得越精越好，肉切得越细越好。的确，食物制作得越精细卫生，越有益于人体健康的消化吸收。

What we drink or eat cannot be absorbed to sustain life until they are accepted and digested by spleen and stomach. Too much eating will increase the burden on the spleen and stomach.

According to Chinese Confucian theories on health preservation, "Grains can never be well-prepared enough, nor can meat be well-minced enough." Indeed, the better foods are prepared, the easier they will be absorbed and digested by the human body.

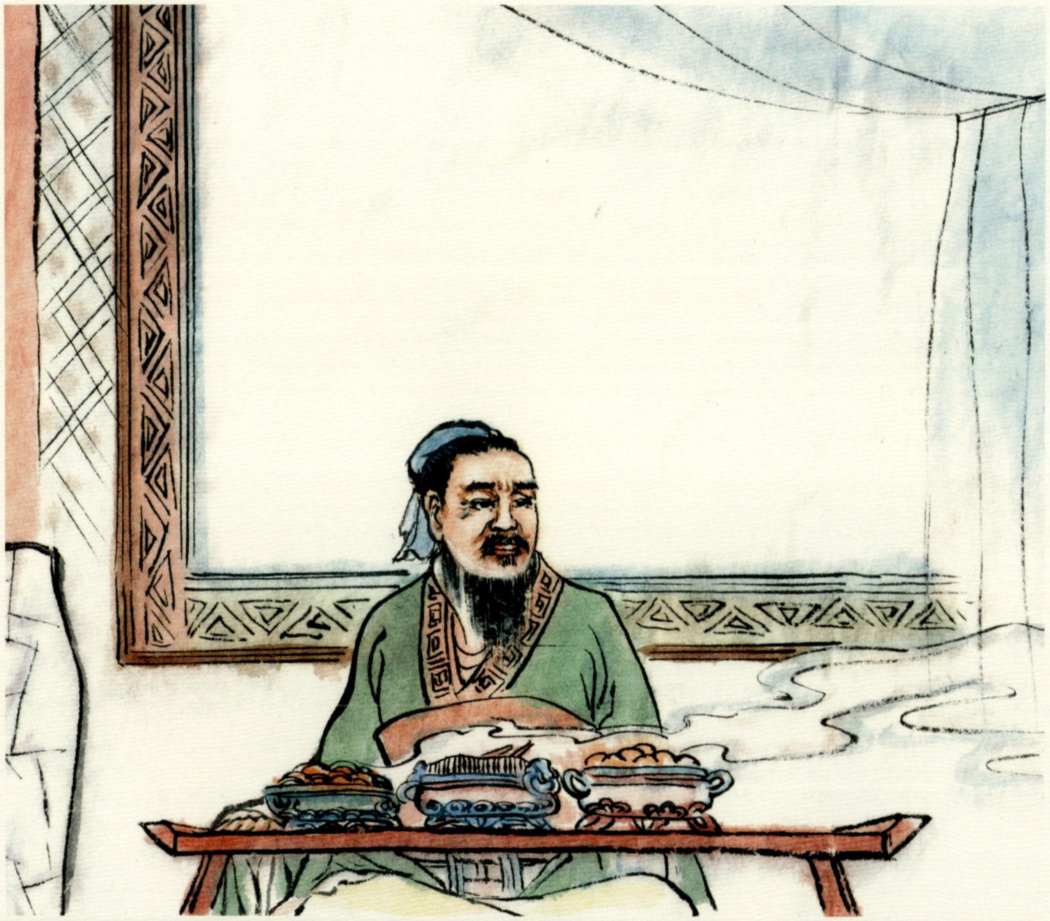

孔子饮食养生图

Confucius's meal

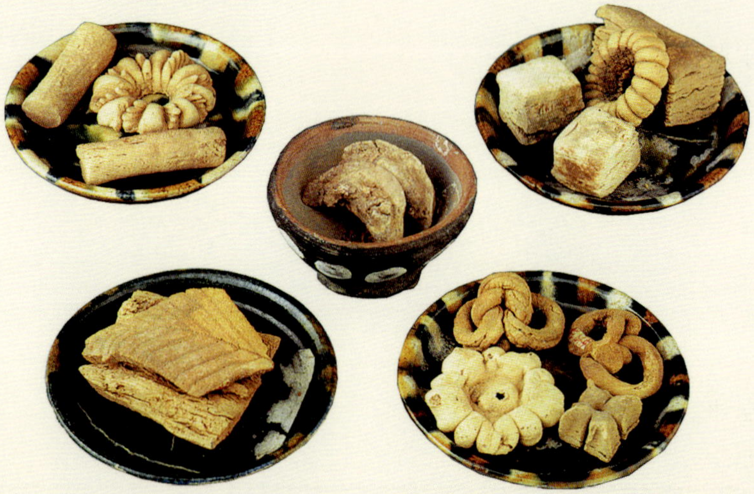

唐代墓葬出土的唐代点心

Dim sum unearthed in a tomb of the Tang Dynasty

催人早衰的物质

Substances inducing premature aging

腌制品

Salted foods

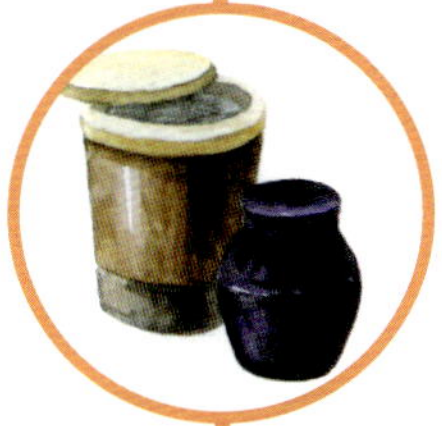

腌制鱼、肉、菜等时，加入的食盐容易转化为亚硝酸盐，在体内生成亚胺类的致癌物质人吃多了易患癌症。

When fish, meat or vegetables are salted, the salt added is prone to isomerize into nitrite. In the human body, it isomerizes into cancer-causing nitrosamines.

含有铝食品

Alluminium-containing foods

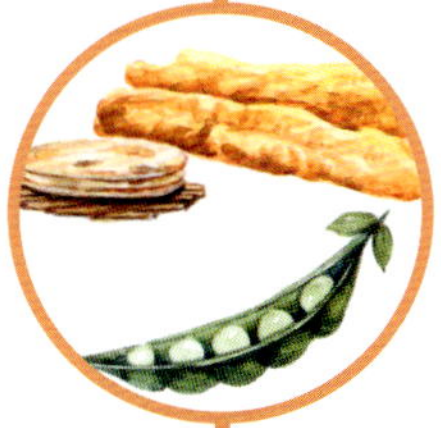

人体摄铝过多，会使脑内肾上腺素、多巴胺的含量大幅降低，造成神经介质传导阻滞，引起记忆力衰退。过多的铝还会直接破坏神经细胞内遗传物质脱氧核糖核酸的功能，使人过早衰老。

Too much aluminum in the human body will reduce the contents of metanephrine and dopamine significantly, which in turn affects the transmission capacity of neurons and thus causes memory to deteriorate. Excessive aluminum may also impair the function of neuron hereditary materials to produce deoxyribonucleic acid (DNA). Consequently, it will cause premature aging.

水垢

Hard water scale

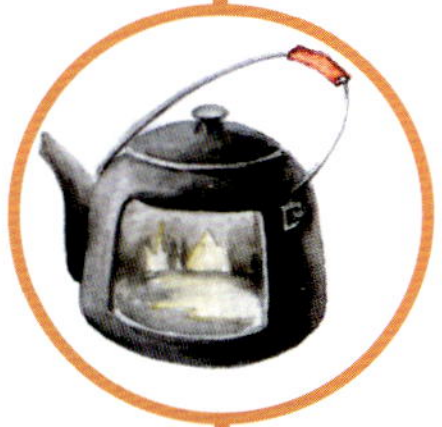

茶具或水具用久后会产生水垢，其中含有较多的有害金属元素，如不及时清除干净，经常饮用会引起消化、神经、泌尿、造血等系统的病变，造成早衰。

Limescale may be seen on tea ware or water vessels that have been used for a long time. It contains maleficent metallic elements. If not removed in time, it will cause diseases to the digestive, nervous, urinary and blood-generating systems and then resulted in premature aging.

高温油烟

High-temperature greasy smoke

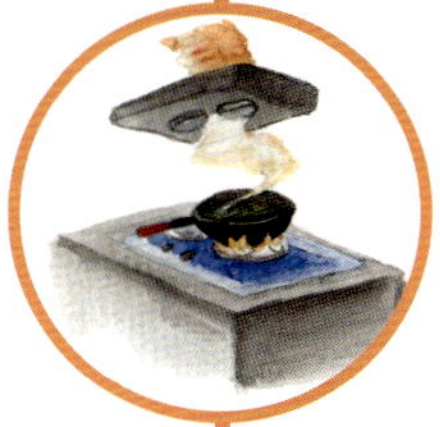

由于食用油在高温下会释放出含有丁二烯成分的烟雾，长期大量吸入这种物质会改变人的遗传免疫功能，催人早衰。

Because, when heated, edible oil may give out smoke containing butadiene, inhaling the material constantly may alter one's hereditary and immune functions and induce premature aging.

酒精饮料

Alcoholics

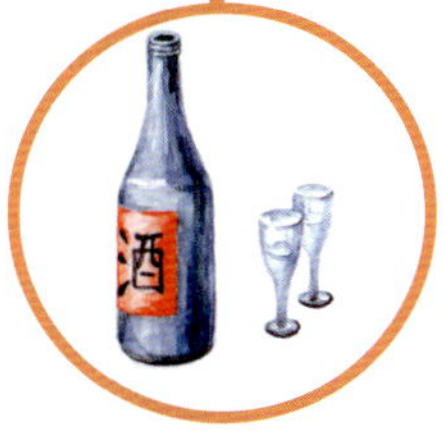

大量饮酒，会导致男性性功能衰退、精子畸形以及女性月经不调、性欲减退等早衰现象。

Drinking excessively may impair a male's sexual capacity and cause the deformation of sperms; it may incur a female's irregular menstruation and sexual apathy.

由于天有日月星辰之推移，时有寒暑昼夜之更替，地有东西南北之分布，人有性别、年龄、体质之不同。因而，正确得当的食养，还必须因人、因时、因地制宜。

As the sun, moon and stars move in the sky, the time changes with day and night, summer and winter, the earth is divided into the east, west, south and north, people are different by gender, age and corporeity. Therefore, diet must be properly adjusted according to the person, time and place.

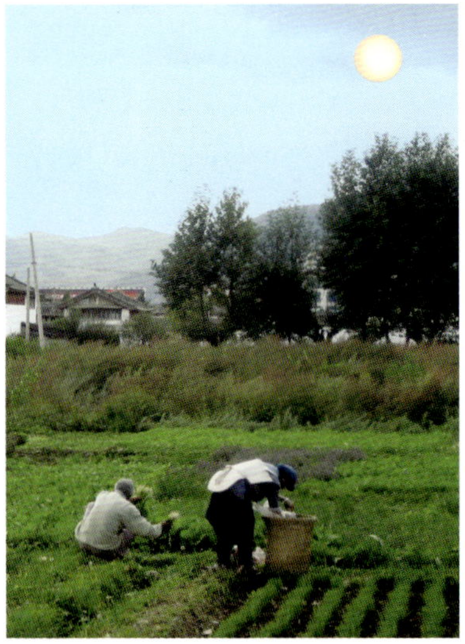

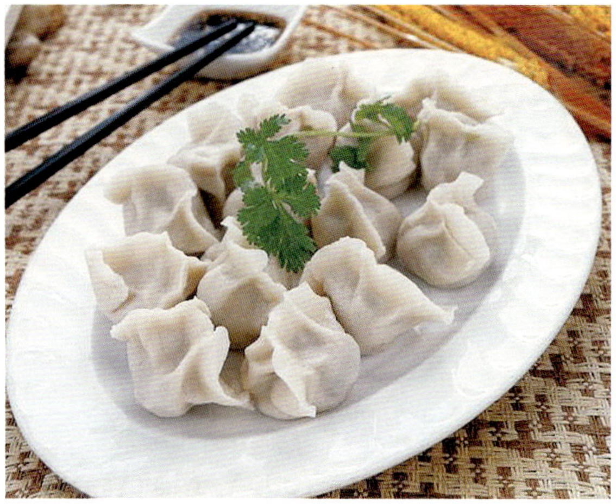

中国北方有句俚语，叫做“头伏饺子二伏面，三伏烙饼摊鸡蛋”。头伏吃饺子是传统习俗，因为每逢伏天，人的胃口就不好，而饺子是营养丰富、开胃解馋的食物。新小麦磨成面粉煮汤吃，吃后出一身汗，新粮营养丰富，发汗亦可以驱病。伏里还可以吃“炒面”。唐代医学家苏恭说，炒面可“解烦热，止泄，实大肠”。

As a saying in northern China goes, “Jiaozi for the first 10-day period of dog days, noodles for the second, and pancakes and fried egg for the third.” It is customary to have jiaozi in the first 10-day period of the dog days. Because when the weather turns very hot, people tend to have a poorer appetite. Jiaozi is a nutritious food that can whet the appetite. Jiaozi often goes with a flour soup made of the newly harvested wheat. After drinking that soup, one will sweat all over. Newly harvested wheat is nutritious. Sweating can prevent diseases. In dog days, people also have chow mein. As Su Gong, Tang Dynasty physician, puts it, the food can “relieve excessive heat, stop diarrhea and fill the large intestine.”

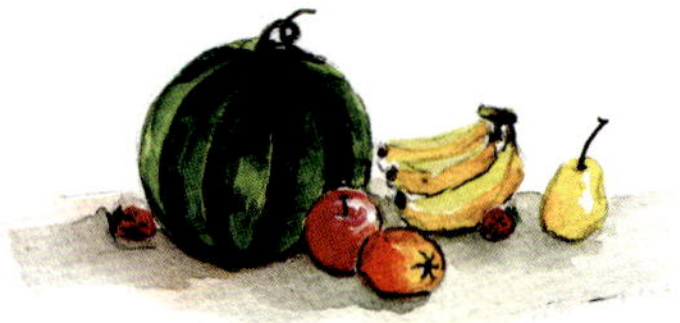

瓜果
Melons and fruits

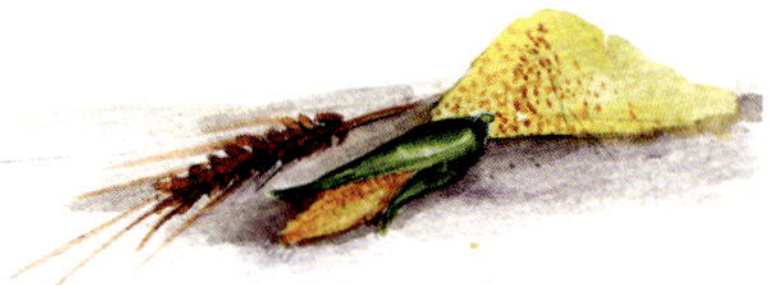

谷类
Cereals

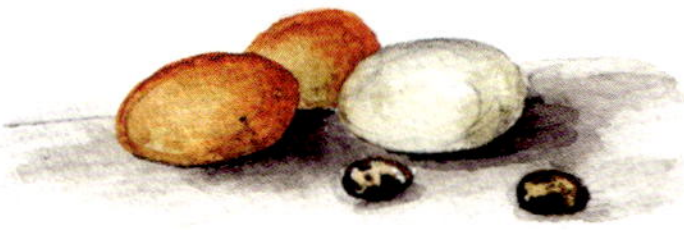

蛋
Eggs

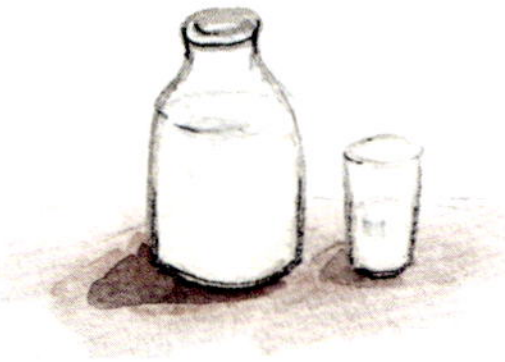

奶
Milk

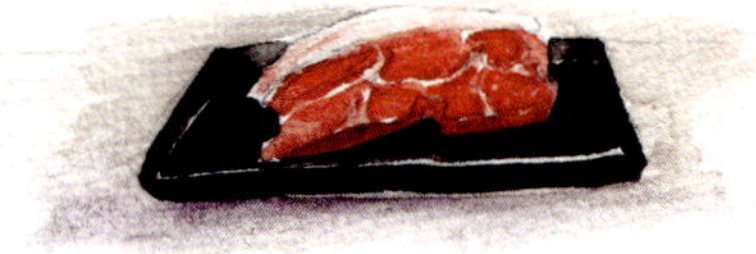

肉类
Meats

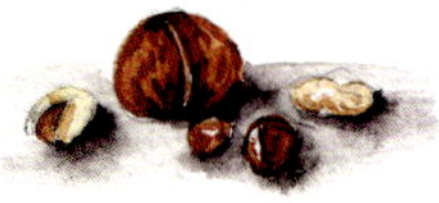

干果
Nuts

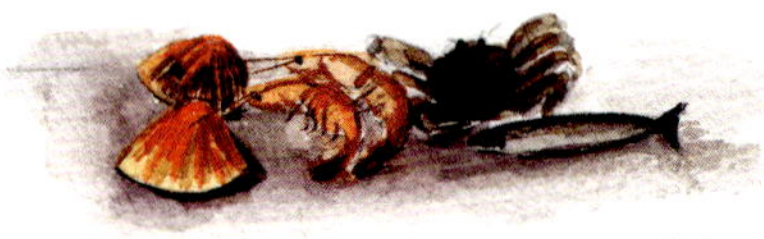

海鲜
Seafoods

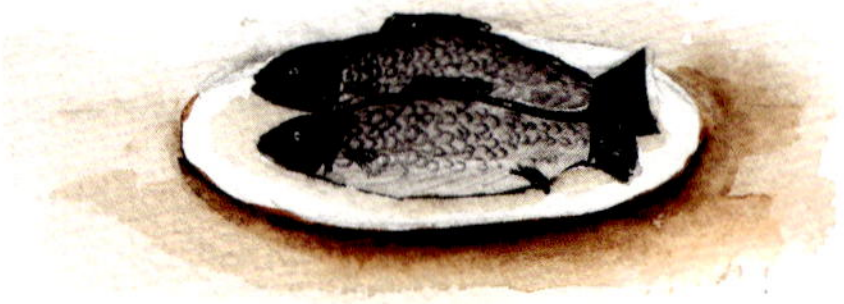

鱼类
Fishes

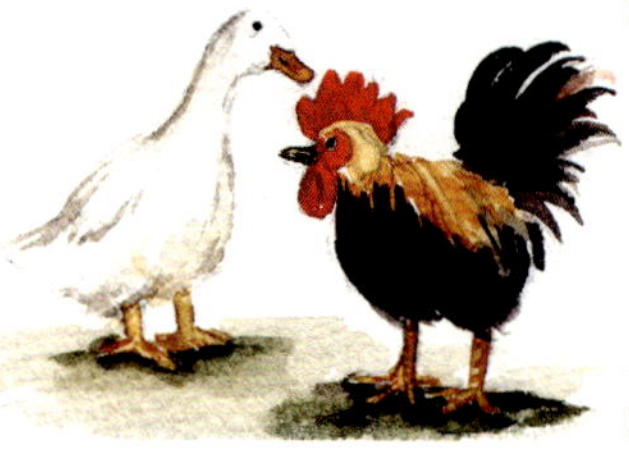

家禽
Domestic fowls

必须注意食品养生之禁忌

Important dietary taboos

食物性味与疾病证候属性有着密切关系，要发挥食物的正确作用就必须根据疾病辨证要求掌握饮食宜忌。一般而言，阳虚、寒证患者，忌生冷寒凉食物；阴虚、热证患者，忌温热性食物；外感未尽或痰湿中满者，忌油腻大补食物。

Food property is closely related to disease syndromes, and therefore, to make good use of the food we must pay attention to the taboos of diet for different diseases. In general, patients of yang deficiency and cold syndrome should not eat raw and cold food, patients of yin deficiency and heat syndrome should not eat high-calorie foods, and patients of colds and phlegm-dampness should not eat too greasy and tonic foods.

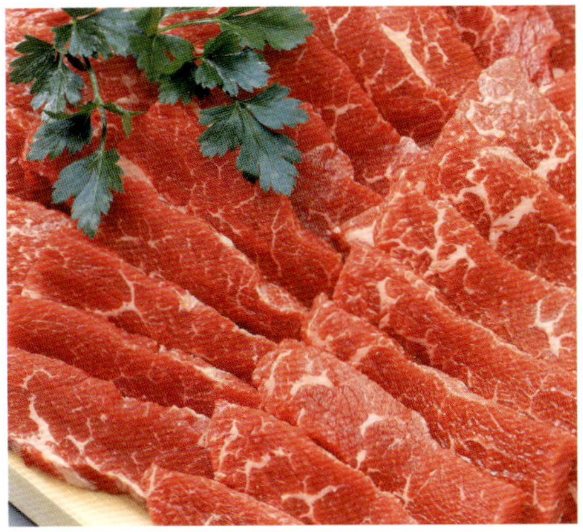

生冷食物不易消化吸收，有肠胃疾病的人群忌吃生冷食物。

Raw and cold foods cannot be easily digested or absorbed. Thus people with intestine or stomach diseases should not have them.

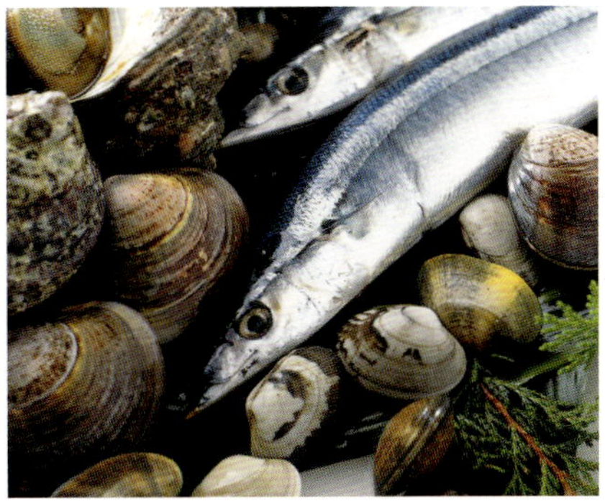

有前列腺、关节炎疾病患者忌多吃海鲜。虾类忌与维生素C同食，海鲜忌与某些水果同食，如柿子、葡萄、石榴、山楂、青果等。

Patients with prostatitis and arthritis should not eat sea food. People should not have shrimps with Vitamin-C, or sea food with fruits like persimmons, grapes, pomegranates, hawthorn fruit, olives etc.

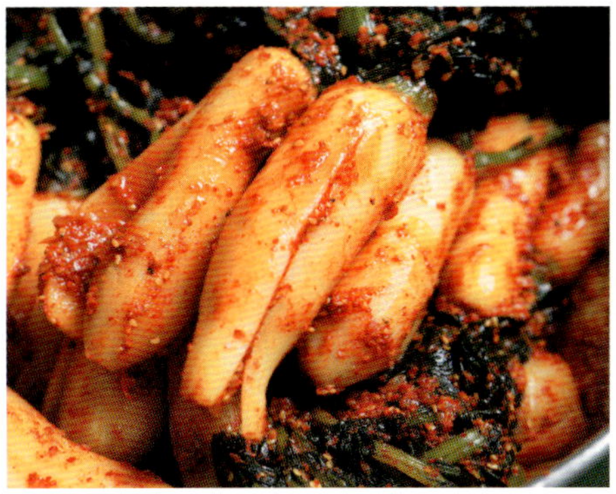

食用含盐量过高的食物，饮食过多会引发高血压，造成肾脏负担过重，并损害胃肠道黏膜。腌制食物的过程中生成的亚硝酸盐还能引起急性中毒。

Too much salt will cause high blood temperature, put too much burden on the kidney and impair the membrane on the walls of the stomach and intestines. Salted food may generate nitrite that gives rise to acute intoxication.

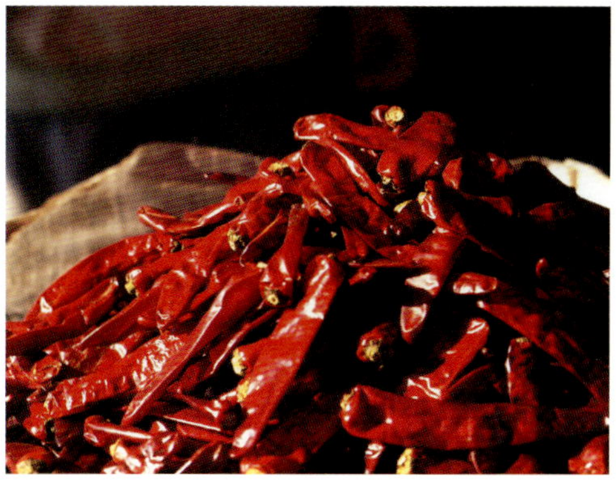

辣椒有发散、活血、健胃消食等功能，但吃多了容易使肺气过盛，导致免疫力降低，引发咽痛、眼赤、鼻热、口干舌痛、牙痛等症状。有胃肠疾病、痔疮、皮炎、慢性气管炎等疾病的人群更应该忌吃辣椒。

Pepper can vent excessive energy, activate blood flow, benefit the stomach and improve digestive capacity. However too much pepper will result in excessive inner energy at the lungs and harm immunity. Then symptoms like a sore throat, pinkeye, hot breath, dry mouth, aching tongue and toothache will appear. People with stomach and intestine diseases, hemorrhoid, skin disease and chronic tracheitis should avoid eating pepper.

饮水

The intake of water

水是人体重要的组成部分，健康儿童体内含水量占体重的80%，成人占65%，可以说，水孕育着生命。进水时间最好是餐前一小时许，最好空腹饮入。应注意饮用符合卫生标准的水，最好不要饮用隔夜水、回锅水。饮用天然饮料“活水”可防病延年。

Water is an important part of human body. Water content in a healthy child accounts for 80% of body weight, and water content in an adult accounts for 65% of body weight. It can be said that water nurses life. The best time to drink water is at about an hour before a meal when the stomach is empty. Drinking water should meet the hygiene standards, and we'd better not drink overnight water or twice-boiled water. Drinking “fresh water” and natural drinks can prevent disease and prolong life.

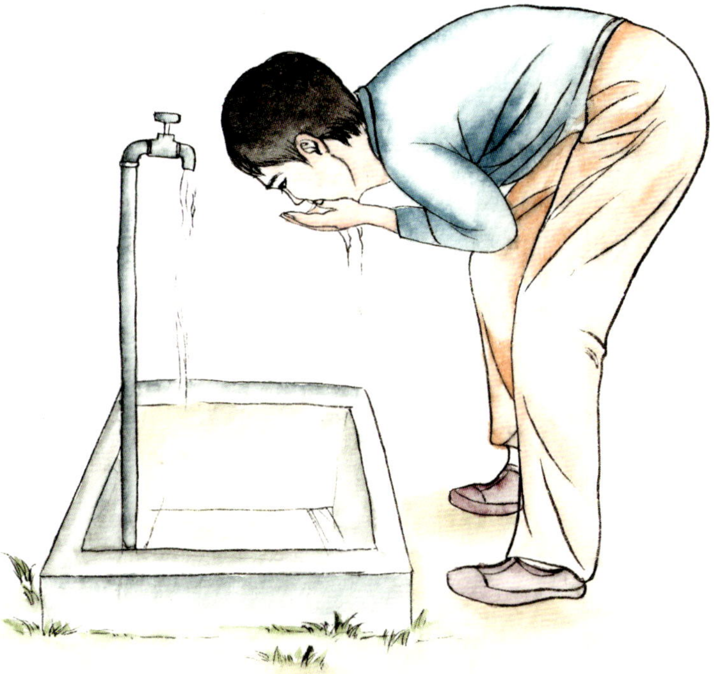

饮用活水

Drink fresh water

《饮膳正要》对饮酒的利害作了较全面的概括，指出“酒味辛甘，大热有毒，主行药势，杀百邪，通血脉，厚肠胃，消忧愁，少饮为佳。多饮伤神折寿，易人本性……饮酒过度，丧生之源”。

Guidance on Drinks and Foods makes a comprehensive summary of the advantages and disadvantages of drinking alcohol, pointing out that “with a strong and sweet flavor, alcohol is rather hot and toxic. It can serve as medicine which can extinguish all kinds of evils, clean arteries and veins, strengthen the stomach and bowels, and relieve one's sorrow. But it is advisable not to drink too much alcohol, since it will do harm to one's nerves, shorten one's life, and change one's character...In short, excessive drinking is a cause of death. ”

中国最著名的诗人李白（右图左）一生创作了很多雄逸奇丽的诗篇，然而因为常年饮酒，晚年疾病缠身。另一位著名田园诗人陶渊明（右图右），一生好酒，晚年穷困潦倒，子嗣都有智力障碍。

Li Bai, most renowned poet in ancient China (left in the right picture), wrote numerous magnificent poems in his life. However, because of excessive drinking, he was eaten up by diseases in his later years. Tao Yuanming, another famous poet known for his idylls (right in the right picture), also had poor health in his later years because of excessive drinking. His offspring all had dysgnosia.

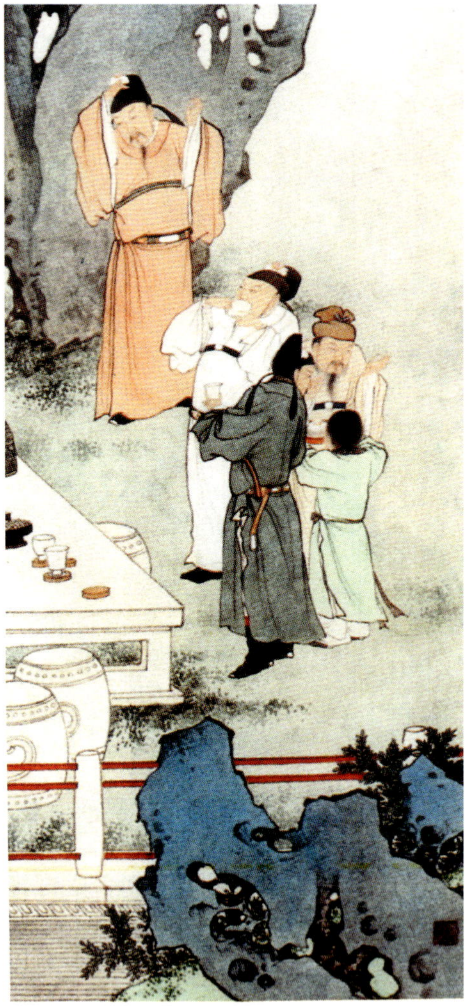

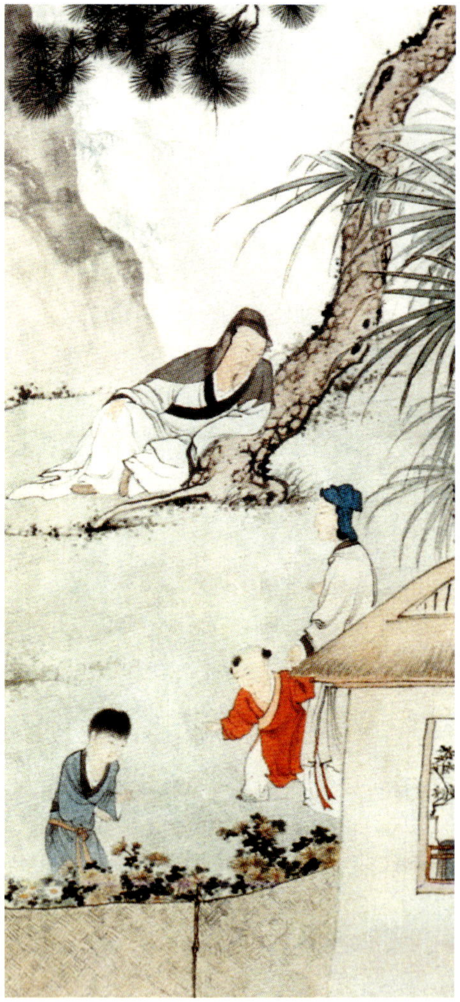

食物——人体的生化之源

Food, the source of energy for the body

中医学认为，食物也具有寒热温凉四气和酸苦辛甘咸五味，而且各有其所主的脏腑和归经，如食物搭配不合理，或者素喜偏食，则有损于人体健康，应该注意食物的合理搭配。

Chinese traditional medicine holds that foods also have four qis: cold, hot, warm, and cool, and five flavors: sour, bitter, pungent, sweet and salty. Each of the qis and flavors corresponds to different organs of the human body. An unbalanced diet or partiality to a particular kind of food is detrimental to one's health. Therefore, we'd better have a healthy diet.

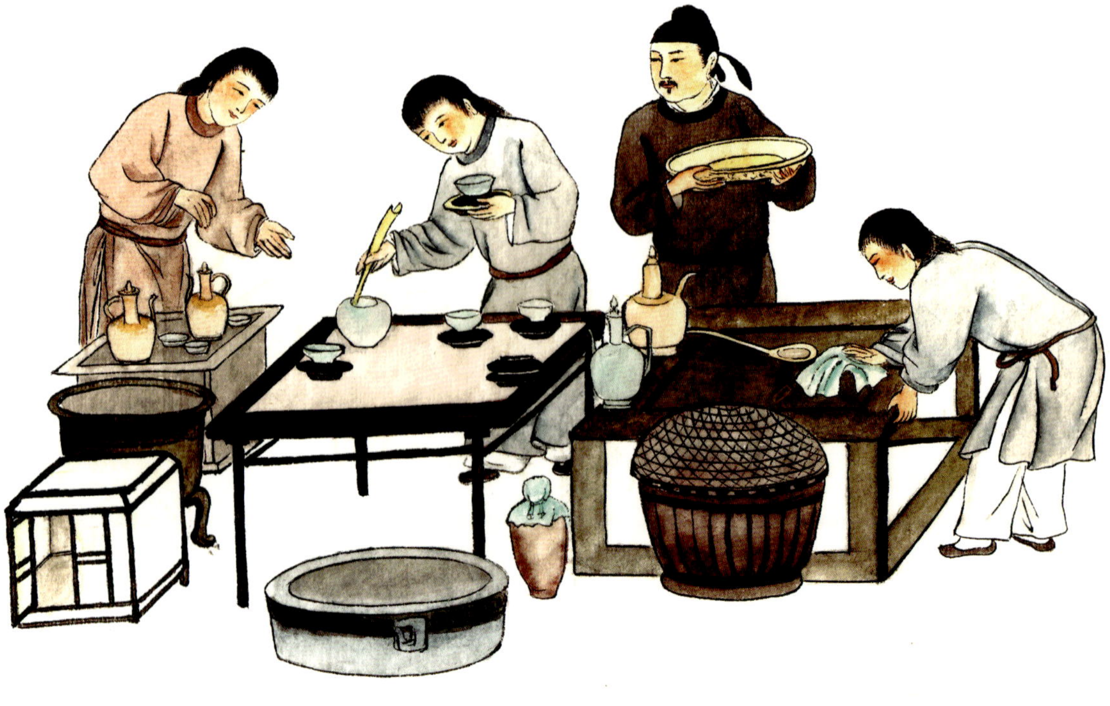

“谨和五味”

Balancing the “five tastes”

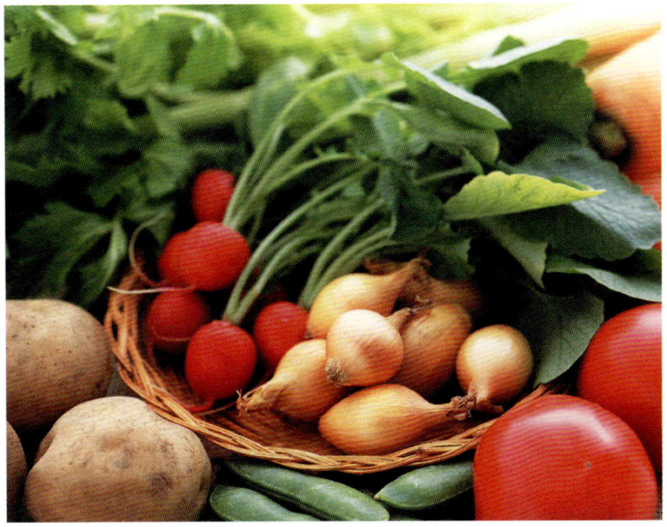

一日三餐的正确分配应该是早餐占全日量的 35~40%，且要保证质量，最好吃牛奶、豆浆、蛋糕一类的食品，午餐占 40~45%，晚餐占 20~25%，而且晚餐应强调多进清淡之品。故民间有谚语云“早吃好，午吃饱，晚吃少，人不老”。如孙思邈指出“不欲极饥而食，食不可过饱”。

The three meals a day should be appropriately arranged as follows: breakfast accounts for 35~40% of the amount of the whole day, and it is best to have high quality food like milk, soybean milk and cake; lunch accounts for 40~45%; dinner accounts for only 20~25%, and plain food is recommended. Just as the saying goes, “Eat best food at breakfast, eat one’s fill at lunch, eat little at supper, and you will not get old.” Sun Simiao also pointed out that people should “not wait until extremely hungry to eat or eat too much.”

科学进餐：一日三餐的习惯，在我国早就形成了，这是科学的。

Dining in a scientific way: the habit of three meals a day was formed in China from ancient times, which has proved to be scientific.

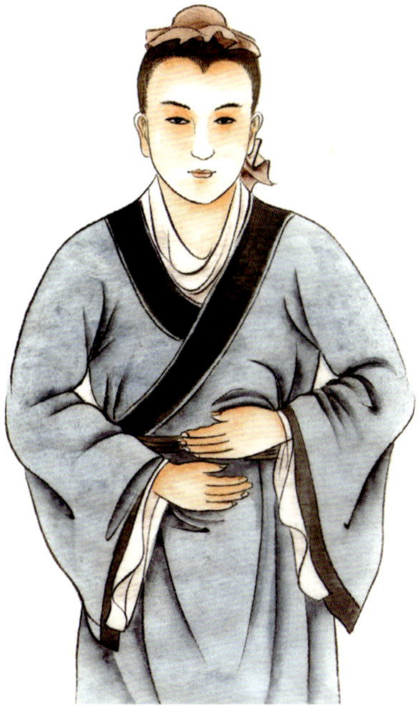

摩腹消食法

Method of abdomen rubbing to aid digestion

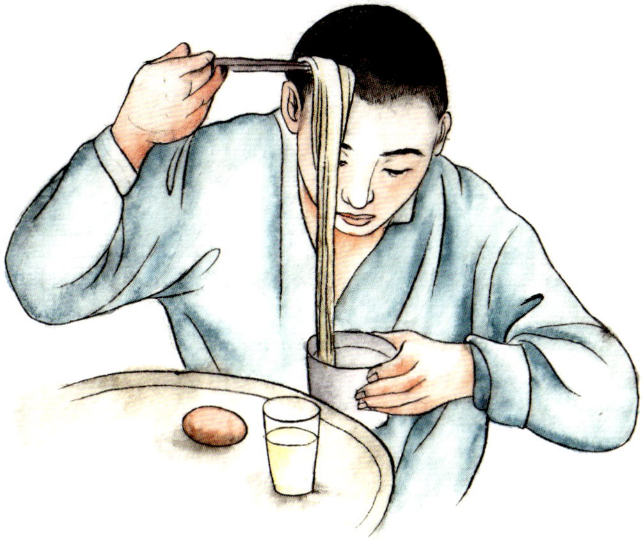

早餐要精，营养要丰富

Breakfast foods should be well-chosen and nutritious.

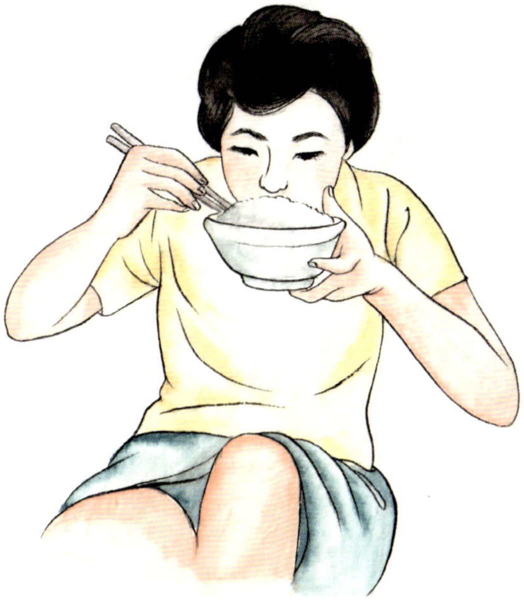

午餐要营养均衡，吃饱无饥饿感即可

Lunch foods should be balanced in nutrition and one should not each much. No feeling of hunger means enough.

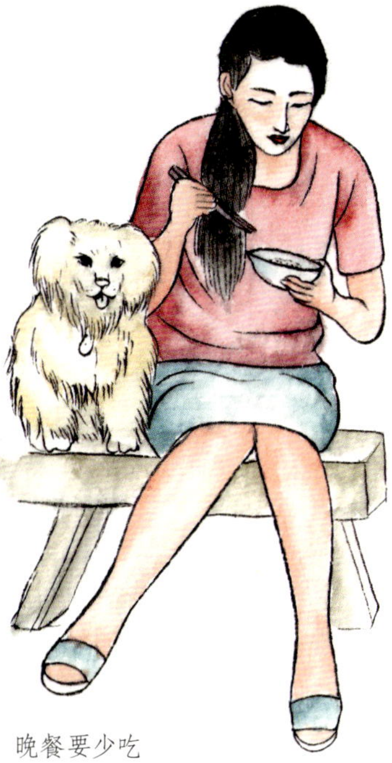

晚餐要少吃

One should eat less for dinner.

茶道养生

The health-preserving effects of tea

饮茶在中国有悠久的历史。《神农本草经》认为“茶味苦，饮之使人益思，少卧、轻身、明目”。

茶具有养生功效，茶可以提神解乏，除脂解腻、促进消化。茶叶中含有较丰富的氟，可以补充钙质、预防龋齿、去除口臭。茶可谓养生的妙药。但茶性寒凉，虚寒之人慎用。

Drinking tea has a long history in China, *Shen Nong's Herbal Classic* believes that “the bitter tea can provoke thinking, reduce sleep and weight, and improve eyesight.”

Tea has hearth-preserving effects. It can refresh the mind, dissolve grease, and aid digestion. Rich in fluorine, it can supplement calcium, prevent tooth decay, and get rid of foul breath. With such properties, it is indeed a wonderful health-preserving substance.

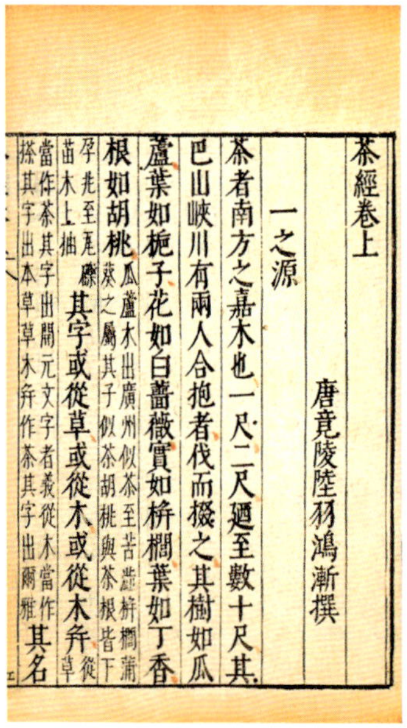

茶經卷上
唐竟陵陸羽鴻漸撰
一之源
茶者南方之嘉木也一尺二尺廼至數十尺其
巴山峽川有兩人合抱者伐而掇之其樹如瓜
蘆葉如梔子花如白薔薇實如栟櫚葉如丁香
根如胡桃

1

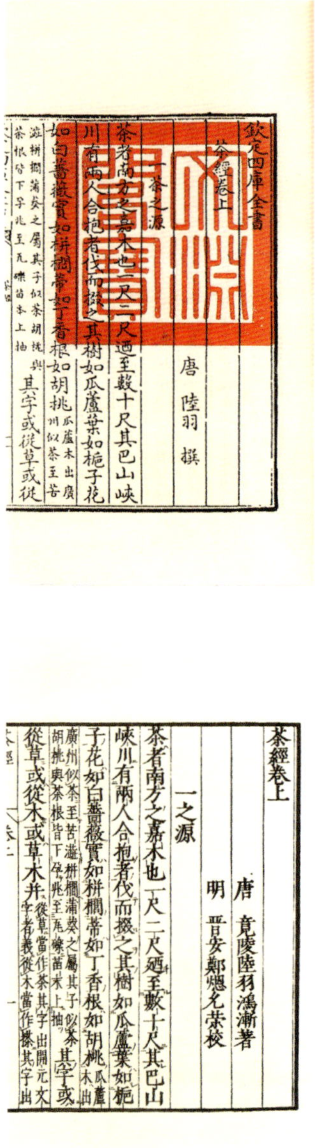

2

1 明 ·《茶经》

1. Ming Dynasty • *Tea Classic*

2 清 ·《四库全书 · 茶经》

2. Qing Dynasty • *Tea Classic in Complete Library of the Four Treasuries*

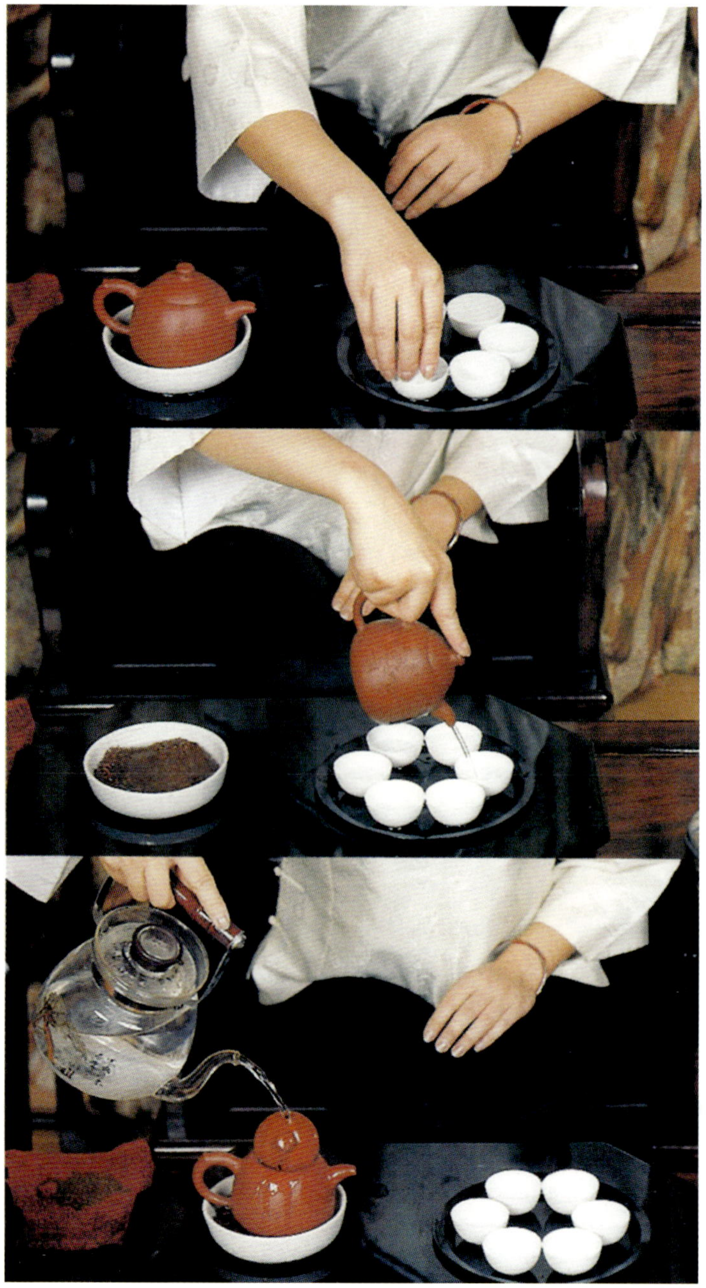

茶艺图

Art of tea drinking

自古有“禅茶一味”之说。禅宗主张明心见性，心胸豁达。茶则使人内心清净、安闲舒适、有节制。人饮茶不光为提神，茶亦有道，僧人们通过饮茶，把禅学与茶道的“静心”、“自悟”相结合，从茶中得到开释。茶和禅有“苦”、”静”、“凡”、“放”四点共通之处。

It has been said since ancient times that Zen and tea have the same taste. Zen advocates developing a broad and enlightened mind, and tea can make one serene, leisurely and temperate. One does not drink only to refresh his mind, for there is Tao in tea. By drinking tea, monks combine Zen philosophy with the ideas of 'serenity' and 'self-enlightenment' in the Tao of Tea (chadao, i.e. tea ceremony) in order to attain true freedom. Tea and Zen have four features in common – bitter taste/suffering (ku), serenity (jing), ordinariness (fan), and detachment (fang).

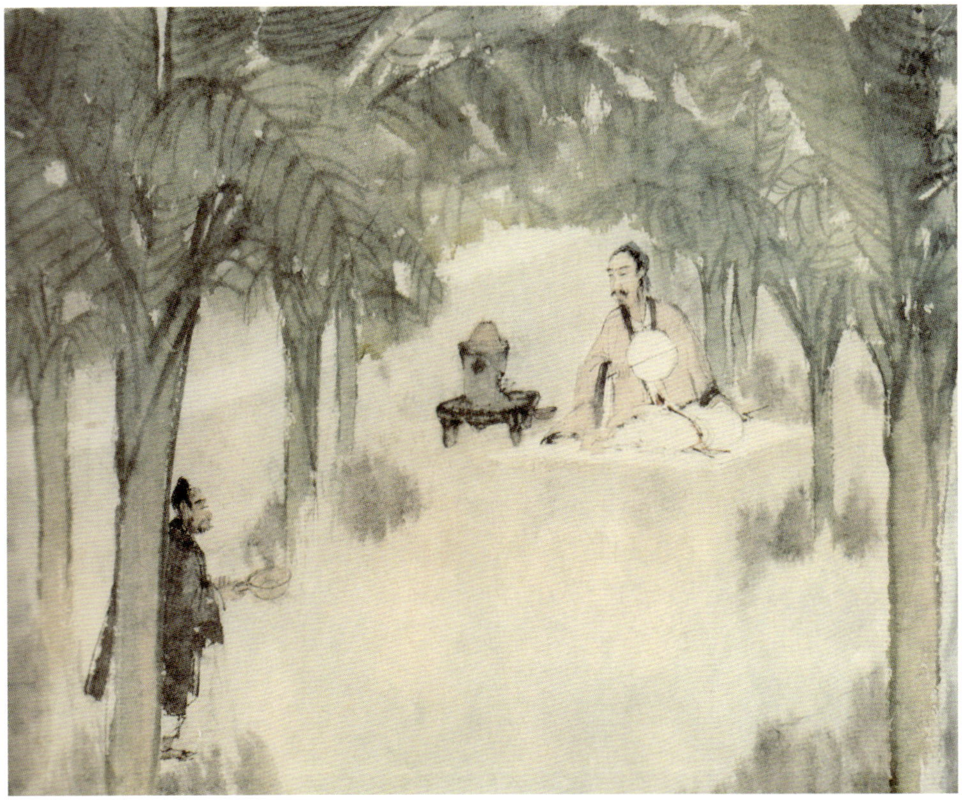

品茶图
Savoring tea

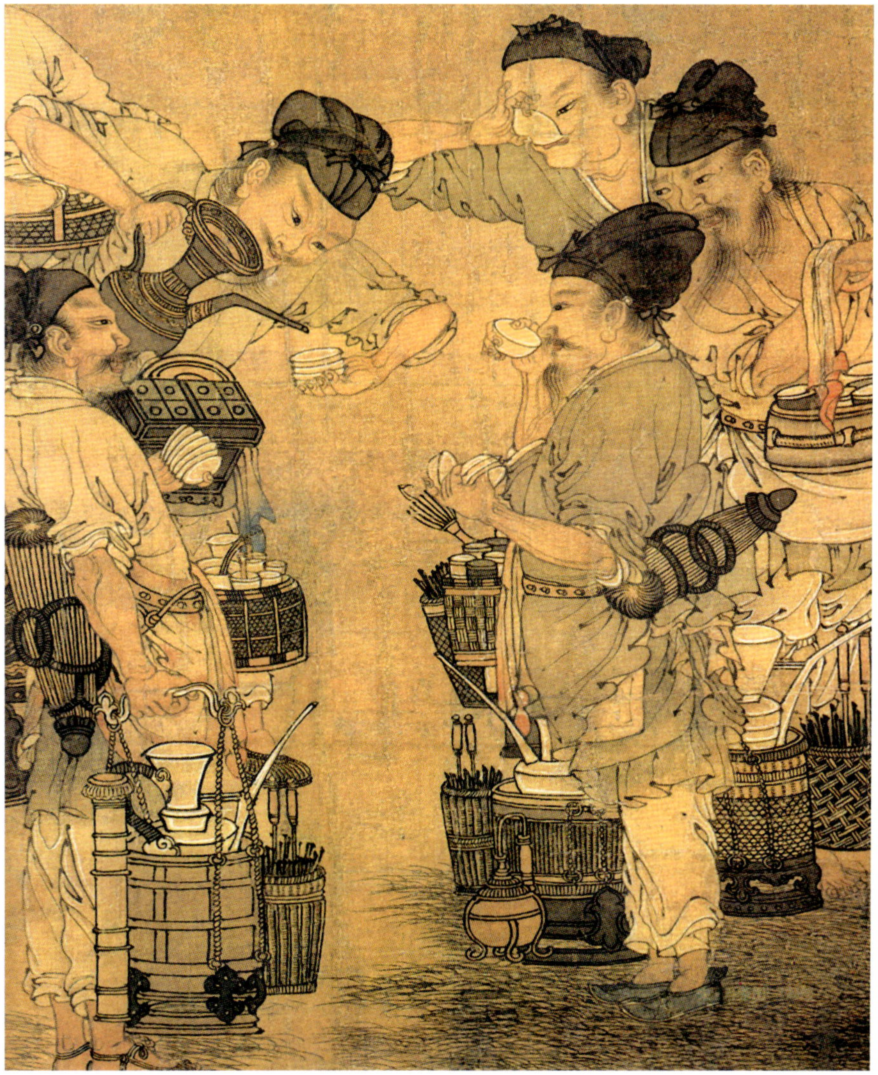

斗茶图
Tea contest

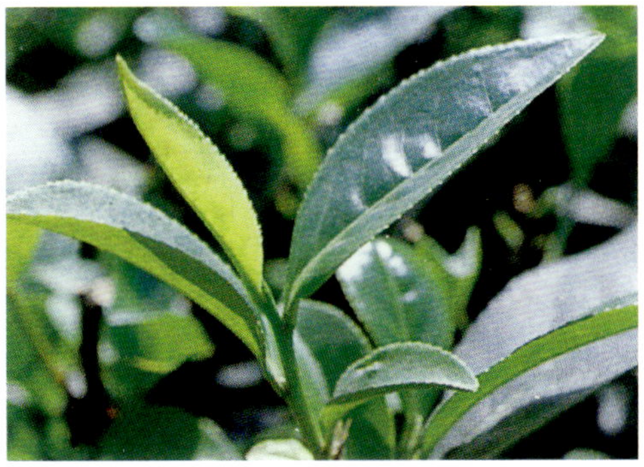

茶
Tea

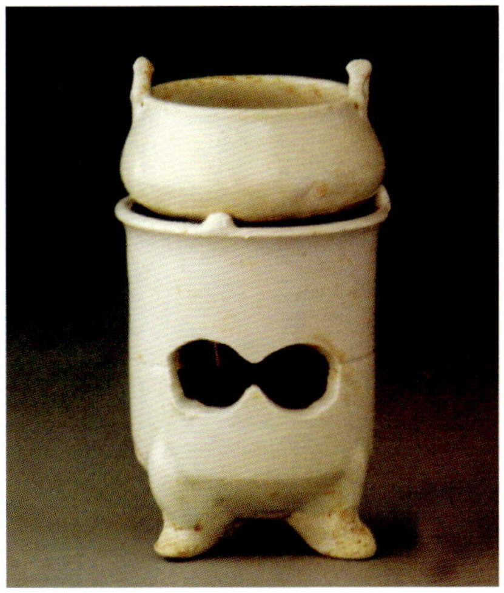

茶具
Tea-drinking utensils

“苦”，佛理以为人有八苦，参禅即是要了悟生死，从“苦”中解脱出来。茶性苦，据《本草纲目》记载，“茶苦而寒，阴中之阴，最能降火，火为百病，火清则上晴矣”。从茶的苦中有书，苦后回比的特性，佛家可以帮助修习佛法的人在品茗时，参破“苦谛”。

Bitter taste/suffering (*ku*): According to Buddhist philosophy, there are eight kinds of sufferings in a person's life, and the purpose of practicing meditation is to gain an insight into life and death and, subsequently, release from suffering. Tea is also *ku* (bitter) by nature. According to *Compendium of Materia Medica*, “Tea is bitter and cold, the most yin of all yin things, and is therefore best for reducing fire. Fire is the origin of many diseases, so the reduction of fire can restore health.” As tea offers delight alongside its bitter taste, it can help a person who practices Buddhism to understand the truth about suffering.

水曹

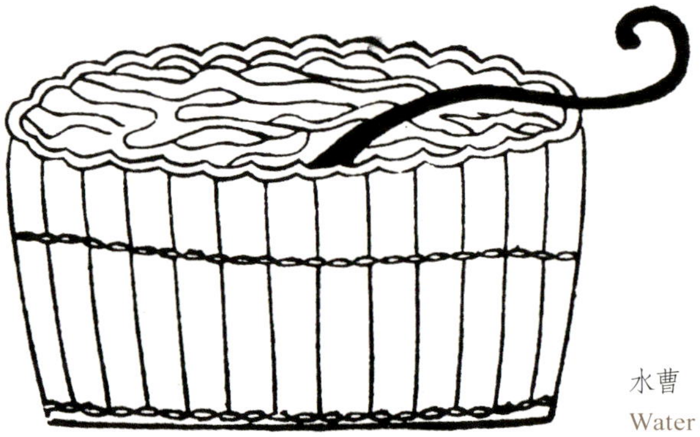

水曹
Water tank

雲屯

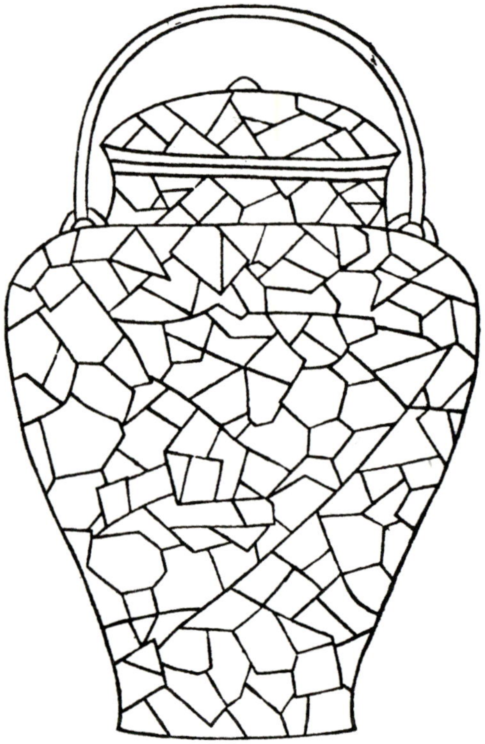

云屯，陶制容器，以盛煎茶用之泉水

Yuntun, a kind of pottery container for spring water used to infuse tea.

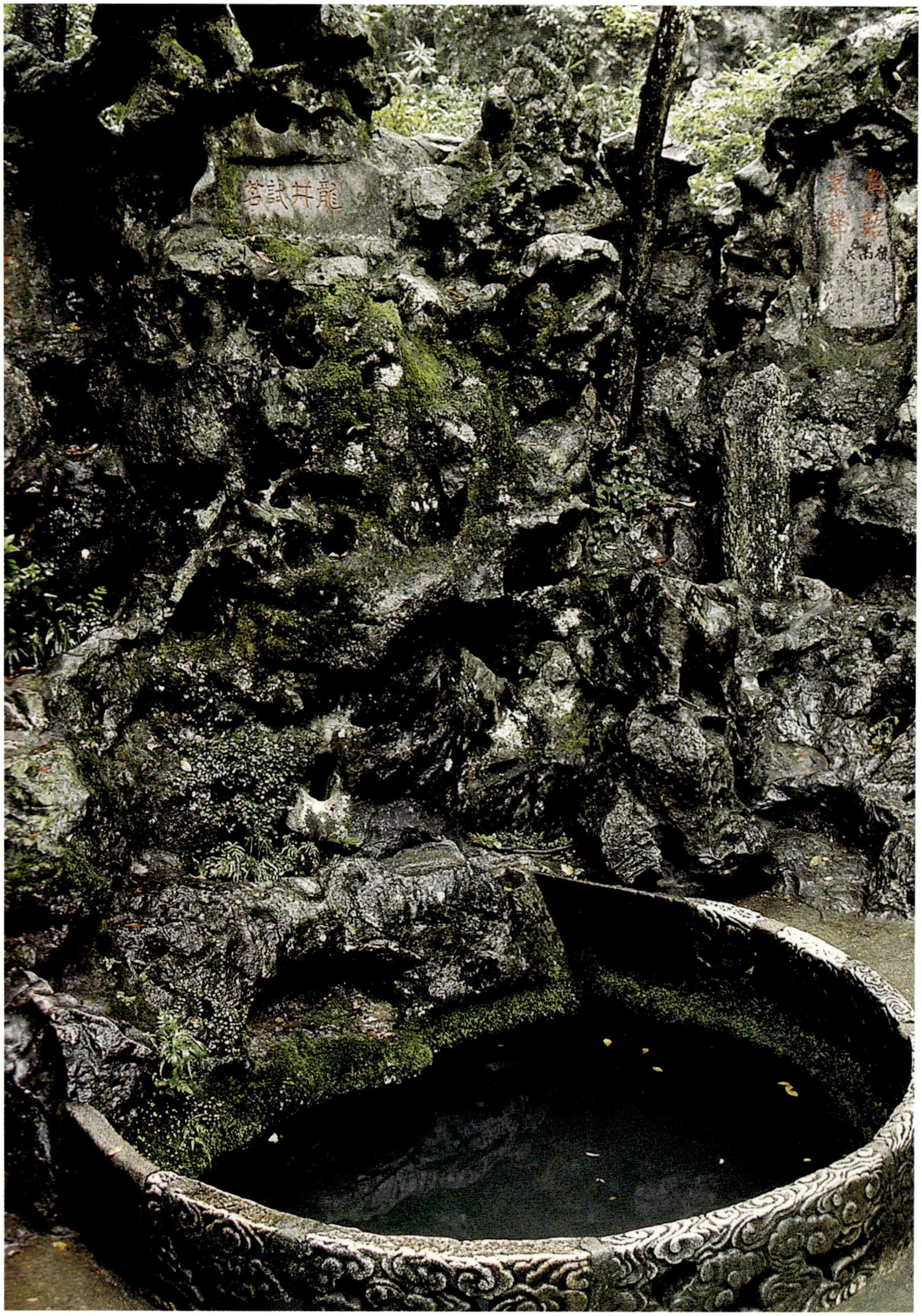

西湖龙井泉
Longjing Spring at the West Lake

"静"，茶道讲究"和静怡真"。禅调五事，即调心、调身、调食、调息、调睡眠以及佛学中的"戒、定、慧"，都是以静为基础。茶恰好能提神益思，帮助人克服静坐静虑中的睡意。

Serenity (*jing*): the Tao of Tea emphasizes "harmony, serenity, delight, and truth". Zen regulates the mind, the body, eating, resting, and sleep. These, as well as *jie-ding-hui* (*sila, dhyana, prajna*, or morality, meditation and wisdom) in Buddhist philosophy, are also based on serenity. Tea can refresh and sharpen the mind, overcoming drowsiness during meditation.

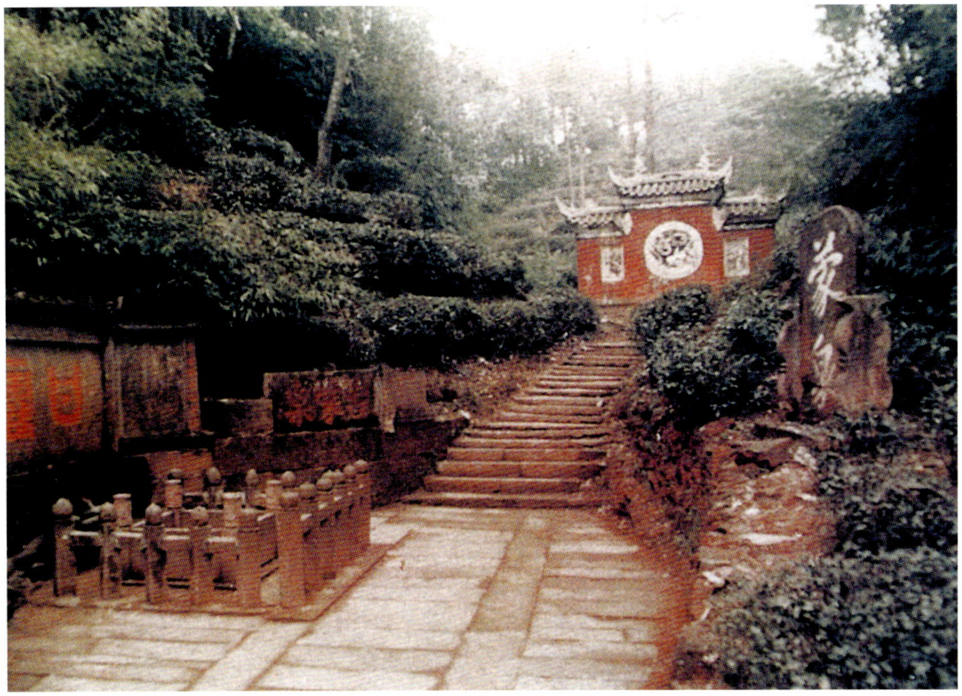

四川蒙山植茶遗址

Relics of cultivating tea trees, Mengshan, Sichuan Prov.

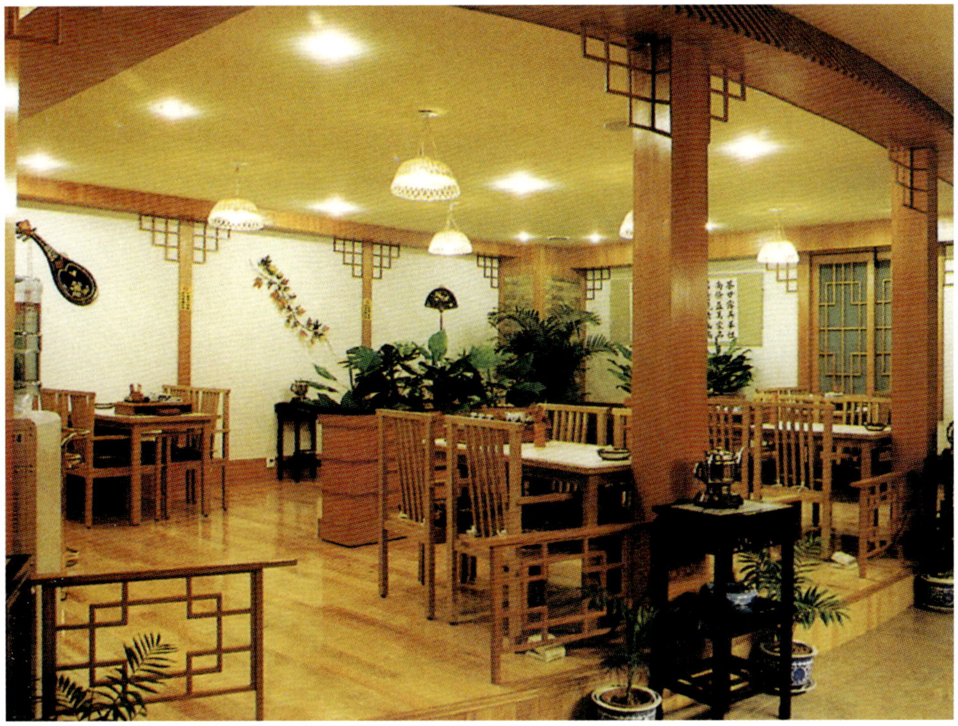

茶馆

Tea house

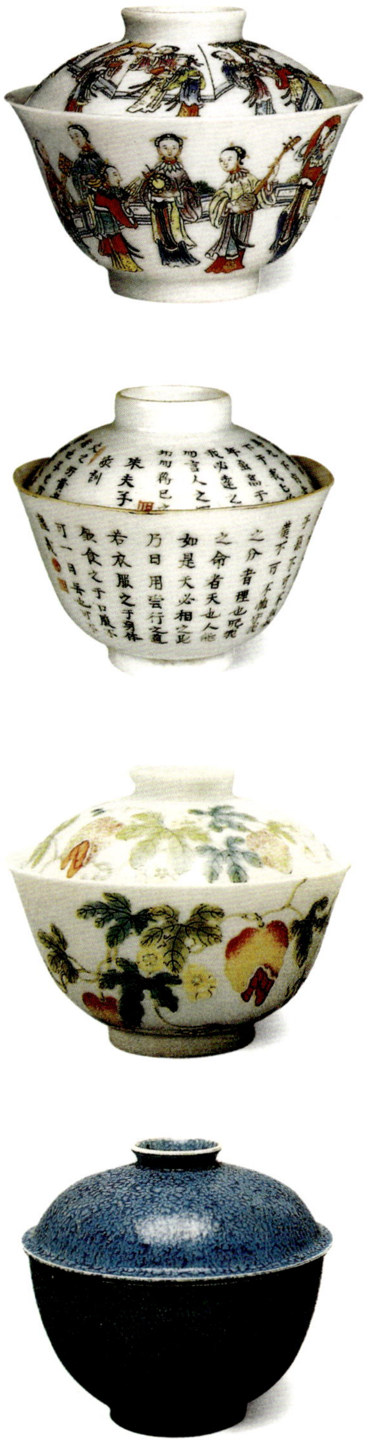

多姿多彩的盖碗

Colorful bowls with lids

“凡”，茶道的本质是从琐碎平凡的生活中感悟自然奥秘和人生哲理。禅则要求人们通过静虑，从平凡的小事中彻悟大道。

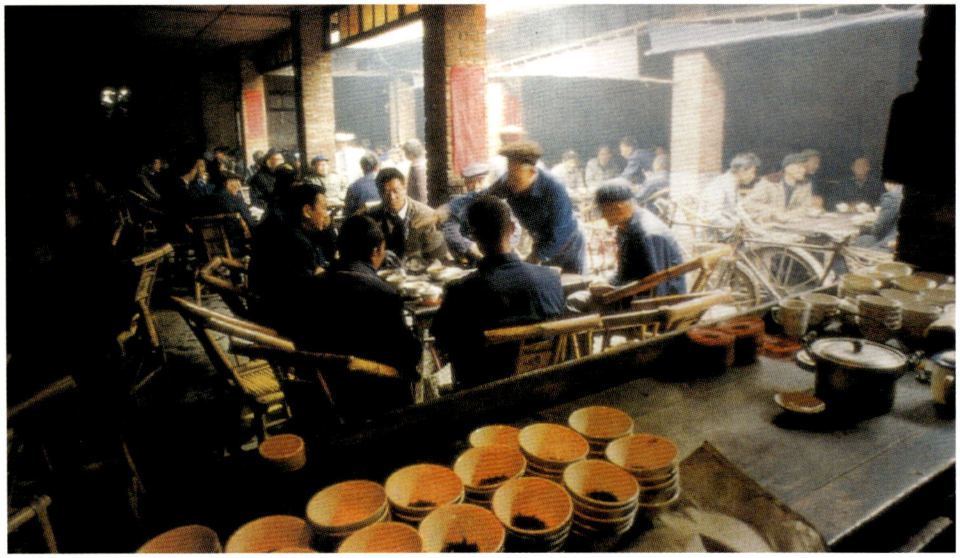

茶室

Tea room

“放”，人的苦恼，归根结底就是“放不下”。佛教修行强调“放下”，品茶也强调茶人无牵挂。

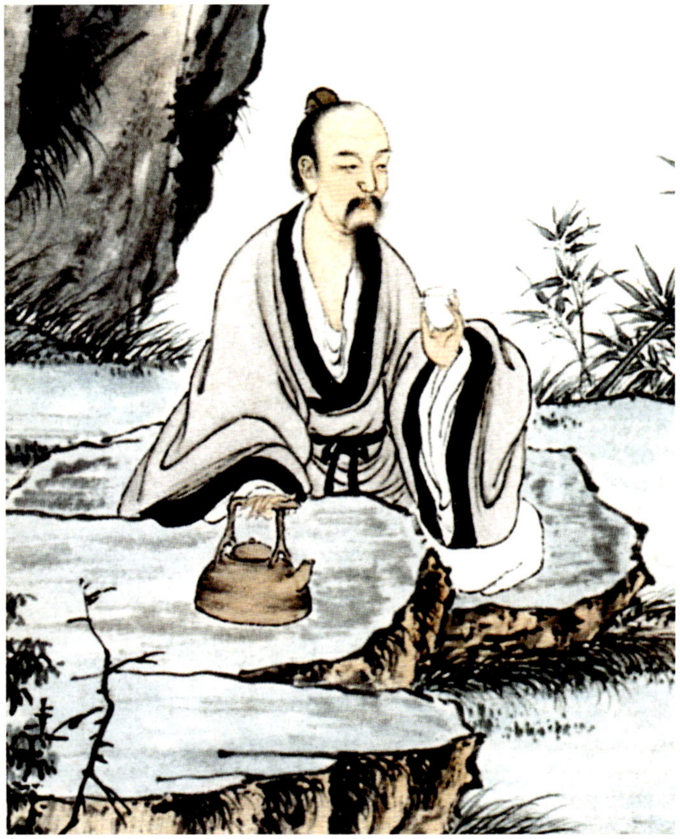

品茗图

Savoring tea

Ordinariness: The essence of the Tao of Tea is to discover philosophical insights into life and nature in trivial and ordinary things. Zen also requires one to find the great Tao in ordinary things through serene thinking.

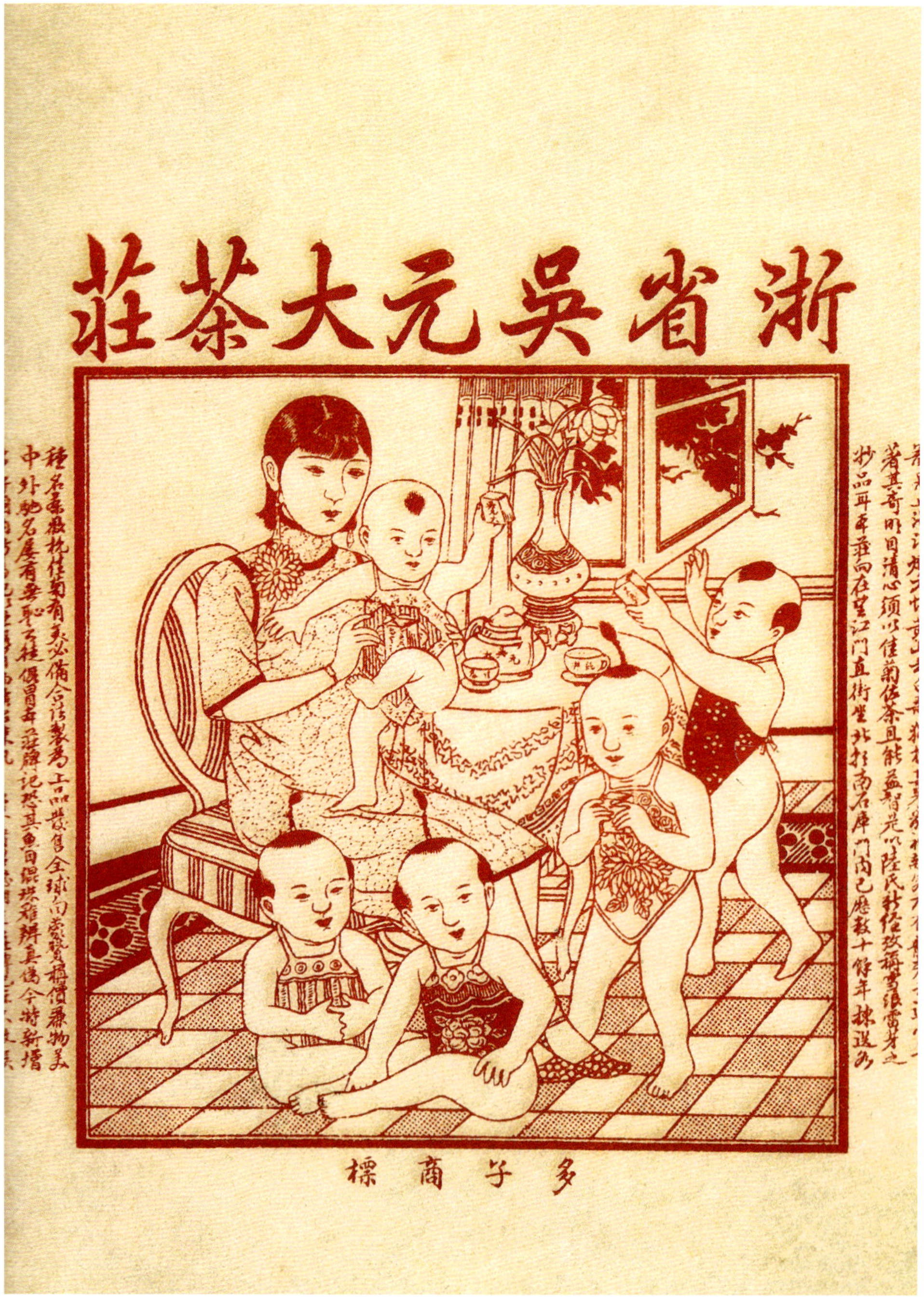

民国茶广告

Tea advertisements during the period of Republic of China

Detachment: The ultimate cause of worries is the inability to detach oneself from the world. Buddhist practice stresses detachment, and the tasting of tea also requires freedom from encumbrances.

名茶珍品

Famous teas

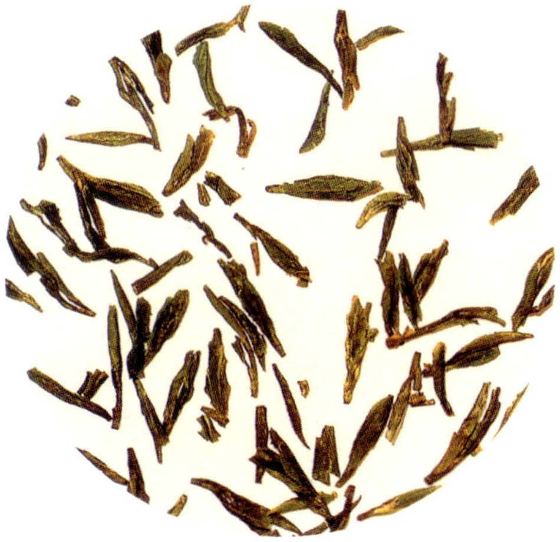

1

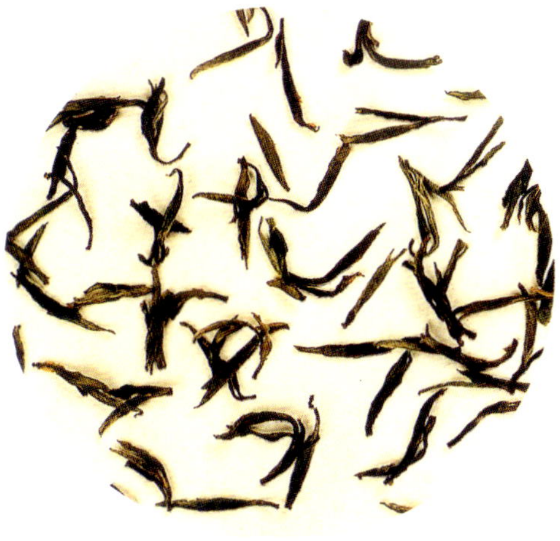

2

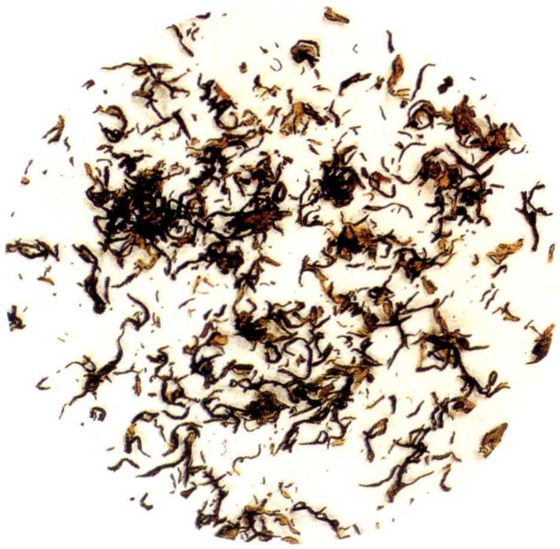

3

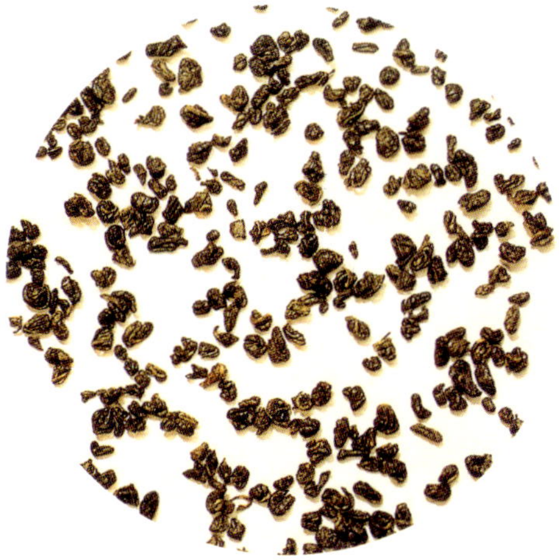

4

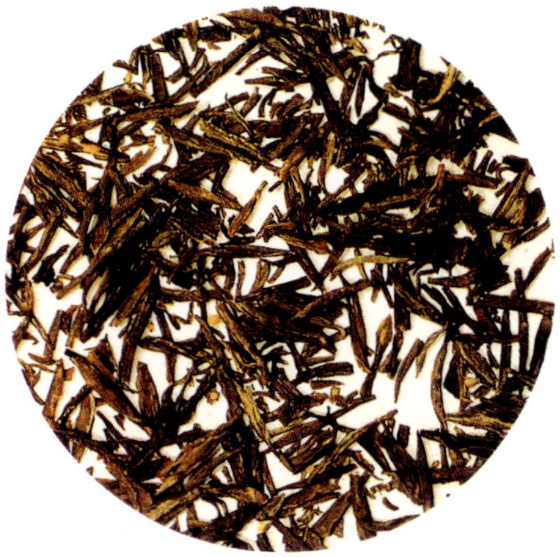

5

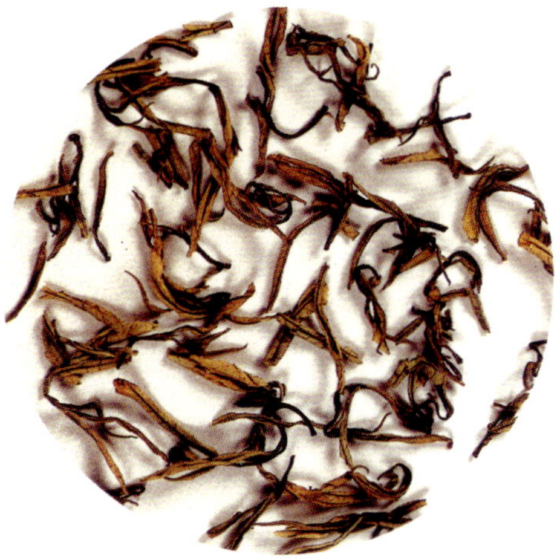

6

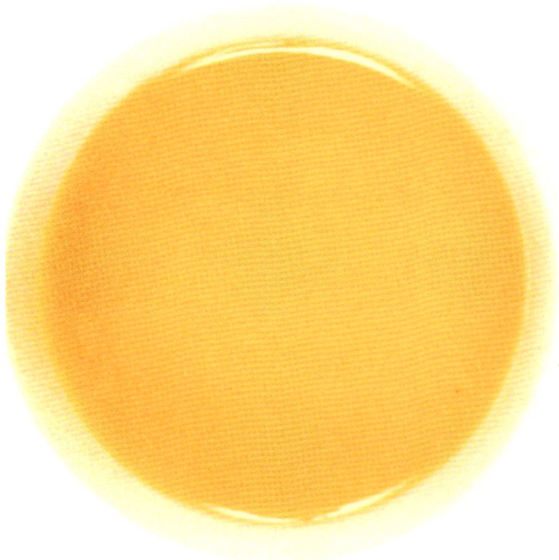

西湖龙井茶汤色

West Lake Longjing tea infusion

1. 西湖龙井
1. West Lake Longjing tea

2. 黄山毛峰
2. Huang Shan Mao Feng tea

3. 洞庭碧螺春
3. Dong Ting Bi Luo Chun

4. 珠茶
4. Gunpowder green tea

5. 竹叶青
5. Zhuyeqing tea

6. 玉凤茶
6. Yufeng tea

捌　房室养生

VIII.　Preserving Health through Sex Life

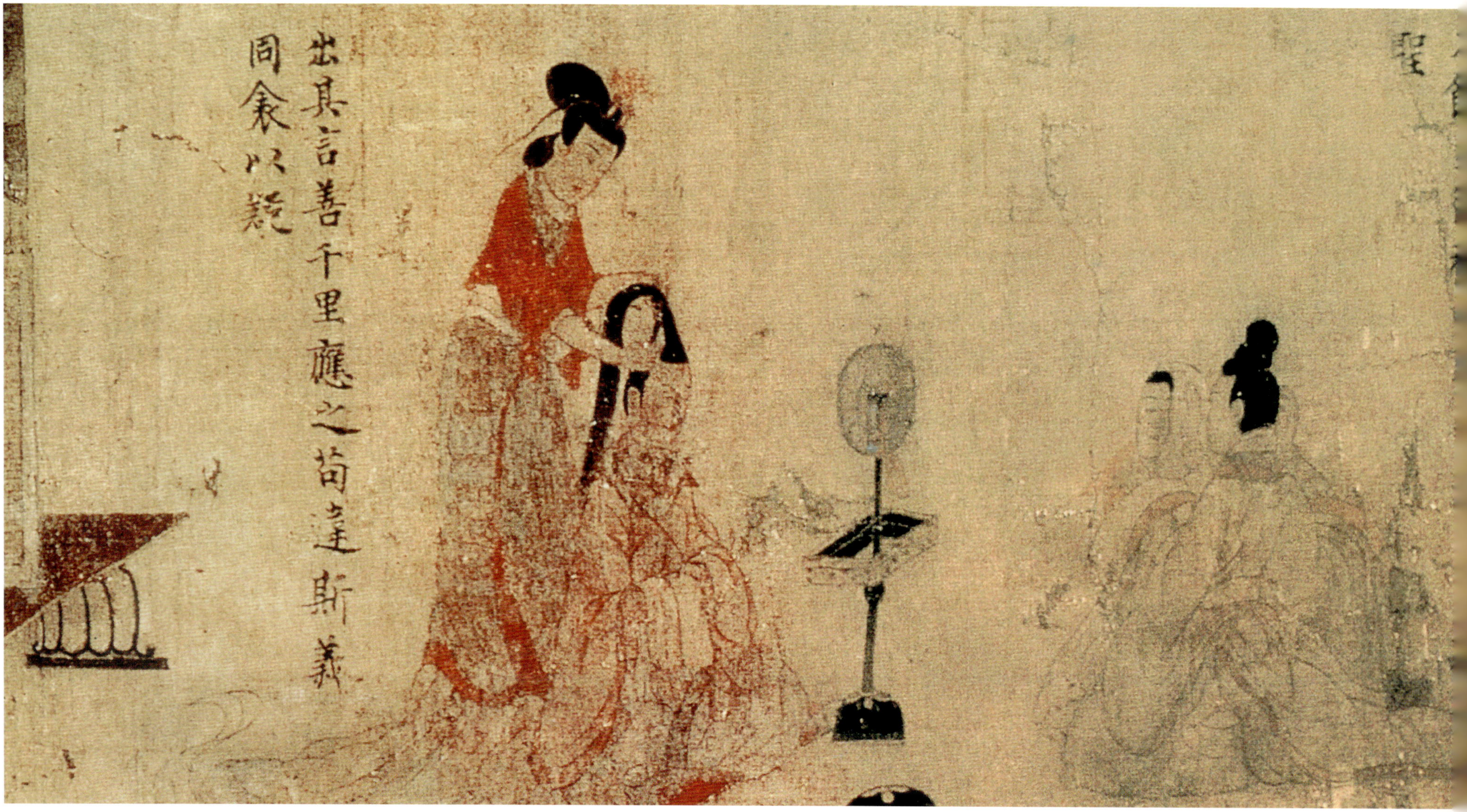

早在春秋时期，先民们已经认识到性生活对人体的影响。《左传》中记载晋侯有病求医，医生诊断为“近女室”，晋侯似有所觉悟说：“女不可近乎？”中国古代养生强调节制一切欲望的，这与后世房中术的放纵观的腐朽庸俗化是不同的。

Chinese people were already aware of the effects of sex life on the human body in the Spring and Autumn Period. *Zuo Zhuan* (the Chronicle of Zuo) records an anecdote of Lord Jin who asked a doctor over to treat his illness. The doctor attributed his illness to ‘indulgence in the bedchamber’. Lord Jin said as if in a sudden enlightenment, ‘So I can not indulge in the bedchamber?’ Ancient Chinese theories on health preservation stress abstinence of desires, which have distinguished from the Bedchamber Art of later times that encourages indulgence in sex life.

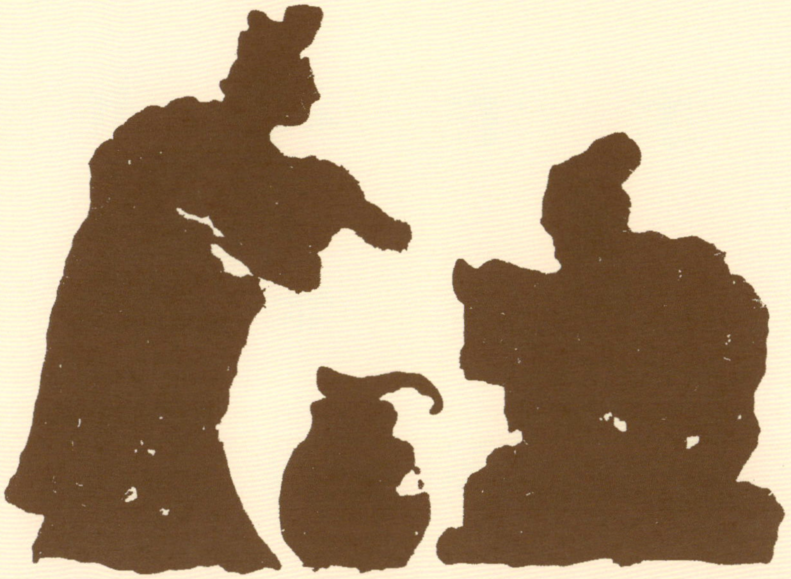

房室养生

Preserving health through sex life

1. 房室养生忌过勤

中医学认为，中老年人气、血渐衰，如果房事不节，则相火妄动，损伤阴精。纵欲的害处，在于损伤人体的精、气、神。历代医学家及现代医学都将纵欲视为中老年房室养生的大忌。

1. Don't have too much sex

According to Chinese traditional medicine, due to the decline in blood and vital energy, middle-aged people who have too much sex will suffer damage to their yin essence from improperly stirred "minister fire". Indulgence in sensual pleasures can weaken one's essence (jing), qi, and spirit (shen). Both ancient and modern medicine see such indulgence as a most serious threat to health for middle-aged and elderly people.

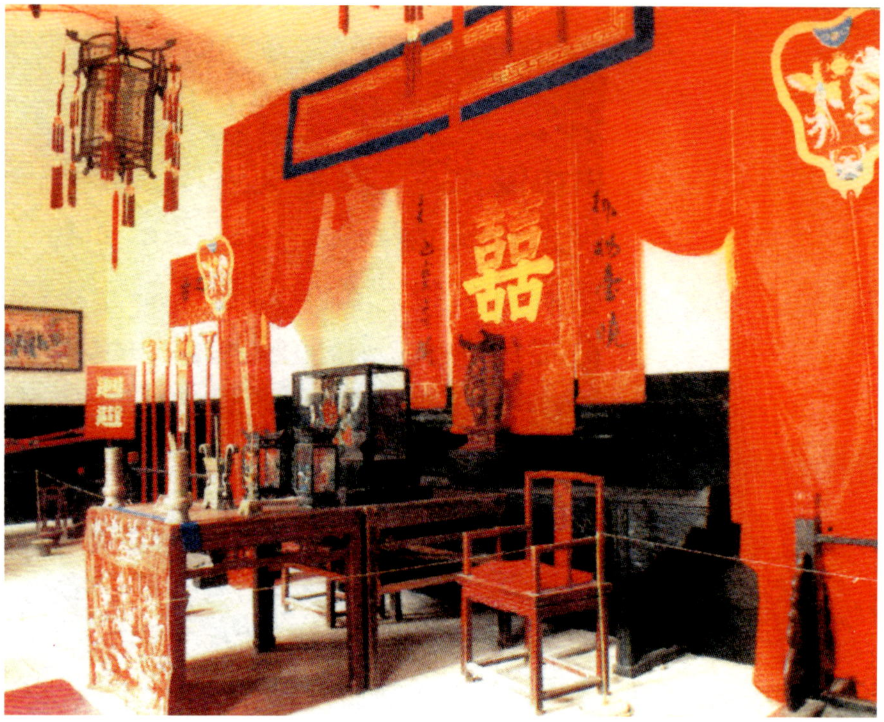

乔家大院喜堂

Qiao family courtyard wedding hall

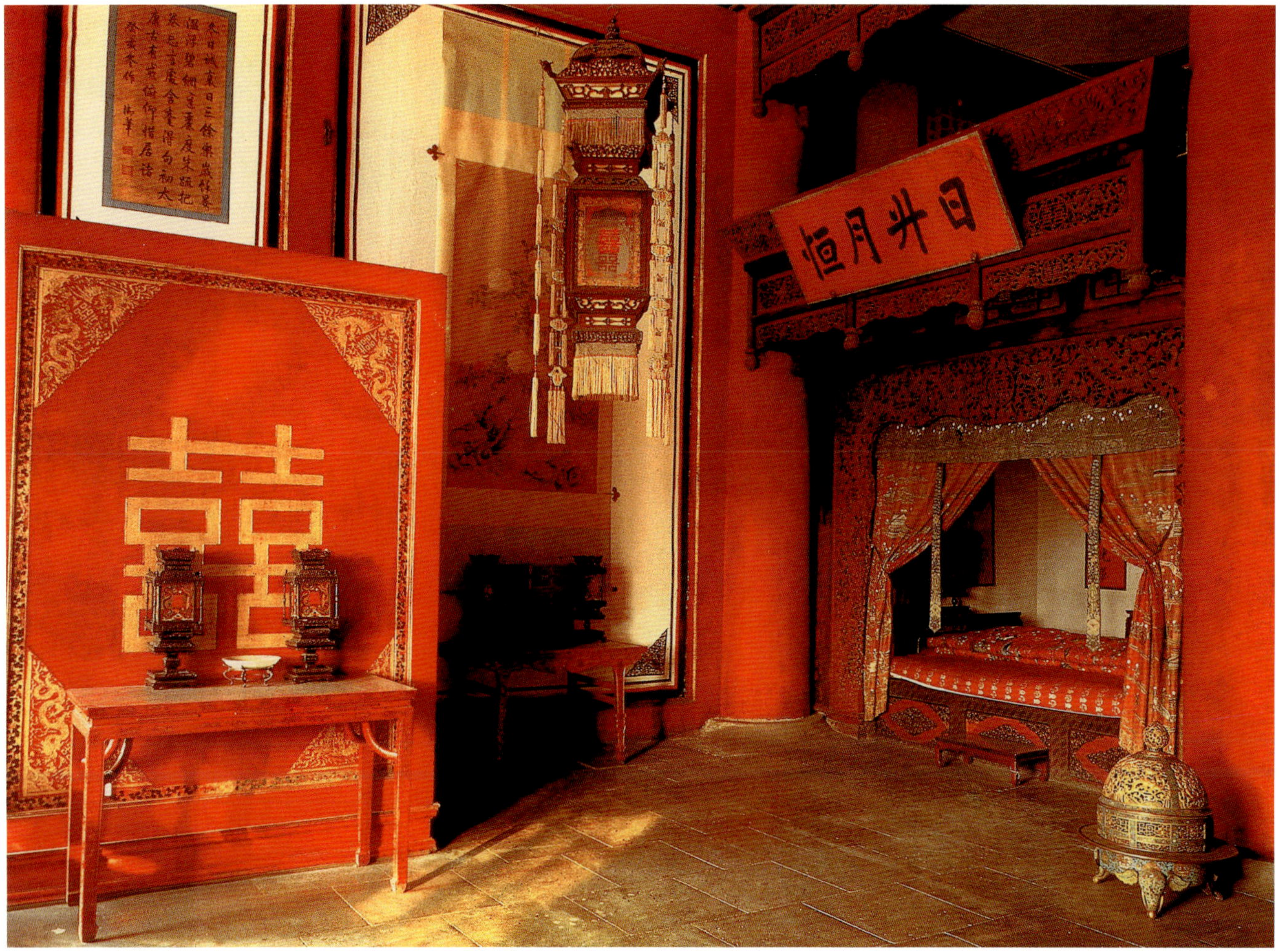

坤宁宫洞房

Bridal chamber in Kunning Gong, the Palace of Earthly Tranquility

2. 房室养生忌男女绝欲

只有适宜地进行性生活，人才能充满活力，身体才会健康。因为人是一个整体，任何一个系统或器官长期不使用，其功能就会衰退，都会导致整个机体的衰老。所谓“用进废退”即是如此。

2. Don’t abstain from sex altogether

One would not be healthy and energetic without regular sex life. Since the human body is an integrated whole, long disuse of any system or organ will cause it to decline in function and consequently lead to the aging of the whole body. This is the natural law that goes, “If you don’t use it, you lose it.”

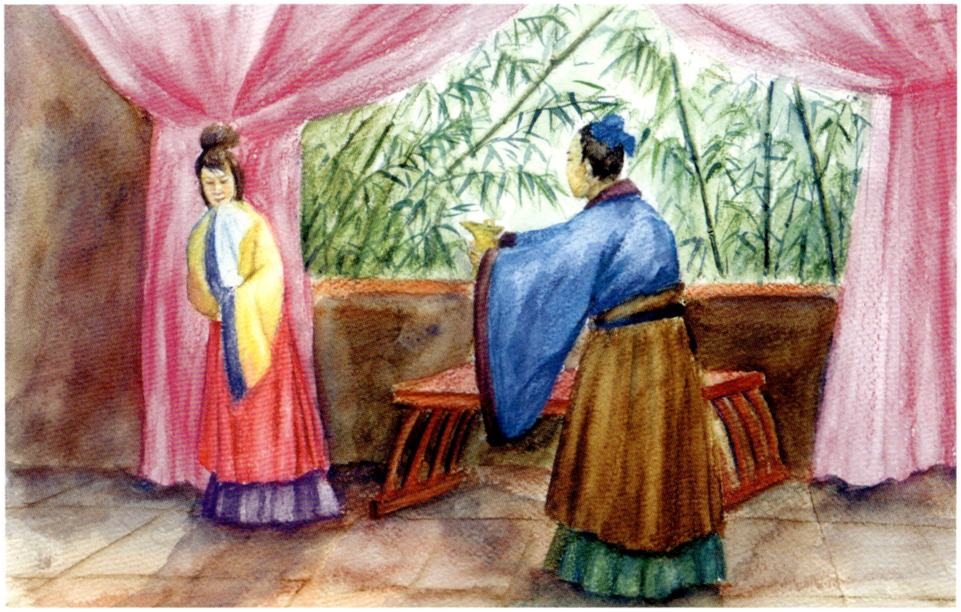

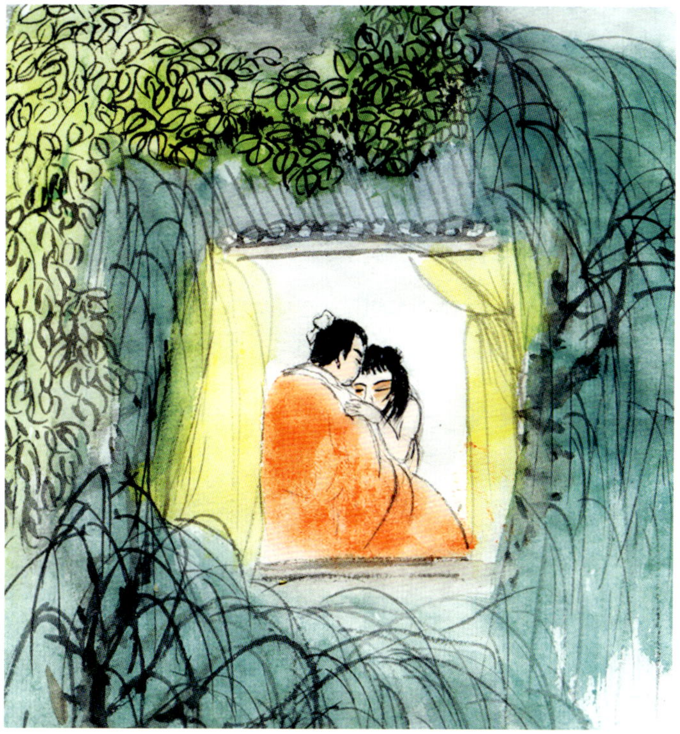

正常的性生活，不但有利于保持健康的心理，而且可以调节人体各个器官的功能，使之保持最佳状态，这样人就不至于过早衰老，相反会延缓衰老。

A normal sex life can not only help to maintain psychological well-being but also regulate the functions of all organs and keep them in the optimal state. Thus aging will be delayed instead of occurring prematurely.

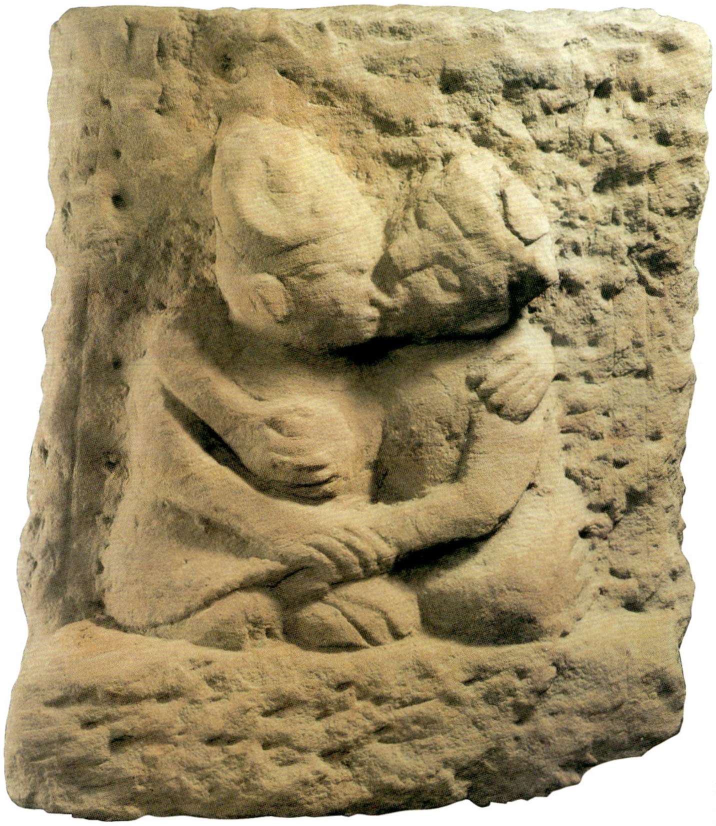

汉代石刻

Stone sculpture of Han Dynasty

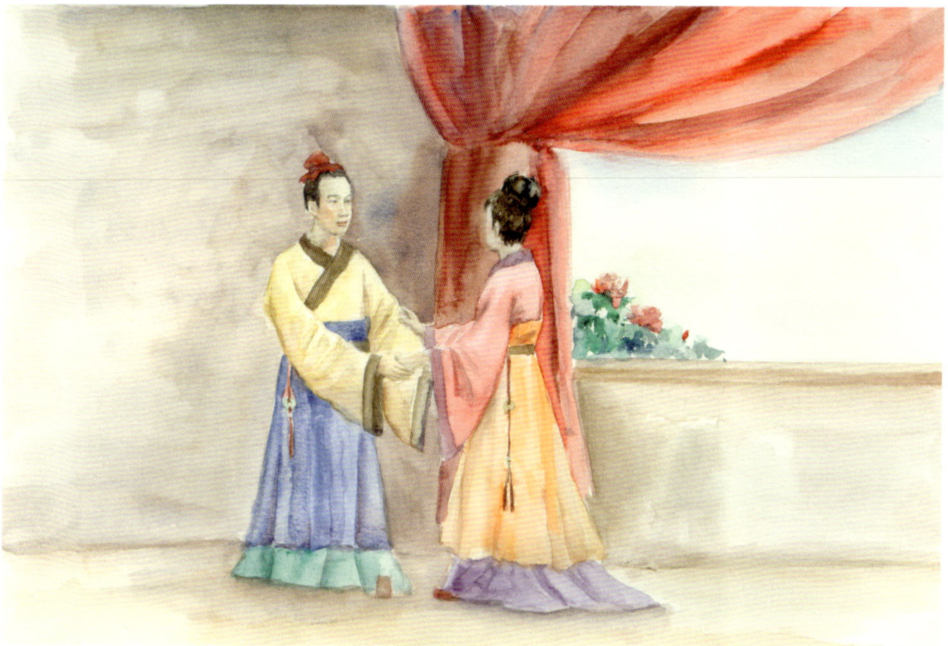

3. 房室养生忌情志过激

性生活要情意调和，不可过分激动。

3. Don't have sex when you are too excited

When having sex, keep a peaceful mind and avoid too much excitement.

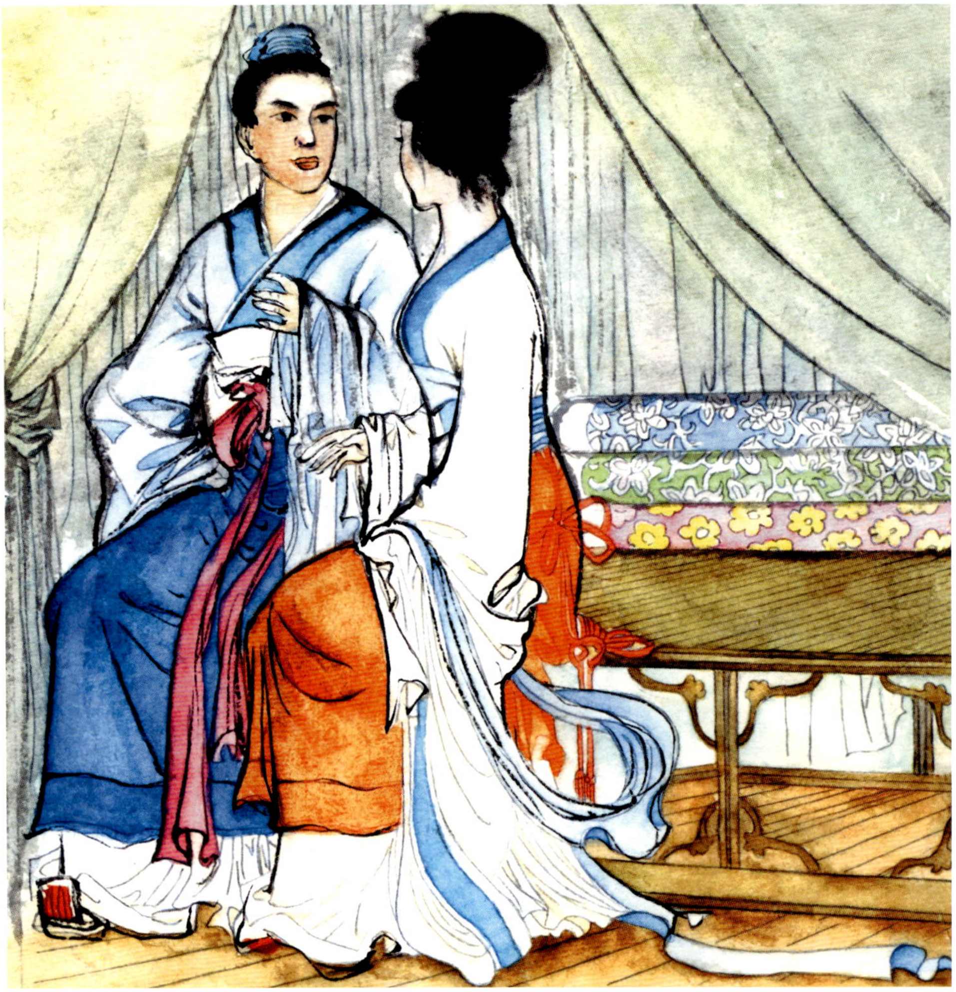

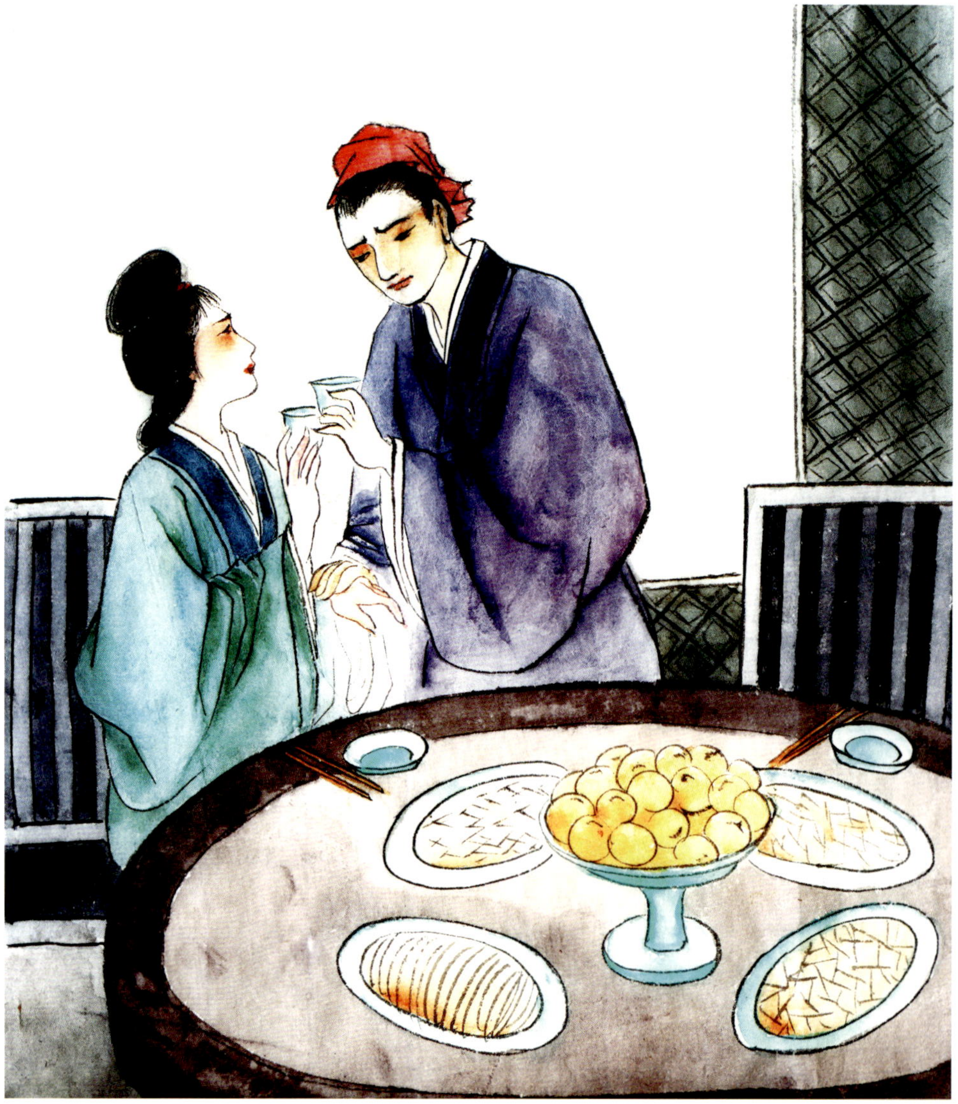

唐代医学家孙思邈说："大喜大悲，皆不可交阴阳。"而且指出："人有所怒，血气未定，因以交合，令人发痈疽。"

《寿世保元》亦指出："恐惧中过性生活，阴阳偏虚，自汗盗汗，积而成劳。"

"Do not have the intercourse of yin and yang in great joy or grief," said Sun Simiao, a Tang medical scientist. He also said, "Having intercourse in anger, which excites blood and vital energy, will cause ulcer."

Preserving Vital Energy for a Long Life notes, "Having sex in fear, which weakens both yin and yang, will cause night sweat and fatigue."

4. 房室养生忌疲劳过度

在身体疲乏、体力和脑力疲惫、精力不足时，应避免房事，否则会损伤肾气，伤害身体。男女双方有一方精力不济，即容易引起早泄，导致性生活草草了事，质量不佳。

4. Don't have sex when you are too tired

Don't have sex when you are tired either mentally or physically. Otherwise it will do harm to your health by weakening your kidney qi. Besides, tiredness in either of a couple is likely to cause premature ejaculation and affect the harmony of sex life.

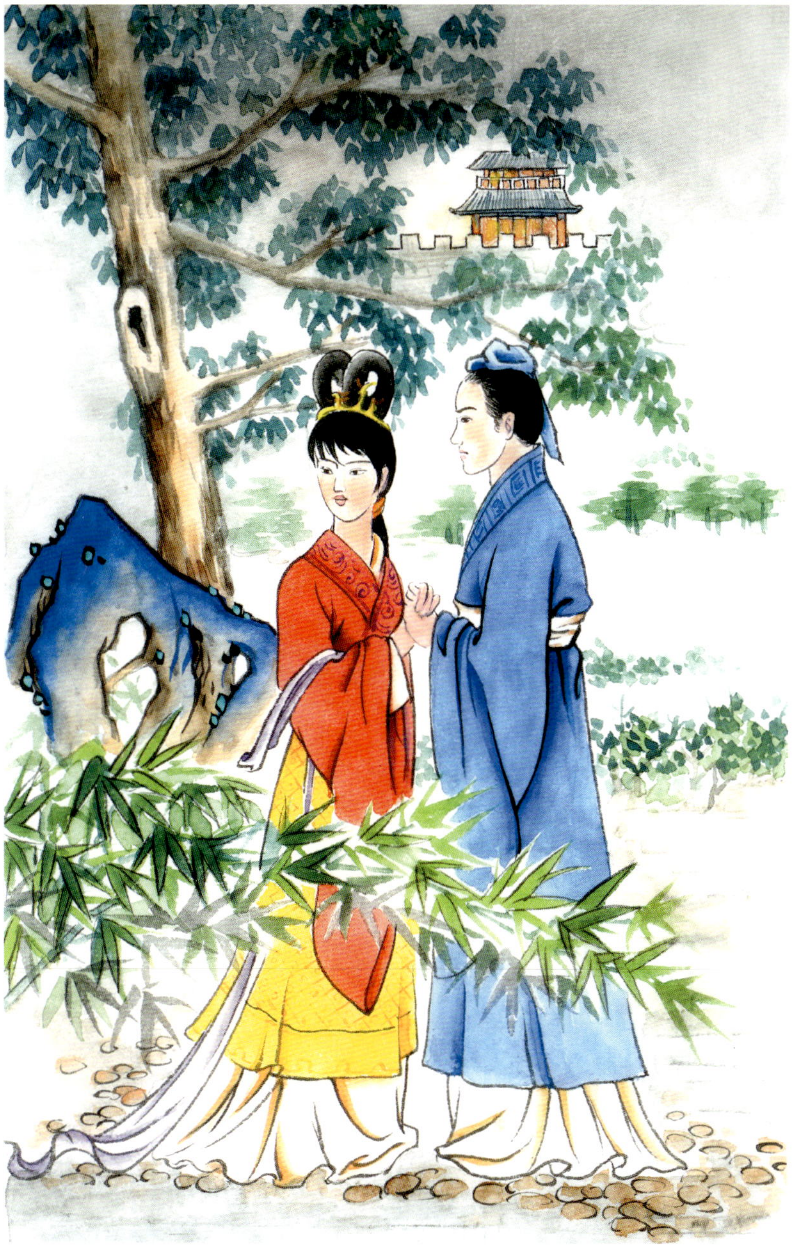

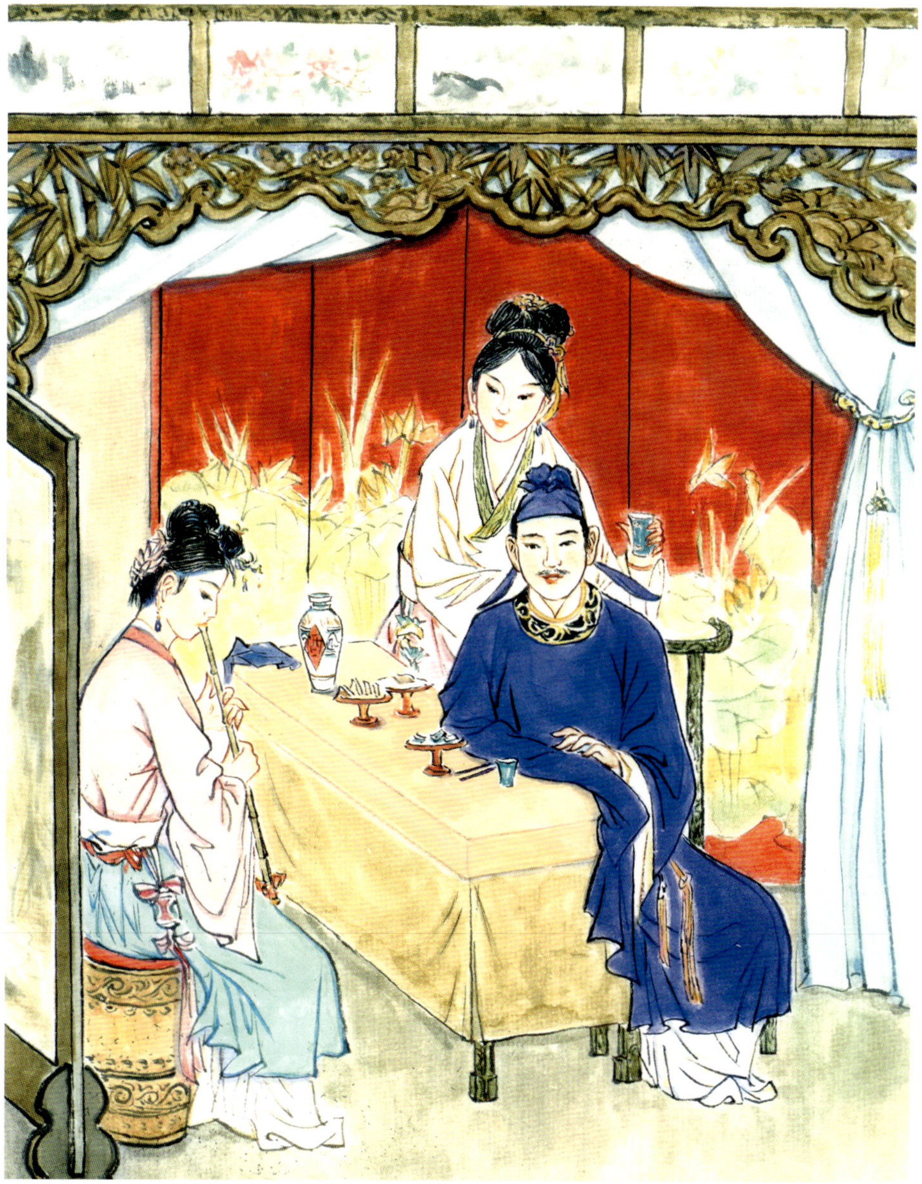

5. 房室养生要顺应四时

自然界的季节年复一年，周而复始地更替变化，这已成了一个规律。正是因为有了四季更替，万物才得以春生、夏长、秋收、冬藏。

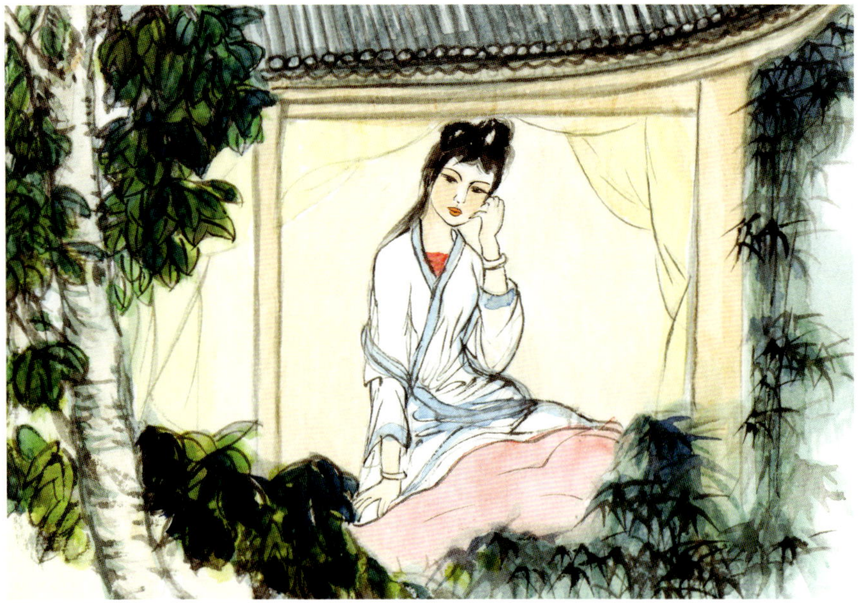

5. Follow the seasons

The cycle of seasons is repeated year in year out. It is the change of seasons that produces the cycle in living things: birth in spring, growth in summer, harvest in autumn, and storage in winter.

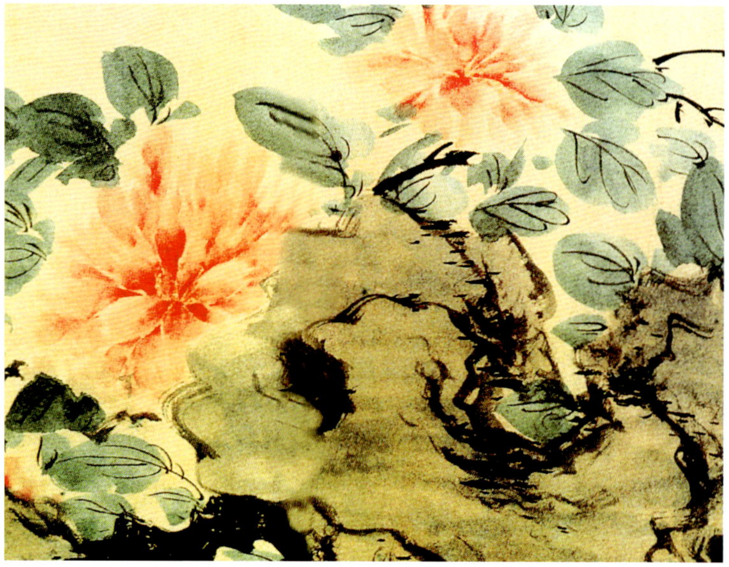

牡丹应时开放

Peonies blooming in good time

6. 房室养生忌浴后过性生活

浴后立即过性生活会引起性功能障碍，对健康有害。因为人体内各个脏器的血液分布是有一定量的，浴后血液大量地存积在皮肤浅表的血管中，易造成性器官供血不足而影响性功能。所以，浴后不宜立即过性生活。

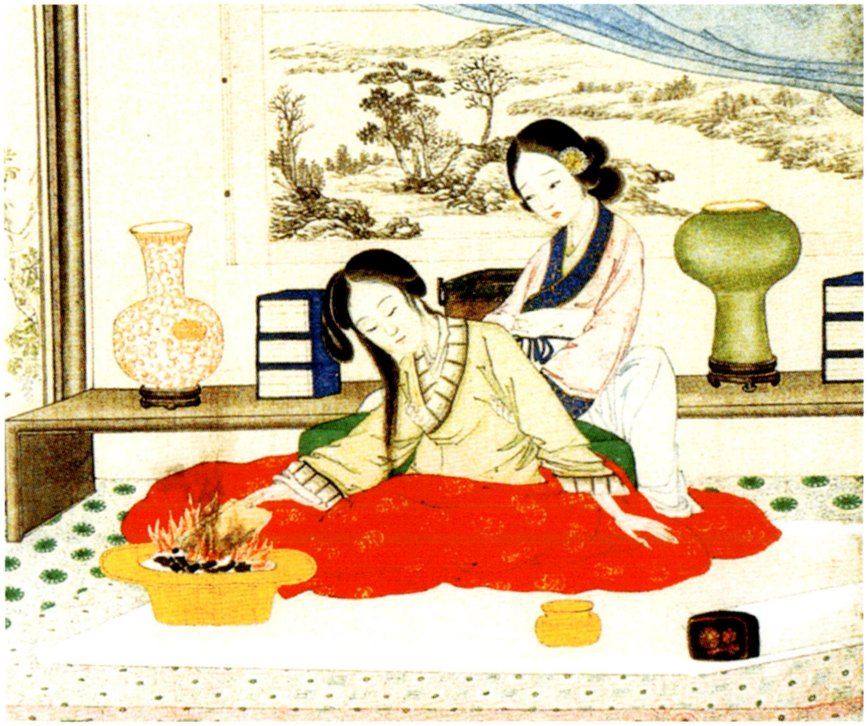

6. Don't have sex immediately after bathing

To have sex immediately after bathing can cause sexual dysfunction or be detrimental to health, for your organs cannot function properly without a certain amount of blood. After bathing, a lot of blood is in the blood vessels right beneath the skin, causing a deficiency in the blood supply to the sexual organs, which will affect their function. That is why it is advisable to have sex when you have just had a bath.

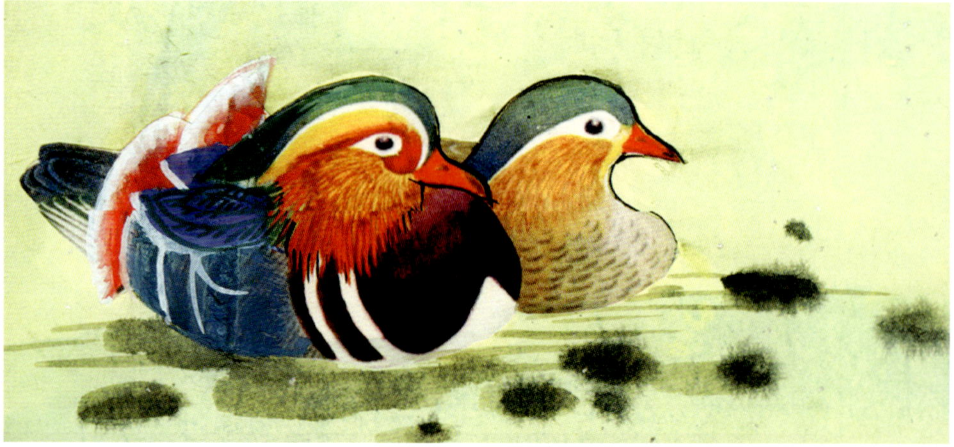

鸳鸯象征和谐

Mandarin ducks symbolize harmony.

7. 房室养生应避“三期”

女性月经期、孕期、产褥期称为“三期”。夫妻性生活对女方“三期”保健是不利的。

7. Avoid the “three periods”

The “three periods” for women refer to menstruation, pregnancy, and puerperium. Having sex is harmful to health for a woman in any of these periods.

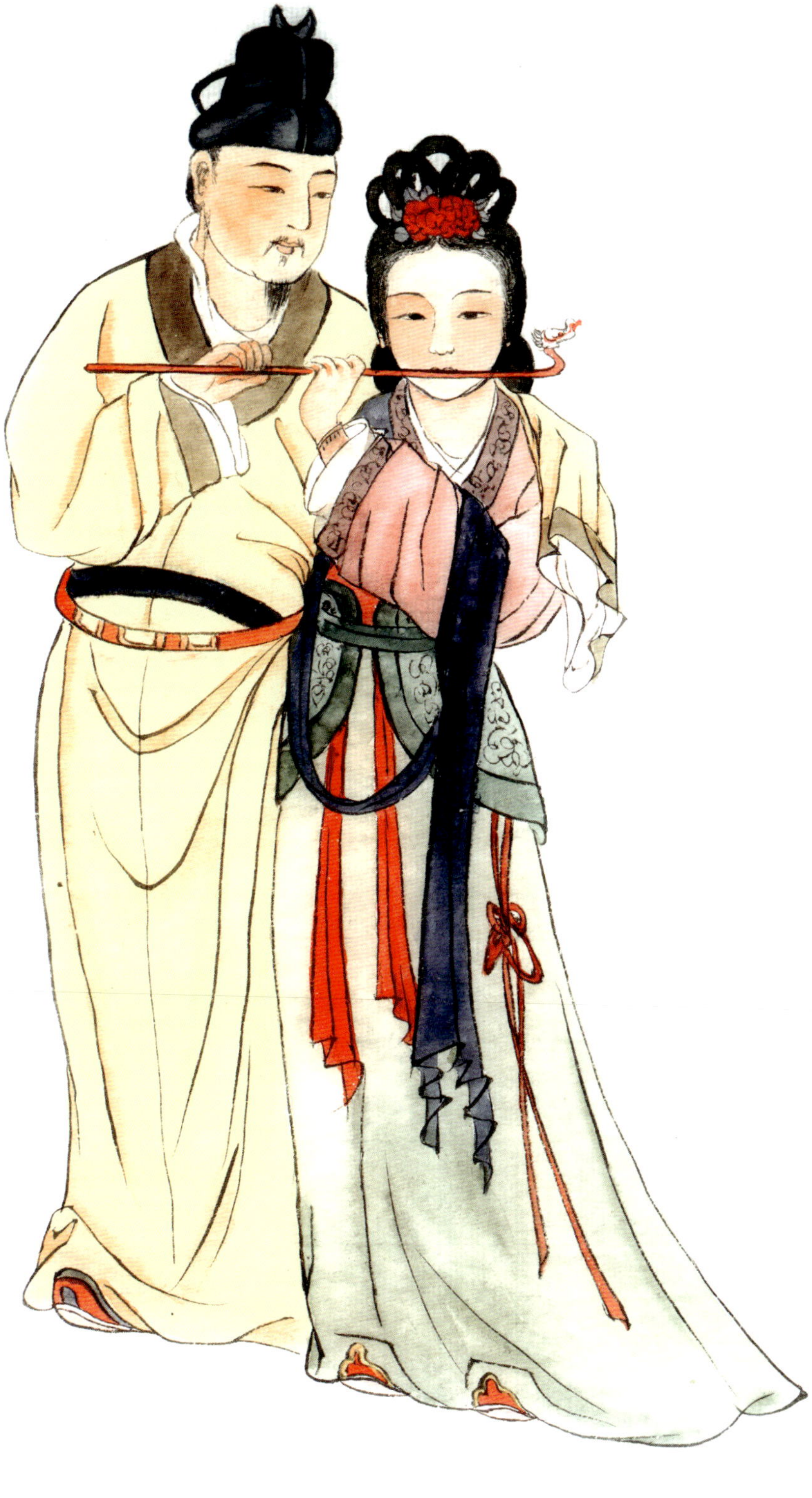

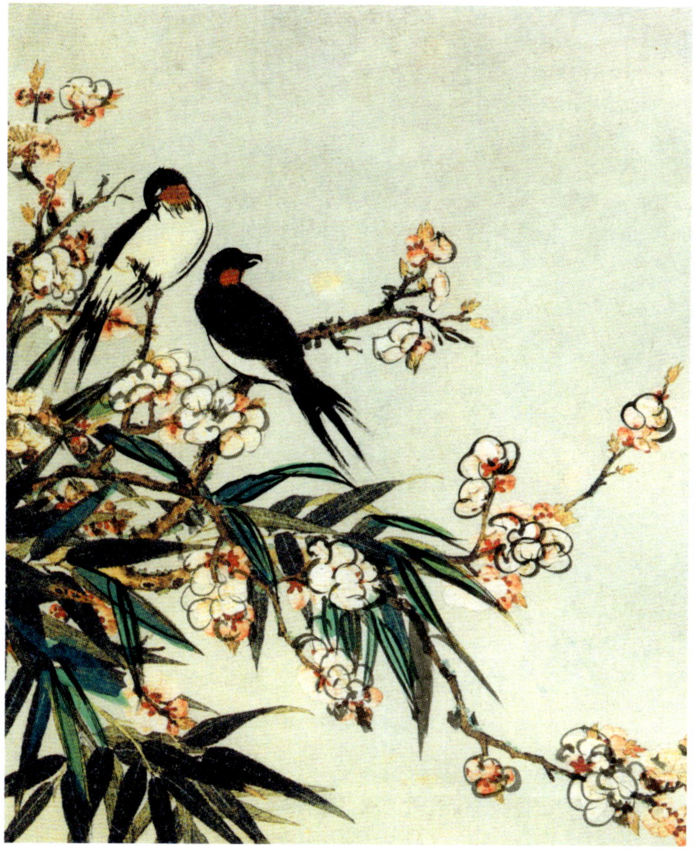

花鸟之乐图

Pleasure of Flowers and Birds

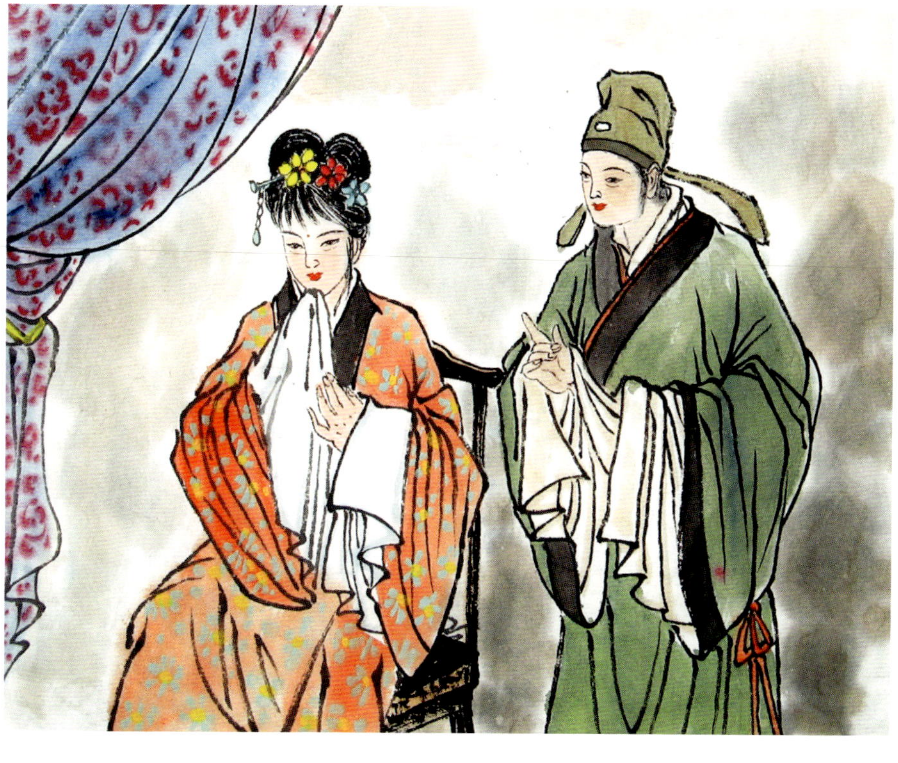

8. 房室生活忌凭借春药

中老年房中之事，应顺其自然。清代医学家徐大椿说："故精之为物，欲动为生，不动则不生，故自然不动者有益，强制者有害，过用衰竭，任其自然而无勉强，则自然之法也。"如果滥用壮阳药，一味增强性欲或提高性生活能力，则犹如杀鸡取卵，更使精竭肾衰。

8. Don't rely on aphrodisiacs

Middle-aged and elderly people should take it easy when having sex. Xu Dachun, a Qing medical scientist, said, "Semen is only generated when desire is aroused. To let desire rest still is beneficial, to activate it by force is harmful, and to use it too much will deplete it. To let it take its own course without intervention is the natural method to follow." To enhance sexual desire or potency with aphrodisiacs, which is comparable to "killing the hen to get the eggs", will drain your semen and enervate your kidney.

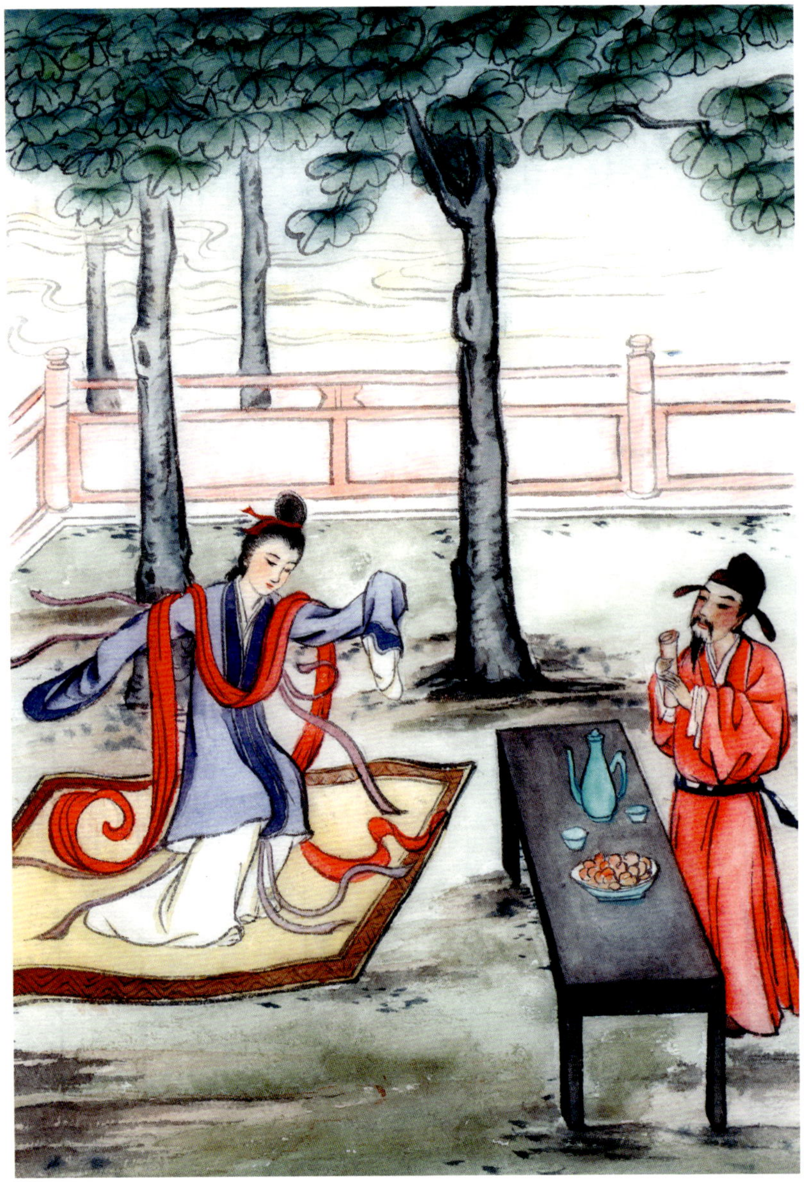

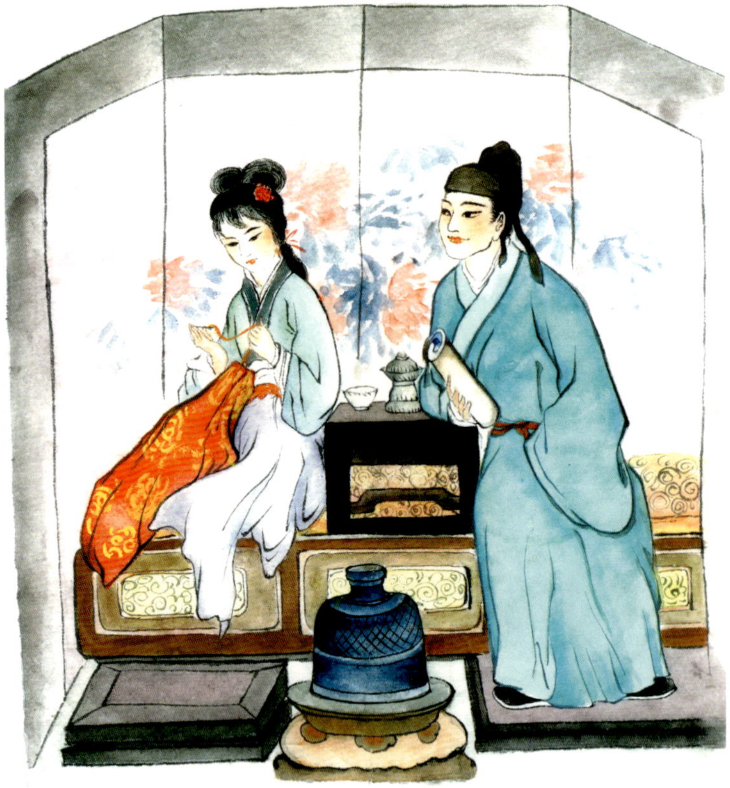

唐代医学家孙思邈也说："贪心未止，兼饵补药，倍力行房，不过半年，精髓枯竭。"

古代皇帝借春药寻欢作乐早夭折寿的故事，便是对这一禁忌的最好说明。

As Tang medical scientist Sun Simiao put it, "If, driven by insatiable greed, one takes drugs and has sex with redoubled efforts, his essence will be drained within six months."

As a case in point, many emperors died an untimely death from the habit of having sex on aphrodisiacs.

9. 房室养生忌过饱或饥饿

中老年人亦不可饱食后过性生活。古人说："饱食过房事，劳伤血气，流溢渗入大肠时，便清血，腹痛，病名肠癖。"老年人胃肠道消化功能降低，如果饮食过量，极易造成胃肠负担过重，出现嗳气、腹胀、腹泻等症状。长此以往可导致肾精化源不足，性功能衰退。

9. Don't have sex when you are full or hungry

Middle-aged and elderly people should not have sex on a full stomach. Ancient people said, "To have intercourse when one is full harms blood and vital energy, which will seep into the large intestine, causing blood in stool and abdominal pain. The name of this disease is changpi." Elderly people tend to be weak in digestion, so eating too much is very likely to put excessive burden on their digestive system, leading to symptoms like belch, abdominal distension, and diarrhea. If this goes on for too long, it can cause deficiency in kidney essence and sexual dysfunction.

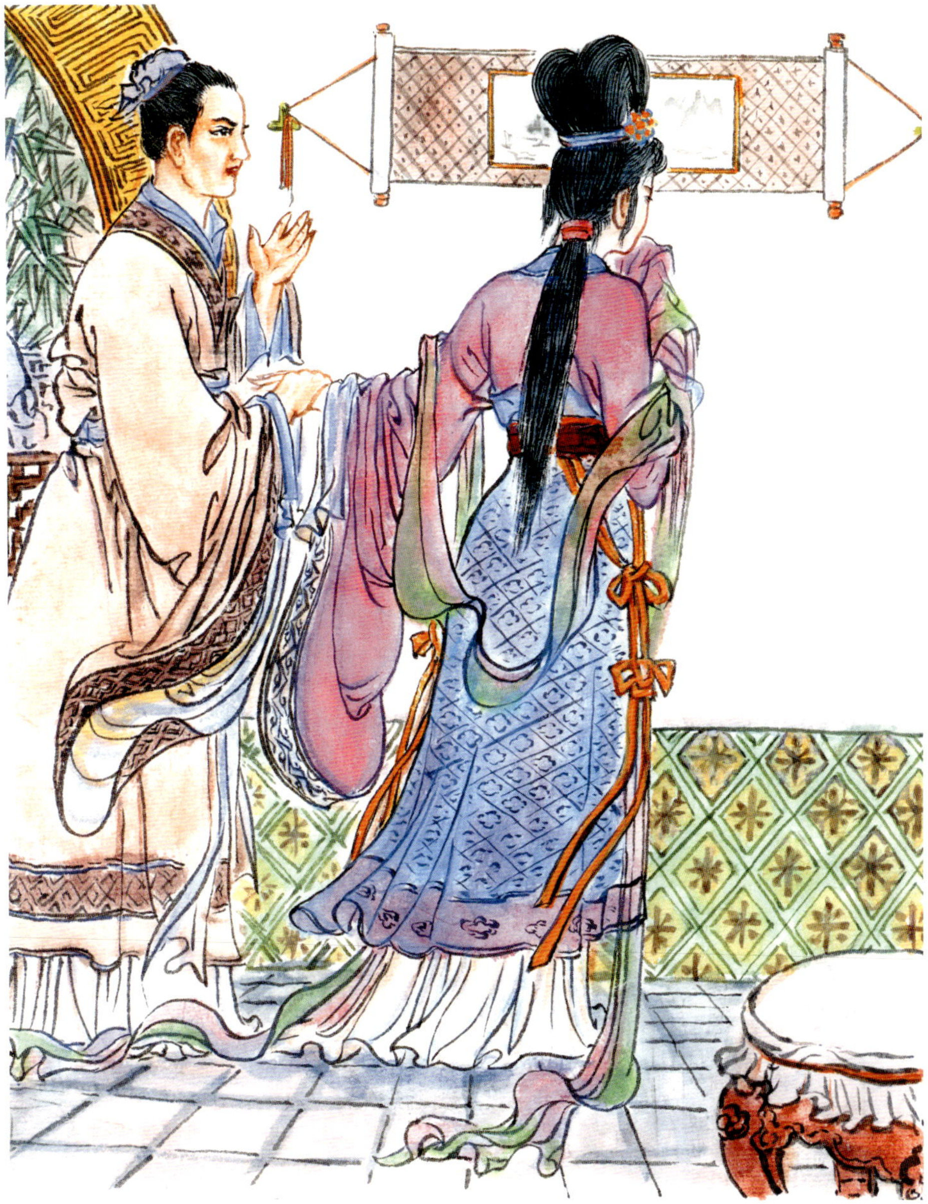

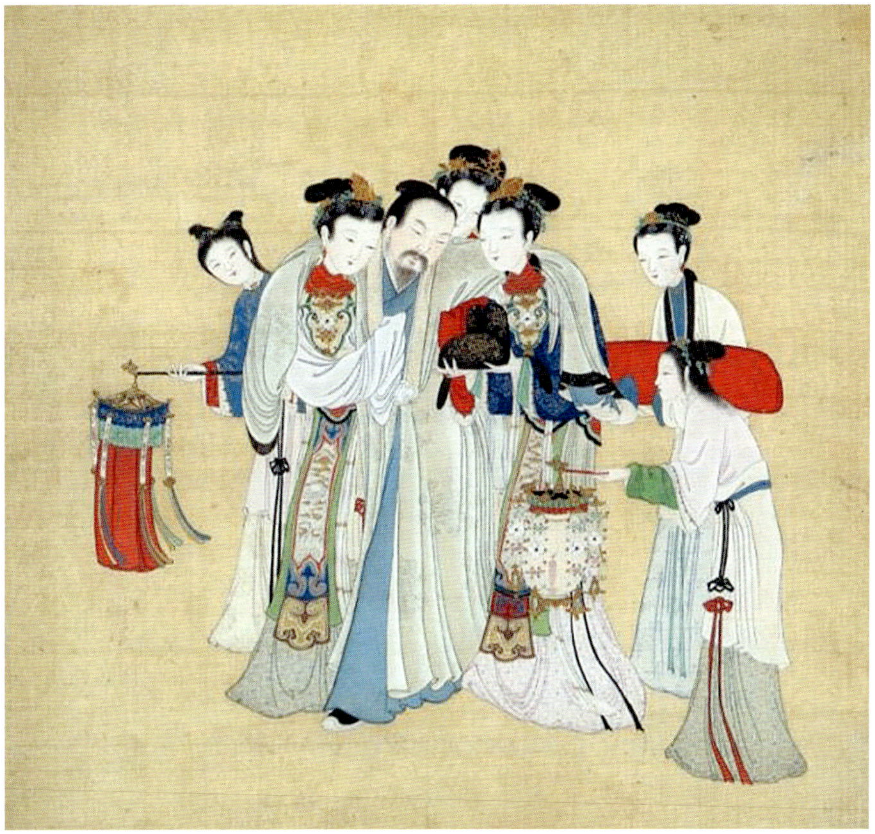

玖　食用本草

IX:　Consumption of Chinese Herbs

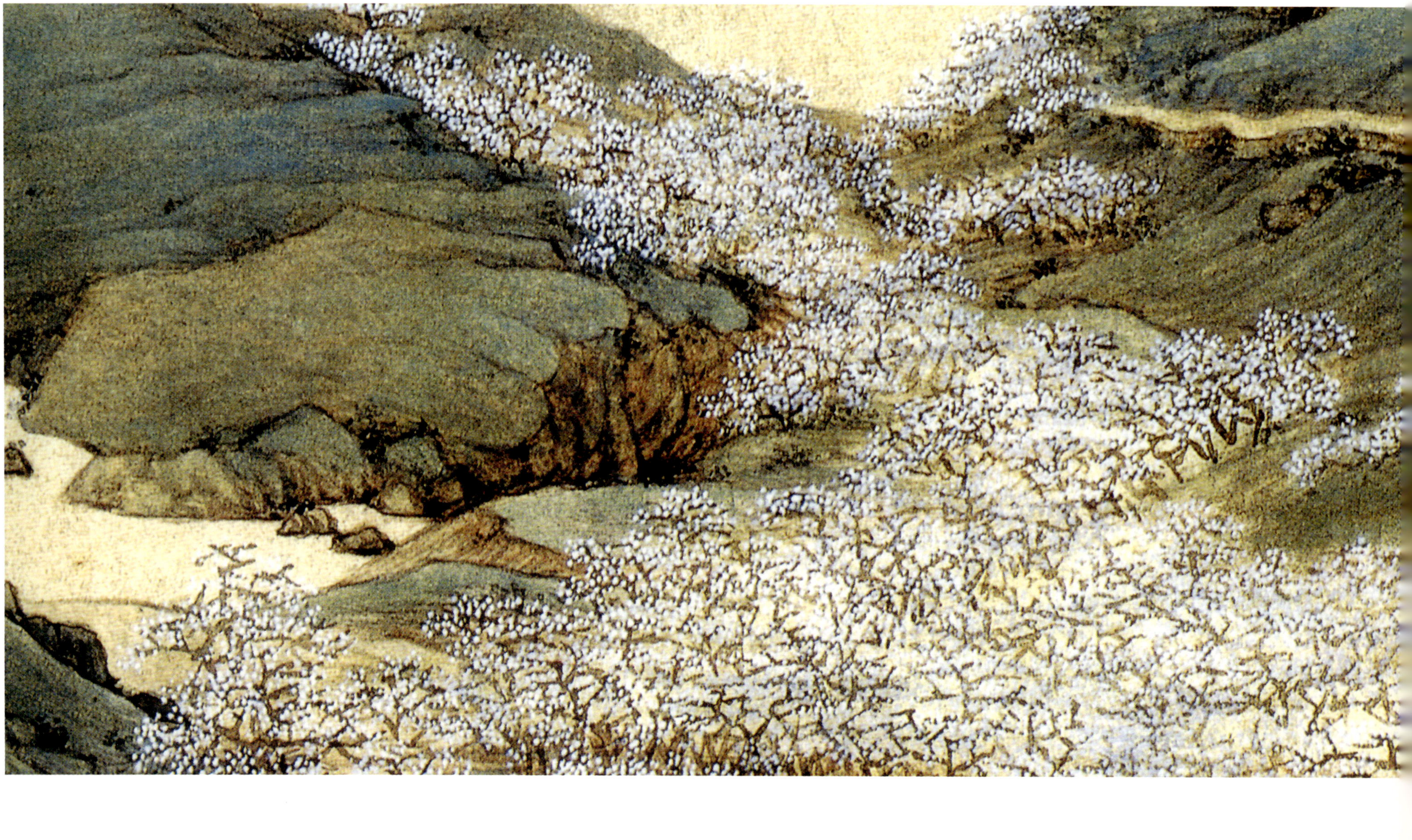

中国医学讲“药食同源”（又称“医食同源”），民间讲“药补不如食补”，就是说许多食物同时也有药用价值，同样能够防病治病，而且食疗是没有副作用的。

本书精选《本草纲目》中常用的食材配以精美手绘插图，附录于此，供可阅读中文者参考。

According to Traditional Chinese Medicine, “medicines and foods are of the same origin”; a folk saying goes, “Kitchen physic is the best physic.” In other words, many foods have medicinal value and can be used to treat diseases. Moreover, dietary therapy has no side effects.

This book selects some common ingredients from the *Compendium of Materia Medica* and provides their illustrations in this annex. Hopefully they may serve as useful reference for the reader.

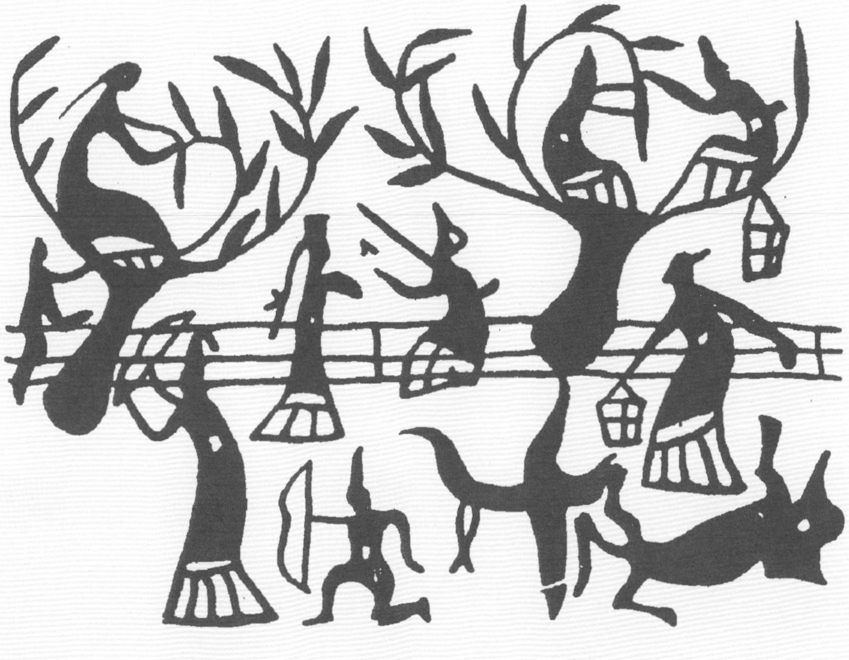

稻

Rice

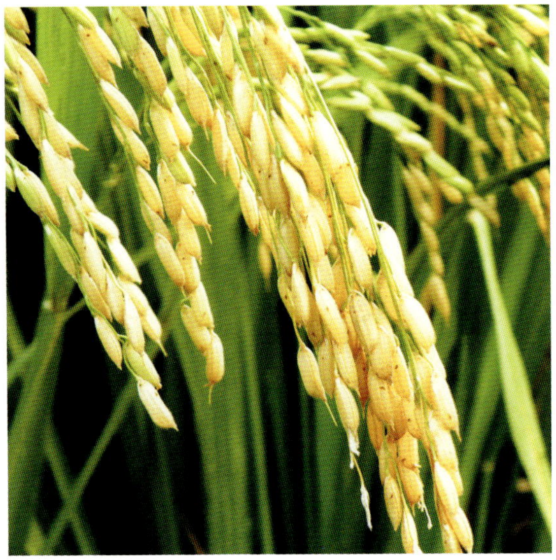

稻米有补中益气的功效。

The rice can strengthen the middle warmer and replenish qi.

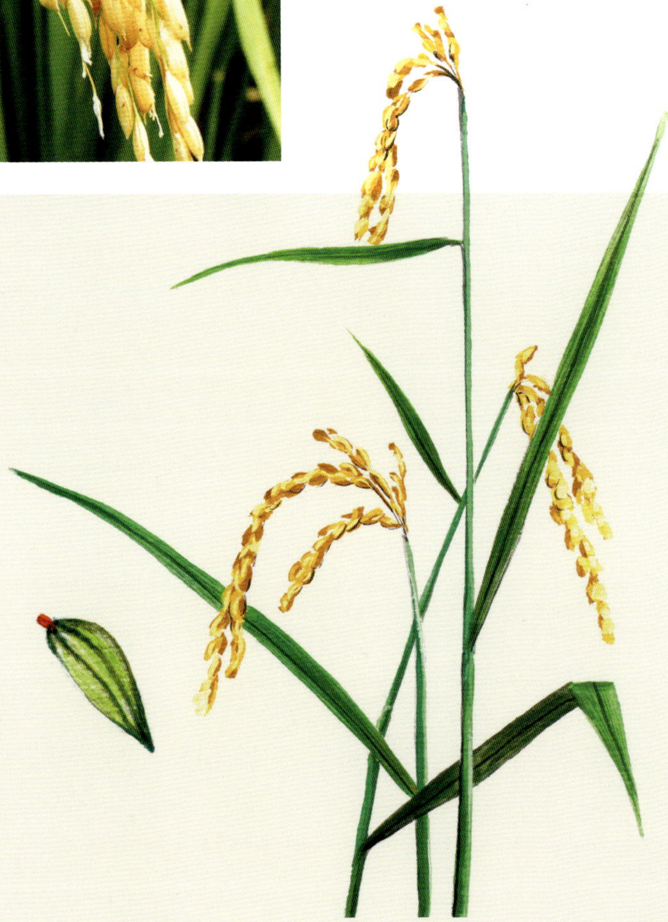

稻米性温 可健脾胃
补中益氣 粥食養生

小麦

Wheat

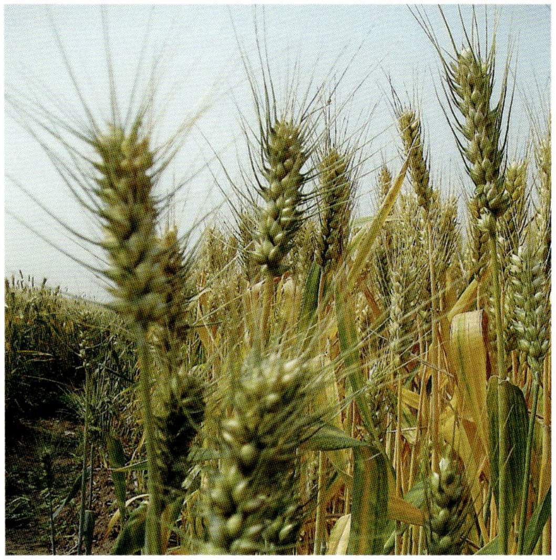

小麦有养心、益肾的功效。

The wheat can nourish the heart and kidney.

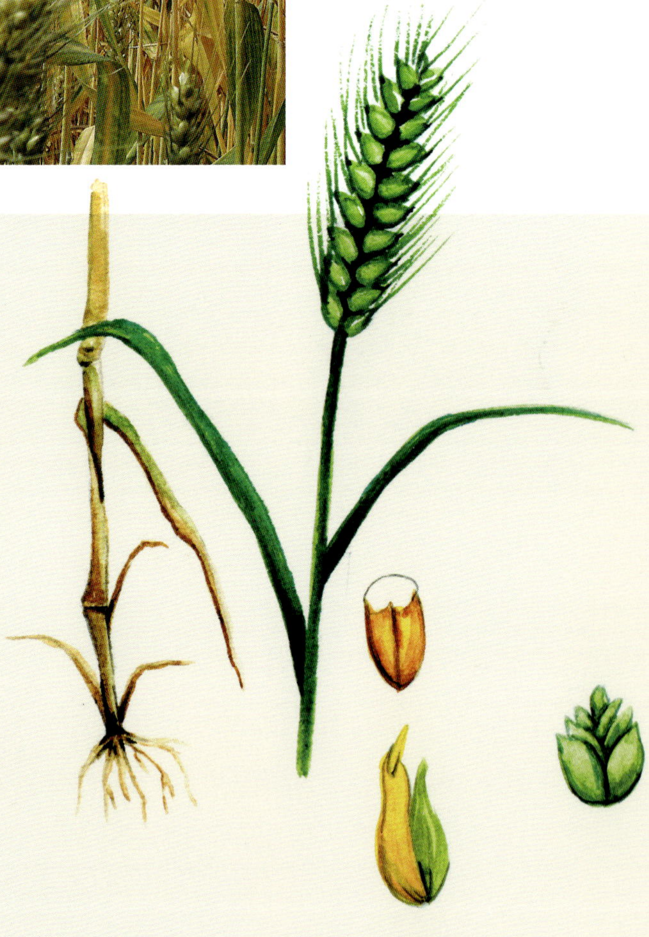

小麦微寒 除熱止渴
養心益腎 饅頭烤食

小米

Millet

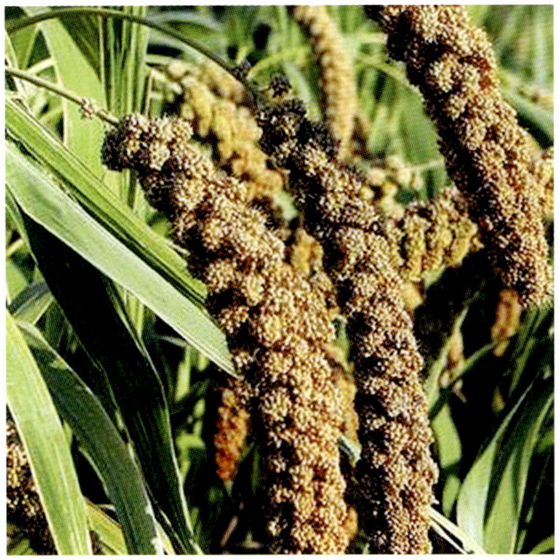

小米可以健胃、和脾、安眠。

Millet can strengthen the stomach, harmonize the spleen, and improve one's sleep.

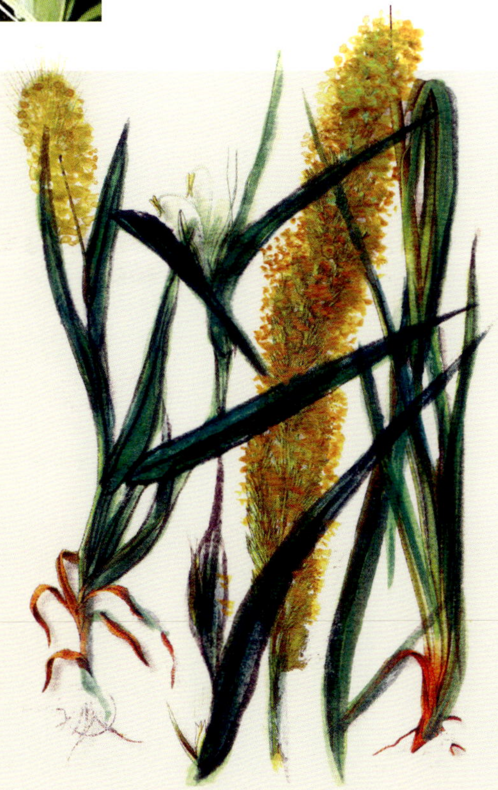

小米谷首 健胃安眠
性質微寒 龍眼紅糖

雀麦

Oat

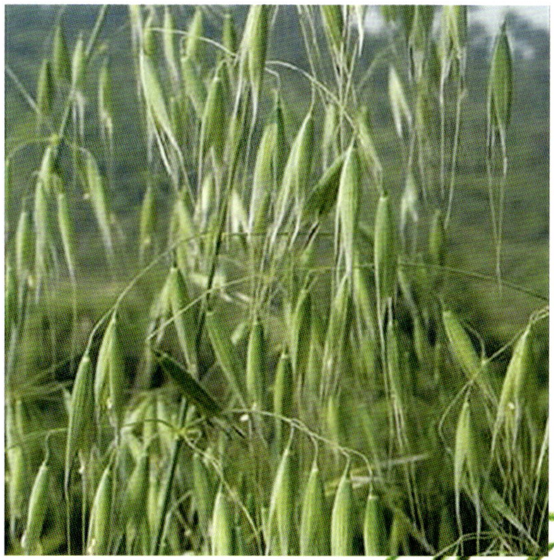

燕麦补益脾胃、降脂降压。

Oat can replenish the kidney and the stomach and reduce blood fat and blood pressure.

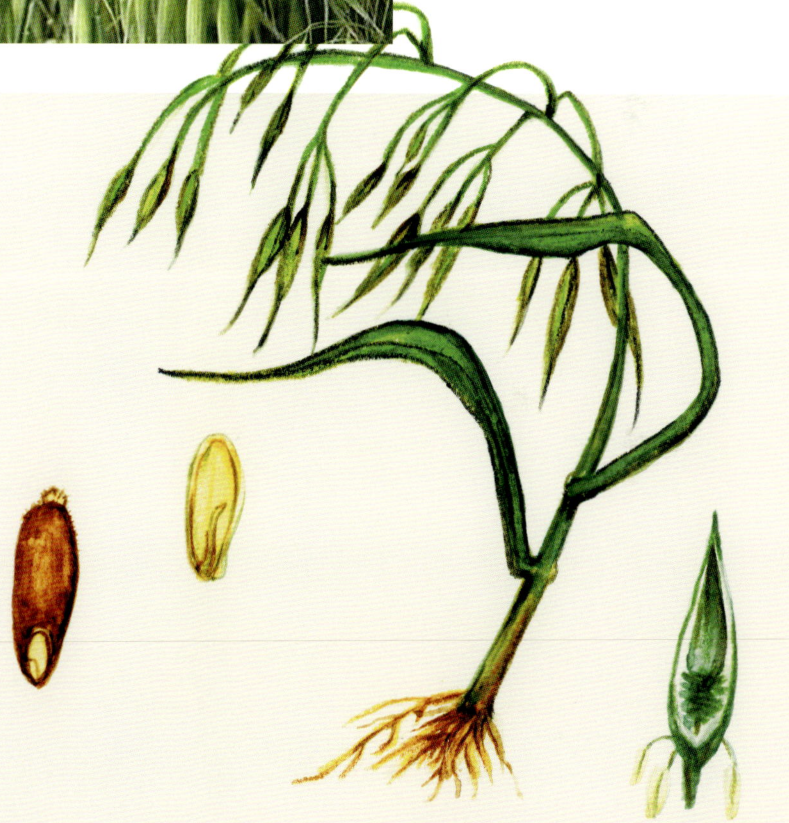

燕麥益脾 降脂降壓
止汗止血 適宜老人

玉米

Maize

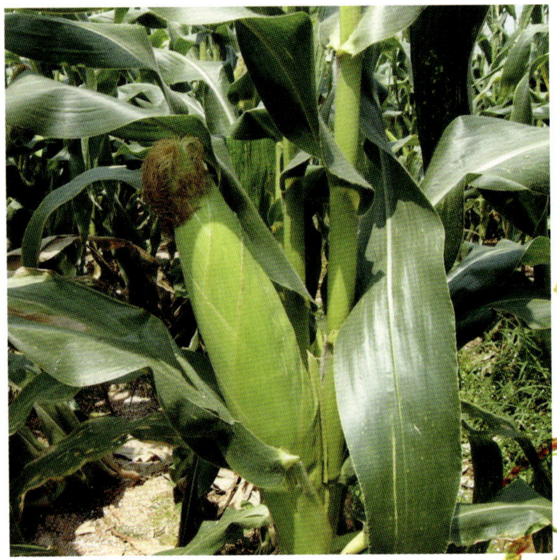

玉米降压、降糖、增人体力。

Maize can reduce blood pressure and blood sugar and increase strength.

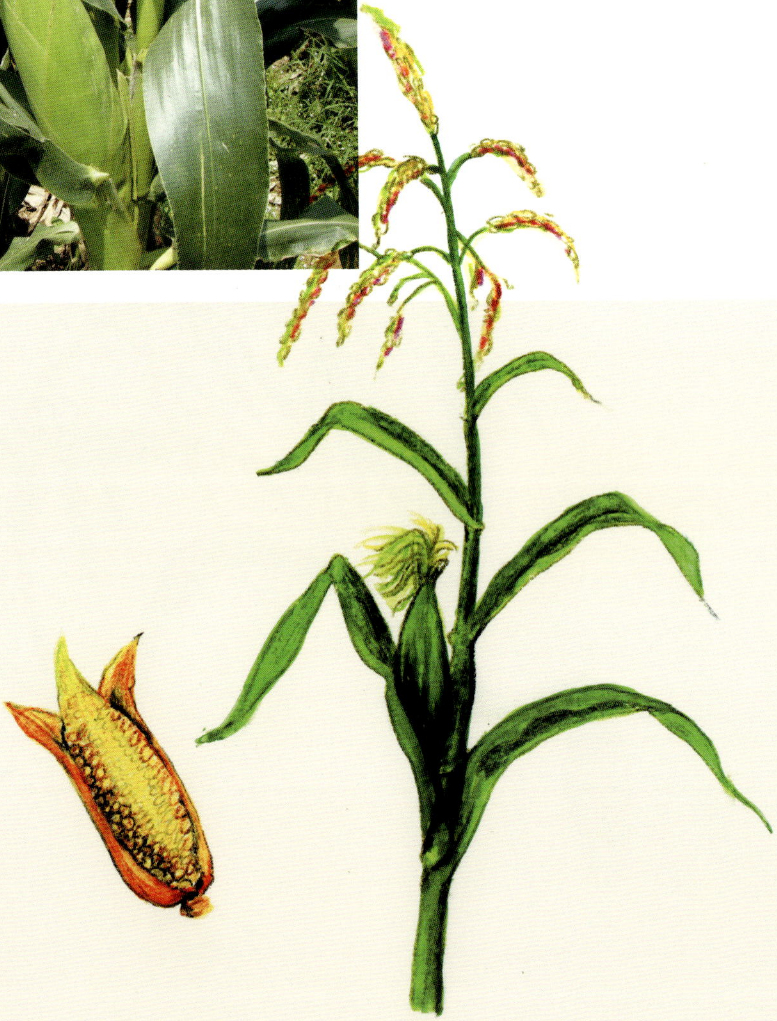

玉米利尿　防治便秘
降糖降壓　增强體力

高粱

Sorghum

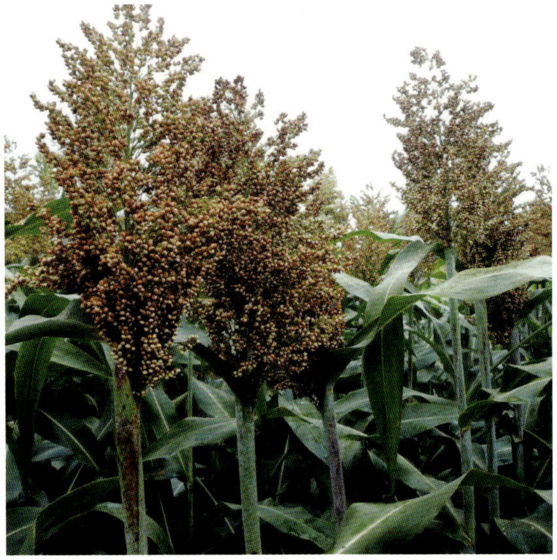

高粱和胃、健脾、凉血。

Sorghum can harmonize the stomach, strengthen the spleen, and cool the blood.

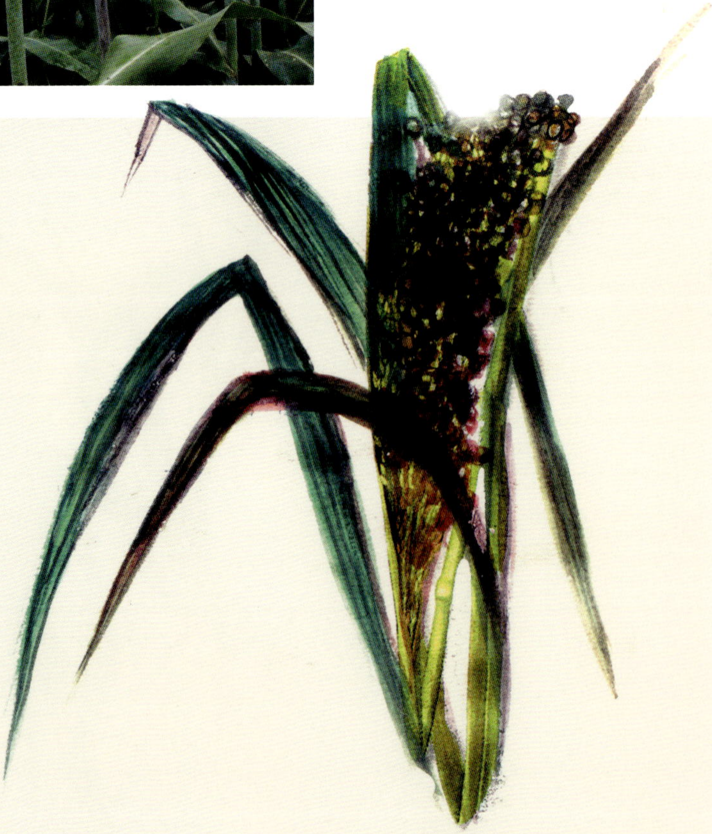

高粱性温　除治積食
和胃健脾　兼治腹瀉

萝卜

Radish

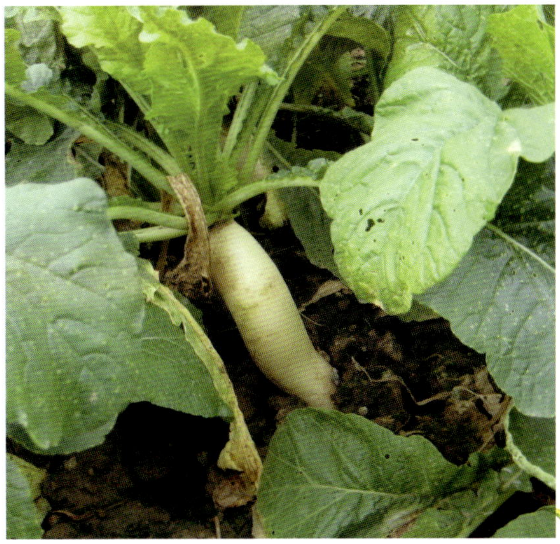

萝卜生食清热，熟食健脾。

Radish can clear away heat when eaten raw and strengthen the spleen when cooked.

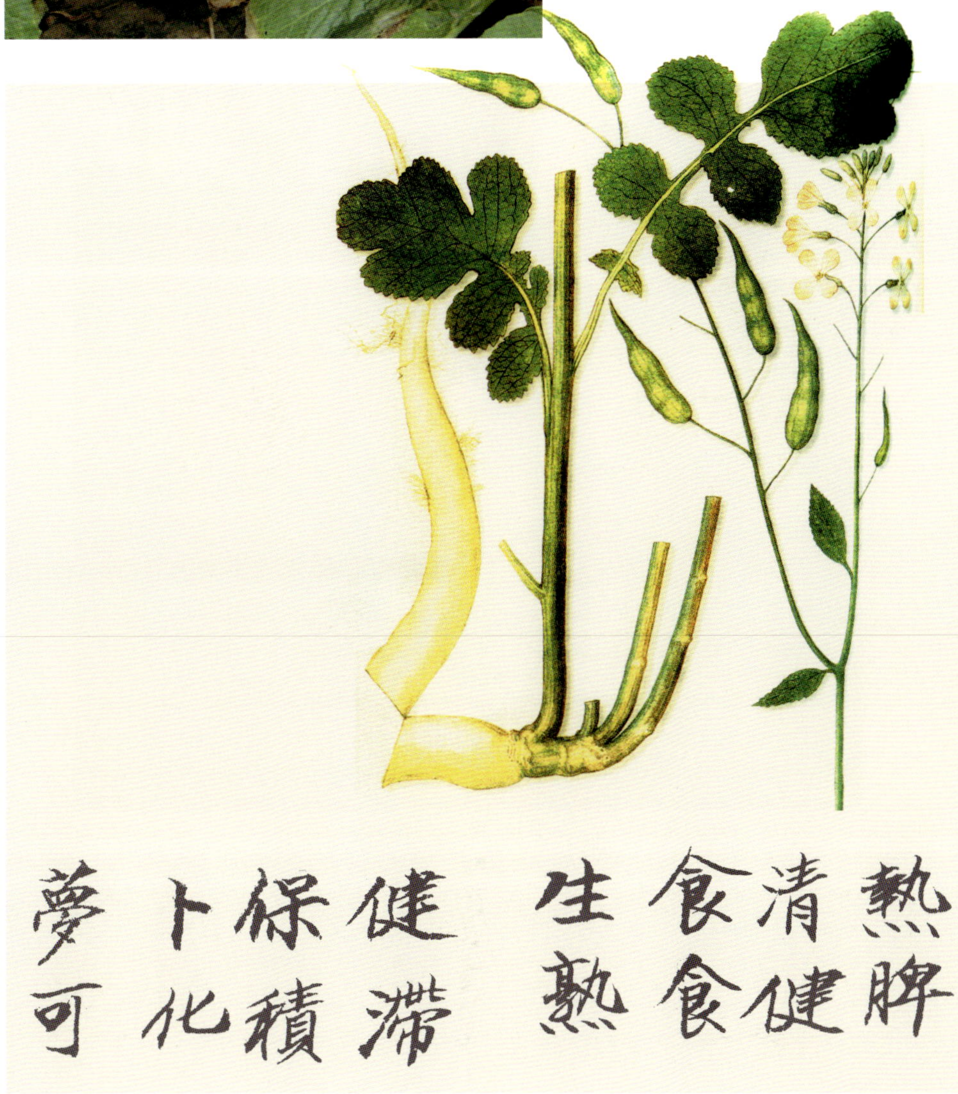

黑豆

Black soybean

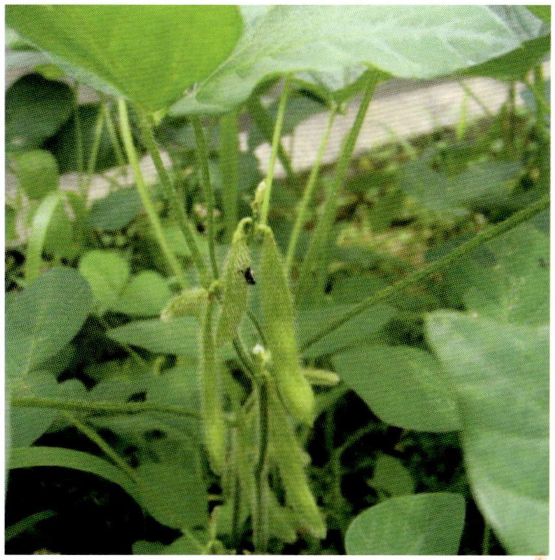

黑豆补肾益精、活血润肤。

Black soybean can replenish the kidney, increase essence, invigorate blood circulation, and moisturize the skin.

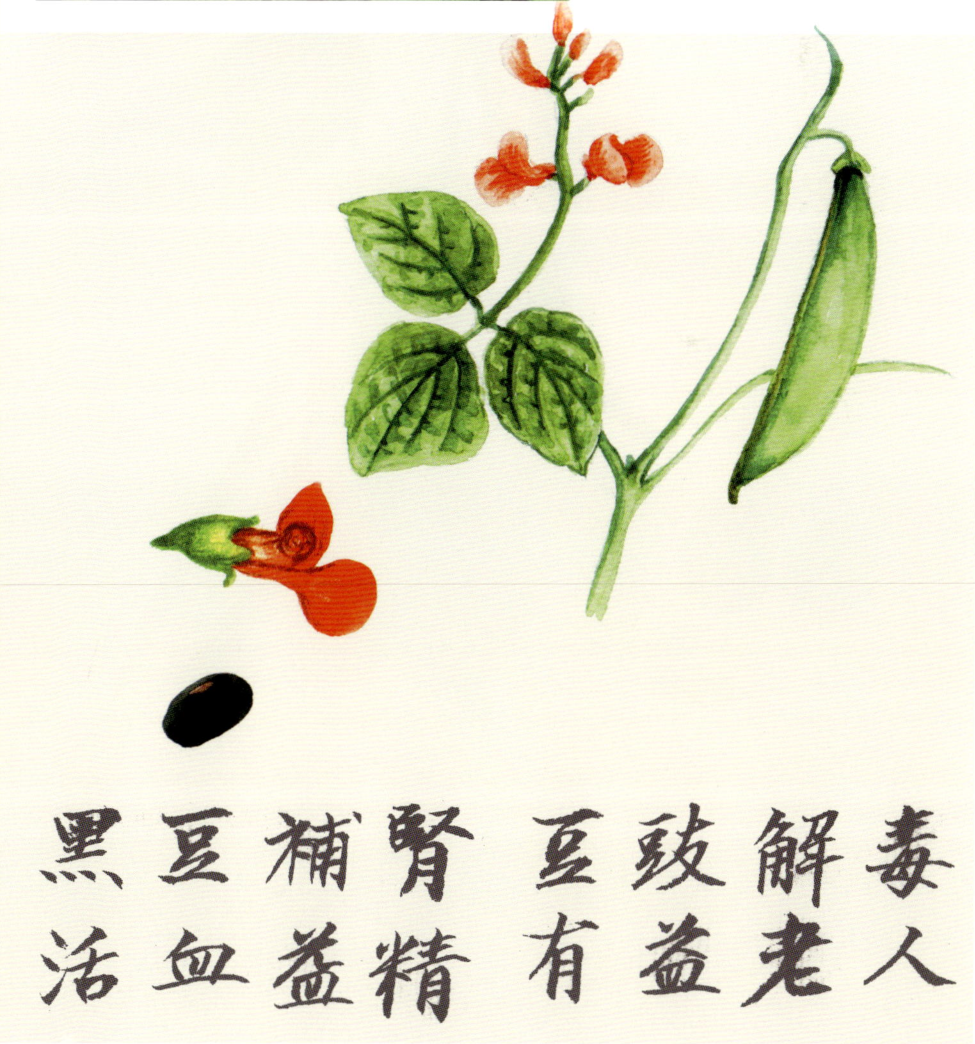

绿豆

Mung bean

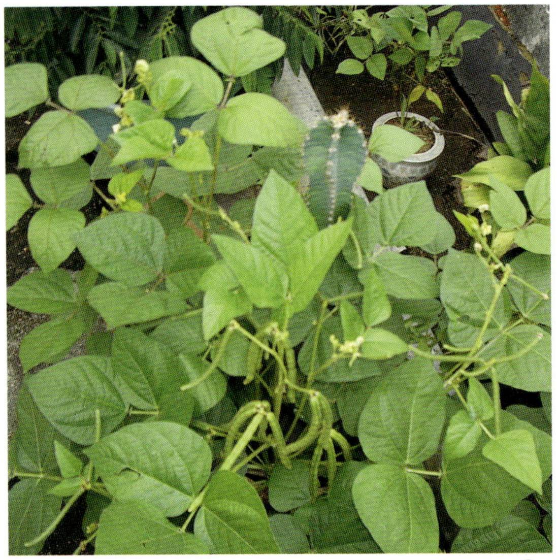

绿豆清热解毒，解暑止渴。

Mung bean can remove heat and toxic elements, clear away summer heat, and quench thirst.

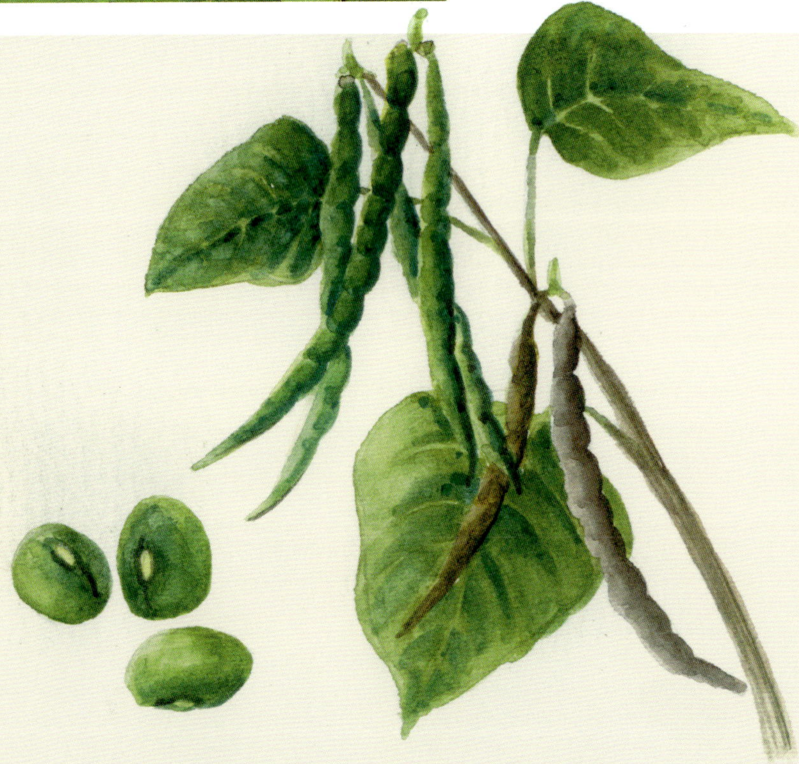

绿豆低脂　解暑止渴
清熱解毒　虚寒不宜

芝麻

Sesame

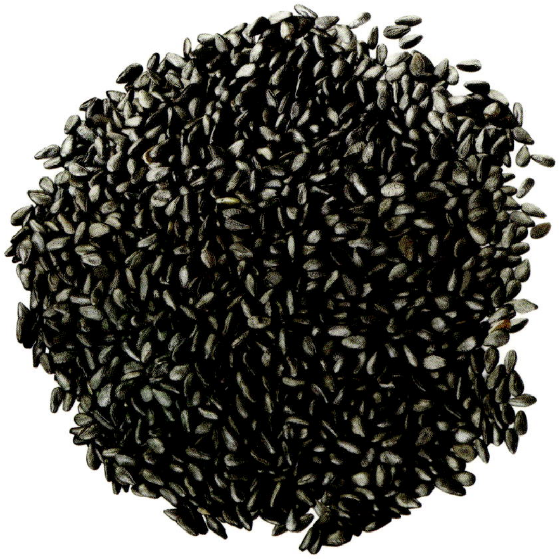

芝麻开胃健脾、和五脏、养血、乌发。

Sesame can whet the appetite, strengthen the spleen, harmonize the internal organs, nourish the blood, and blacken the hair.

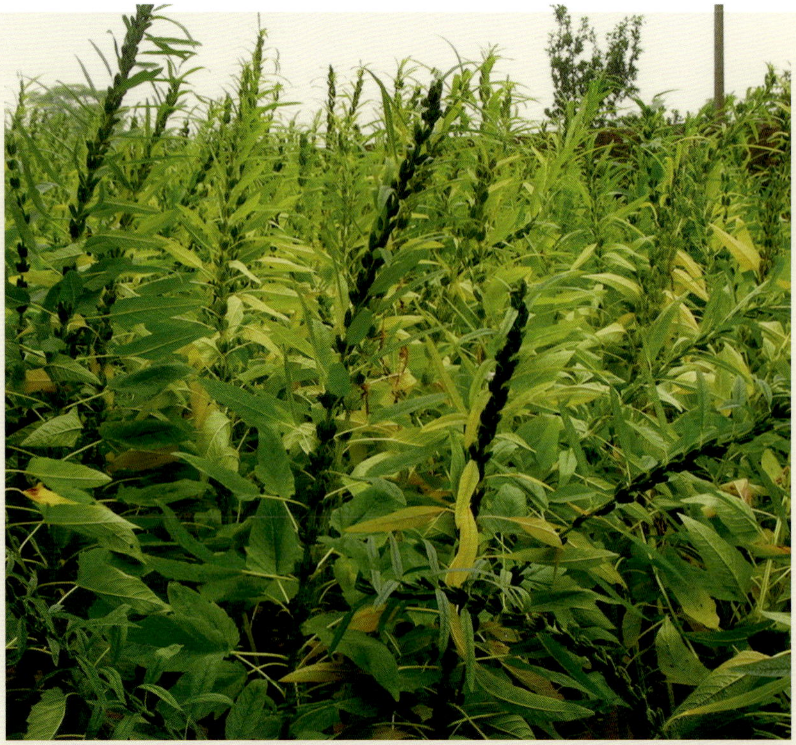

芝麻和人　益肝補腎
開胃健脾　養血潤燥

白菜

Chinese cabbage

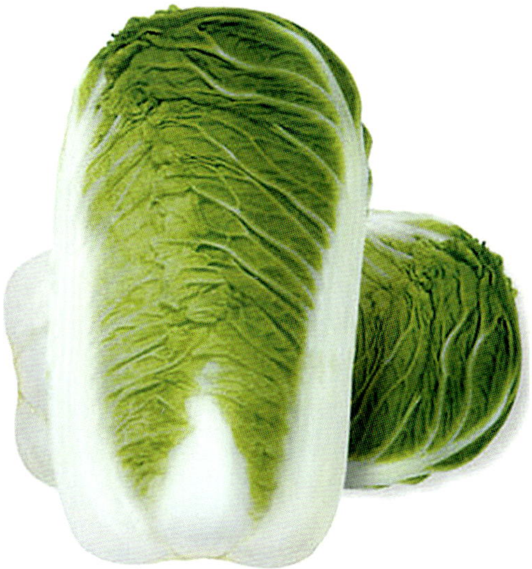

白菜养胃、降脂、清热、防癌。

Chinese cabbage can nourish the stomach, reduce blood fat, clear away heat, and prevent cancer.

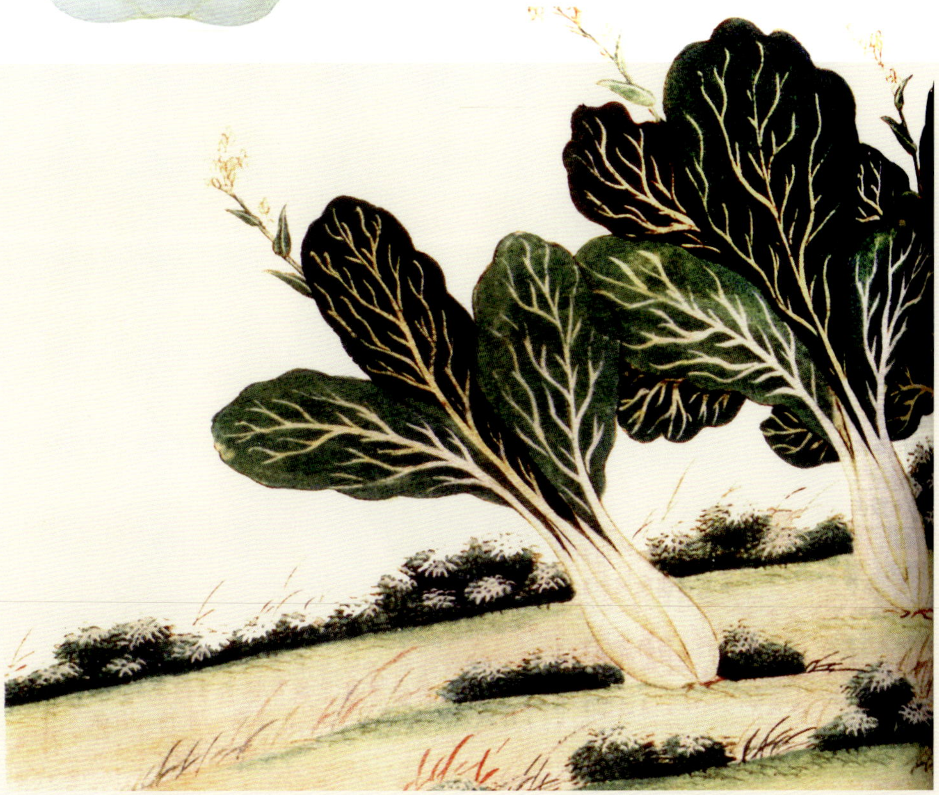

白菜菜王 降脂防癌
養胃利腸 清熱除煩

韭菜

Leek

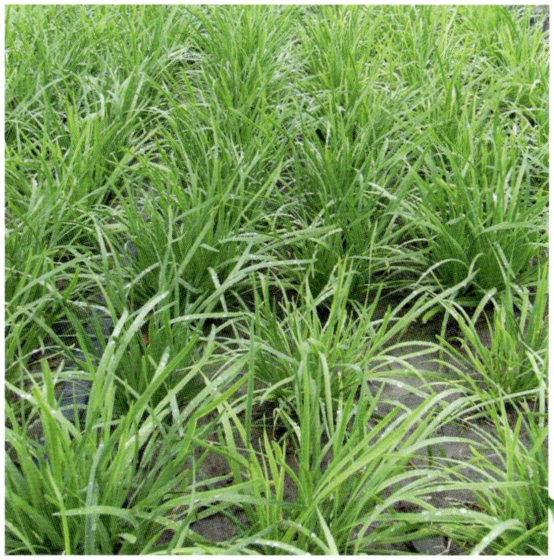

韭菜温补肝肾，助阳固精。

Leek can warm and replenish the liver and the kidney, reinforce yang, and prevent premature ejaculation.

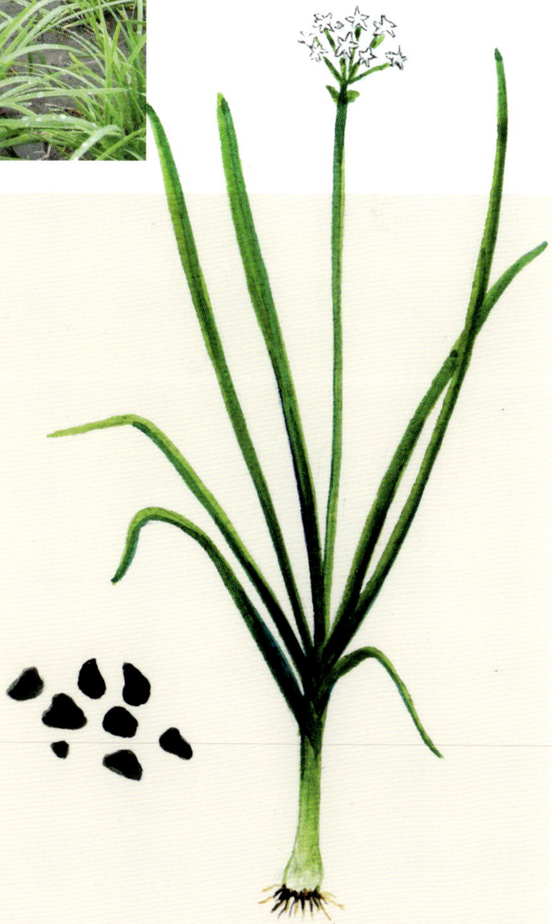

韭菜潤腸 補肝防癌
固精助陽 春食最好

芹菜

Celery

芹菜可预防糖尿病、通便、明目、止咳。

Celery can prevent diabetes, improve vision, and arrest cough.

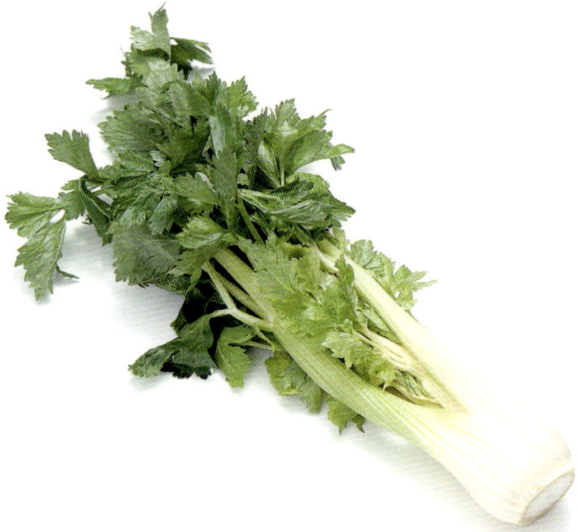

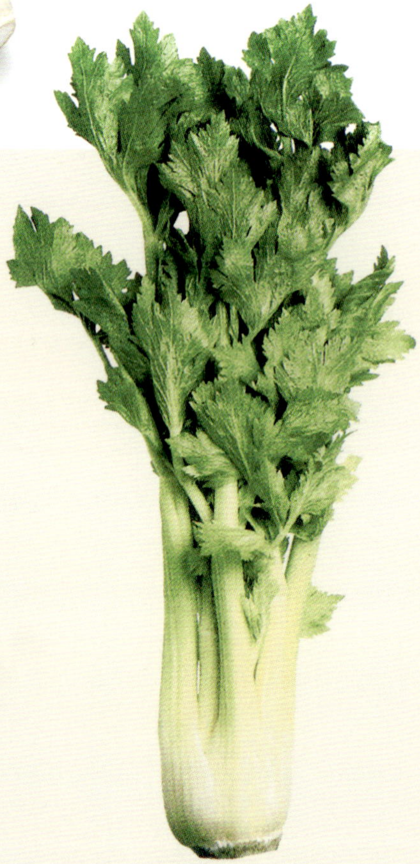

芹菜助消 降壓減脂

預防消渴 清熱解毒

菠菜

Spinach

菠菜可以生血，护肤。

Spinach can generate blood and protect the skin.

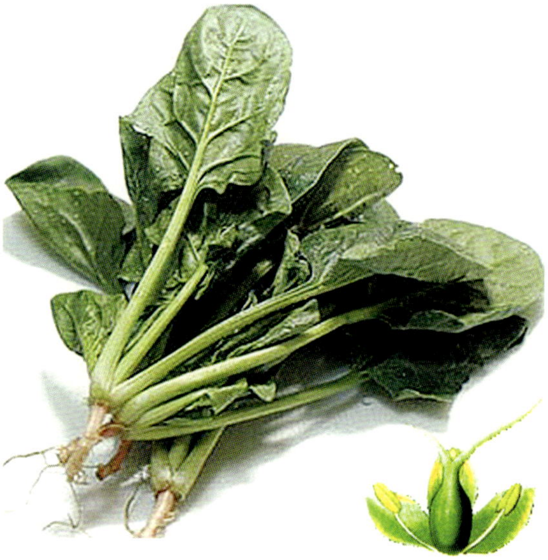

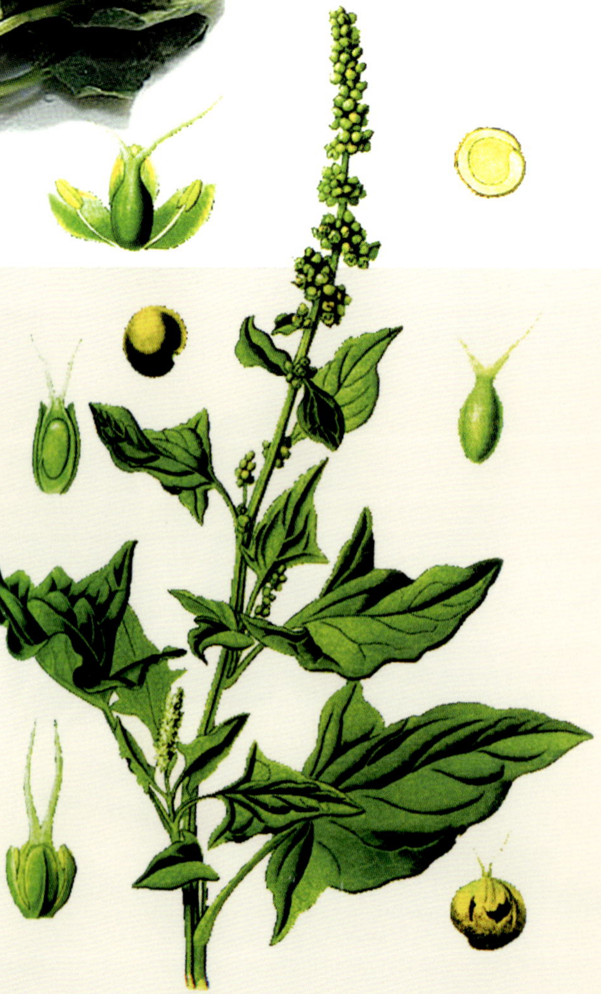

菠菜生血 緩解便秘

保護皮肤 消渴忌食

黄瓜

Cucumber

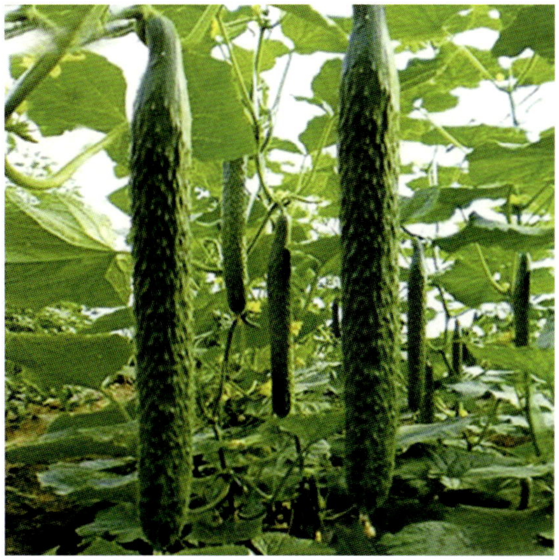

黄瓜可以降脂，利尿。

Cucumber can reduce blood fat and increase the discharge of urine.

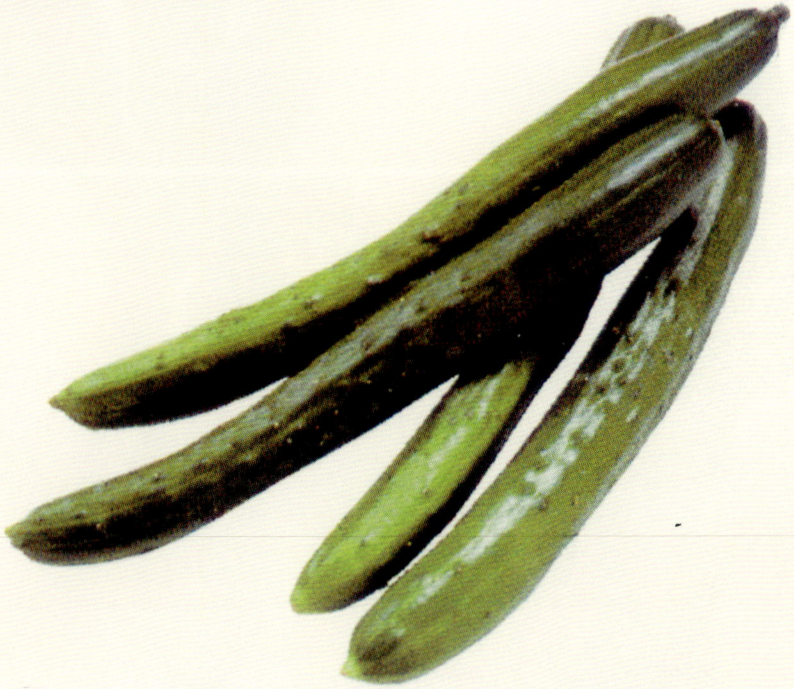

黄瓜降脂 除濕鎮痛
利尿减肥 忌同花生

茄子

Eggplant

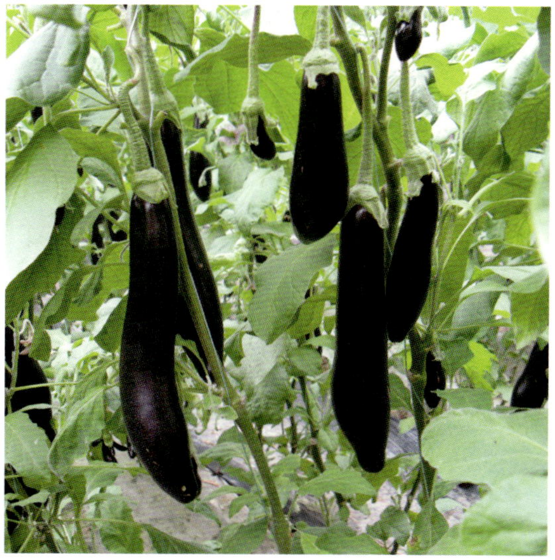

茄子可以降脂、活血、通脉。

Eggplant can reduce blood fat, promote blood circulation, and invigorate vital energy.

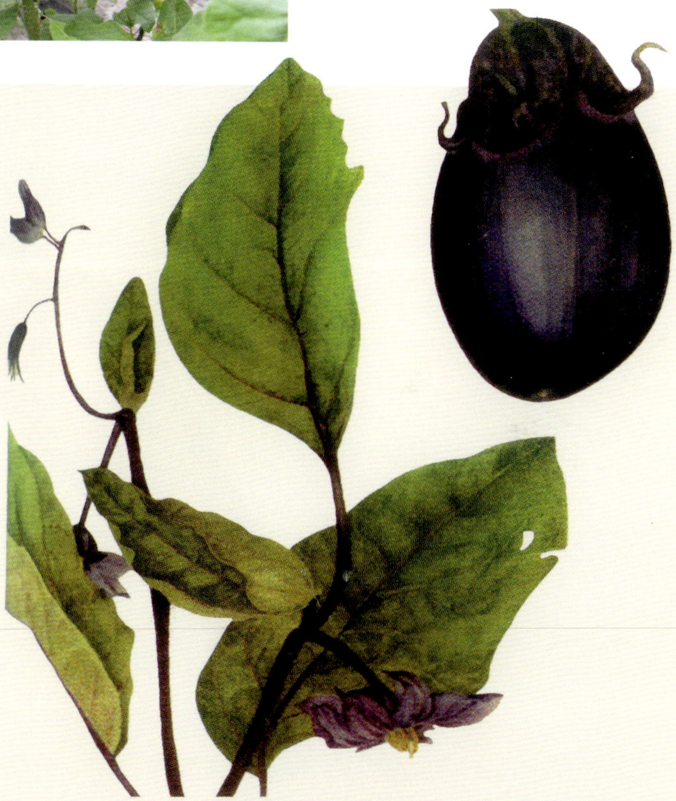

茄子活血 皮肤去斑
通脉抗癌 减少血栓

胡萝卜

Carrot

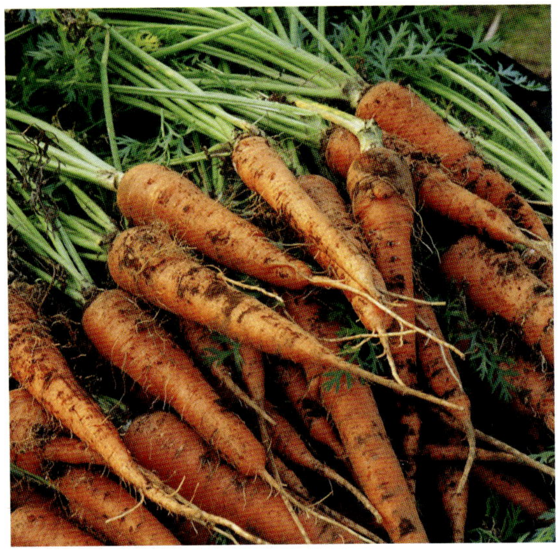

胡萝卜护发美容，增强记忆力。

Carrot can protect the hair, beautify the face, and improve memory.

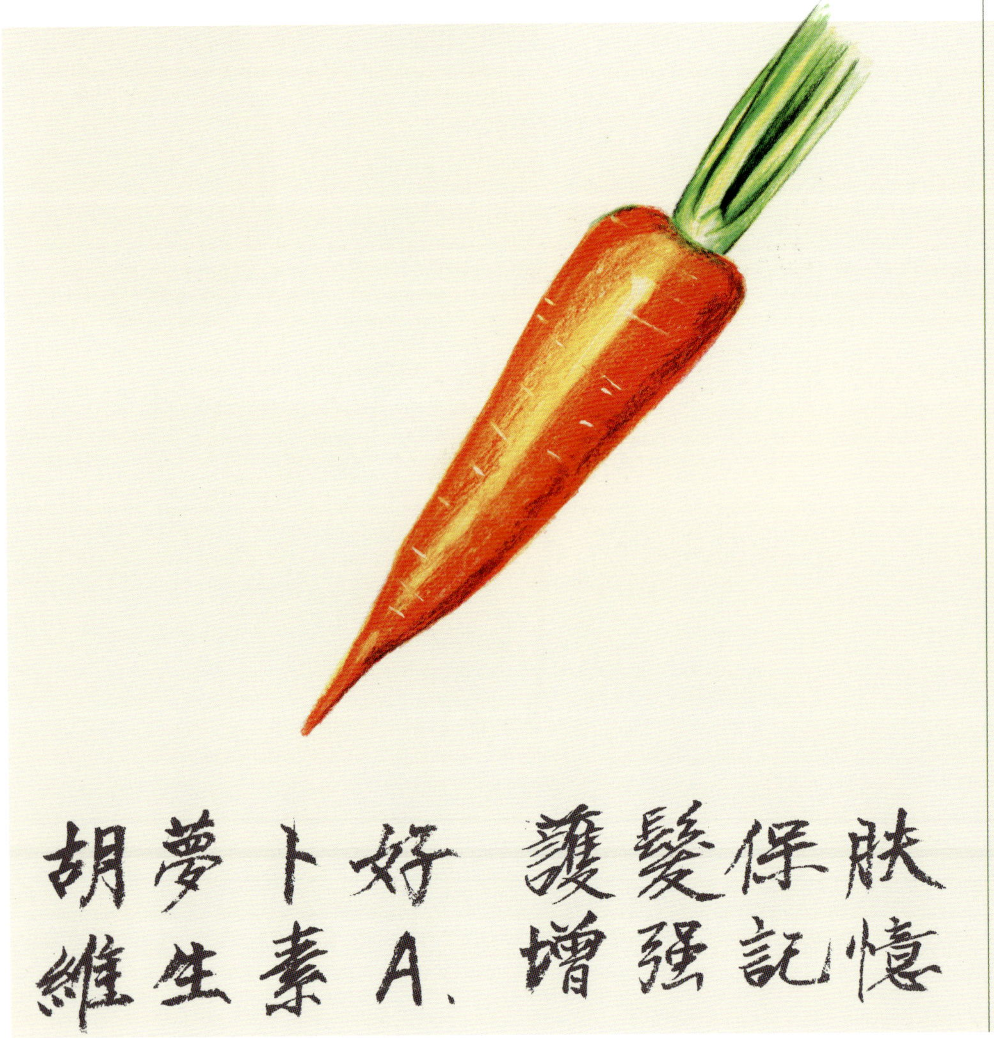

莴笋

Lettuce

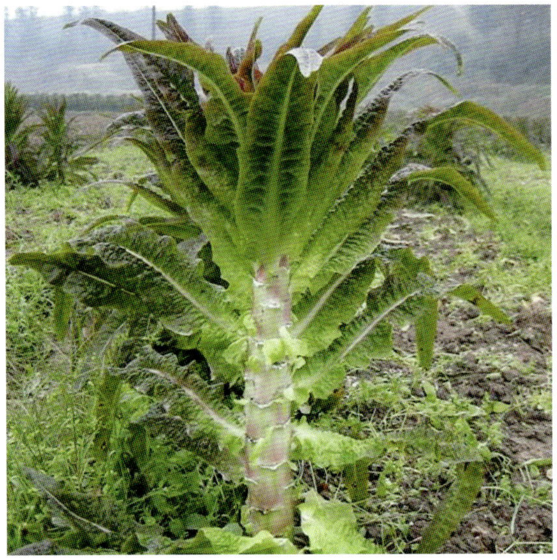

莴笋益齿助消化。

Lettuce can strengthen teeth and aid digestion.

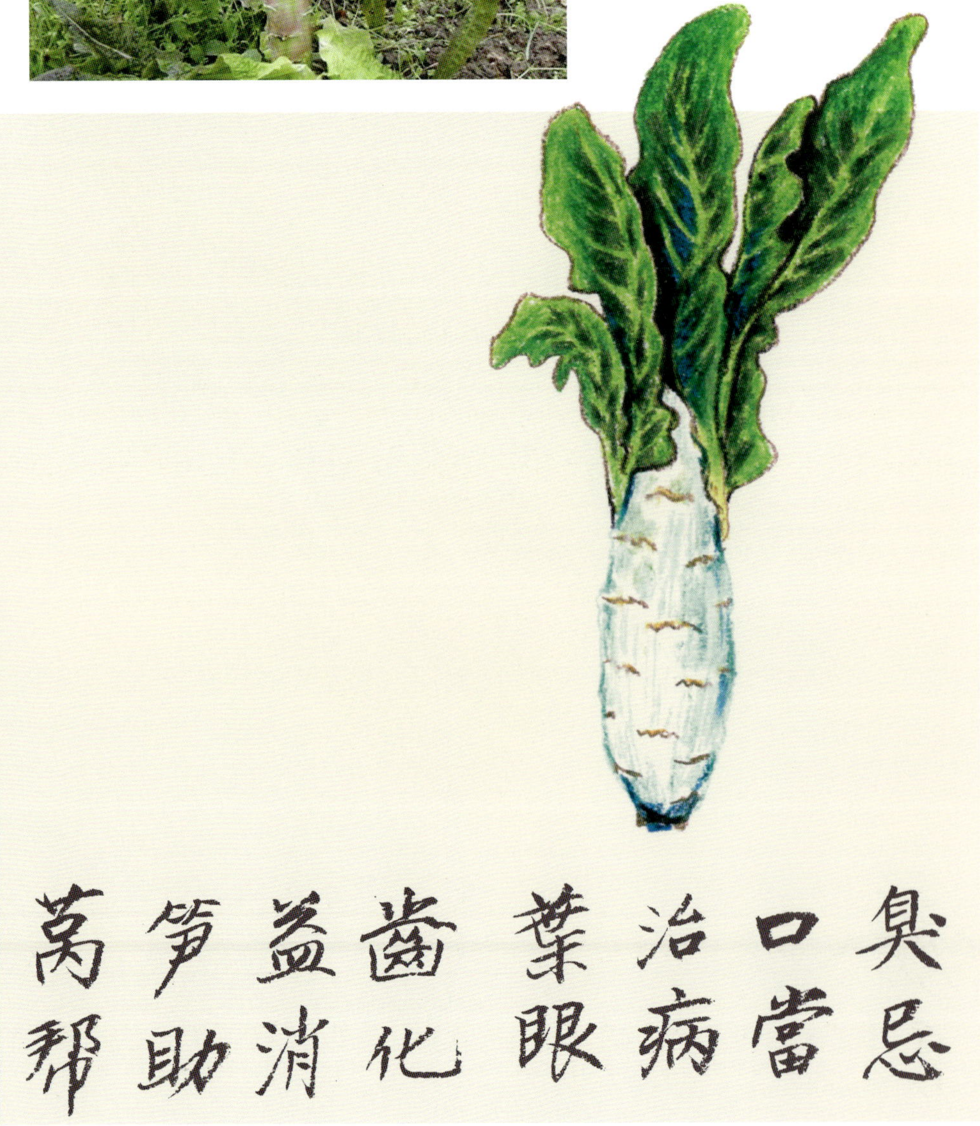

木耳

Black fungus

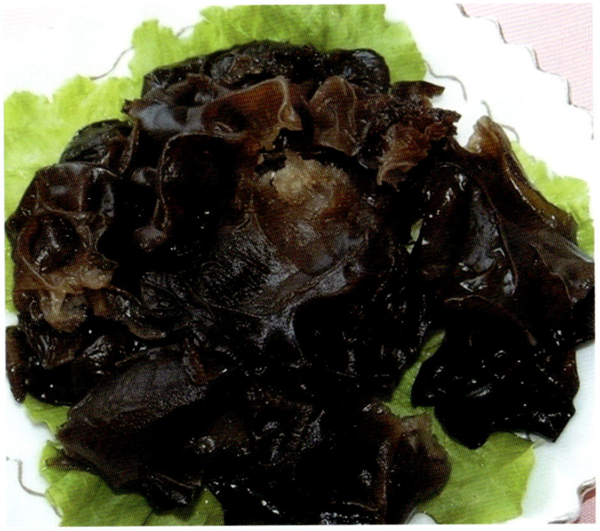

木耳活血，消化杂物。

Black fungus can invigorate blood circulation and aid digestion of miscellaneous food.

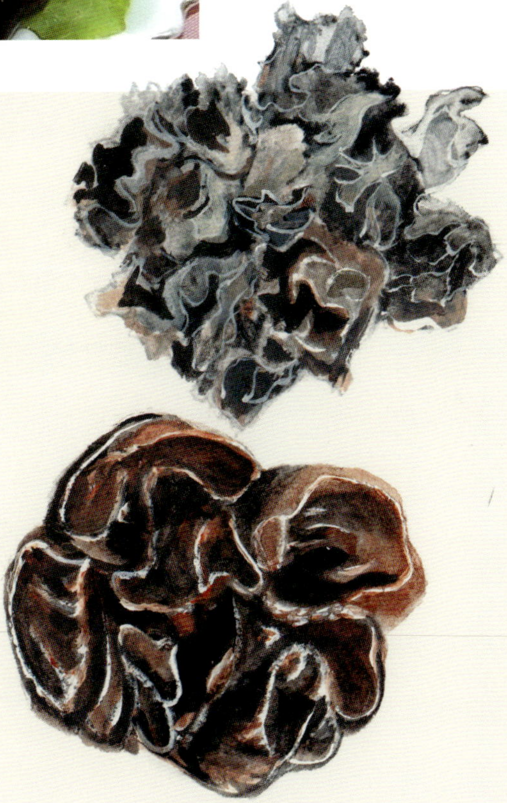

蘑菇免疫降低血糖
防止貧血兼治乏力

山药

Yam

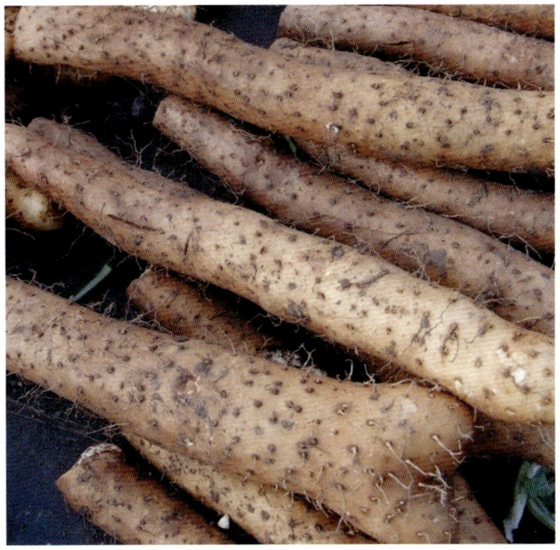

山药滋补身体，健胃益肾。

Yam can nourish the body, strengthen the stomach, and invigorate the kidney.

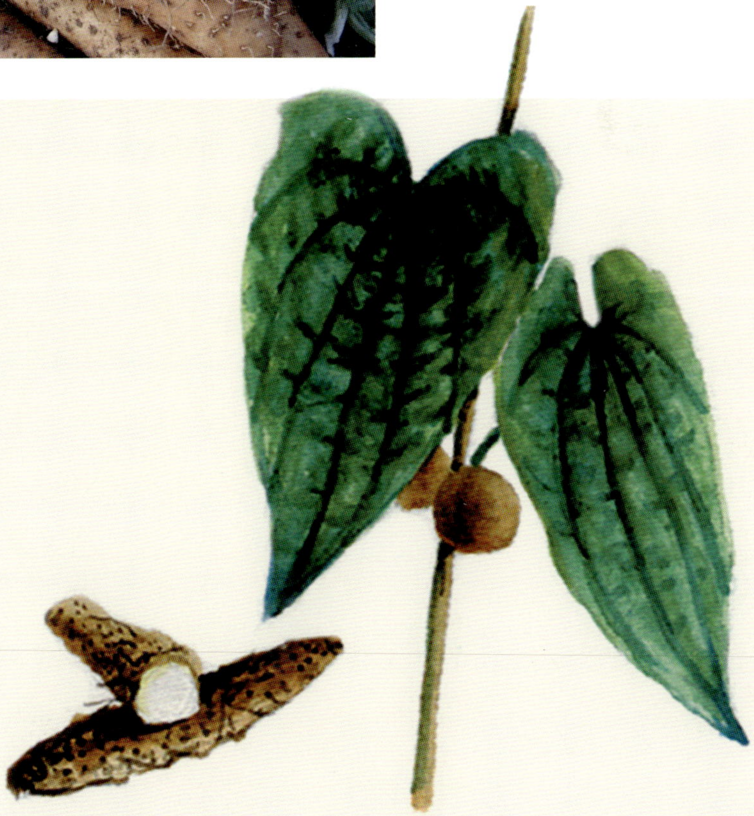

山藥滋補健胃益腎
可葷可素補肺治喘

大葱

Scallion

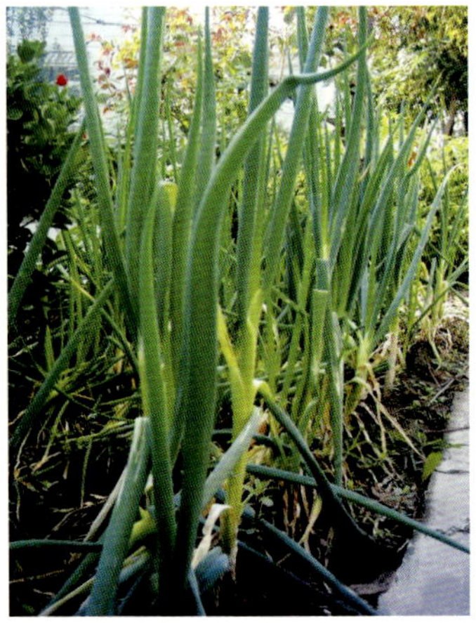

大葱杀菌，发汗解表。

Scallion can kill bacteria, induce perspiration, and relieve exterior syndrome.

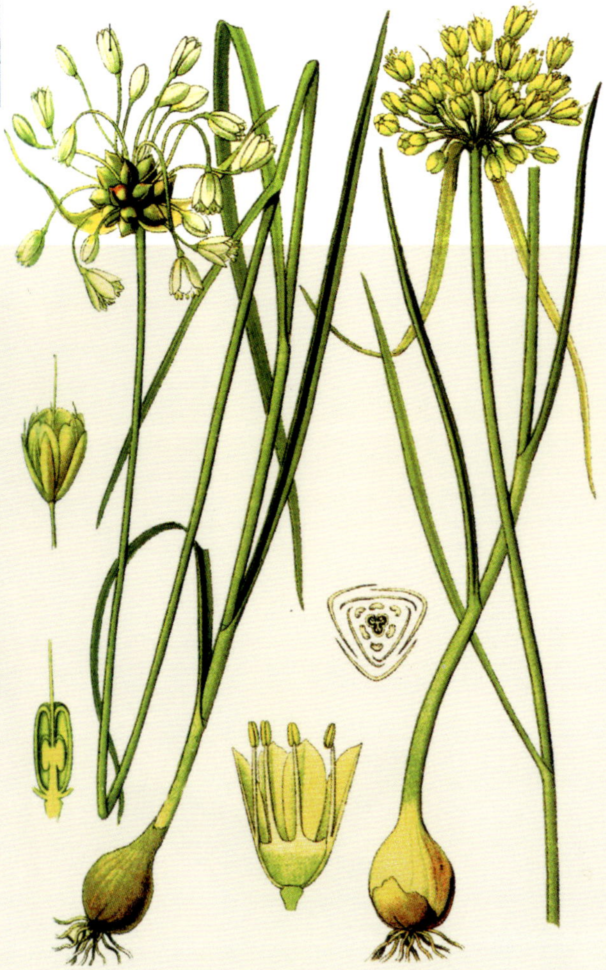

大葱杀菌　降脂健胃
發汗解表　忌同蜂蜜

姜

Ginger

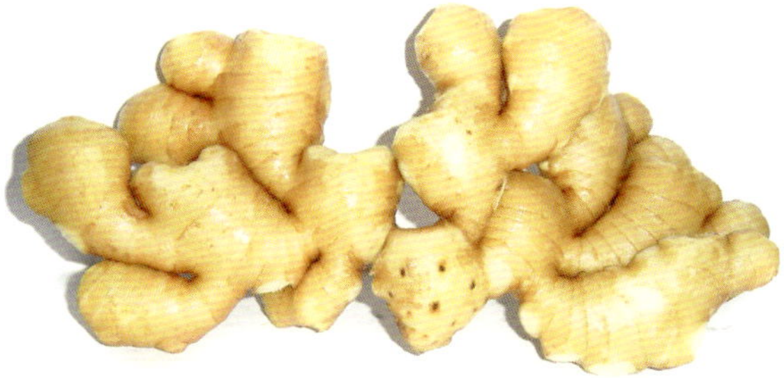

姜能健胃，发汗解毒。

Ginger can strengthen the stomach, induce perspiration, and clear away toxic substance.

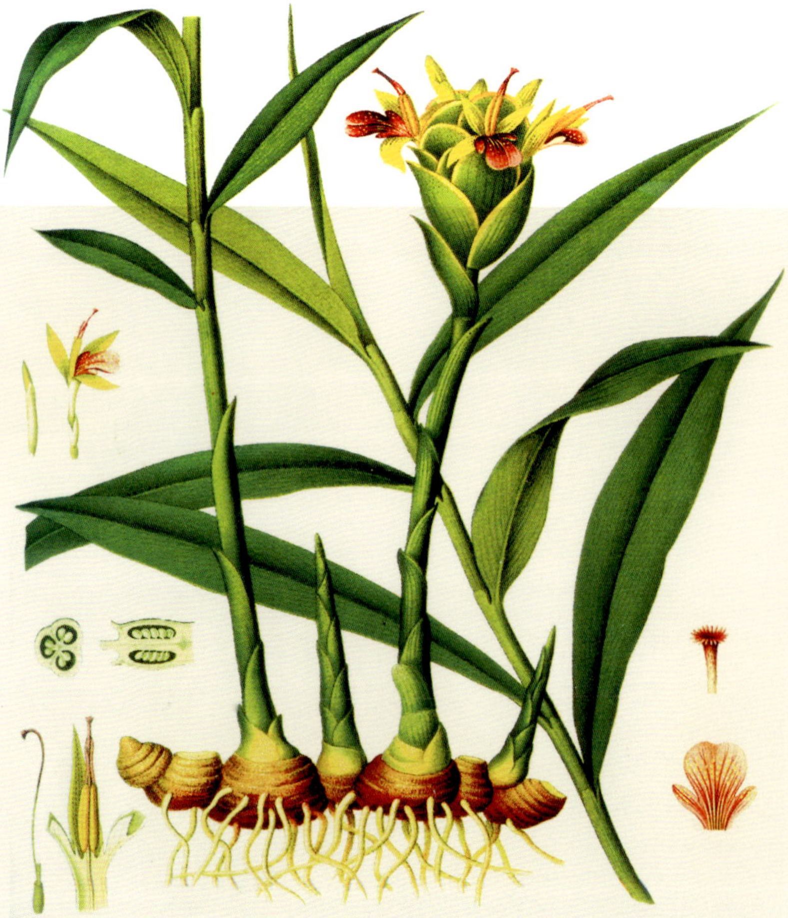

姜能健胃　助人消化
發汗去濕　亦可救毒

番茄

Tomato

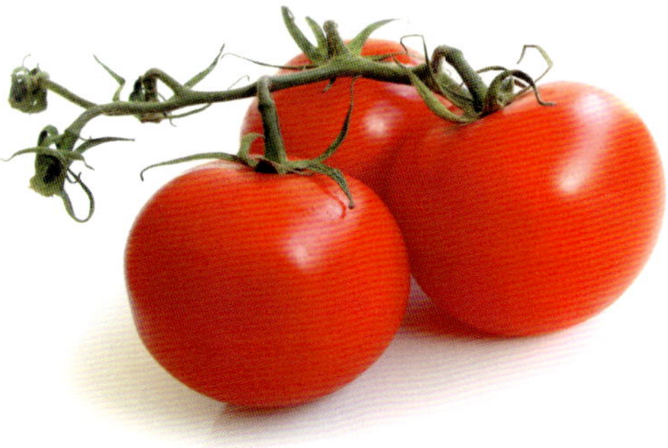

番茄可以助消化，清热生津。

Tomato can aid digestion, clear away heat, and help to generate saliva.

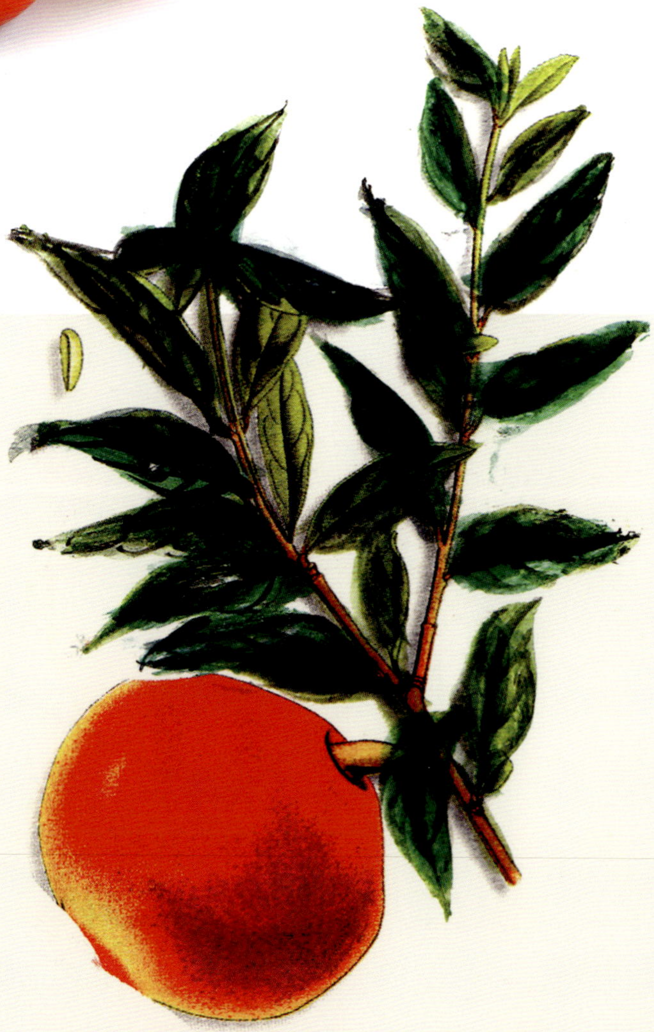

番茄防癌　消化肉食
清熱生津　空腹不宜

番薯

Sweet potato

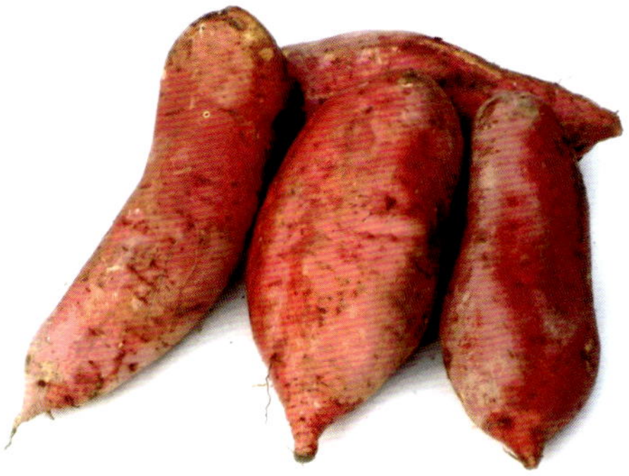

番薯能保持人体酸碱平衡，有助于减肥。

Sweet potato can maintain acid-base balance and help to lose weight.

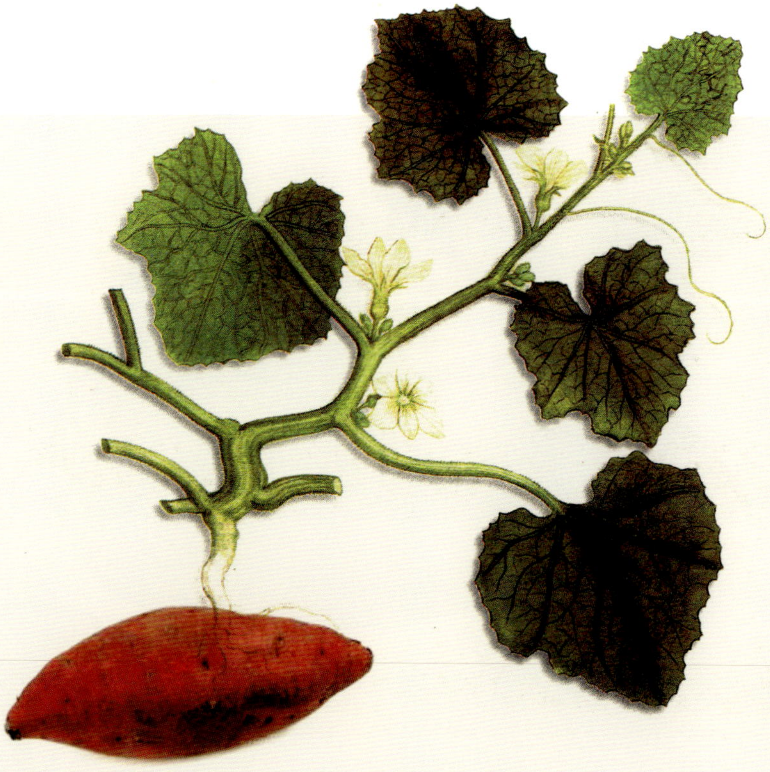

番薯降脂　酸碱平衡
减肥抗癌　胸悶忌食

冬瓜

Wax gourd

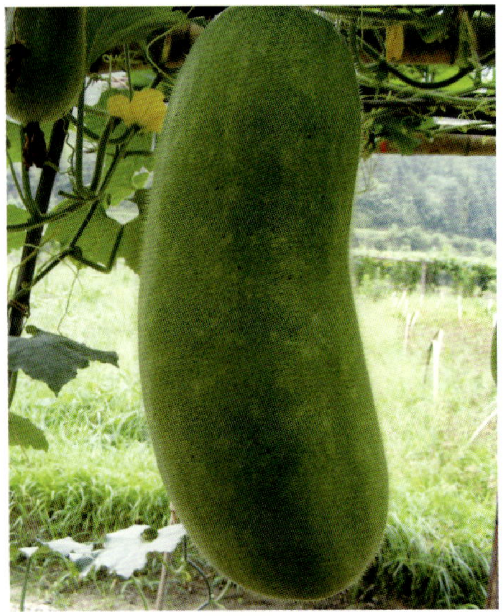

冬瓜利尿，减肥。

Wax gourd can increase the discharge of urine and help to lose weight.

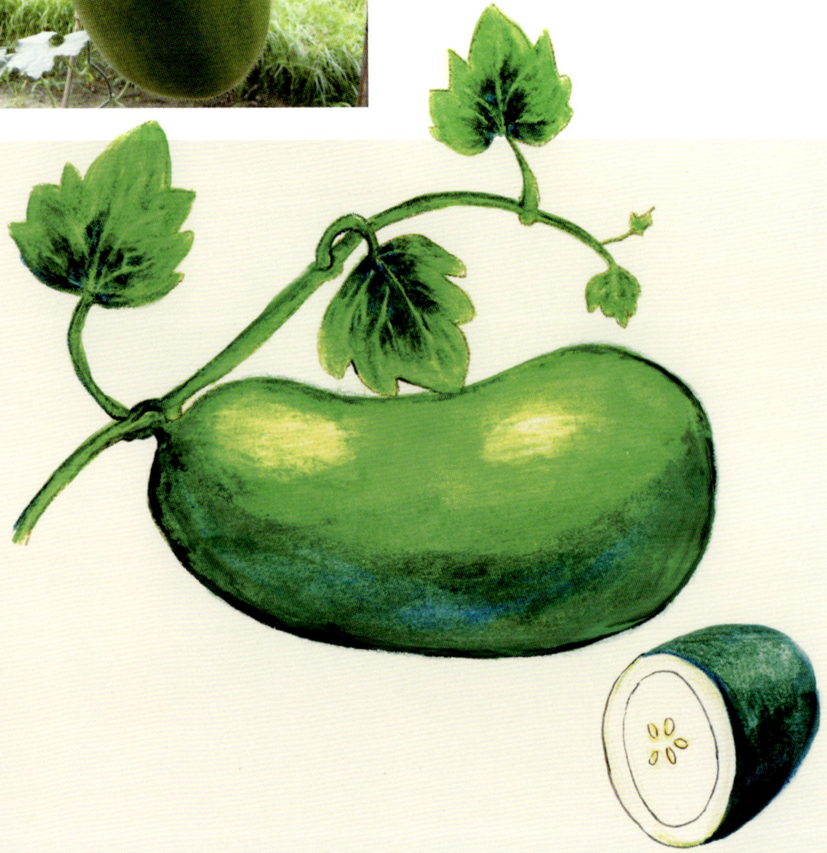

冬瓜利尿 不含脂肪

消除水肿 健脾减肥

豆腐

Tofu

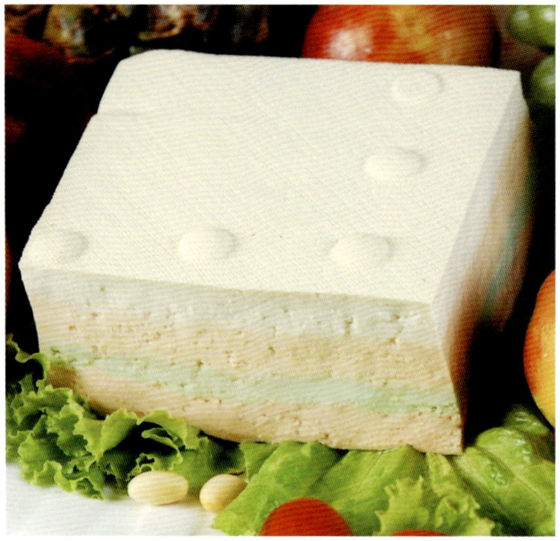

豆腐补虚益气。

Tofu, or bean curd, can treat the deficiency syndrome and supplement qi.

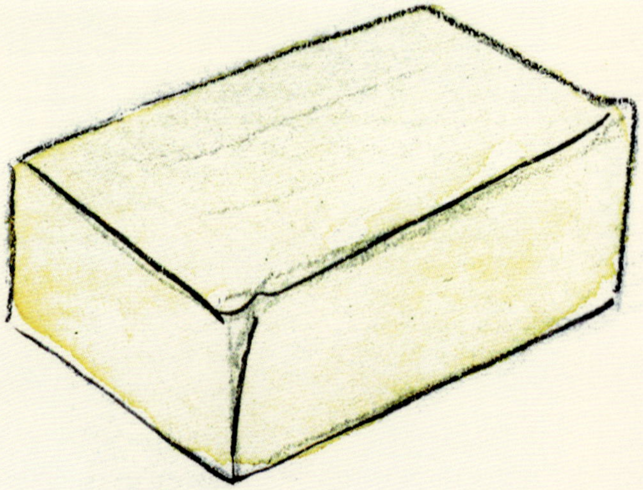

豆腐益氣 有益少年

補虛保肝 又益老人

洋葱

Onion

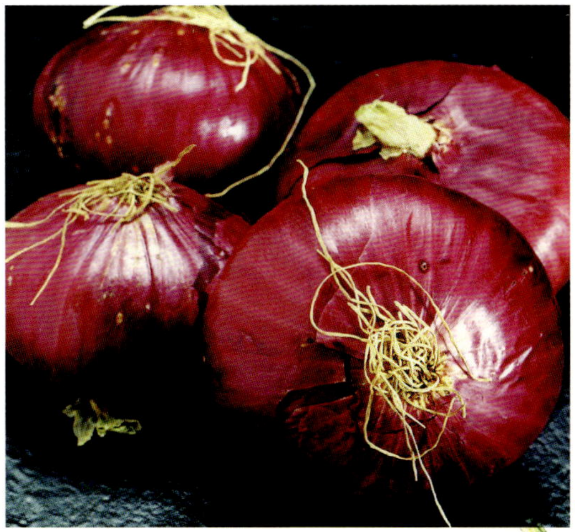

洋葱生食可以预防动脉硬化。

Eaten raw, onion can prevent arteriosclerosis.

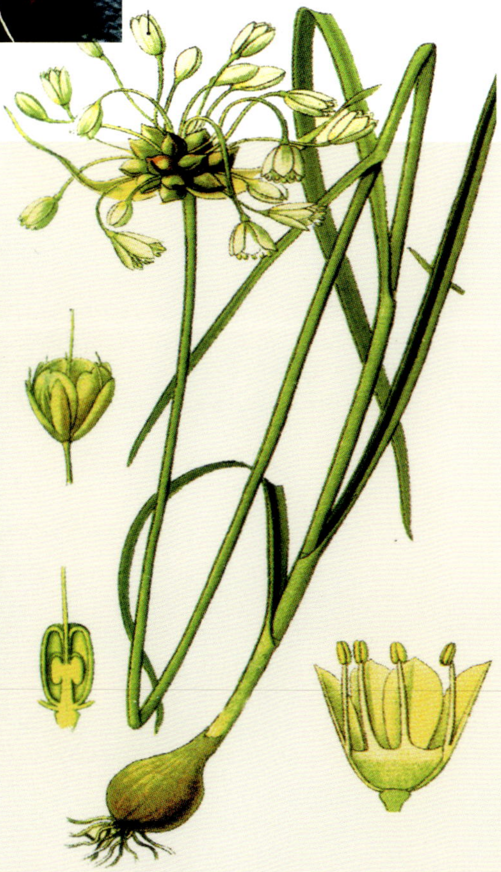

洋葱圓葱 生食可治

降脂降壓 動脈硬化

鸡蛋

Eggs

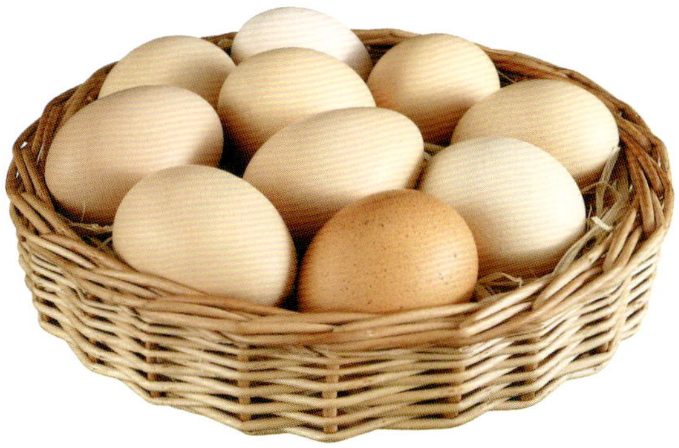

鸡蛋养人，益肝防癌。

Eggs can strengthen the liver and prevent cancer, nourishing the body.

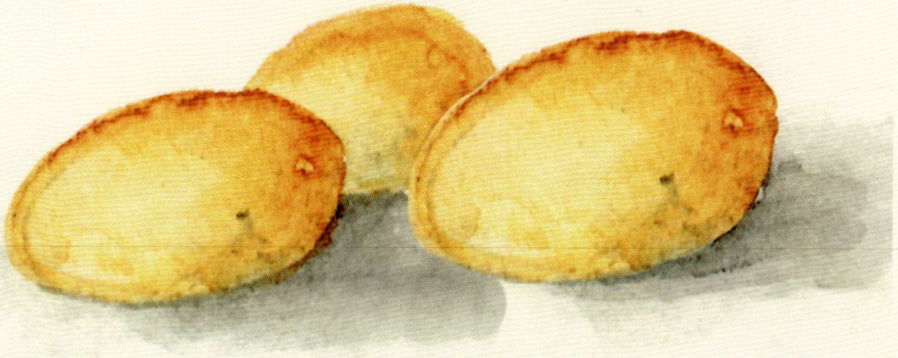

鷄蛋養人 增强记憶

益肝防癌 胆固醇高

藕

Lotus root

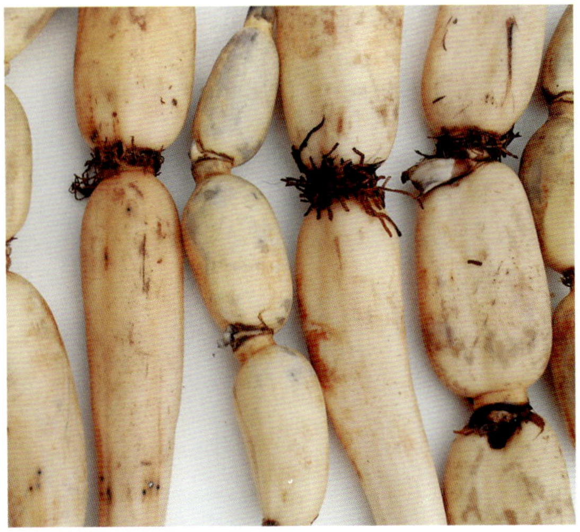

藕清热，开胃。

Lotus root can clear away heat and whet appetite.

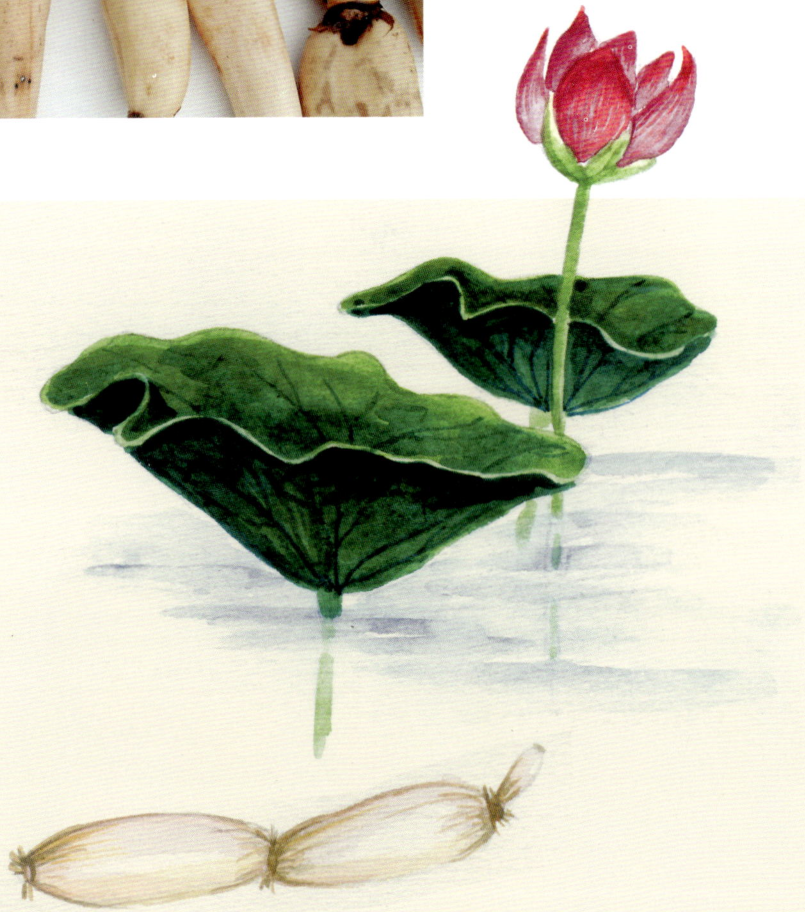

藕能清熱　健脾開胃

潤肺涼血　止瀉固精

海带

Kelp

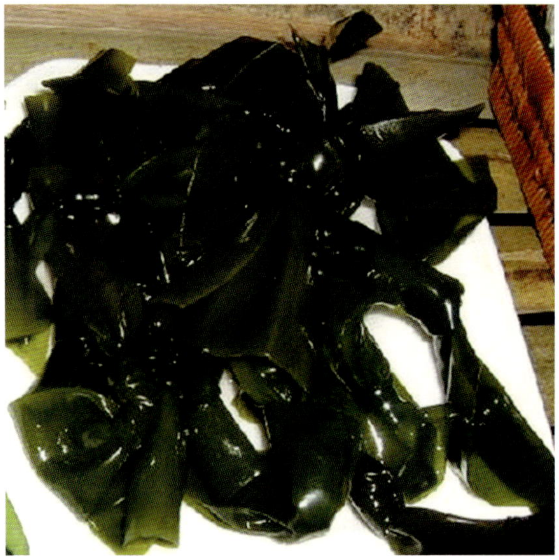

海带降压，乌发。

Kelp can reduce blood pressure and blacken the hair.

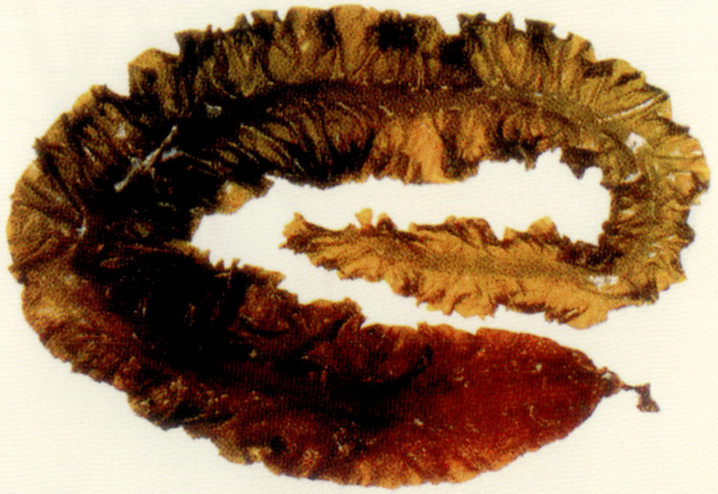

海帶碘多　降壓烏髮

營養豐富　兼能防癌

苹果

Apple

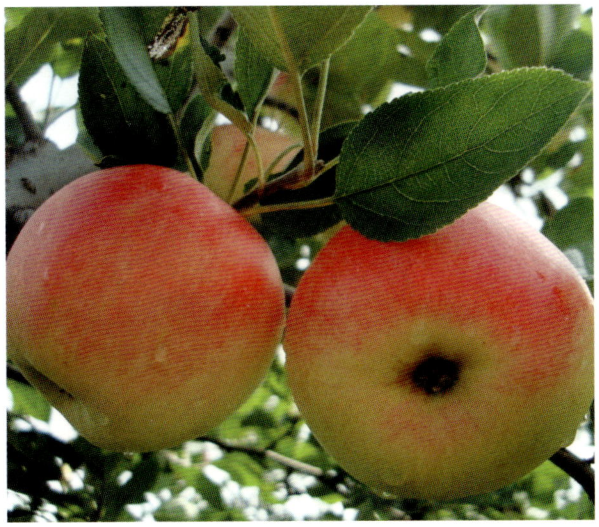

苹果益人，调理生理。

Apple is beneficial to health and capable of physiological regulation.

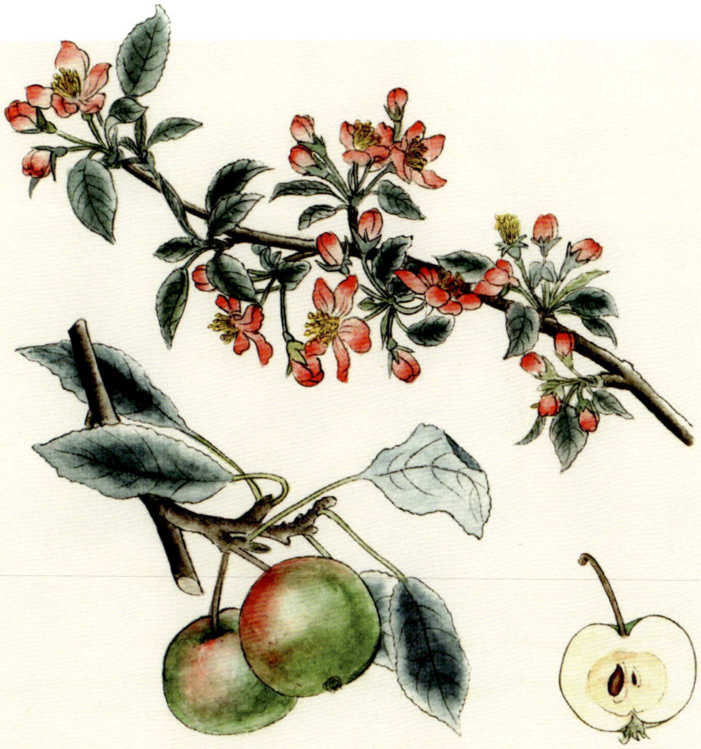

苹果益人　降脂潤腸
調理生理　食後漱口

梨

Pear

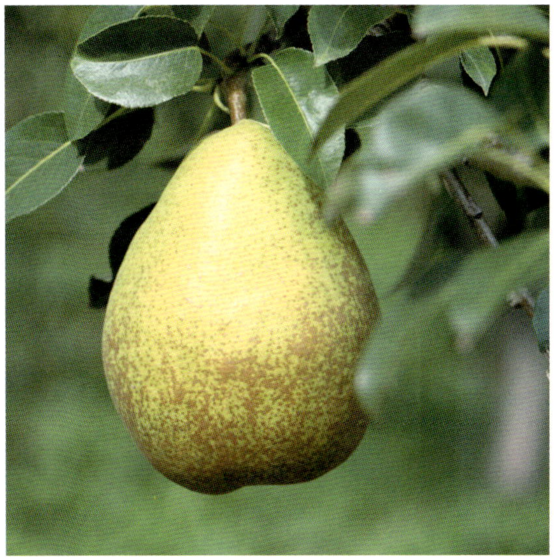

梨能润肺，消痰降火。

Pear can moisten the lungs, remove phlegm, and reduce excessive internal heat.

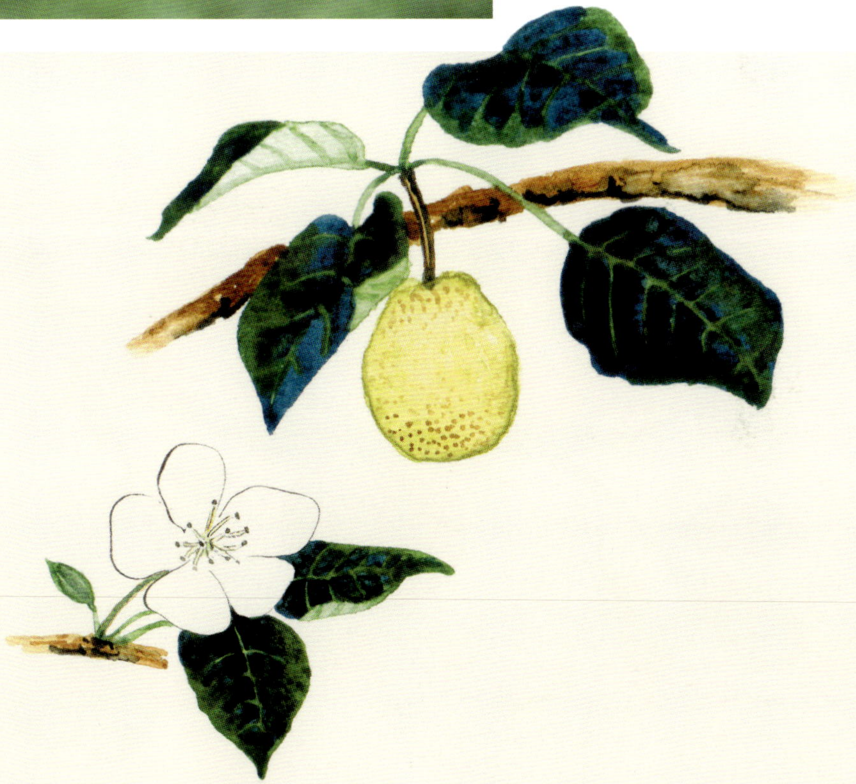

梨能潤肺　預防便秘
消痰降火　多食傷脾

柑

Tangerine

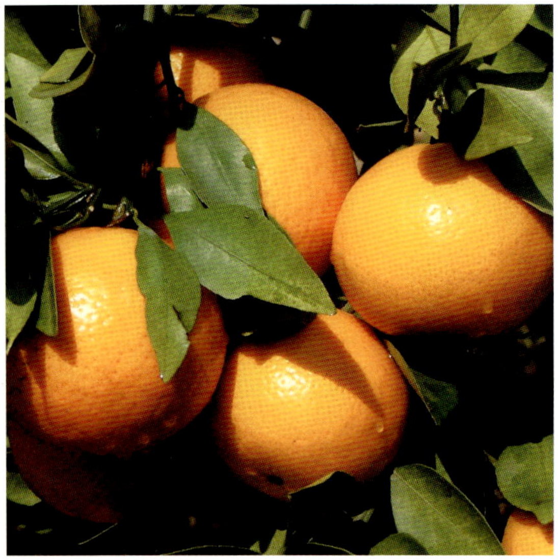

柑可滋养，健脾润肺。

Tangerine can strengthen the spleen and moisten the lungs, nourishing the body.

桃子

Peach

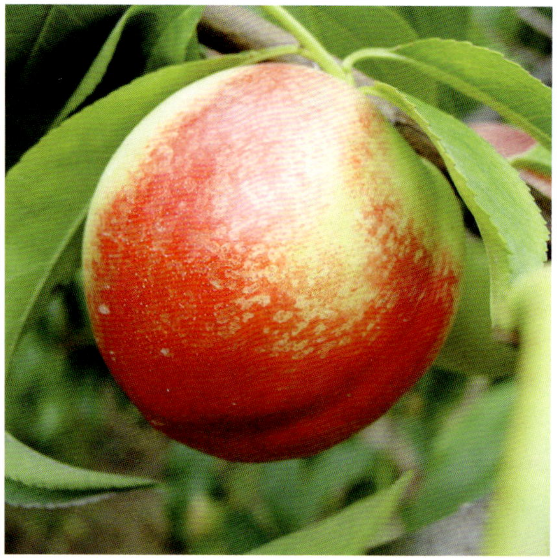

桃子养人，补气益血。

Peach can nourish the body by replenishing qi and blood.

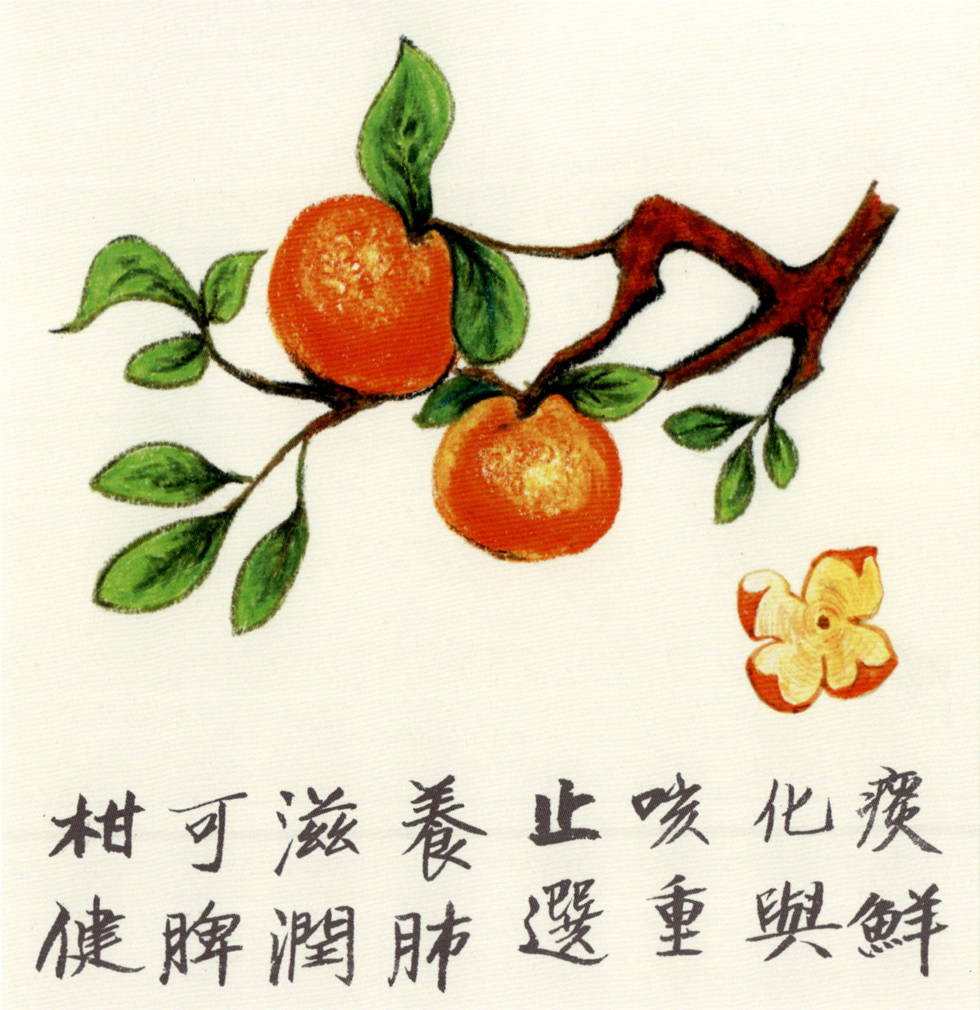

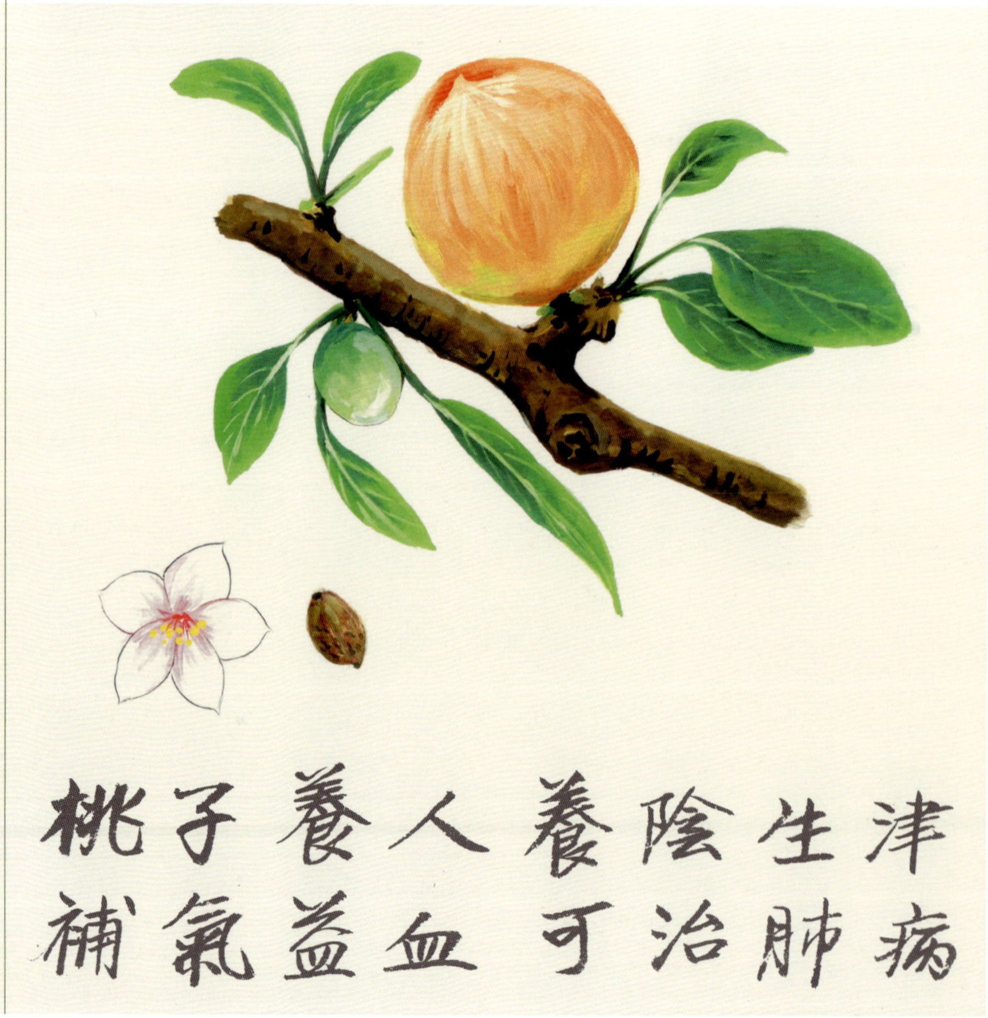

葡萄

Grape

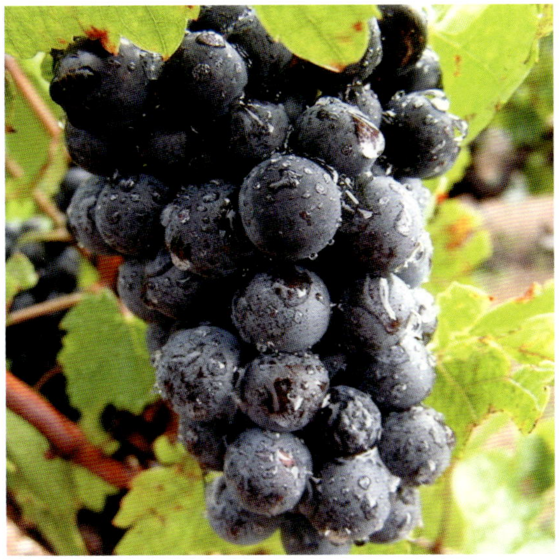

葡萄补虚，有益身体。

Grape can treat the deficiency syndrome.

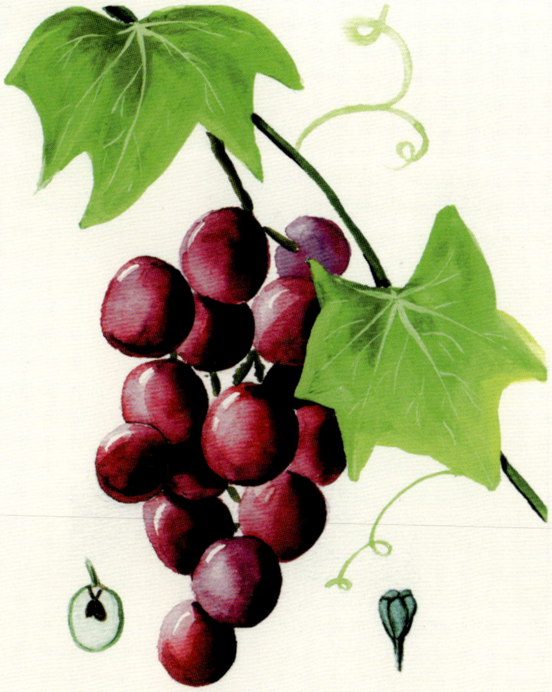

葡萄補虛 利在五臟

有益身體 長人壽命

香蕉

Banana

香蕉性寒，清热生津。

Banana, which has a cold nature, can clear away heat and help to generate saliva.

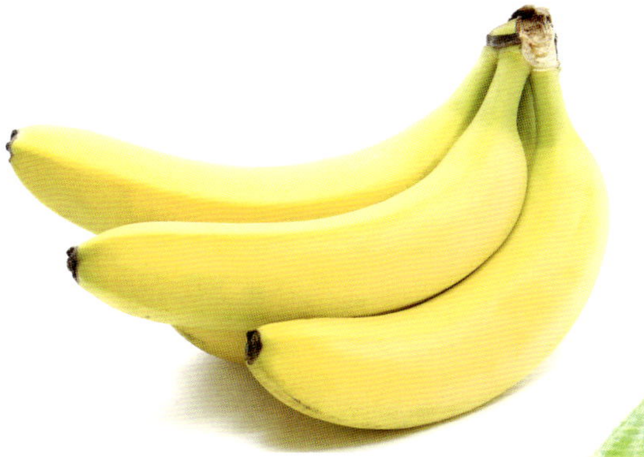

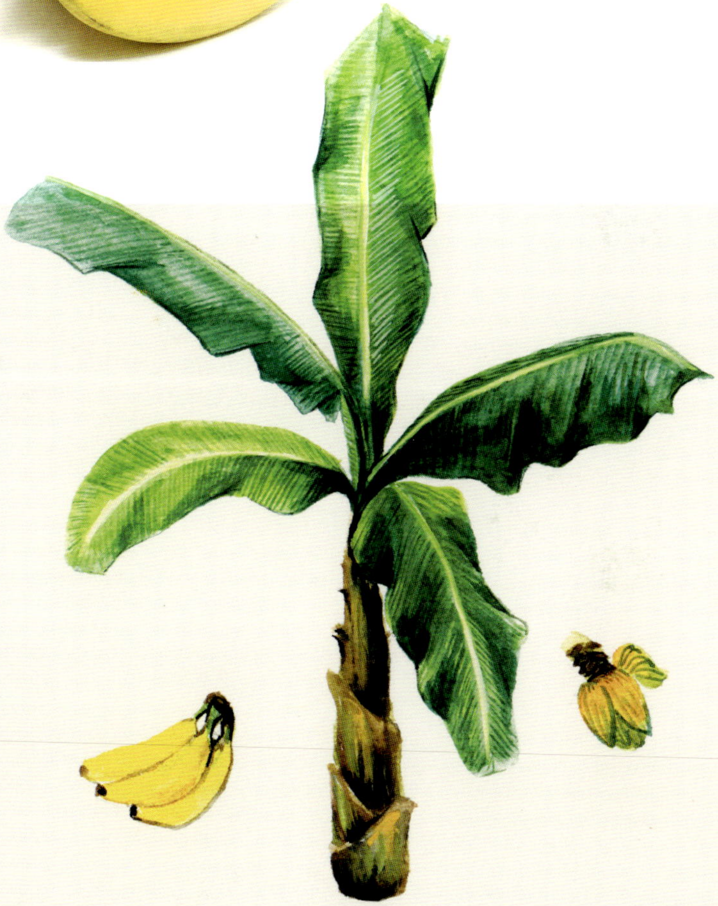

香蕉性寒 潤肺養陰

清熱生津 潤腸通便

西瓜

Watermelon

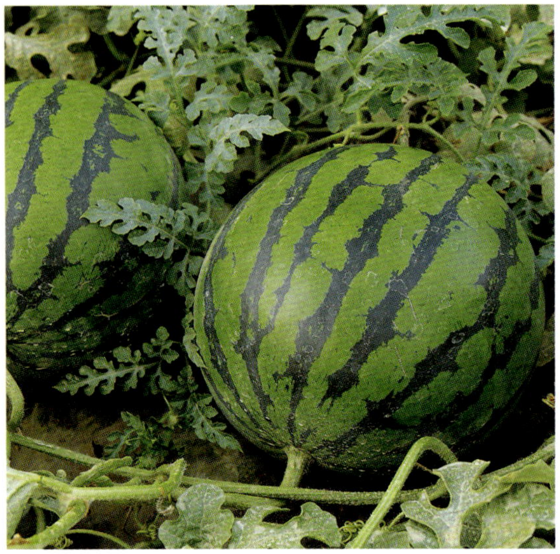

西瓜寒瓜，清热解暑。

Watermelon, which has a cold nature, can clear away summer heat.

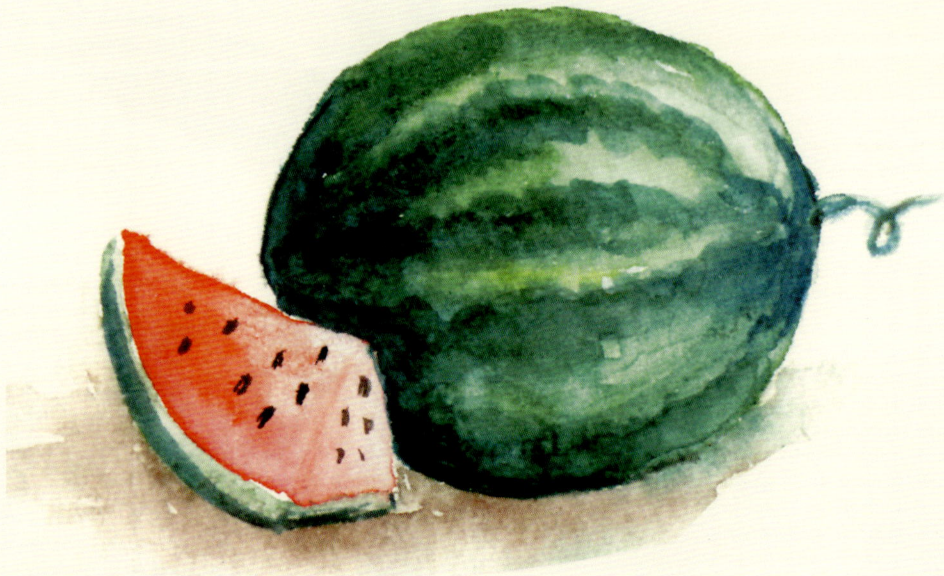

西瓜寒瓜　生津止渴
清熱解暑　并可利尿

荔枝

Litchi

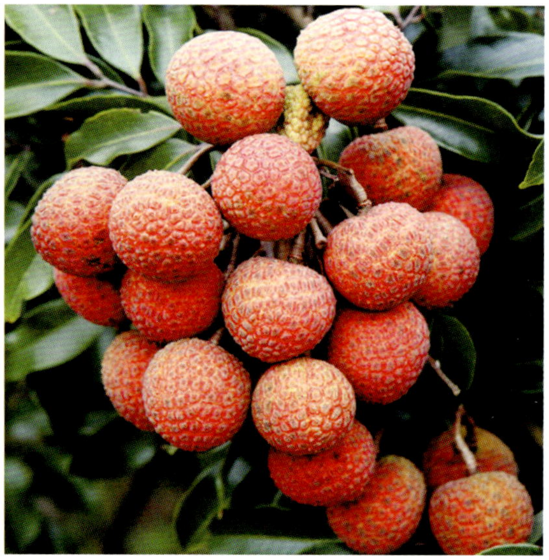

荔枝佳品，补脑健身。

Litchi can tonify the brain and improve health.

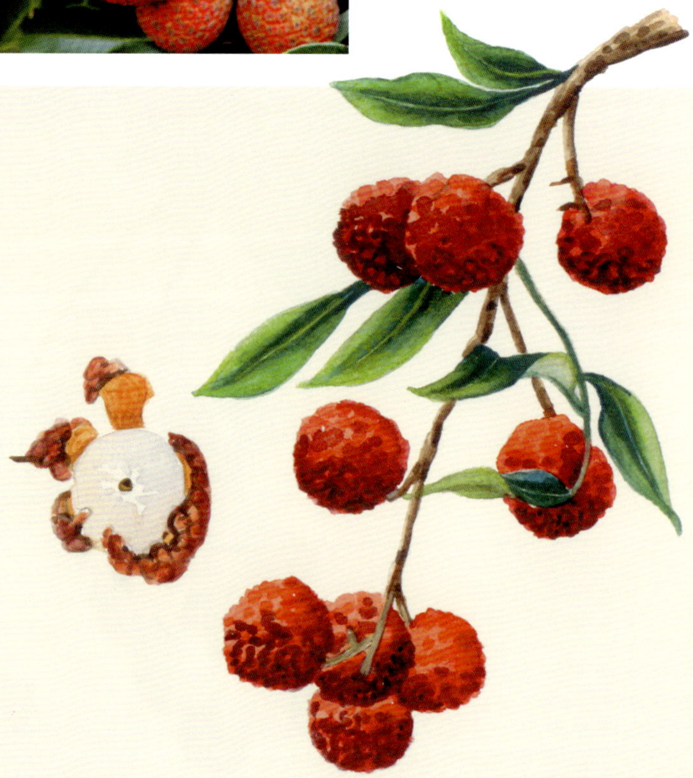

荔枝佳品　强心益智
補腦健身　多食上火

栗子

Chestnut

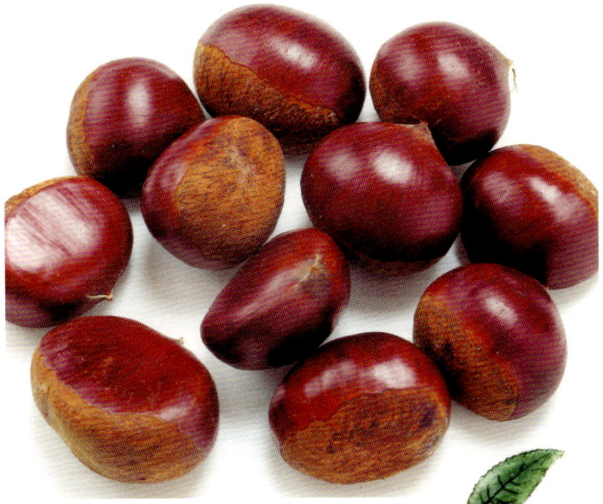

栗子补益，滋养肾气。

Chestnut can nourish and replenish kidney qi.

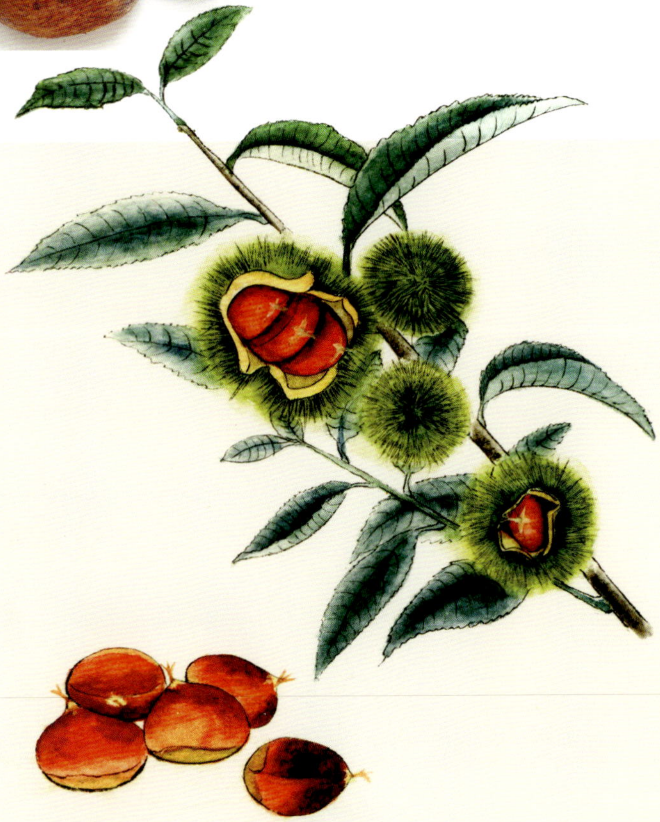

栗子補益 滋養腎氣
厚人腸胃 令人耐飢

枣

Date

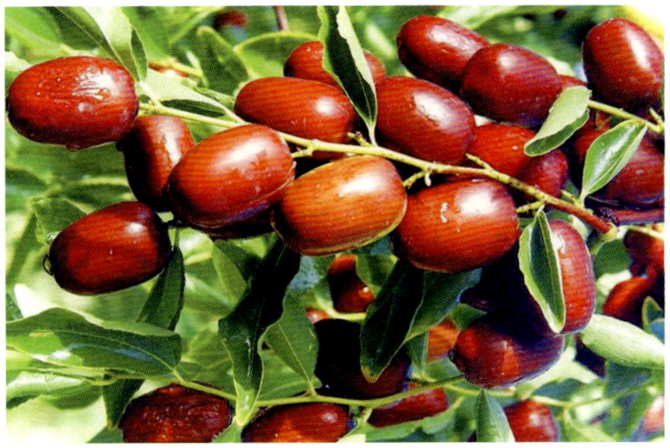

枣能安中，养血安神。

Date can harmonize the stomach and the spleen, nourish blood, and soothe the nerves.

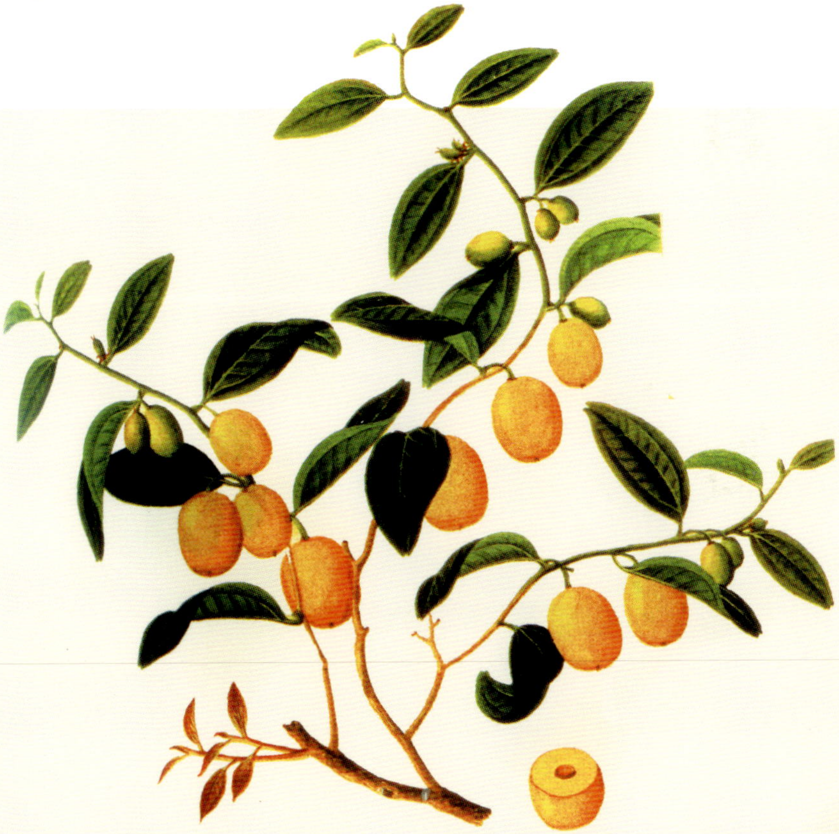

枣能安中 養血安神
補中益氣 多食生熱

猪肉

Pork

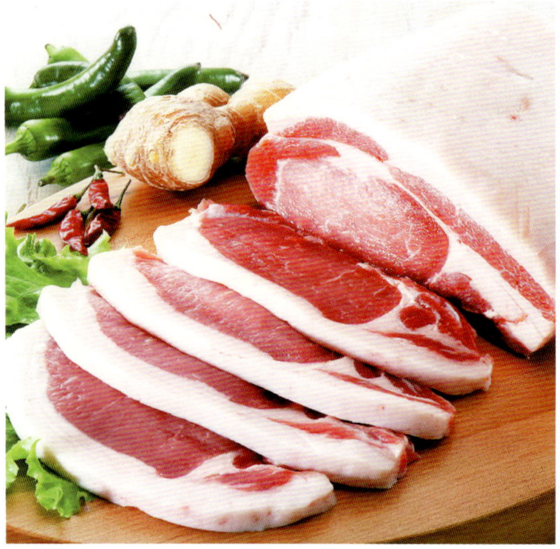

猪肉补益，增人气力。

Pork can nourish the body and increase strength.

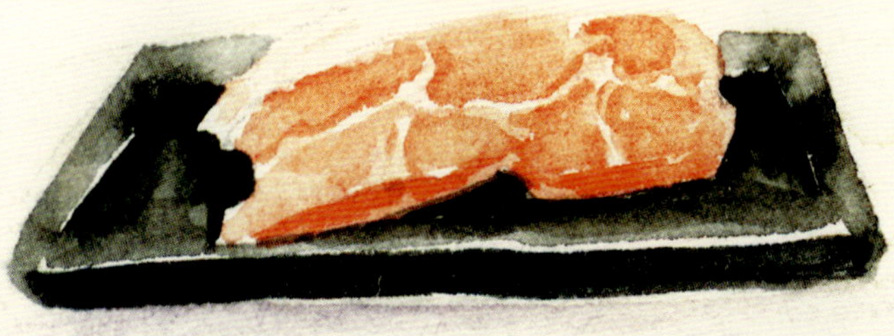

猪肉補益　猪臟多用

增人氣力　猪血清廢

牛肉

Beef

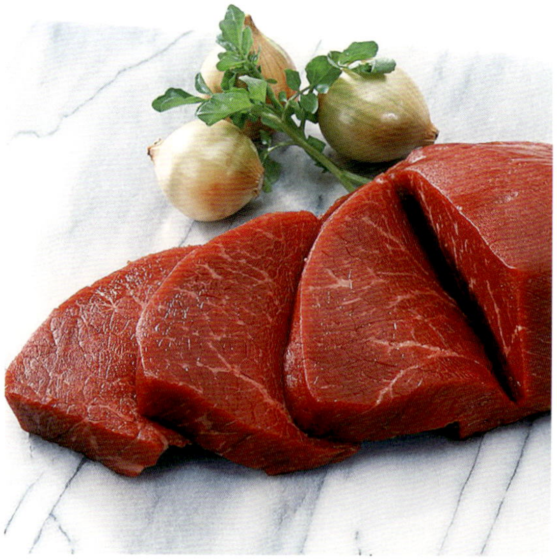

牛肉强身，补益气血。

Beef can strengthen the body and supplement qi and blood.

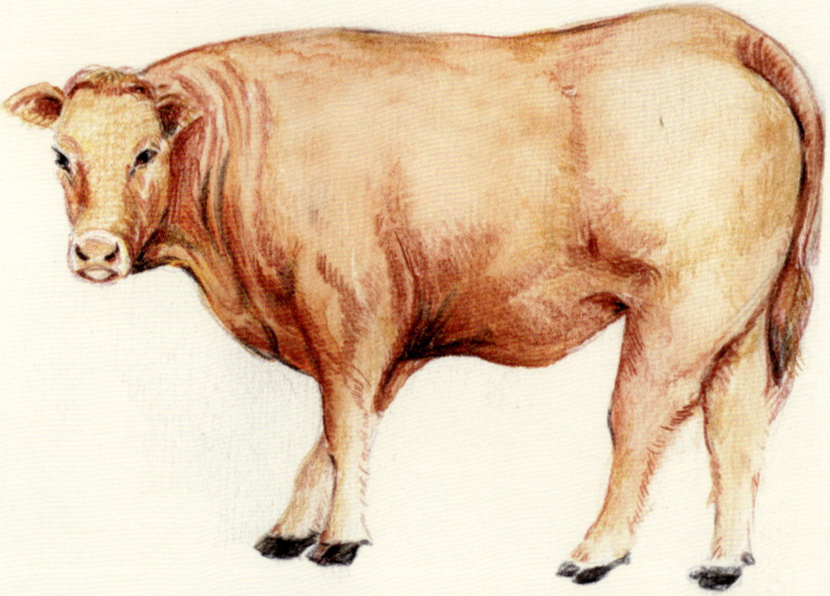

牛肉强身　强壮筋骨

補益氣血　治虚防弱

羊肉

Mutton

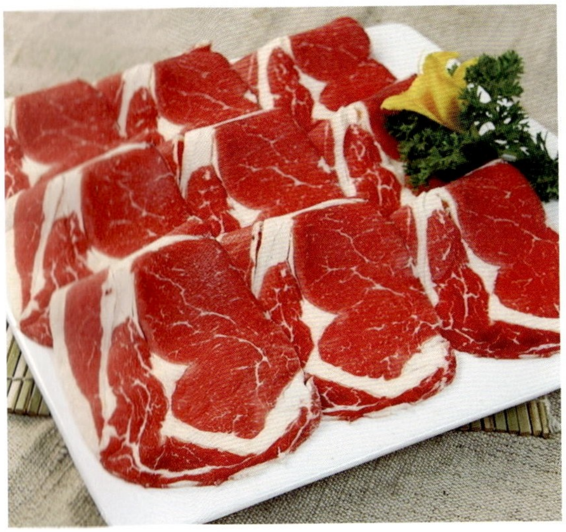

羊肉暖肾，补气养血。

Mutton can warm the kidney, replenish qi, and nourish blood.

鸡肉

Chicken

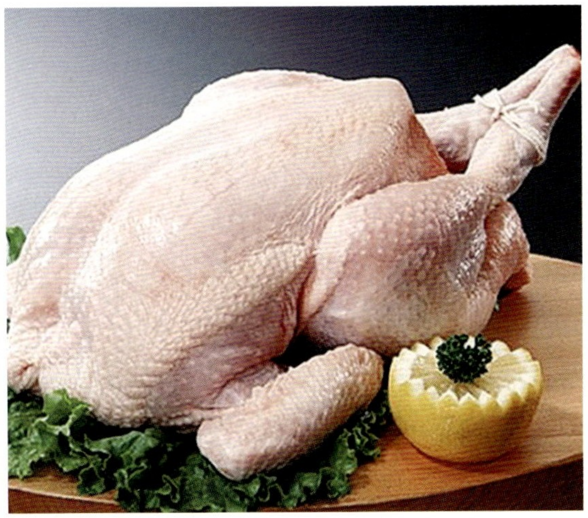

鸡肉温中，益气补精。

Chicken can warm the stomach and the spleen, supplement qi, and replenish essence.

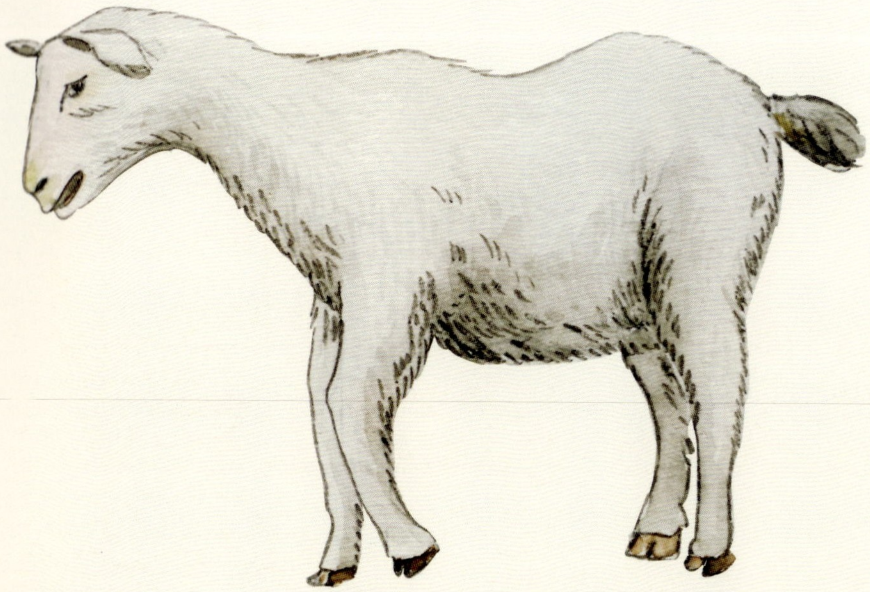

羊肉暖腎 脾胃虛冷
補氣養血 治虛防痿

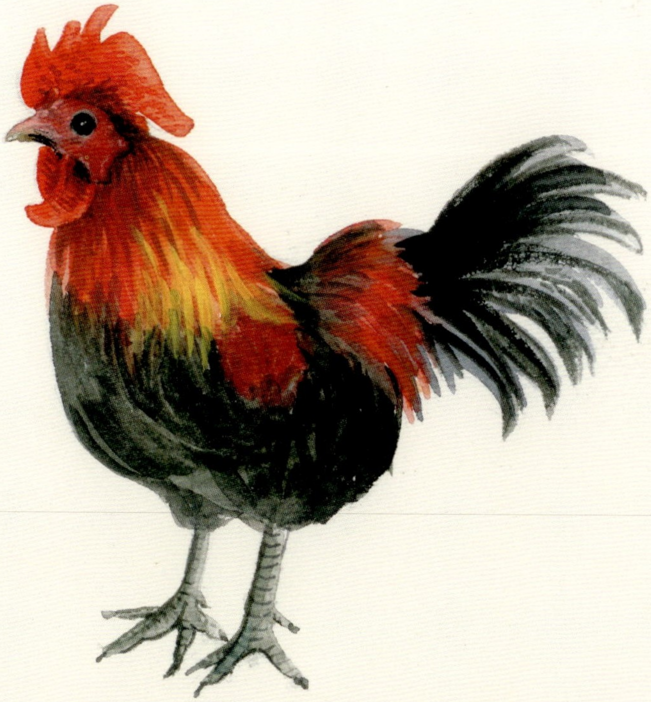

鷄肉温中 防治虛弱
益氣補精 葯用養陰

后记

Afterword

这是“文明中华”系列图册的殿军之作。增强体质，增进健康，提高生活品质已经成为富裕起来的中国人民的重要追求之一。中华民族有着源远流长的养生文化。为了向世界简明扼要地介绍中华养生，摄影家沈家兴先生策划本书的原则是：介绍中华养生经典理论和历史公认的养生方法，不走偏，不信邪，让中华养生学得到科学解释。本图册由任犀然编写，徐芳博士等英译。

编　者

2012 年 3 月 25 日

This is the last of the series of 'Chinese Civilization' illustrated books. To build up the body and improve health has been one of the major pursuits of Chinese people who have grown wealthy. The Chinese nation has time-honored traditions in health preservation. To introduce them to the world briefly, when planning this book, Mr. Shen Jiaxing, a distinguished photographer, has adhered to the following principles: introduce the classical theories and universally acknowledged practices of Chinese health preservation; do not include unproven or preposterous theories; and try to provide scientific explanations. This illustrated book is compiled by Ren Xiran and translated into English by Xu Fang, et al.

Editors

March 25, 2012

羊肉

Mutton

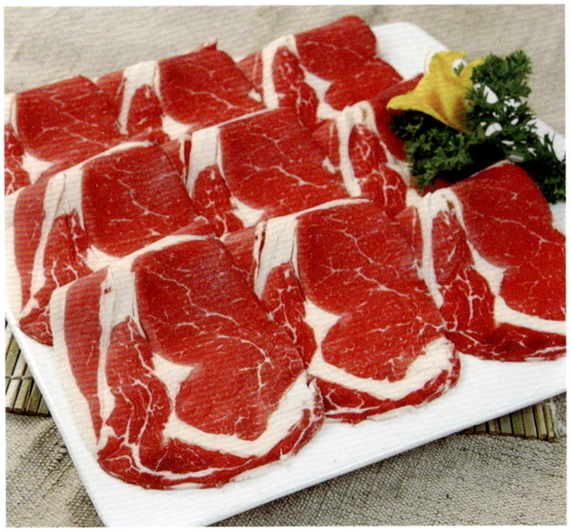

羊肉暖肾，补气养血。

Mutton can warm the kidney, replenish qi, and nourish blood.

鸡肉

Chicken

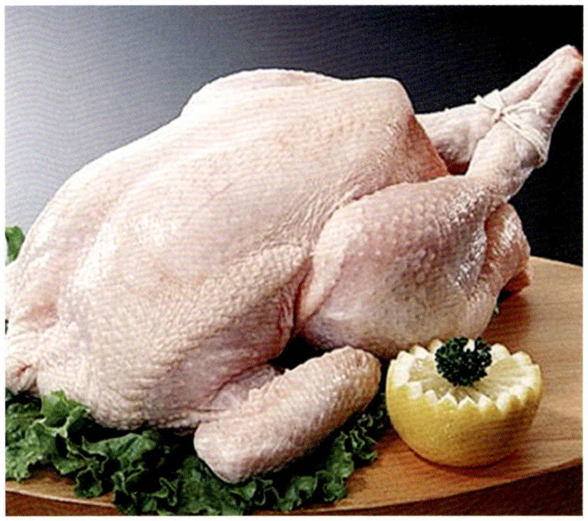

鸡肉温中，益气补精。

Chicken can warm the stomach and the spleen, supplement qi, and replenish essence.

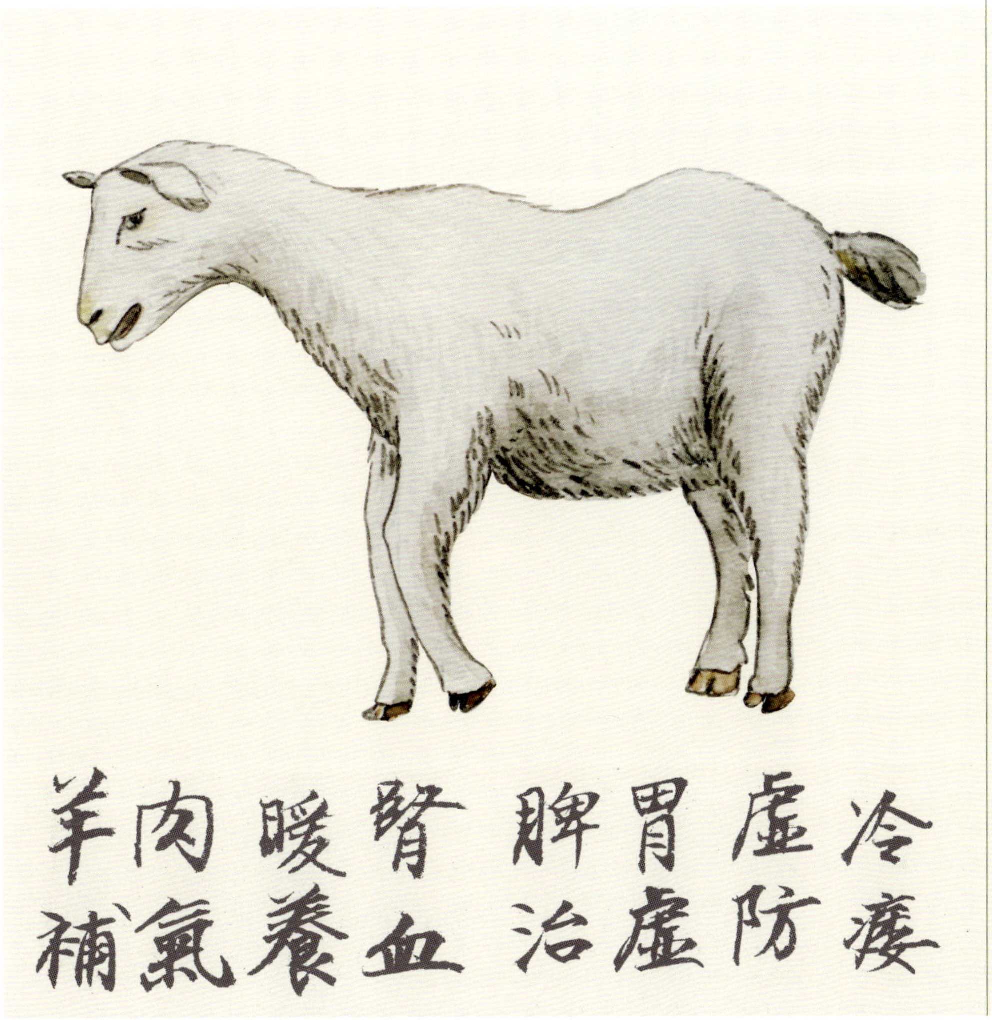

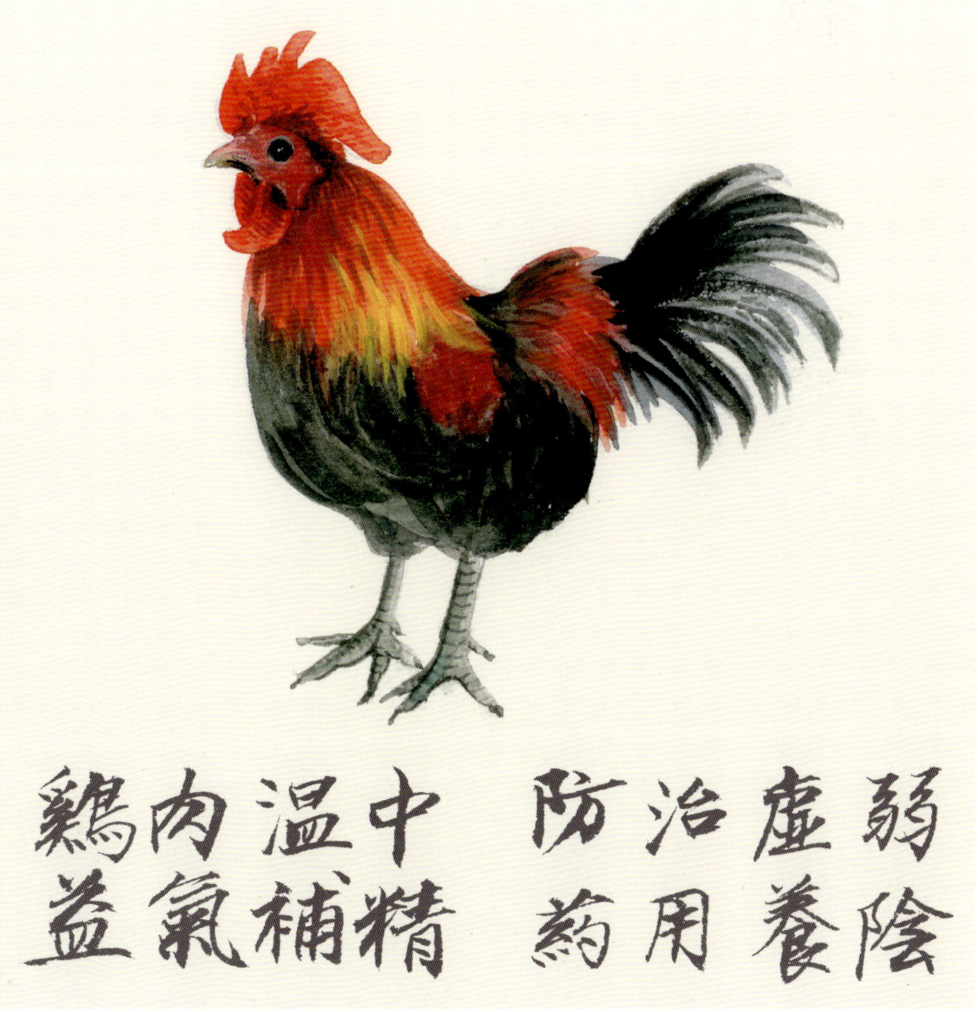

后记

Afterword

这是“文明中华”系列图册的殿军之作。增强体质，增进健康，提高生活品质已经成为富裕起来的中国人民的重要追求之一。中华民族有着源远流长的养生文化。为了向世界简明扼要地介绍中华养生，摄影家沈家兴先生策划本书的原则是：介绍中华养生经典理论和历史公认的养生方法，不走偏，不信邪，让中华养生学得到科学解释。本图册由任犀然编写，徐芳博士等英译。

编　者
2012年3月25日

This is the last of the series of ‘Chinese Civilization’ illustrated books. To build up the body and improve health has been one of the major pursuits of Chinese people who have grown wealthy. The Chinese nation has time-honored traditions in health preservation. To introduce them to the world briefly, when planning this book, Mr. Shen Jiaxing, a distinguished photographer, has adhered to the following principles: introduce the classical theories and universally acknowledged practices of Chinese health preservation; do not include unproven or preposterous theories; and try to provide scientific explanations. This illustrated book is compiled by Ren Xiran and translated into English by Xu Fang, et al.

Editors
March 25, 2012